CASE REVIEW

Emergency Radiology

Series Editor

David M. Yousem, MD, MBA
Professor of Radiology
Director of Neuroradiology
Russell H. Morgan Department of Radiology Science
The Johns Hopkins Medical Institutions
Baltimore, MD

Other Volumes in the CASE REVIEW Series

Brain Imaging, Second Edition
Breast Imaging
Cardiac Imaging
Gastrointestinal Imaging, Second Edition
General and Vascular Ultrasound, Second Edition
Genitourinary Imaging, Second Edition
Head and Neck Imaging, Second Edition
Musculoskeletal Imaging, Second Edition
Nuclear Medicine
Obstetric and Gynecologic Ultrasound, Second Edition
Pediatric Imaging
Spine Imaging, Second Edition
Thoracic Imaging
Vascular and Interventional Imaging

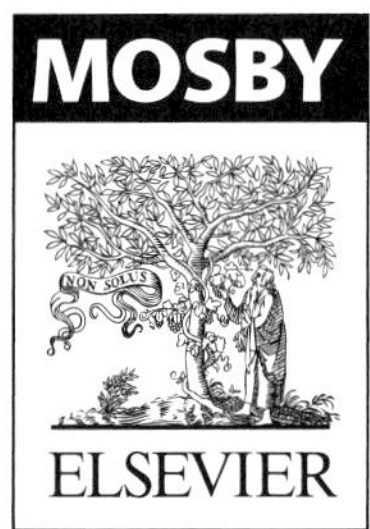

Stuart E. Mirvis, MD, FACR
Professor of Diagnostic Radiology and Nuclear Medicine
University of Maryland School of Medicine
Associate Vice Chairman for Medical Affairs
Director, Trauma/Emergency Radiology
University of Maryland Medical Center
Baltimore, Maryland

Kathirkamanathan Shanmuganathan, MD
Professor of Diagnostic Radiology and Nuclear Medicine
University of Maryland School of Medicine
University of Maryland Medical Center
Baltimore, Maryland

Lisa A. Miller, MD
Assistant Professor of Diagnostic Radiology and Nuclear Medicine
University of Maryland School of Medicine
University of Maryland Medical Center
Baltimore, Maryland

Clint W. Sliker, MD
Assistant Professor of Diagnostic Radiology and Nuclear Medicine
University of Maryland School of Medicine
University of Maryland Medical Center
Baltimore, Maryland

CASE REVIEW

Emergency Radiology

CASE REVIEW SERIES

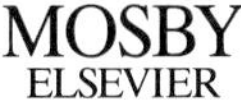

1600 John F. Kennedy Boulevard
Suite 1800
Philadelphia, PA 19103-2899

EMERGENCY RADIOLOGY: CASE REVIEW ISBN: 978-0-323-04957-3

NOTICE

Knowledge and best practice in this field are constantly changing. As new research and experience broaden our knowledge, changes in practice, treatment and drug therapy may become necessary or appropriate. Readers are advised to check the most current information provided (i) on procedures featured or (ii) by the manufacturer of each product to be administered, to verify the recommended dose or formula, the method and duration of administration, and contraindications. It is the responsibility of the practitioner, relying on thier own experience and knowledge of the patient, to make diagnoses, to determine dosages and the best treatment for each individual patient, and to take all appropriate safety precautions. To the fullest extent of the law, neither the Publisher nor the Authors assume any liability for any injury and/or damage to persons or property arising out or related to any use of the material contained in this book.

The Publisher

Library of Congress Cataloging-in-Publication Data
Emergency radiology/Stuart E. Mirvis ... [et al.]. – 1st ed.
p. ; cm. – (Case review series)
Includes bibliographical references.
ISBN 978-0-323-04957-3
1. Diagnosis, Radioscopic- -Case studies. 2. Radiography, Medical–Case studies. 3. Emergency medicine–Case studies. 4. Medical emergencies–Imaging–Case studies. I. Mirvis, Stuart E. II. Series.
[DNLM: 1. Emergencies–Case Reports. 2. Radiography–methods–Case Reports. 3. Critical Care–methods–Case Reports. 4. Emergency Medical Services–methods–Case Reports. 5.Wounds and Injuries–radiography–Case Reports. WN 200 E532 2010]
RC78.E5827 2010
616.07′57–dc22
2008032281

Acquisitions Editor: Rebecca S. Gaertner
Project Manager: Bryan Hayward
Design Direction: Steven Stave
Marketing Manager: Nancy Ciliberti

Printed in the United States of America.

Last digit is the print number: 9 8 7 6 5 4 3 2 1

To my wife, Linda R. Mirvis, for her love and tireless help.
—Stuart E. Mirvis

To my sister, Nalayini Shan, who is always available for moral support and advice when required.
—Kathirkamanathan Shanmuganathan

To my mother, Vivian A. Miller, for her love and support.
—Lisa A. Miller

To my wife, Lisa, and my children, Lauren, Kelly, and Christopher, thank you for the love, patience, and caring that motivate me to work hard every day.
—Clint W. Sliker

To our Chairman, Reuben Mezrich, MD, PhD, for supporting the growth of our section.
—Stuart E. Mirvis, Kathirkamanathan Shanmuganathan, Lisa A. Miller, and Clint W. Sliker

One of the most recent recognized subspecialties of radiology is Emergency Radiology. While some opine that this should not be recognized as a separate entity itself, delving into many already established subspecialties of radiology, I disagree. Those who practice Emergency Radiology have to be so much better versed in issues related to trauma, acute stroke care, acute abdomens, painful acute pelvic conditions, and cardiopulmonary emergencies. The development of teleradiology nighthawk services and 24/7 radiology makes mastery of this arena of radiology a necessity. This is a niche job opportunity that requires special training and knowledge.

In Baltimore, the University of Maryland Shock Trauma Center is the primary referral locale for patients in serious motor vehicle accidents and/or catastrophes. The Center has a stellar reputation in part because of the quality of the imaging and the service provided by the radiology group led by Stuart Mirvis. The material at Dr. Mirvis's disposal is outstanding in terms of quantity and quality. When I was asked to suggest an author for this Case Review Series, there was only one candidate I wanted to enlist . . . Stuart Mirvis. He and his team have created a wonderful new first edition to the series that will be valuable worldwide even as some of the practice of emergency radiology becomes a global endeavor.

As the reader undoubtedly knows by now, this series is set up such that there are gradations of difficulty so that the reader can assess his or her proficiency and can use this self-evaluation to guide continued education. By referencing THE REQUISITES textbook, the reader can "bone up" on a topic if a weakness is perceived. Since each case in the book is distinct, this is the kind of text that you can pick up and review at any time in your day, in your career.

Drs. Mirvis, Shanmuganathan, Miller, and Sliker have written a fantastic book that I recommend for all radiologists reviewing ED studies. I welcome "Emergency Radiology" to the Case Review Series. Don't leave home without it!

David M. Yousem, MD, MBA

In the past two decades, Emergency Radiology has emerged as a specialty that continues to grow in importance. An ever-increasing number of our patients enters the hospital via the emergency department (ED), usually not during routine working hours. The need to provide quality radiology interpretation for these patients, whenever they arrive, is, in part, responsible for the development of this specialty. The recognition that Emergency Radiology encompasses a special and well-defined body of clinical and imaging knowledge has fostered development of the specialty, as well.

Regardless of their areas of specialization, most practicing and training radiologists will, at some time, provide emergency radiology coverage. The ED is a place where diagnostic decisions must often be made rapidly and where the workload fluctuates in an unpredictable manner. Familiarity with the common and some less common diagnoses is necessary both to move patients efficiently through the typically very busy ED and, more important, to promote rapid, appropriate treatment of acute illness.

This case review book is meant to provide an opportunity to rapidly familiarize the reader with the classic appearance of a range of emergent imaging pathology and key points concerning these diagnoses. The Trauma and Emergency Radiology section of the University of Maryland provides 24/7 coverage for both a busy urban ED and a major level 1 trauma center. These venues provide us with plenty of "raw material" from which to select our cases. In preparing these cases, we sought to be comprehensive with the topics covered while providing a range of difficulties for case interpretation. Hopefully, we have accomplished these goals.

Obviously, we are big fans of Emergency Radiology and enjoy the opportunity to share our material with the radiology community at large; we hope you benefit from its review. As we prepared these cases, we heightened our awareness of less familiar entities and refreshed our knowledge of those more familiar to us. In so doing, we and, by extension, our patients benefited. If review of these cases fosters in you a sense of why we enjoy Emergency Radiology and helps you provide better care to your ED patients, we certainly have succeeded in our efforts.

Stuart Mirvis, MD, FACR
K. Shanmuganathan, MD
Lisa Miller, MD
Clint Sliker, MD

CASE REVIEW
Emergency Radiology

Color Plates

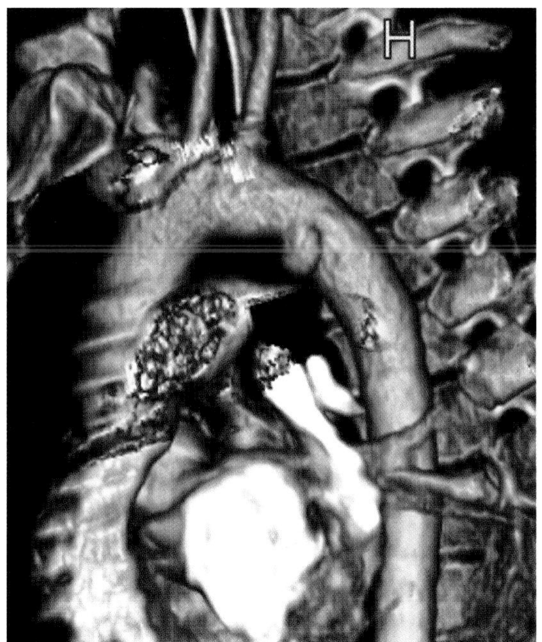

Case 3 (see page 7).

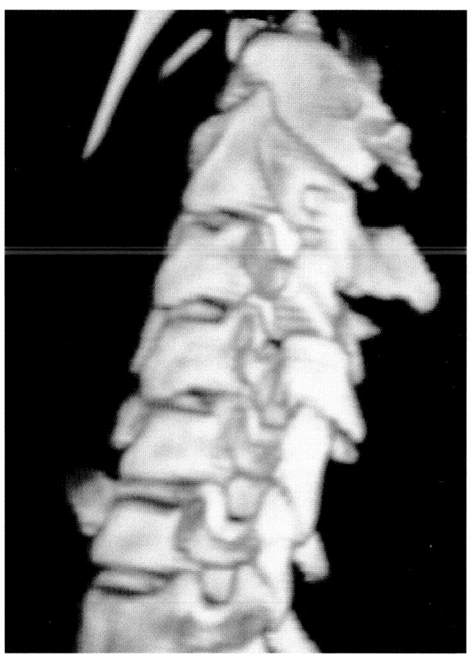

Case 6 (see page 13).

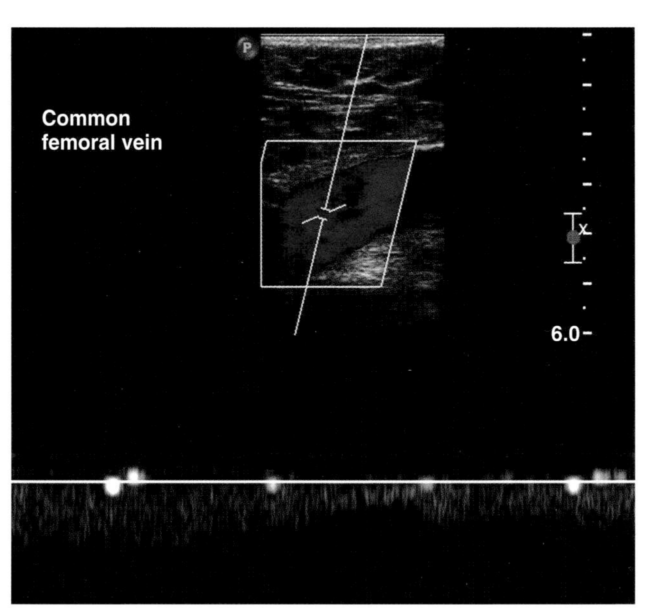

Case 4 (see page 7).

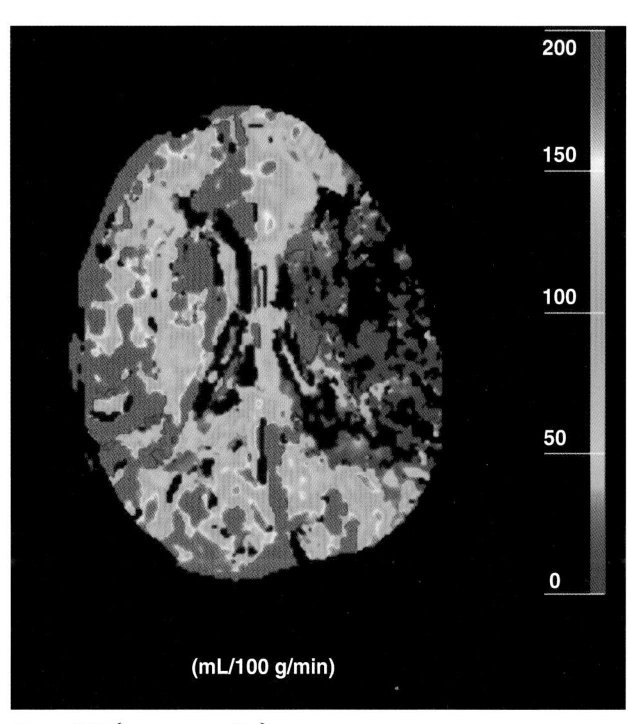

Case 13 (see page 27).

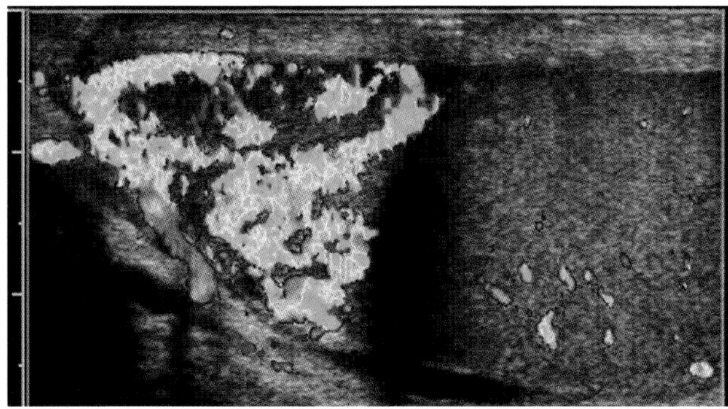

Case 47 (see page 95).

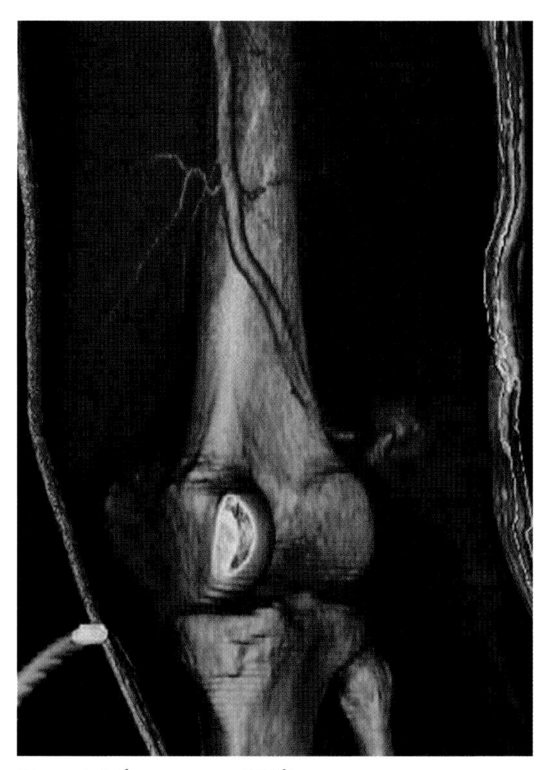

Case 51 (see page 103).

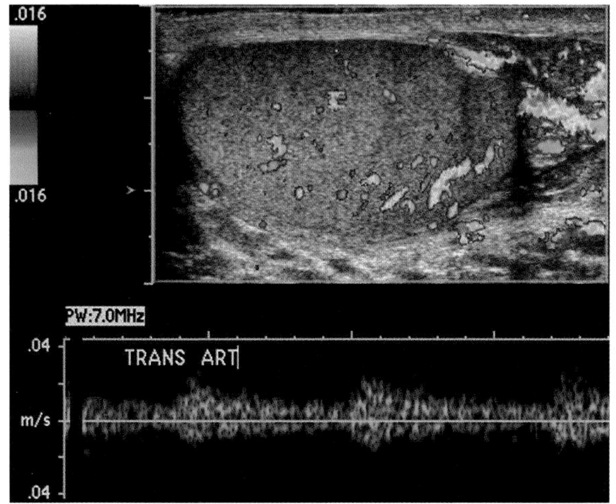

Case 47 (see page 95).

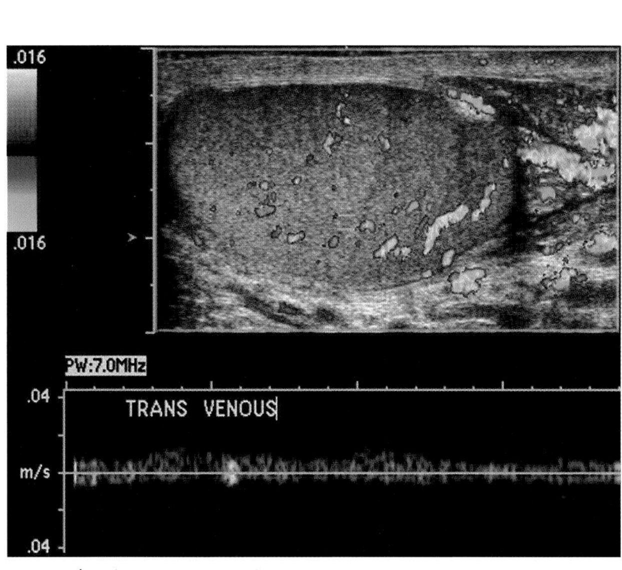

Case 47 (see page 95).

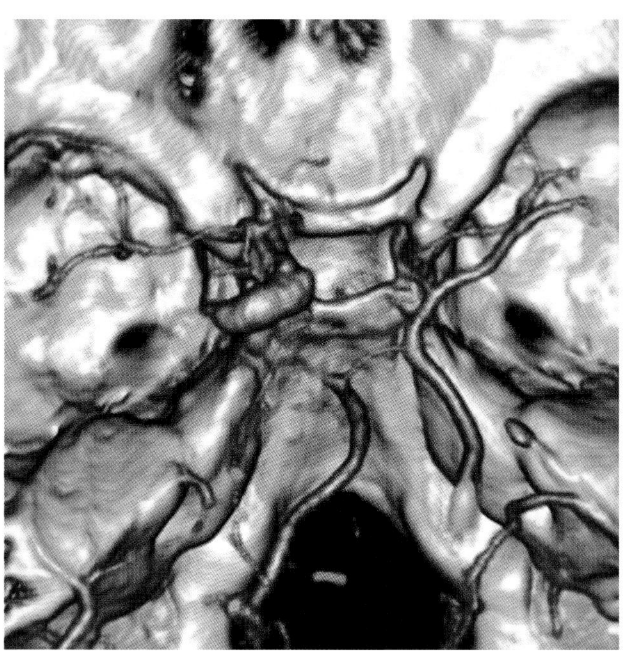

Case 58 (see page 117).

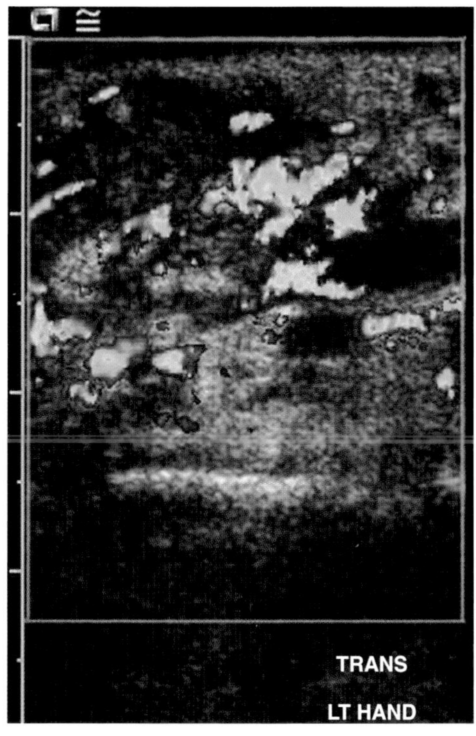

Case 59 (see page 119).

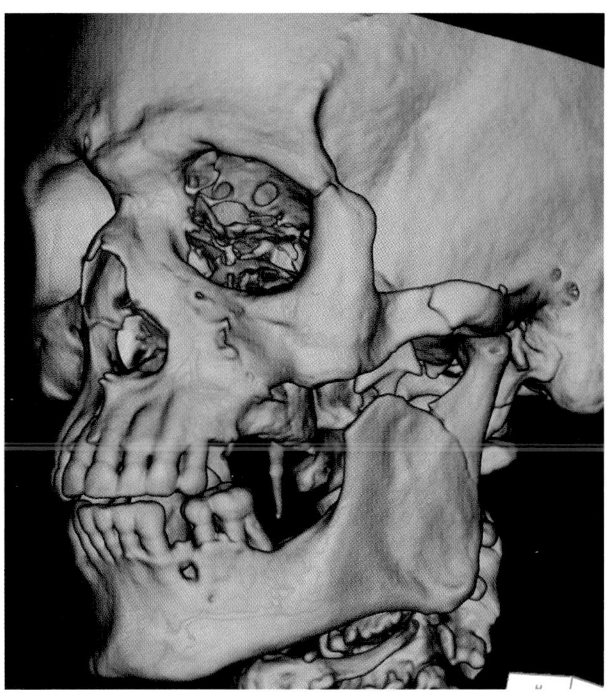
Case 63 (see page 127).

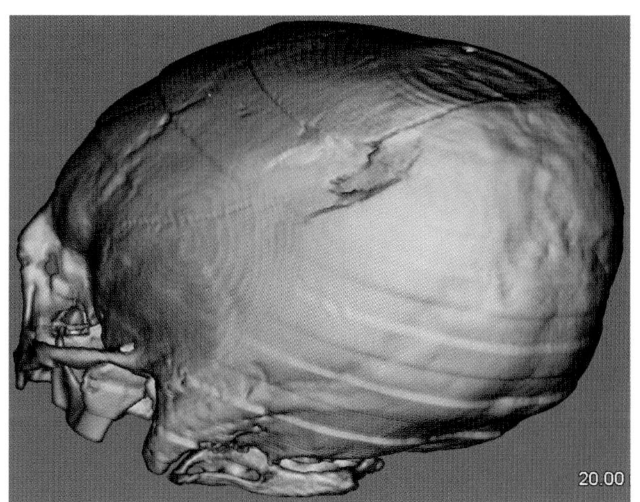

Case 62 (see page 125).

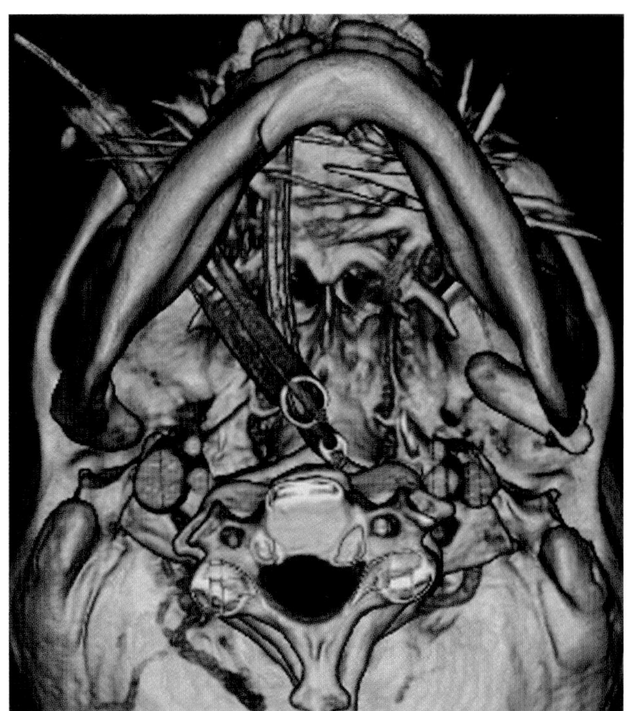
Case 64 (see page 129).

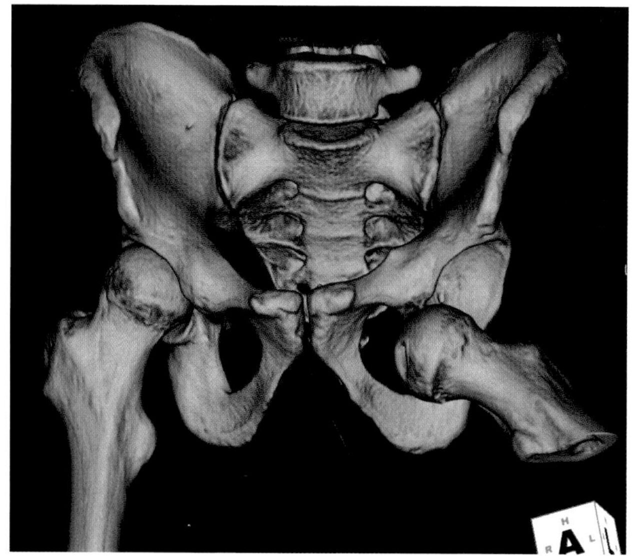

Case 66 (see page 133).

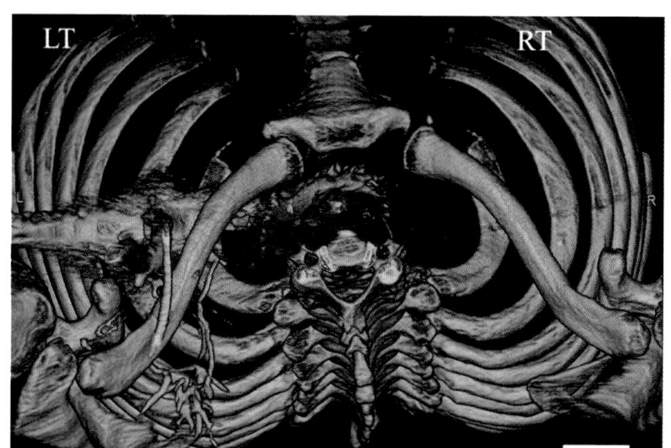

Case 67 (see page 135).

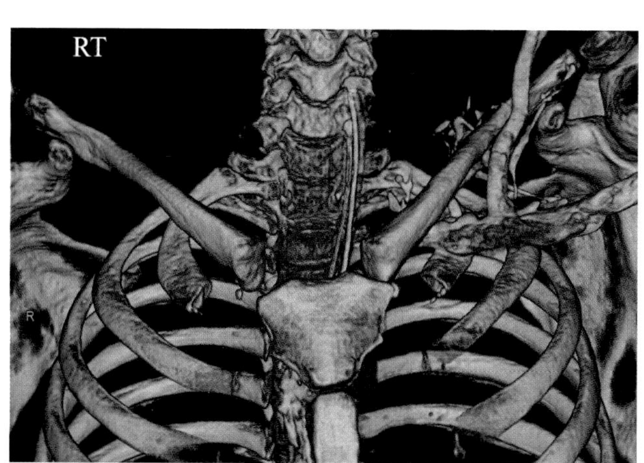

Case 67 (see page 135).

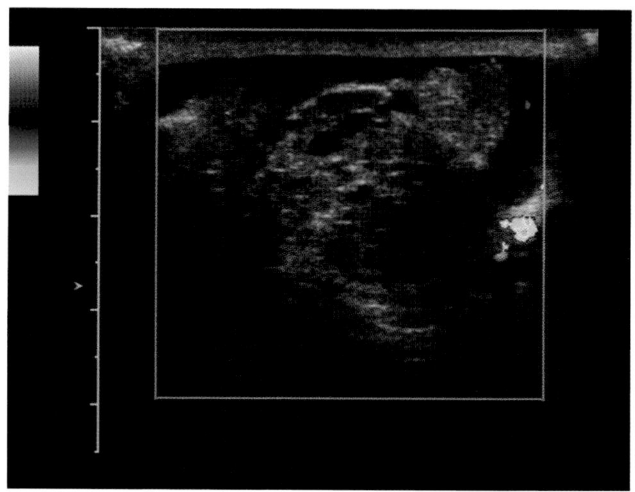

Case 97 (see page 197).

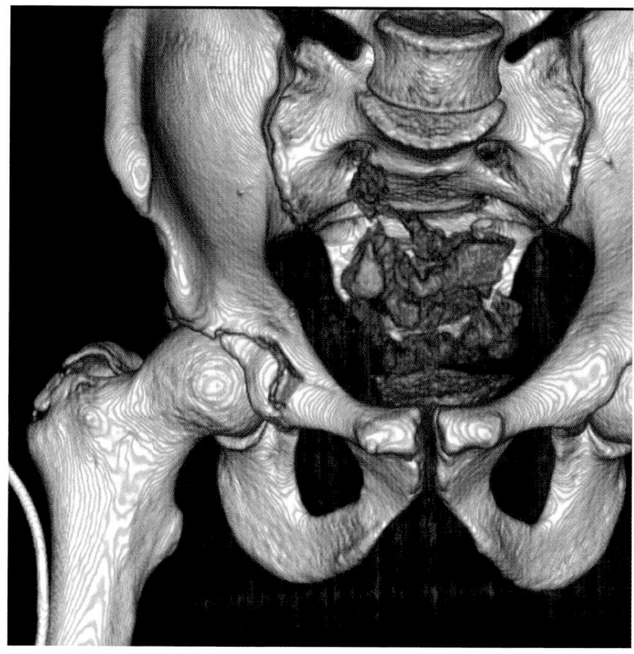

Case 114 (see page 231).

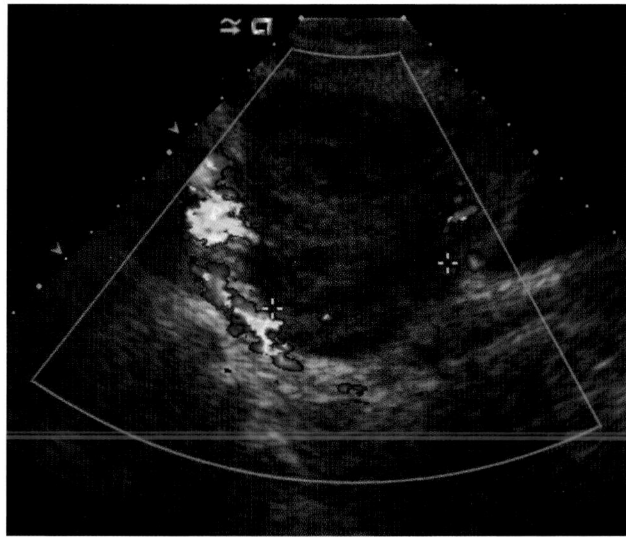

Case 119 (see page 241).

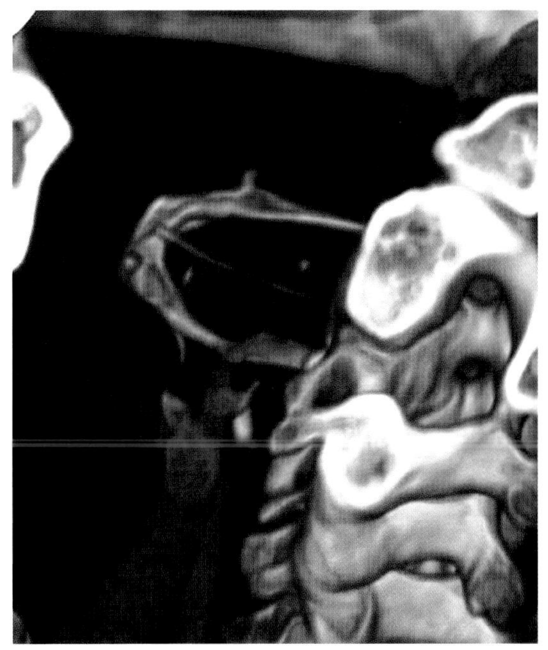

Case 121 (see page 245).

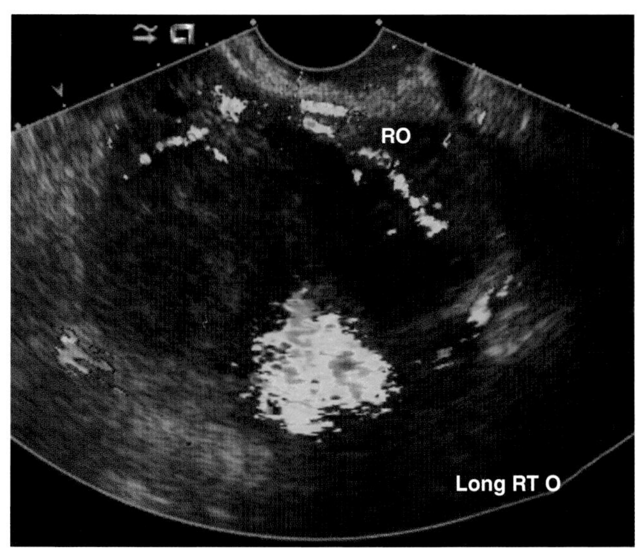

Case 119 (see page 241).

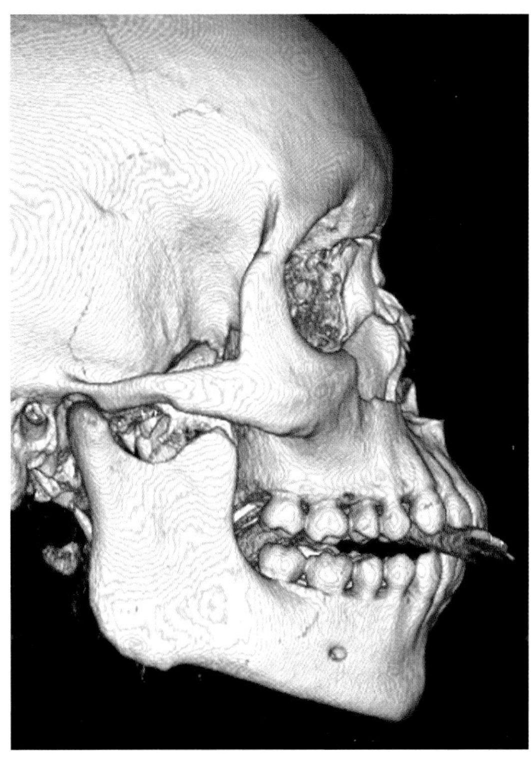

Case 125 (see page 253).

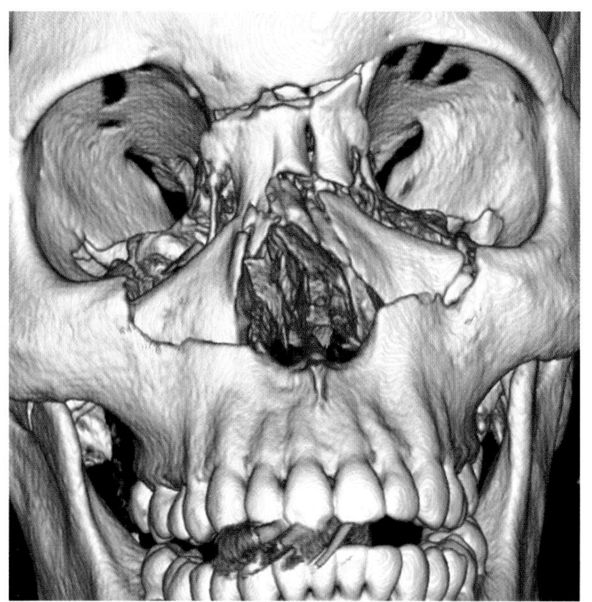

Case 125 (see page 253).

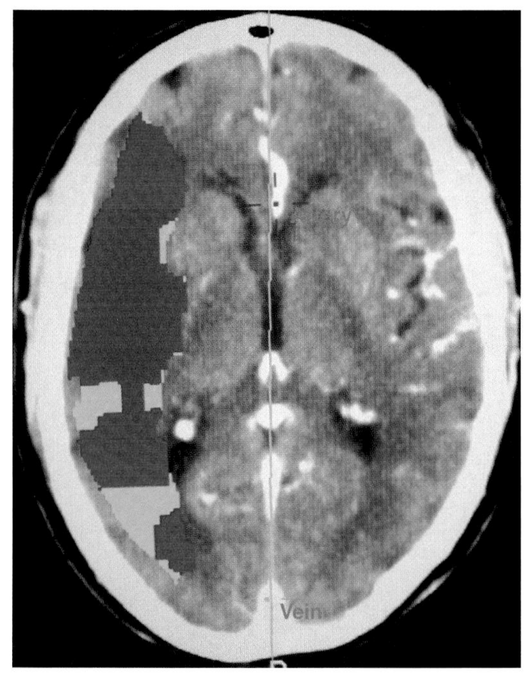

Case 136 (see page 275).

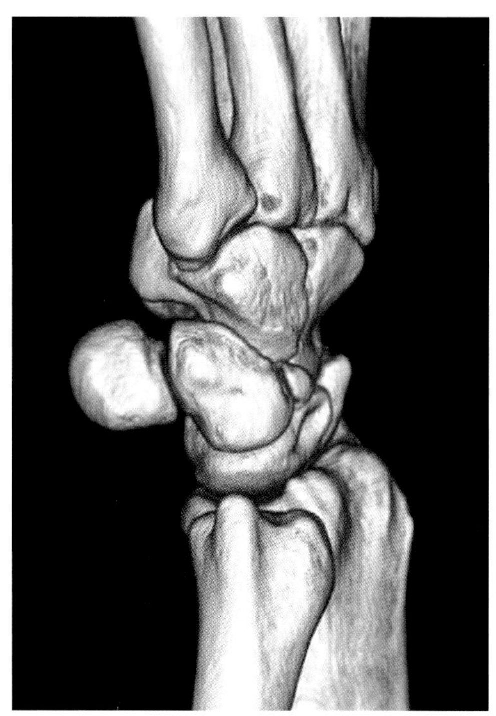

Case 128 (see page 259).

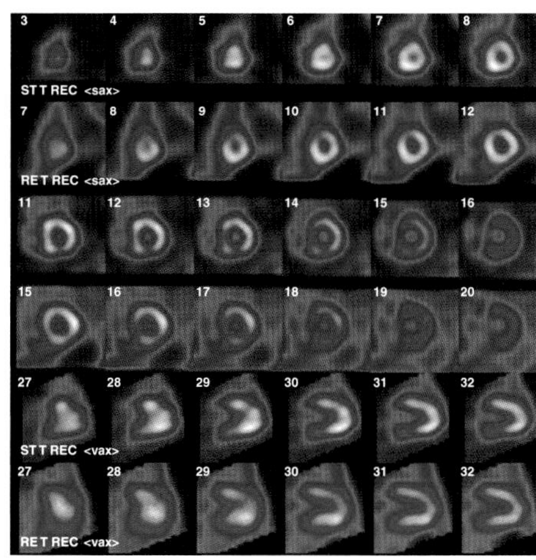

Case 142 (see page 287).

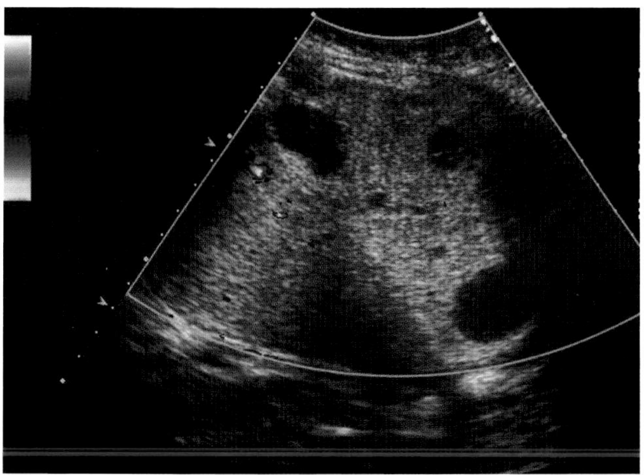

Case 158 (see page 321).

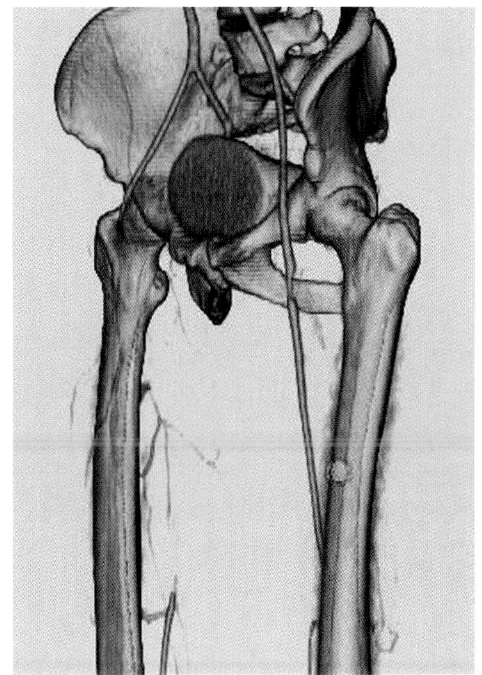

Case 174 (see page 353).

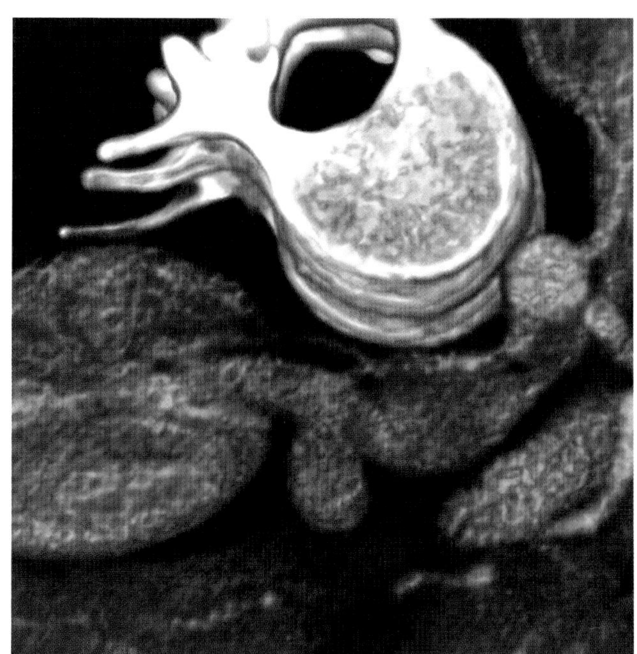

Case 162 (see page 329).

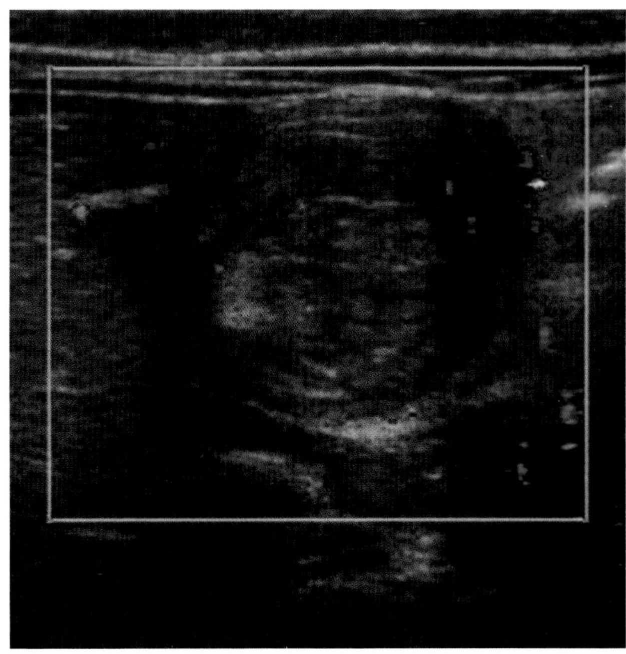

Case 180 (see page 365).

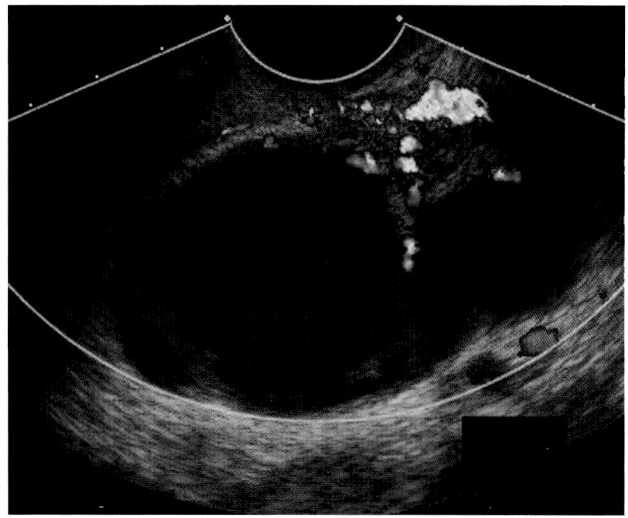

Case 185 (see page 375).

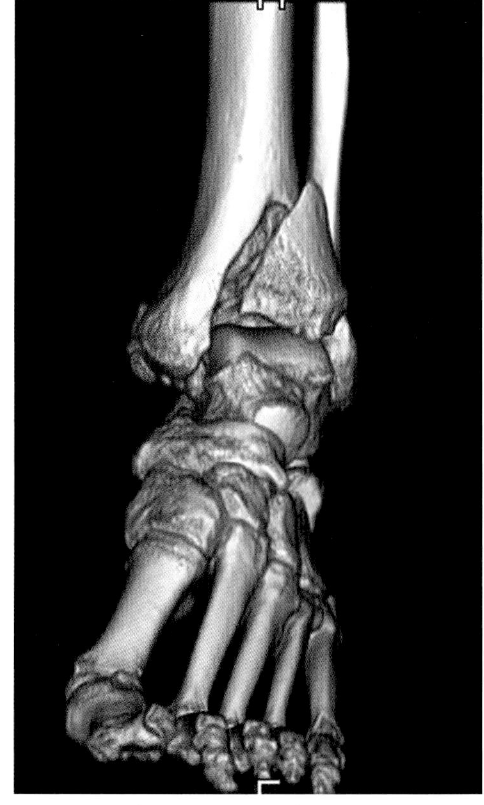

Case 197 (see page 399).

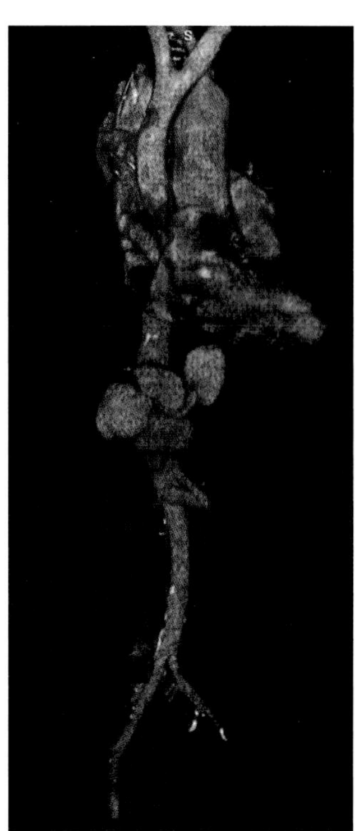

Case 186 (see page 377).

Opening Round

CASE 1

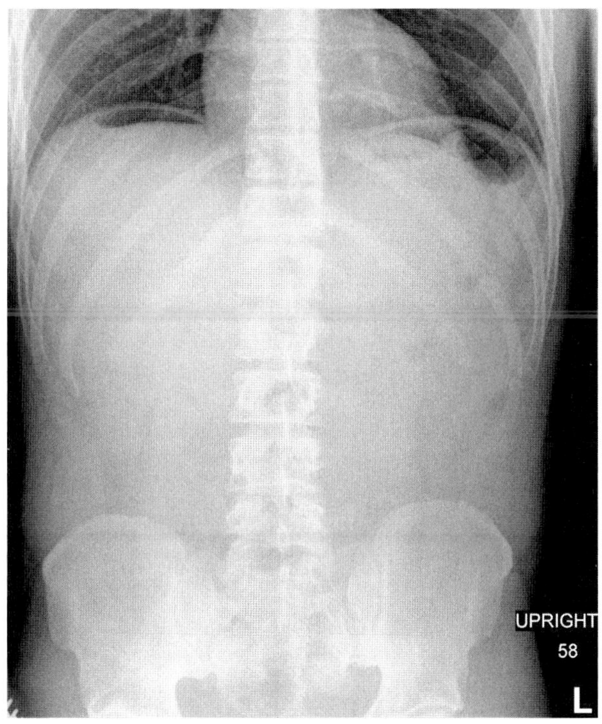

1. What is the radiographic abnormality, and where is it located?
2. Is this the most sensitive radiographic projection for identifying this radiographic abnormality? If not, what projection is?
3. What is the most common cause of this abnormality?
4. Is surgery always necessary to treat patients who manifest this abnormality?

CASE 1

Pneumoperitoneum

1. Pneumoperitoneum located in both subphrenic spaces.
2. Erect chest radiograph.
3. Recent surgery.
4. No.

References

Cho KC, Baker SR: Extraluminal air. Diagnosis and significance, *Radiol Clin North Am* 32:829–844, 1994.

Mularski RA, Ciccolo ML, Rappaport WD: Nonsurgical causes of pneumoperitoneum, *West J Med* 170: 41–46, 1999.

Cross-Reference

Emergency Radiology: THE REQUISITES, pp 95, 305.

Comment

Pneumoperitoneum refers to free intraperitoneal gas collections. The most frequent cause of free peritoneal gas is recent abdominal surgery or other iatrogenic causes of peritoneal violation. Among the pathologic causes of pneumoperitoneum, the most common are spontaneous visceral perforations, with up to 85% of patients exhibiting pneumoperitoneum. Foremost among the visceral sources are perforating gastroduodenal ulcers followed both small- and large-bowel perforations secondary to various causes that include bowel obstruction, infection, and infarction.

Acute appendicitis and colonic diverticulitis are common causes of perforation, yet they are not common causes of pneumoperitoneum, because either the volume of gas in the perforated organ is small (e.g., appendicitis) or the gas is localized to the site of perforation by inflammatory reaction (e.g., diverticulitis). Spontaneous pneumoperitoneum without visceral perforation is an uncommon yet well-recognized clinical-radiologic entity. The many causes of "nonsurgical pneumoperitoneum" include, but are not limited to, barotrauma, asthma and other causes of elevated intrathoracic pressure, collagen vascular disease, pneumatosis cystoides intestinalis, jejunal and sigmoid diverticulosis, and gynecologic sources that include pelvic examinations, vaginal douching, and coitus.

Erect posteroanterior (PA) chest and left lateral decubitus abdominal radiographs have been considered the most sensitive radiographic projections for identifying pneumoperitoneum, although erect lateral chest radiographs have been promoted as more sensitive than erect PA chest radiographs. Although properly exposed radiographs can identify as little as 1 to 2 mL of free gas, the sensitivity of radiographs relies on maintaining the patient in the desired position for 10 to 20 minutes prior to image acquisition in order to allow gas to migrate to nondependent positions in the peritoneum. However, the time constraints inherent a busy emergency department, coupled with difficulties positioning and maintaining acutely ill patients into the necessary positions, can reduce the ability of radiography to detect such small volumes of pneumoperitoneum. In difficult cases in which clinical suspicion for perforated viscus is high but there are no peritoneal signs or other clear indications for immediate surgical exploration, computed tomography (CT) may be a useful diagnostic tool as it may identify small collections of peritoneal gas missed by radiography. Still, even CT may fail to identify pneumoperitoneum in the presence of perforated viscus, and, at times, the only abnormality demonstrated by CT may be peritoneal free fluid.

When radiographs demonstrate pneumoperitoneum and the clinical picture is compatible with perforated viscus, there is no need for additional imaging. However, when patient history and atypical clinical presentation suggest the possibility of nonsurgical pneumoperitoneum, additional or follow-up imaging may be useful to exclude lesions requiring surgical intervention, as long as close clinical monitoring is maintained.

Notes

CASE 2

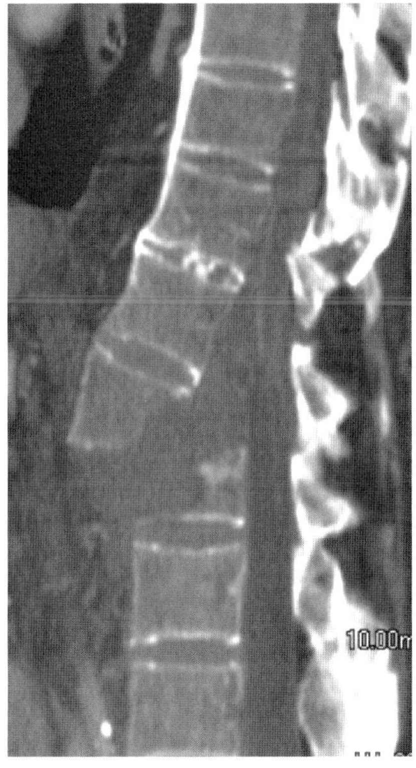

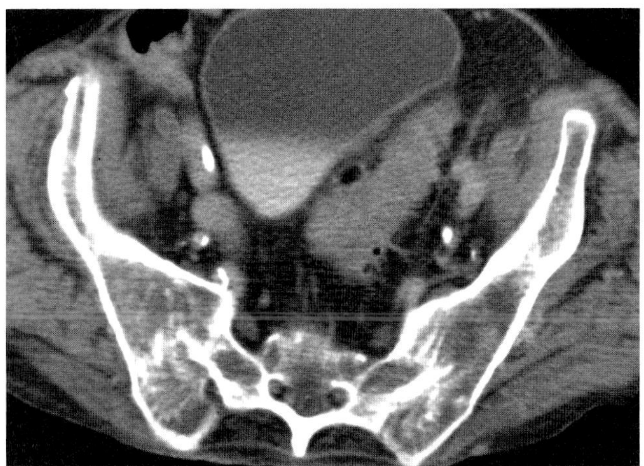

You are shown images of a blunt trauma patient.

1. What is the diagnosis?
2. What predisposes the patient to spinal injury?
3. What are other features of this disease?
4. What is the most common mechanism producing this injury?

CASE 2

Spinal Extension Fracture-Dislocation in Ankylosing Spondylitis

1. Low thoracic spine fracture-dislocation—ankylosing spondylitis.
2. Fusion of vertebrae by syndesmophytes and disc calcification/ossification creating spinal rigidity.
3. Sacroiliitis, peripheral arthritis, apical lung lesions, inflammatory spinal pain, chest wall pain, peripheral enthesitis, dactylitis, conjunctivitis, uveitis, and aortic incompetence with conduction disturbances.
4. Hyperextension.

Reference

Wang YF, Teng MM, Chang CY, et al: Imaging manifestations of spinal fractures in ankylosing spondylitis, *Am J Neuroradiol* 26:2067–2076, 2005.

Cross-Reference

Emergency Radiology: THE REQUISITES, pp 221, 223.

Comment

Patients with ankylosing spondylitis (AS) are prone to sustain spinal fractures, often with minimal trauma. The rigidity of the spine does not allow bending which would normally dissipate impacting force. The rigid spine usually fractures along a single line which may involve the vertebral body, disc level, or both. Usually, the injuries occur from extension force and involve all three spinal columns leading to instability. In some cases the injuries may be very subtle, particularly radiographically, yet still unstable. Patients with AS admitted with blunt trauma should be regarded with a high level of suspicion for spinal fractures involving any part of the spine and at multiple levels. In these cases thin-section computed tomography is the study of choice to detect subtle fracture lines. Injuries heal by pseudoarthrosis predisposing the patient to further vertebral displacement and cord injury. Magnetic resonance imaging (MRI) is also useful in documenting the extent of ligament disruption, assessing the degree of cord compression, and detecting epidural hematomas, to which these patients are prone.

It should be recognized that patients with similar spinal rigidity, including diffuse idiopathic skeletal hyperostosis and severe hypertrophic osteoarthritis, are also at greater risk of spinal column injury from a given force than is the general population, and should be investigated with a similar degree of caution after sustaining blunt trauma.

Notes

CASE 3

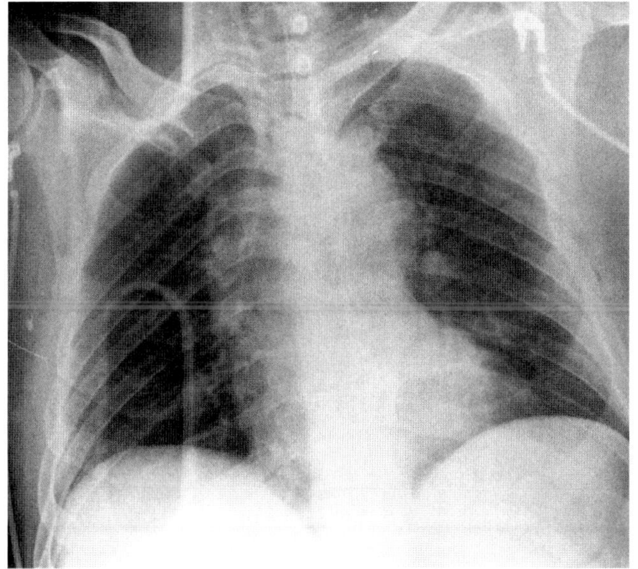

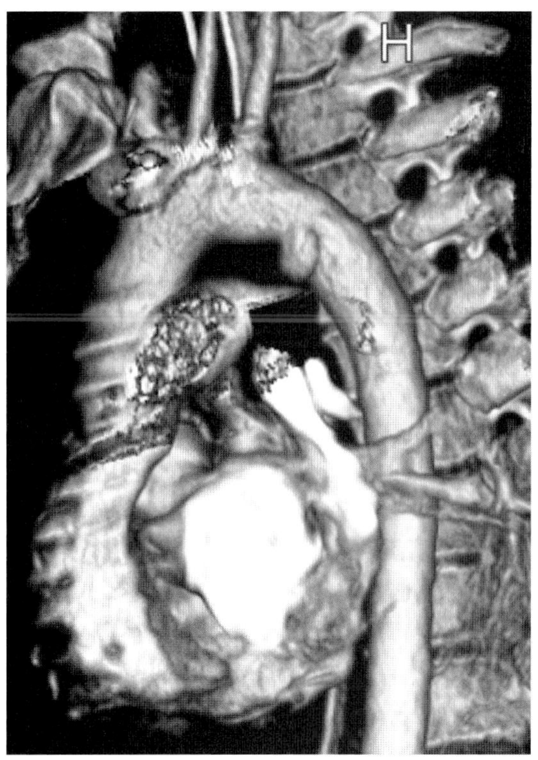

See also Color Plate

You are shown images of a blunt trauma patient.

1. What radiographic abnormalities are present?
2. What computed tomographic angiographic abnormality is present?
3. What treatment options should be considered?
4. What is the next most common site of this injury seen clinically?

CASE 3

Traumatic Aortic Pseudoaneurysm

1. Abnormal contour of the mediastinum and loss of aortic shadow. Mild displacement of trachea to the right, but partially accounted for by patient rotation.
2. Traumatic aortic injury.
3. Surgical repair, stent graft, blood pressure control (usually temporary).
4. The ascending aorta is the next most common site, but few of these patients survive. The aortic arch is the next most common clinically observed site of injury.

Reference

Mirvis SE: Thoracic vascular injury, *Radiol Clin North Am* 44:181–197, 2006.

Cross-Reference

Emergency Radiology: THE REQUISITES, pp 62–64, 323–326.

Comment

Traumatic aortic injury (TAI) accounts for up to 16% of deaths in motor vehicle collisions and has about 40% in-hospital mortality within 24 hours if untreated. The diagnosis is usually suspected on the basis of an abnormal mediastinal contour on admission chest radiograph and includes signs such as tracheal/nasogastric tube deviation to the right, widened paraspinal stripes, loss of the aortic outline, and depression of the left mainstem bronchus. These are all signs of mediastinal hemorrhage that may or may not be associated with major vascular injury. In general, radiographs are sensitive, but quite nonspecific for TAI.

Currently, multidetector-row CT is the next study performed and is being used more routinely in screening for chest pathology in blunt trauma. CT findings of TAI include pseudoaneurysm, sudden change in aortic diameter or contour, periaortic hemorrhage, decreased diameter of the lower thoracic and abdominal aorta, intimal flaps, and intraluminal thrombus. Additional injuries to the aorta or proximal great vessels must be sought. Use of multiplanar, angioscopic, and volume-rendered views assists in CT diagnosis. In rare cases when CT is equivocal, angiography or transesophageal echocardiogram may be useful for further assessment.

Treatment usually consists of blood pressure control (usually temporary) and surgical repair. Increasingly, endovascular stents are used to manage these injuries when anatomically feasible.

Notes

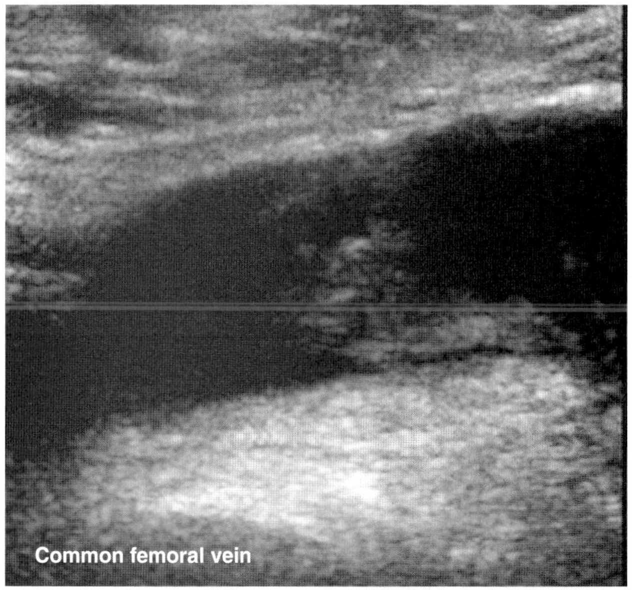

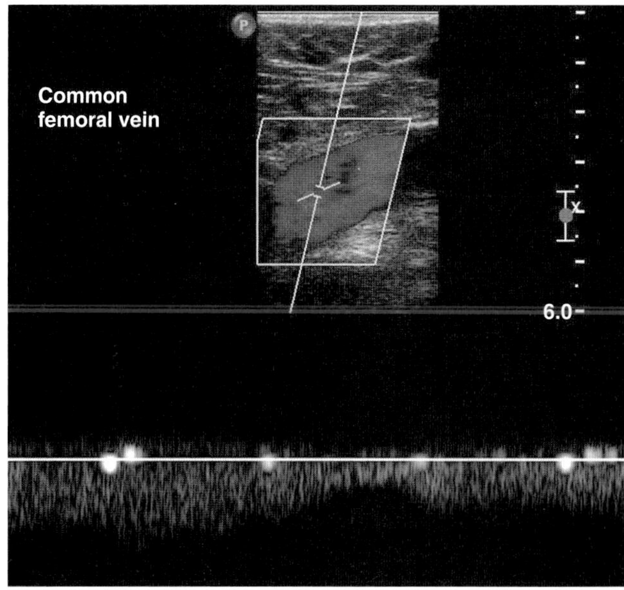

See also Color Plate

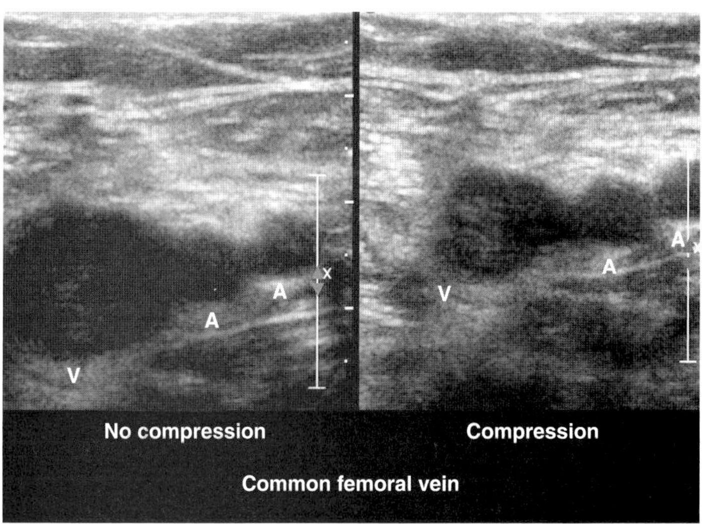

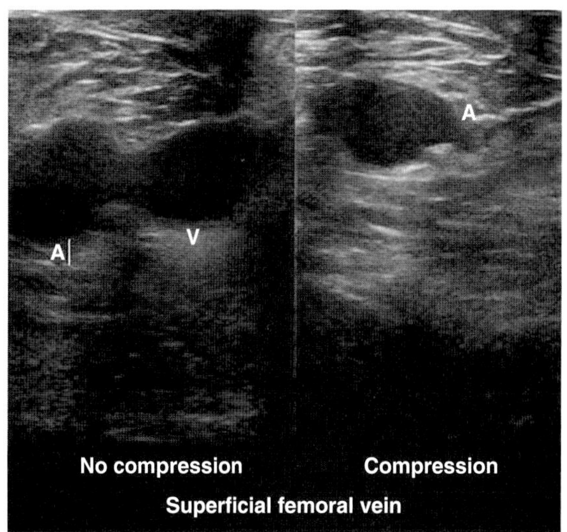

1. What is the diagnosis?
2. How does color Doppler interrogation further characterize the abnormality?
3. What maneuver performed during the sonographic examination is vital for maximizing the accuracy of ultrasound for detecting this abnormality?
4. What percentage of patients will have this diagnosis confirmed by sonography when it is suspected clinically?

CASE 4

Common Femoral Vein Deep Venous Thrombosis

1. Common femoral vein deep venous thrombosis.
2. It demonstrates flow around the thrombus thereby indicating it is nonocclusive.
3. Compression of the vein with the transducer.
4. 50%

References

Cronan JJ, Dorfman GS, Scola FH, et al: Deep venous thrombosis: US assessment using vein compression, *Radiology* 162:191–194, 1987.

Hamper UM, DeJong MR, Scoutt LM: Ultrasound evaluation of the lower extremity veins, *Radiol Clin North Am* 45:525–547, 2007.

Cross-Reference

Emergency Radiology: THE REQUISITES, p 240, 357–358.

Comment

Acute deep venous thrombosis (DVT) is common. The most important consequence of DVT is pulmonary embolism, which can complicate 50% to 60% of cases. Most DVTs originate in the deep veins of the legs and pelvis. Risk factors for DVT include hypercoagulability, venous stasis, malignancy, orthopedic surgery, trauma, oral contraceptive pills, and pregnancy. Signs and symptoms of lower extremity DVT include leg swelling, pain, edema, and tenderness. Reflecting the nonspecific nature of these clinical signs and symptoms, it has been shown that only 50% of patients who manifest them will be diagnosed with DVT. Moreover, acute DVT can be identified in asymptomatic patients.

Sonography is the current standard for diagnosing leg DVT. The sensitivity and specificity of ultrasound (US) for detecting leg DVTs are 89% to 95% and 92% to 100%, respectively. Importantly, US can demonstrate alternative diagnoses in 10% of patients with suspected acute DVT during normal venous examinations.

During grayscale US examination, acute thrombi can be identified as hyperechoic or hypoechoic intraluminal structures within the vein, although they are frequently anechoic and indistinguishable from the blood-filled venous lumen. Because of the varied echogenicities of acute thrombi, high accuracy of the US examination is facilitated by the use of compression sonography, whereby the vein is compressed by the transducer held along the axial plane of the vessel lumen. During compression, a thrombus prevents complete collapse of the vessel lumen. Conversely, complete collapse of the vessel lumen during compression effectively excludes DVT, even when relatively slow-flowing blood results in intraluminal echoes that may mimic a thrombus. At times, compression cannot be reliably performed because of either pain and swelling in the extremity or body habitus.

Other sonographic signs can be used to either diagnose or suggest DVT. Color Doppler imaging demonstrates absent flow in the presence of an occlusive thrombus, whereas flow will be reduced (i.e., it will not fill the venous lumen) if the thrombus is nonocclusive. Spectral analysis may show diminished augmentation of venous flow proximal to a thrombus when the calf is compressed during Doppler interrogation. Respiratory phasicity of the Doppler spectrum at the common femoral vein can be blunted by a more proximal occlusive venous thrombus, although it can also be seen if there is compression of the vein by a mass, hematoma, and so on. Expansion of the venous diameter by less than 50% following a Valsava maneuver also suggests a proximal DVT. When identified at the common femoral vein, the latter two signs can be used to suggest a pelvic DVT.

Notes

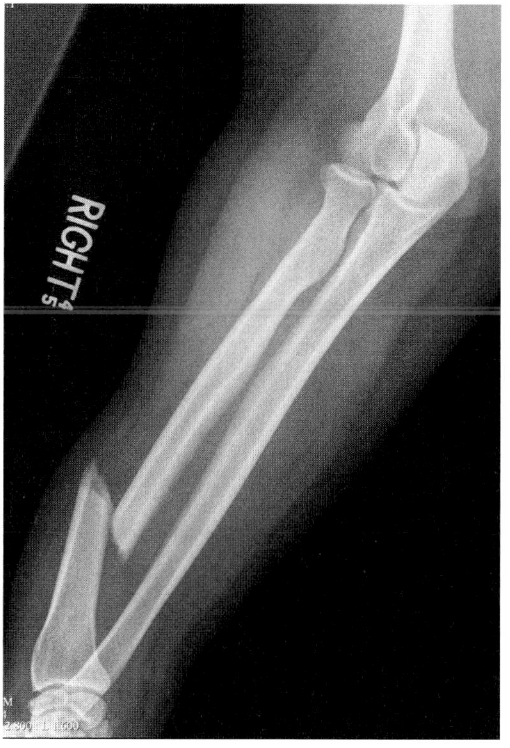

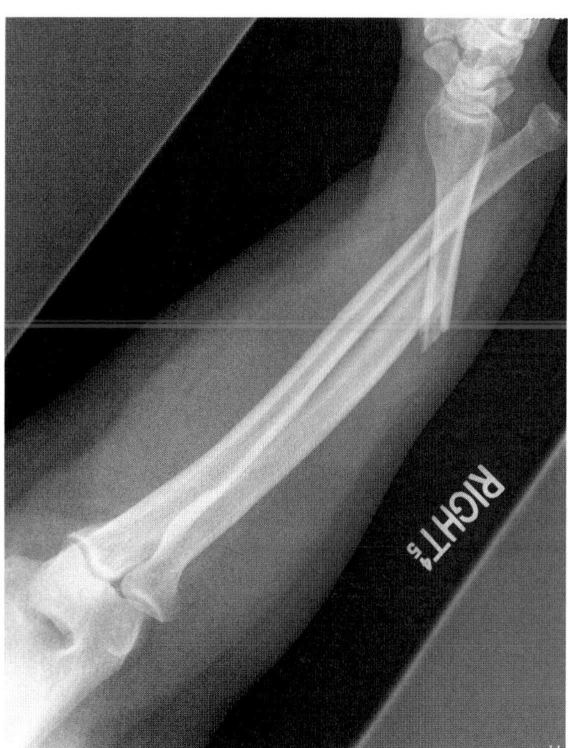

1. What injury is demonstrated?
2. Describe two mechanisms that can produce the injury.
3. In treating the injury in adults, is reduction maintained by internal or external fixation?
4. Is this injury pattern or an isolated radial fracture more common?

CASE 5

Galeazzi Fracture-Dislocation

1. Galeazzi fracture-dislocation (also referred to as "reverse" Monteggia fracture).
2. Fall on outstretched pronated hand or direct blow to dorsal lateral wrist.
3. Injury is unstable and requires open reduction and internal fixation.
4. An isolated radial fracture is a more common injury.

References

Giannoulis FS, Sotereanos DG: Galeazzi fractures and dislocations, *Hand Clin* 23:153–163, 2007.

Ring D, Rhim R, Carpenter C, Jupiter JB: Isolated radial shaft fractures are more common than Galeazzi fractures, *J Hand Surg Am* 31:17–21, 2006.

Cross-Reference

Emergency Radiology: THE REQUISITES, p 126.

Comment

The Galeazzi fracture was first described in 1934. The fracture typically occurs between the middle and distal thirds of the radius just above the level of the proximal border of the pronator quadratus muscle. The radial fracture is dorsally angulated. It is important to look for an associated injury to the distal radioulnar joint. The ulna is typically displaced dorsally, but can be palmar. In addition, there may be disruption of the triangular fibrocartilage complex with or without an ulnar styloid fracture. In children, the distal ulnar epiphysis may be separated.

The action of the pronator quadratus muscle on the palmar aspect of the distal radial fragment tends to rotate the fragment toward the ulna and pulls it in a proximal and palmar direction. The dorsal displacement of the ulna (ulnar plus variance) permits radial shortening. Shortening that exceeds 10 mm indicates complete disruption of the interosseous membrane and complete instability of the radioulnar joint. Complications of the injury include nonunion, delayed radial union, or malunion (residual instability). Open reduction and internal fixation with plate and screw fixation of the radial diaphyseal fracture and K-wire fixation of the distal radial-ulnar articulation are required to treat unstable injuries.

Notes

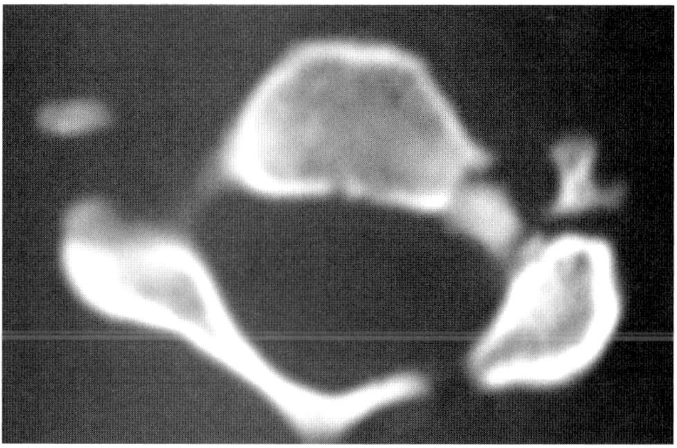

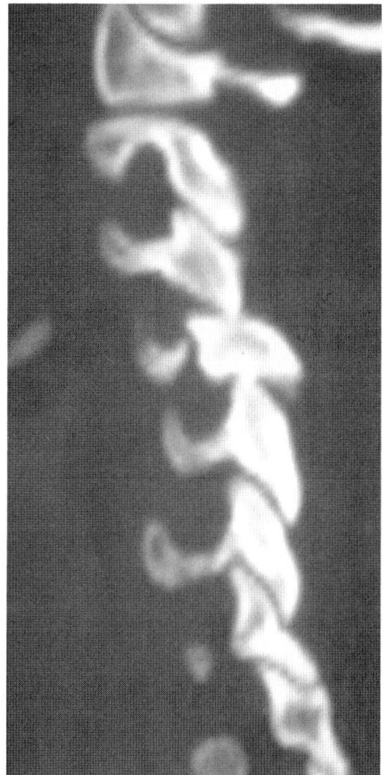

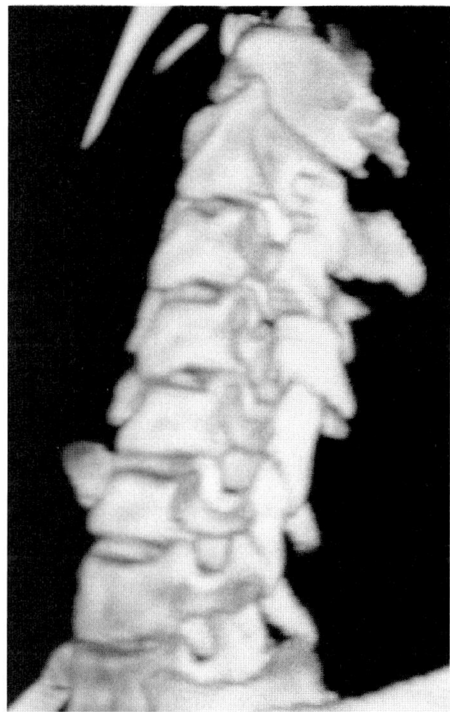

See also Color Plate

You are shown images of a blunt trauma patient.

1. What is the diagnosis?
2. Is this injury due primarily to a flexion or extension force?
3. Is this injury mechanically stable or unstable?
4. What complication should be sought in association with this injury pattern?

CASE 6

Isolated Articular Pillar (Lamino-pedicular Separation)

1. Isolated articular pillar.
2. Flexion force.
3. Unstable.
4. Ipsilateral vertebral artery injury from transforaminal fracture course.

Reference

Shanmuganathan K, Mirvis SE, Dowe M, Levine AM: Traumatic isolation of the cervical articular pillar: imaging observations in 21 patients, *AJR Am J Roentgenol* 166:897–902, 1996.

Cross-Reference

Emergency Radiology: THE REQUISITES, p 221.

Comment

The isolated articular pillar fracture, or lamino-pedicular separation, is created with combined ipsilateral laminar and pedicle fractures. There is simultaneous disruption of the facet joints above and below the injury. This pattern permits the entire articular pillar to rotate freely. The forces acting on the pillar rotate the anterior aspect of the pillar caudally and the posterior portion cephalad. This motion changes the orientation of the facets, which are normally angled 35 degrees to the horizontal plane, to a zero degree angle. On an anteroposterior radiograph of the cervical spine, the joint space above and below the rotated pillar can be visualized directly.

While some researchers have suggested that the injury mechanism is compressive extension, more recent studies have indicated that flexion forces are far more commonly associated with the isolated pillar. Often the injury is seen concurrently with other flexion injuries such as the unilateral facet dislocation or subluxation, articular pillar fracture-subluxation, or bifacet dislocation. The flexion injury produced appears to depend on the vector and duration of flexion, flexion rotation, and flexion-loading forces acting on the spine. The injury is considered mechanically unstable and requires three-level fixation. Another important feature of the injury is a tendency for the fracture lines to extend across the foramen transversarium and injure the adjacent vertebral artery.

Notes

CASE 7

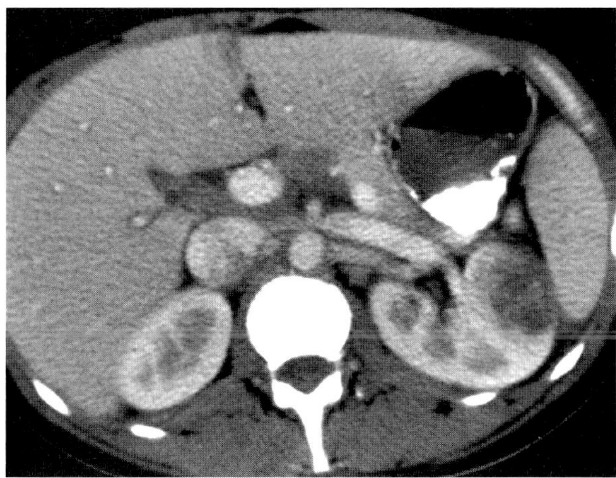

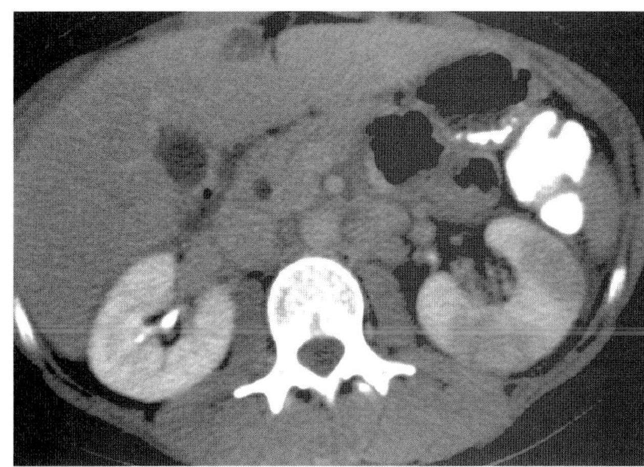

You are shown images of a patient with nontraumatic left flank pain.

1. What pathologic process is shown?
2. What is the most common etiology?
3. What signs and symptoms are likely to be present?
4. Is computed tomography or sonography the most sensitive and specific means of diagnosis?

CASE 7

Focal Bacterial Acute Pyelonephritis (Acute Lobar Nephronia)

1. Focal bacterial acute pyelonephritis (lobar nephronia).
2. Gram-negative rods (*E. coli*).
3. Fever, flank pain, pyuria, leukocytosis, bacteriuria.
4. Computed tomography.

Reference

Kawashima A, LeRoy AJ: Radiologic evaluation of patients with renal infections, *Infect Dis Clin North Am* 17:433–456, 2003.

Cross-Reference

Emergency Radiology: THE REQUISITES, pp 299–300.

Comment

Acute lobar nephronia (ALN) is a localized and nonliquefactive renal infection that involves one or more lobes. It is believed to represent a stage of infection between pyelonephritis and renal abscess. While most patients present with fever, flank pain, leukocytosis, and pyuria, the presentation may be atypical with minimal symptoms such as vague flank or abdominal pain, malaise, fever, and negative urine cultures, and without specific urinary tract symptoms. Many patients who develop ALN have urine reflux or congenital urinary tract abnormalities, but the condition also can arise in patients with normal urinary systems. In almost all cases gram-negative bacteria, usually *E. coli*, are the etiologic organisms.

Three pathologic forms of ALN have been described including focal or diffuse wedge-shaped lesions, focal masslike lesions, and multiple diffuse masslike lesions, the latter having the worst prognosis. Most patients respond well to a prolonged course of antibiotics, about 3 weeks.

The diagnosis is usually established by sonography or computed tomography (CT). On sonography the kidney is usually enlarged with an irregular mass that disrupts the corticomedullary junction. The mass is usually hypoechoic, but may appear iso- or hyperechoic as well. Generally, sonography is the preferred initial study for suspected pediatric cases to avoid X-ray exposure, but may require CT when results are uncertain. On intravenous contrast-enhanced CT, ALN appears as hypodense round or wedge-shaped areas with focal or diffuse renal swelling.

Overall, CT scanning is considered to be the most sensitive and specific means of diagnosing ALN. A voiding cystourethrogram should be done to rule out reflux as an underlying cause. Usually lesions resolve within 1 to 3 months after treatment and sonography is appropriate for follow-up to confirm resolution. Misdiagnosis of masslike ALN as abscess or renal tumor, which it may simulate, can lead to inappropriate surgical or interventional therapy.

Notes

CASE 8

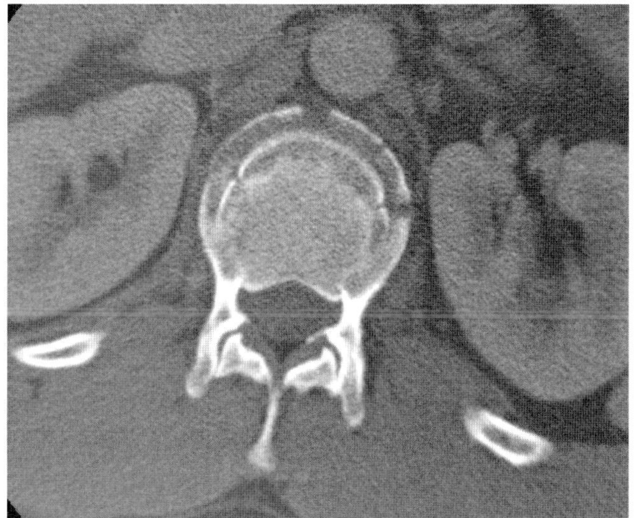

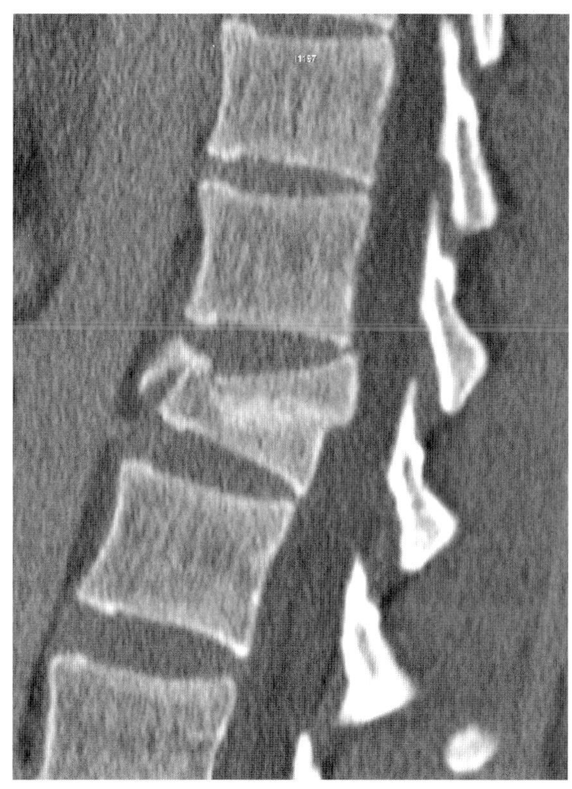

You are shown images of a blunt trauma patient.

1. What is the spinal injury shown?
2. Is it a stable or unstable injury?
3. What is the most common level of the injury?
4. What other nonspinal fractures should be sought with this injury?

CASE 8

Lumbar Burst Fracture

1. Lumbar burst fracture.
2. Unstable.
3. L1.
4. Pelvic and calcaneal fractures.

Reference

Bensch FV, Kiuru MJ, Koivikko MP, Koskinen SK: Spine fractures in falling accidents: analysis of multidetector CT findings, *Eur J Radiol* 14:618–624, 2004.

Cross-Reference

Emergency Radiology: THE REQUISITES, pp 223, 225.

Comment

The burst fracture is an axial loading injury with flexion. It primarily affects the lower thoracic and upper lumbar spine from T4 to L5 and constitutes 14% of spinal column injuries. Burst fractures differ from anterior compression fractures by the greater loss of anterior column height (>40%), the loss of posterior column height with disruption of the posterior cortical line, a common mid-sagittal vertebral body split, retropulsion of posterior vertebral fragments typically from the superior aspect of the body, and fractures of the posterior spinal elements. Concurrent spinal fractures, both contiguous and noncontiguous, occur in up to 40% of patients.

Since there is disruption of the anterior and middle spinal columns and potential disruption of the posterior ligaments, the injury should be regarded as mechanically unstable with about 50% of patients demonstrating neurologic deficits. The incidence of neurologic deficits increases the more cephalad the level of spinal injury and the greater the area of canal compromise, but the severity of any neurologic deficit is not reliably predictable in individual cases. A variant of this injury is the "chance burst" which can involve more than 40% of burst fractures and combines features of both injury patterns (horizontally oriented posterior element and pedicle fractures). This variant is associated more commonly with concurrent abdominal pathology as occurs with the flexion-distraction mechanism.

Notes

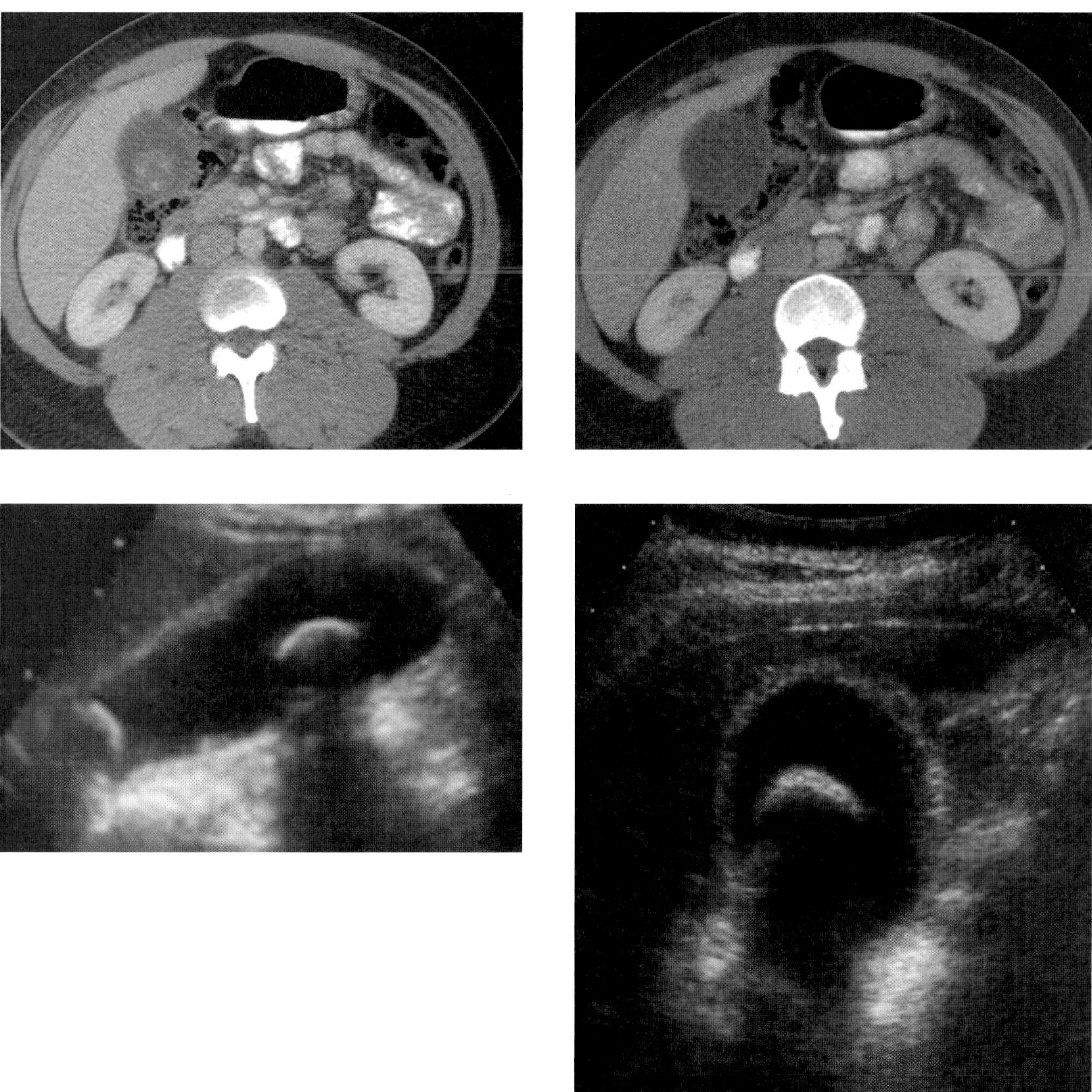

You are shown images of a patient with nontraumatic upper abdominal pain.

1. What is the diagnosis?
2. What cross-sectional imaging findings suggest the diagnosis?
3. What complications can develop from this illness?
4. Which imaging study is typically the first choice to establish this diagnosis?

CASE 9

Acute Calculus Cholecystitis

1. Acute cholecystitis.
2. Gallbladder hydrops (rounded distension, diameter > 5 cm), gallstones, wall thickening > 3 mm, subserosal or pericholecystic edema, pericholecystic fat infiltration, sludge, sonographic Murphy's sign.
3. Abscess, empyema (purulent fluid in lumen), gangrene, perforation, cholecystoenteric fistula.
4. Sonography.

Reference

Hanbidge AE, Buckler PM, O'Malley ME, Wilson SR: Imaging evaluation for acute pain in the right upper quadrant, *Radiographics* 24:1117–1135, 2004.

Cross-Reference

Emergency Radiology: THE REQUISITES, pp 294–296.

Comment

Acute cholecystitis occurs in approximately one third of patients with gallstones and is caused by obstruction of the cystic duct by an impacted calculus in 90% to 95% of cases. This results in gallbladder wall inflammation which may lead to infection and necrosis. The illness occurs more commonly in women (75%) aged 40 to 60 years. The incidence is higher with advancing age and in races with a higher incidence of gallstones, including Native Americans and persons of Chinese or Japanese descent. The main symptom is abdominal pain, particularly after a fatty meal, located in the right upper quadrant (RUQ) and occasionally accompanied by nausea, vomiting, and low-grade fever. Palpation may reveal a RUQ mass representing the distended gallbladder and Murphy's sign (sudden suspension of inspiration with manual compression in right subcostal region).

Hepatobiliary scintigraphy with technetium-99m (^{99m}Tc IDA) is 92% to 95% accurate and is an excellent method to confirm the diagnosis based on nonvisualization of the gallbladder. Cross-section imaging by sonography or computed tomography (CT) is indicated when a broader differential diagnosis is under consideration, with sonography typically the first choice. CT is preferred when factors limit sonography (open wounds, surgical dressings, obesity) or when complications are suspected. Sonography is sensitive and specific with a 92% positive predictive value. Positive findings include gallstones, gallbladder (GB) wall thickening (>3 mm), a "halo sign" or GB wall lucency (subserosal edema), GB hydrops when anteroposterior diameter is greater than 5 cm, a sonographic Murphy's sign, and pericholecystic fluid. CT shows these same findings and is the single best study to identify more general pathology in the RUQ as well as other positive findings such as sloughed mucosal membranes, high attention bile, and inflammatory changes in the pericholecystic fat. CT is advantageous in detecting complications such as GB perforation, empyema, pericholecystic abscess, and gangrene (suggested by irregular wall ulcers, intraluminal hemorrhage, wall or intraluminal air, and hyperechoic foci within GB wall microabscesses).

Notes

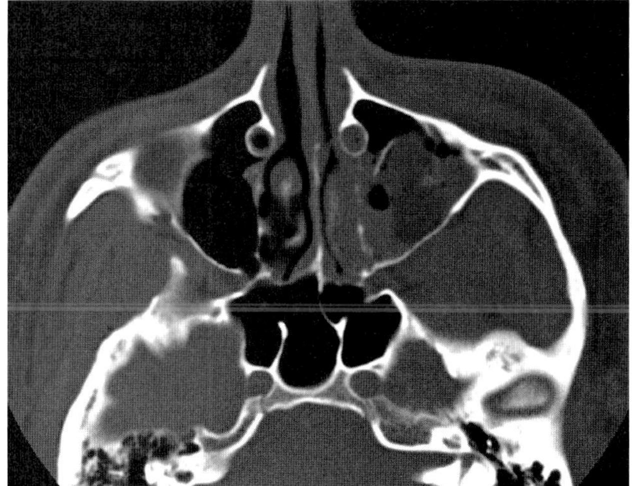

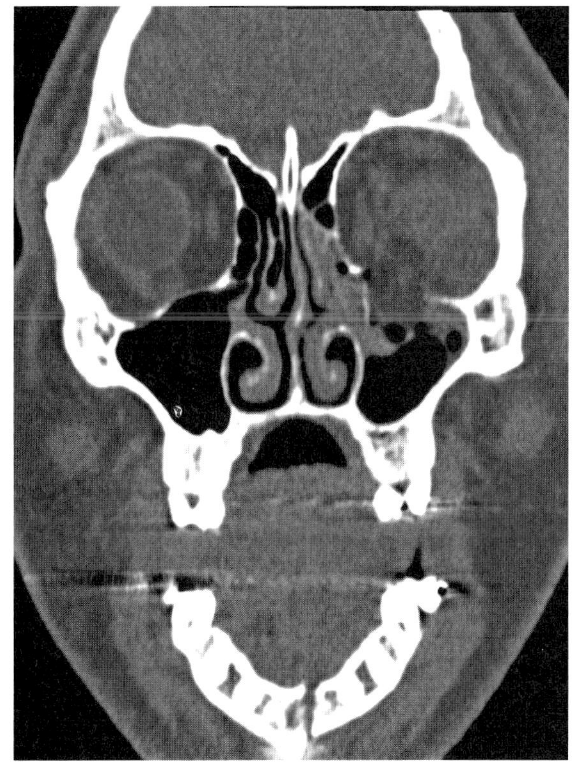

You are shown images of a patient with blunt trauma and left facial swelling.

1. What is the facial injury shown?
2. What are the potential associated complications?
3. What is the most common concurrent fracture?
4. What is the difference between the "pure" and "impure" form of this injury?

CASE 10

Orbital Blow-out Fracture

1. Orbital floor "blow-out" fracture with orbital fat herniation.
2. Diplopia, enophthalmos (usually delayed), hypoesthesia or dysesthesia of cheek, upper lip, anterior maxillary teeth.
3. An inferior medial orbital wall fracture (20%–40%).
4. The pure fracture involves the orbital floor only; the impure also involves the inferior orbital rim and is more likely with mid-facial fractures.

Reference

Rhea JT, Rao PM, Novelline RA: Helical CT and three-dimensional CT of facial and orbital injury, *Radiol Clin North Am* 37:489–513, 1999.

Cross-Reference

Emergency Radiology: THE REQUISITES, pp 38–39.

Comment

Orbital floor fractures are one of the more common blunt trauma facial injuries resulting from direct impact to the orbit by an object larger than the orbital diameter. Fractures of the thin osseous plates surrounding the orbit and the orbital fat help absorb impacting energy, decompress intraorbital pressure, and preserve the integrity of the globe. Complications of the injury usually include diplopia resulting from numerous causes (orbital hematoma, extra-ocular muscle (EOM) contusion, EOM herniation-entrapment, oculomotor nerve branch contusion) and injury to the inferior orbital nerve as it runs along the floor of the orbit. Most causes of diplopia resolve within 1 to 2 weeks, but care must be taken to identify entrapment of the inferior rectus muscle or tethered orbital fat. Entrapment requires surgical release. Inferior rectus entrapment is typically associated with small orbital floor fractures, descent of the muscle below the plane of the floor, and distortion of muscle contour. Large orbital floor fractures or concurrent orbital wall fractures may lead to delayed enophthalmos due to increased orbital volume. Direct axial imaging of the orbit with 2-mm images and coronal reformation is usually adequate to diagnose significant injuries, without irradiating the orbit in the direct coronal plane.

Notes

CASE 11

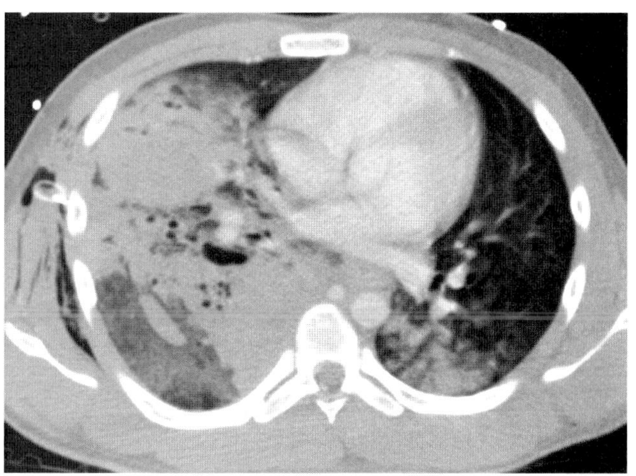

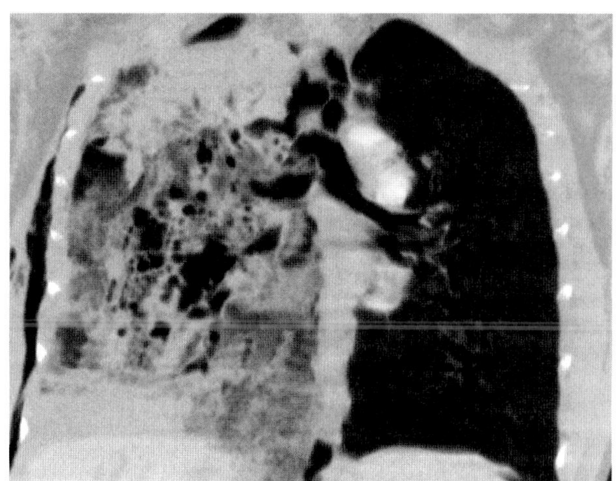

You are shown images of a blunt trauma patient.

1. What is the diagnosis?
2. What are potential complications of this pathology?
3. Does the absence of rib fractures alter the likely diagnosis?
4. Is the condition seen more commonly in the perihilar or peripheral lung?

CASE 11

Pulmonary Contusions and Lacerations

1. Pulmonary contusions and lacerations.
2. Infection, abscess, bronchopleural fistula, hemorrhage, enlarging traumatic pulmonary pseudocyst.
3. No; in young patients with pliable chest walls, rib fractures are frequently absent.
4. Usually involves the periphery in a nonsegmental distribution.

Reference

Mirvis SE: Diagnostic imaging of acute thoracic injury, *Semin Ultrasound CT MR* 25:156–179, 2004.

Cross-Reference

Emergency Radiology: THE REQUISITES, pp 65–66.

Comment

Pulmonary contusions commonly accompany blunt chest trauma. The location and shape of lung contusions reflect the location and shape of the impacting object so contusions tend to be nonsegmental and nonlobar in distribution and typically are peripheral lung opacities. Computed tomography (CT) is far more sensitive than radiography in demonstrating the injury and accurately depicting its extent. Most contusions appear as areas of lung consolidation often partly composed of small rounded areas of hematoma formation. Almost all nonminor contusions are associated with lacerations of the lung, which may be linear or rounded (traumatic pneumatoceles), may be either air-filled or fluid-filled, or may contain air–fluid levels. Air-bronchograms are infrequently seen with lung contusions due to filling of the small airways with blood. Rib fractures are usually present in older adult patients, but children and young adults, with compliant chest walls, may not have concurrent rib fractures.

The diagnosis of pulmonary contusion by CT alone, with a normal chest radiograph, implies the injury will make no significant contribution to morbidity. Uncommonly, complications related to major contusion and lacerations, including lung abscess formation and bronchopleural fistula, and enlarging traumatic pulmonary pseudocyst compressing the adjacent lung can develop and can cause significant morbidity. The volume of injured lung appears to correlate positively with the likelihood of developing subsequent acute respiratory distress syndrome (ARDS). Contusions may appear to undergo some radiologic resolution as soon as 2 to 3 days after injury. Persistence or progression of density raises questions of bleeding, aspiration, atelectasis, ARDS, and superimposed pneumonia.

Notes

CASE 12

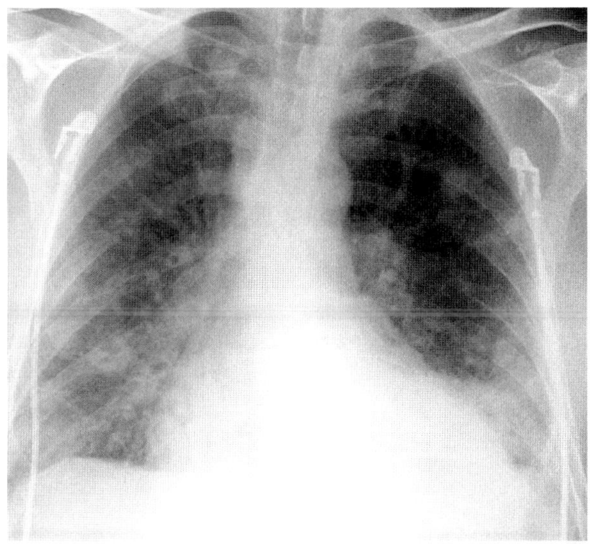

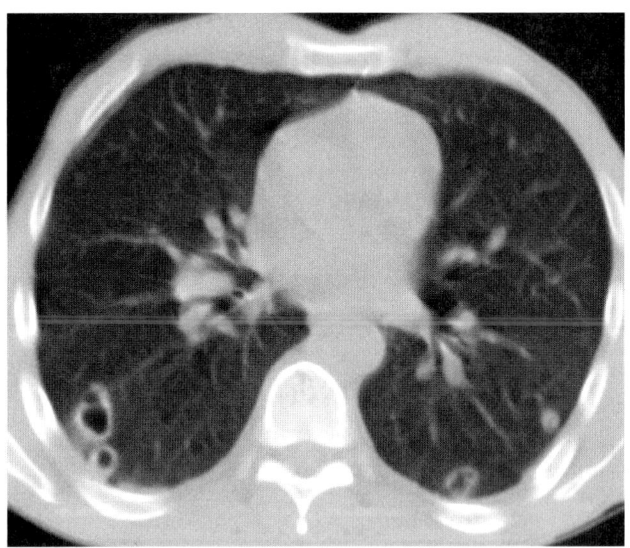

You are shown images of a nontrauma patient with fever and cough.

1. What is the most likely diagnosis?
2. What are some alternative diagnoses?
3. What diagnosis study should be performed to appropriately evaluate the patient?
4. What are some etiologies of this condition?

CASE 12

Septic Pulmonary Emboli

1. Septic pulmonary emboli.
2. Potentially a long list, but some other considerations are cystic metastasis, pneumocystitis carinii pneumonia, Langerhan's histiocytosis, lymphangioleiomyomatosis, and peripheral bronchiectasis.
3. Echocardiography to assess tricuspid and pulmonic valves for vegetations and cardiac and valve function.
4. Long-term indwelling catheters, pacemakers, chronic infection such as osteomyelitis, liver abscess, septic jugular venous thrombosis (Lemierre's syndrome), intravenous drug abuser, periodontal disease.

References

Kulman JE, Fishman EK, Teigen BA: Pulmonary septic emboli: diagnosis with CT, *Radiology* 174:211–213, 1990.

Natuhara A, Harada H, Kubota Y, et al: Spiral CT findings in septic pulmonary emboli, *Eur J Radiol* 37: 190–194, 2001.

Comment

Septic pulmonary embolism (SPE) is an uncommon entity and may be insidious in its clinical presentation. Symptoms include fever, dyspnea, pleuritic chest pain, cough, and hemoptysis. A variety of infectious sources are responsible such as long-term central venous catheters, prosthetic cardiac valves, pacemaker wires, and chronic infections such as osteomyelitis, otitis media, or chronic abscesses. A history of intravenous drug abuse is often present.

Immunocompromised patients are also at increased risk. Staphylococcus is the most common pathogen. Chest radiographic findings may be nonspecific showing patchy infiltrates, but can also show well-demarcated rounded peripheral opacifications, some with cavitation strongly suggesting the diagnosis. Computed tomography (CT) findings include peripheral and subpleural nodule opacifications of varying size usually ranging from 10 to 20 mm in diameter, wedge-shaped lesions, or nonspecific infiltrates. The extent of disease usually appears greater on CT than on radiographs. Some nodules will have necrotic centers and some demonstrate a central "feeding" artery, although this finding is less common than previously thought based on high-resolution multidetector CT findings. It is important to perform echocardiography to assess for valve vegetations (typically tricuspid) and function.

Notes

CASE 13

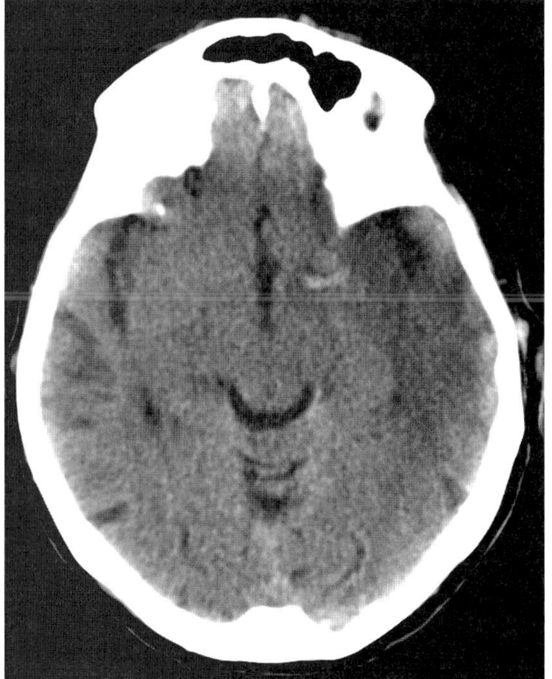

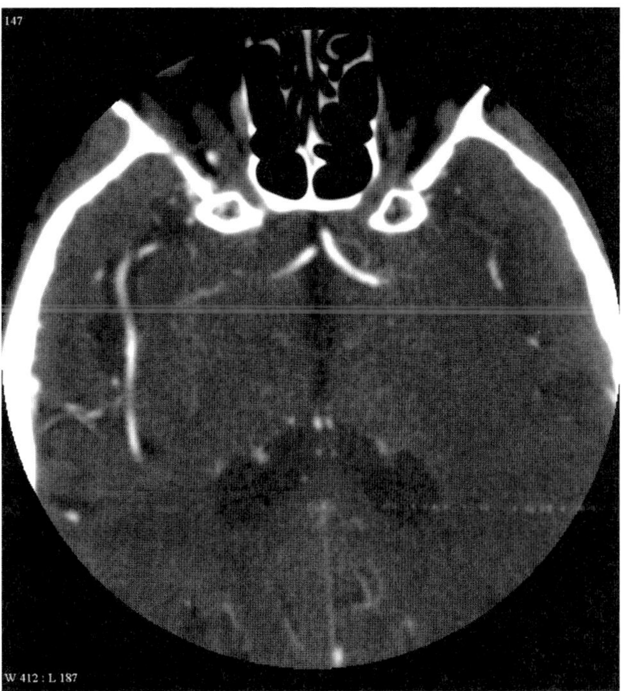

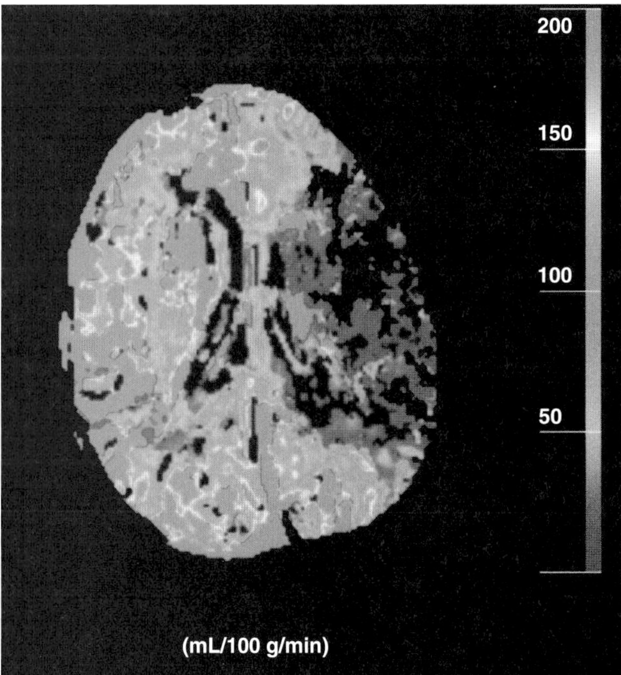

See also Color Plate

You are shown images of a nontrauma patient with right-sided weakness.

1. What computed tomography (CT) sign is observed on the nonenhanced brain CT?
2. Which other CT findings may be seen within the first 6 hours of this condition?
3. What entities could mimic the CT sign displayed in the nonenhanced CT?
4. Is the perfusion CT finding one that would be expected in an acute cerebrovascular accident?

CASE 13

Hyperdense Middle Cerebral Artery Sign

1. A left hyperdense middle cerebral artery sign.
2. Loss of grey-white junction along insula (insular ribbon sign), obscured lentiform nucleus borders, effacement of cortical sulci, swelling of cortical gyri (cellular edema).
3. Atherosclerotic calcification, elevated hematocrit, prior administration of intravenous contrast material.
4. Yes, diminished cerebral blood flow is expected due to occluded middle cerebral artery.

References

Beauchamp NJ, Barker PB, Wang PY, vanZijl PCM: Imaging of acute cerebral ischemia, *Radiology* 212: 307–324, 1999.

Somford DM, Nederkoorn PJ, Rutgers DR, et al: Proximal and distal hyperattenuation middle cerebral artery sign at CT: different prognostic implications, *Radiology* 223:667–671, 2002.

Cross-Reference

Emergency Radiology: THE REQUISITES, pp 12–14.

Comment

The hyperdense middle cerebral artery (MCA) sign is a thrombus in the M1 segment of the middle cerebral artery. Unlike some relatively early CT signs of ischemic stroke, this sign may be present at the time of ictus. The density is due to thrombus within the vessel which should have a density clearly exceeding that of the contralateral MCA and basilar artery. The clot is identified because of both the transverse course of the M1 segment along the plane of the CT section and the low-attenuation cerebrospinal fluid around the vessel. False positive findings can occur due to vascular calcification of atherosclerosis or an elevated hematocrit. In both cases one would expect the density of the M1 segment to be elevated bilaterally. The MCA sign has a prevalence of 17.5% to 50% and the prevalence appears to be higher the earlier the CT scan is performed after the ictus.

While the MCA sign has a specificity approaching 100%, the sensitivity is much lower, at about 54% (negative predictive value 71%), so its absence in no way excludes the diagnosis of stroke. Because the thrombosis occurs proximally in the MCA, patients usually sustain a large and deep MCA distribution infarct, and the finding is believed to predict a worse prognosis than for patients with a more distal M2 or M3 segment thrombosis. Confirmation of vascular occlusion can be by CT angiography and evidence of diminished regional cerebral blood flow can be documented by perfusion CT. However, in most cases MRI is best suited to verify ischemia based on elevation of signal on diffusion weighted scans accompanied by decreased signal on apparent diffusion coefficient maps.

The MCA "dot sign" is a variant of the hyperdense MCA sign in which a more distal branch of the MCA (M2 or M3) is seen as a focal hyperdensity. The hyperdense dot typically corresponds to a vertical MCA branch coursing in the Sylvian fissure, appearing as a bright dot in CT cross-section. Since the more distal thrombus results in ischemia to a smaller volume of cerebral tissue it is believed to predict a better neurologic outcome than the typical MCA sign. Again, the "dot sign" is quite insensitive to stroke at 38%, but also has specificity approaching 100%.

Notes

CASE 14

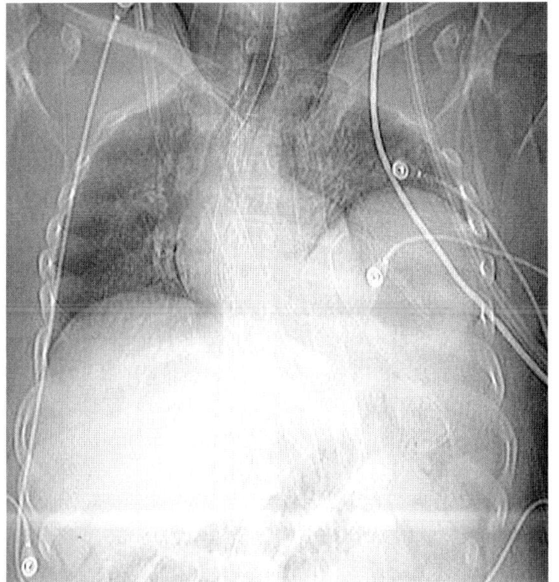

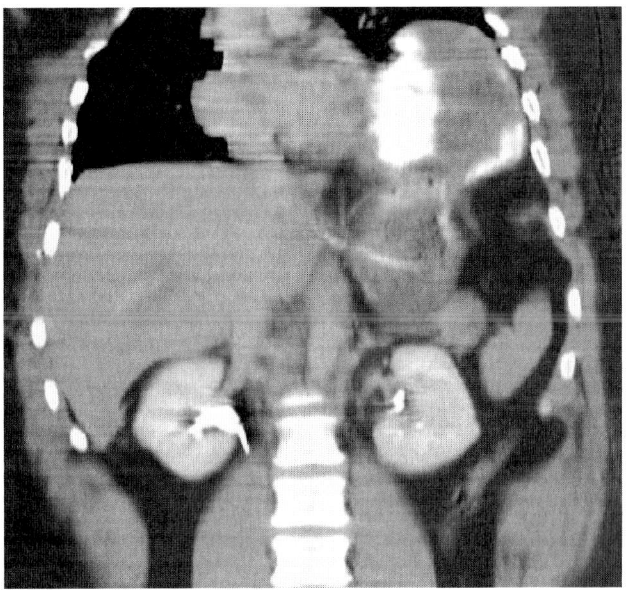

You are shown images of a blunt trauma patient.

1. What is the diagnosis?
2. What are three diagnostic computed tomography findings of this injury?
3. What three entities can mimic this diagnosis?
4. Which side is involved more commonly and why?

CASE 14

Left Hemidiaphragm Rupture and Gastric Herniation into Thorax

1. Ruptured left hemidiaphragm and gastric herniation into thorax.
2. Computed tomography "collar" sign, direct visualization of torn diaphragm edges, "dependent viscera" sign.
3. Diaphragm eventration, lower lobe atelectasis, phrenic nerve palsy.
4. Left side; thinner than right, line of weakness at fusion of costal and lumbar portions, liver protects right hemidiaphragm.

Reference

Sliker CW: Imaging of diaphragm injuries, *Radiol Clin North Am* 44:199–211, 2006.

Cross-Reference

Emergency Radiology: THE REQUISITES, pp 70–74.

Comment

Left hemidiaphragm tears are more common than right-sided injuries, as cited earlier, with about 75% occurring on the left. These injuries commonly result from sudden increases in intraperitoneal pressure transmitted throughout the abdominal cavity tearing the relatively weak and exposed left hemidiaphragm. Shearing forces and tears from rib fractures also can be etiologic. Usually tears are 10 cm or more beginning posterolaterally and extending medially toward the central tendon. The initial chest radiograph is diagnostic in up to two thirds of cases showing clear herniation of abdominal viscera into the chest. Suspicious radiographic findings include elevated hemidiaphragm, irregular contour or nonvisualized hemidiaphragm, mass effects on the heart and mediastinum, and lower lobe atelectasis and effusion.

The diagnosis of right-sided rupture is less commonly made radiographically, as the liver often prevents herniation. The liver is the most likely organ to herniate in right-sided rupture and produces a "humplike" contour in the apparent right hemidiaphragm. Thin-section computed tomography (CT) with sagittal and coronal reformations assists in making the diagnosis in uncertain cases.

The "dependent viscera" sign is present when the herniated structure is in direct contact with the posterior chest wall on CT of the supine patient. A torn diaphragm and waistlike constriction of the herniated structure ("collar" sign) are other diagnostic CT findings. Concurrent lower rib fractures and other chest and abdominal injuries are relatively common. The negative pressure gradient between the pleural and peritoneal cavity increases the likelihood of herniation, and this effect can be negated for patients on positive pressure ventilatory support. Postextubation films in such cases are important to detect delayed herniation. MRI serves as a third-line diagnostic study when CT is not definitive and relies mainly on T1-weighted sagittal and coronal views.

Notes

CASE 15

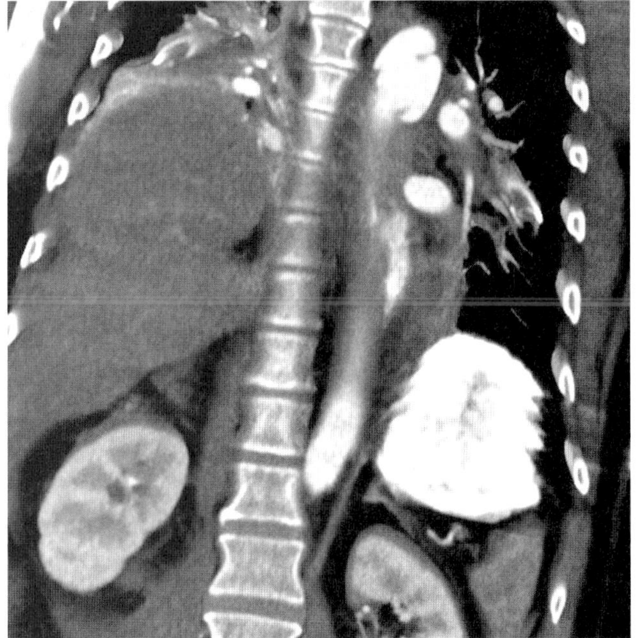

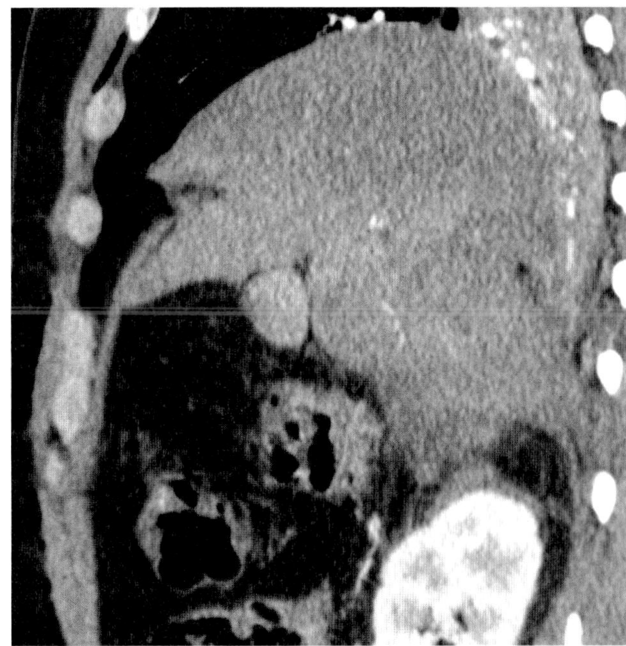

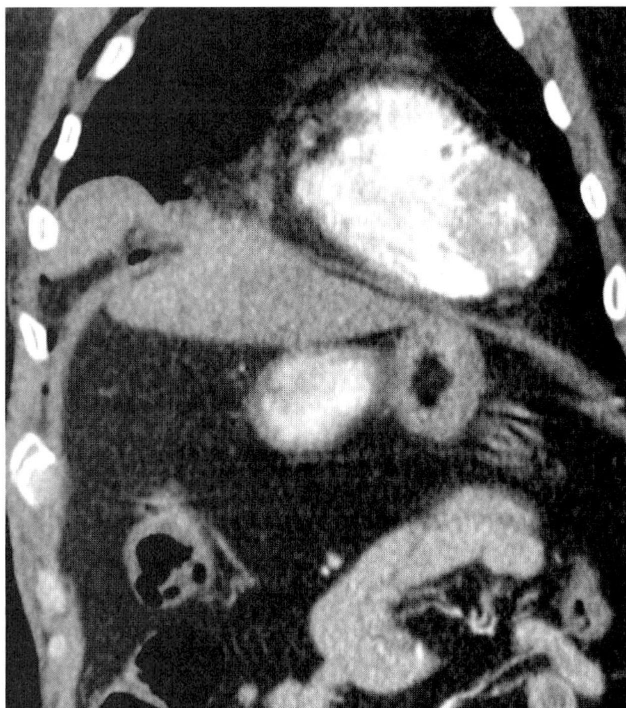

You are shown images of a blunt trauma patient.

1. What is the diagnosis?
2. What major computed tomography signs can establish the diagnosis?
3. Why is this diagnosis more common on the left side?
4. What entities can mimic this diagnosis on imaging studies?

CASE 15

Rupture of the Right Hemidiaphragm with Liver Herniation

1. Rupture of the right hemidiaphragm with liver herniation.
2. "Collar" sign, direct diaphragm tear visualization, dependent viscera sign, "bump" sign ("humplike" configuration of herniated liver segment), "band" sign (linear low attenuation across constricted part of liver at level of diaphragm).
3. The left diaphragm is congenitally weaker than the right, and the liver mass protects the right hemidiaphragm.
4. Eventration of the right hemidiaphragm, right lower lobe atelectasis, phrenic nerve injury, foramen of Bochdalek hernia.

References

Iochum S, Ludig T, Walter F, et al: Imaging of diaphragmatic injury: a diagnostic challenge? *Radiographics* 22:103–111, 2002.

Rees O, Mirvis SE, Shanmuganathan K: Multidetector-row CT of right hemidiaphragmatic rupture caused by blunt trauma: a review of 12 cases, *Clin Radiol* 60:1280–1289, 2005.

Cross-Reference

Emergency Radiology: THE REQUISITES, pp 70–74.

Comment

Diaphragmatic injuries occur in 0.8% to 8% of patients after blunt trauma. Rupture of the right hemidiaphragm occurs less commonly than left-sided rupture due to the greater strength of the right hemidiaphragm and absorption of energy by the liver protecting the diaphragm. Even when right hemidiaphragm ruptures occur, the bulk of the liver may prevent herniation unless the tear is substantial in length. In surgical series of blunt abdominal trauma, the diagnosis of right hemidiaphragm injury is more commonly established than by imaging since the diaphragm tear can be directly visualized. In surgical series right-sided injury accounts for about one third of total diaphragm injuries, which is a higher percentage than typically seen in imaging series. The diagnosis usually requires herniation of the liver or other abdominal structures into the right hemithorax before the imaging diagnosis can be established.

Radiography, computed tomography (CT), sonography, and magnetic resonance imaging all have the potential to diagnose this injury. In the setting of blunt trauma, elevation of the apparent right hemidiaphragm 4 cm or more above the left hemidiaphragm by chest radiography should be regarded with suspicion for the injury. The herniated portion of the liver may have a "humplike" shape due to the contour imposed by the residual intact diaphragm. CT is the most useful modality to establish the diagnosis. The "collar" sign, created by the edges of the diaphragm, direct visualization of the torn diaphragm edges, herniation of abdominal content into the hemithorax, and direct contact of the posterior liver and posterior chest wall in the supine patient (dependent viscera sign) all establish the diagnosis. The application of coronal and sagittal reformations is particularly useful to visualize these findings and improves diagnostic accuracy. Not surprisingly, there are typically concurrent injuries in the lower right hemithorax and liver. Overall mortality exceeds that in patients with left-sided ruptures, probably indicating the greater energy level required to produce the injury.

Notes

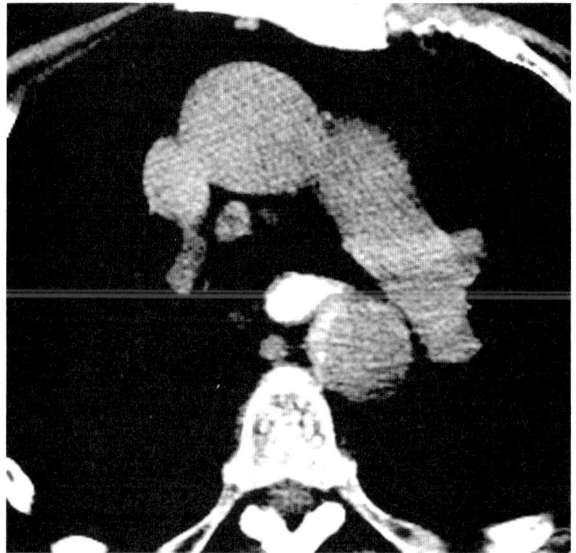

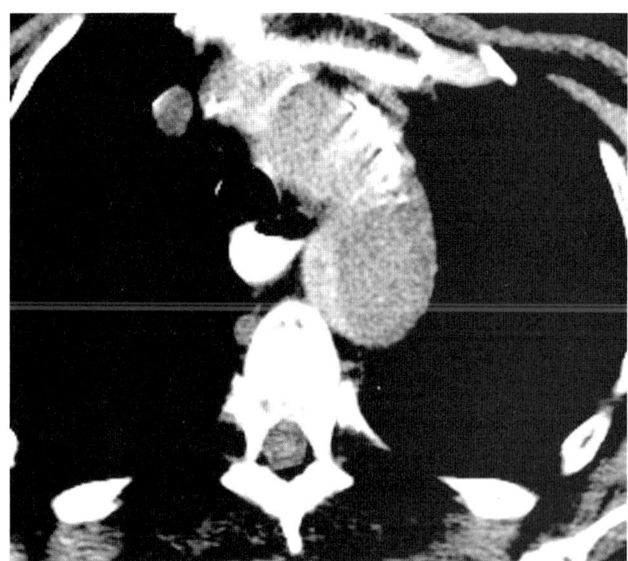

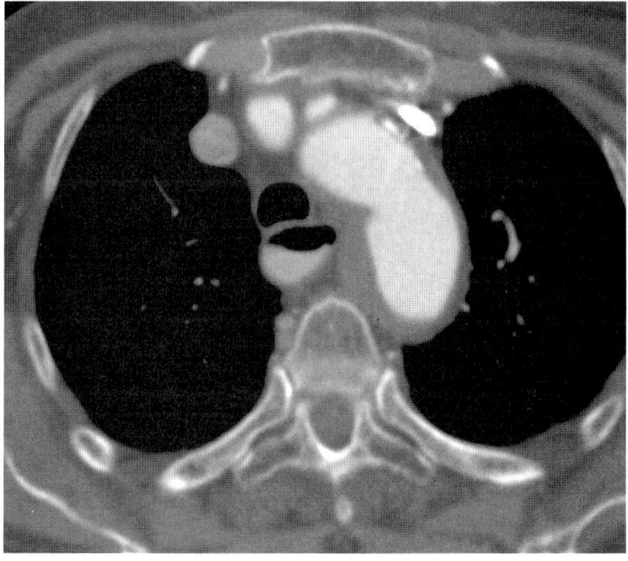

1. What is the diagnosis?
2. What is the typical clinical presentation?
3. What conditions can develop with progression of this lesion?
4. What computed tomography features favor likely progression of this lesion?

CASE 16

Intramural Aortic Hematoma

1. Intramural aortic hematoma.
2. Chest and/or back pain.
3. Aortic dissection, aortic aneurysm, aortic rupture.
4. Location in the ascending aorta (type A), ascending aorta diameter greater than 5 cm, descending aortic diameter greater than 4 cm (type B), thick hematoma compressing lumen.

Reference

Castañer E, Andreu M, Gallardo X, et al: CT in nontraumatic acute thoracic aortic disease: typical and atypical features and complications, *Radiographics* 23: S93–S110, 2003.

Cross-Reference

Emergency Radiology: THE REQUISITES, pp 249–250.

Comment

Intramural hematoma (IMH) is one of three entities that are considered non-traumatic acute aortic pathologies; the other two entities are aortic dissection and penetrating aortic ulcer. These conditions are usually found in patients with a history of hypertension and who present with acute chest and/or back pain. IMH results from bleeding of the vaso vasorum, producing a localized wall hematoma. Since contrast material in the aortic lumen can obscure the hyperdense blood within the wall, all patients with suspected acute aortic syndrome must undergo non-enhanced chest computed tomography (CT) initially. In the majority of cases IMH appears as a crescent-shaped area of attenuation in the aortic wall typically greater than 4 mm thick, corresponding to a hematoma in the medial layer; occasionally the hematoma is concentric. Hematoma may or may not compress the aortic lumen. Intimal calcifications also may be displaced by IMH.

IMH is divided into types A and B in the same manner as the Stanford system for aortic dissections. IMH in either location can progress to frank dissection, aneurysm, or aortic rupture. Initial IMH accounts for approximately 13% of the prevalence of acute aortic dissection. Progression of IMH is more likely with an ascending aortic location, a thick hematoma with luminal compression, and an aortic diameter greater than 5 cm in the ascending and greater than 4 cm in the descending aorta. Since IMH of the ascending aorta (type A) is at high risk for early progression, undelayed surgical repair is often performed. Careful follow-up after the initial diagnostic CT is important to assess for progression using CT or MRI.

Notes

CASE 17

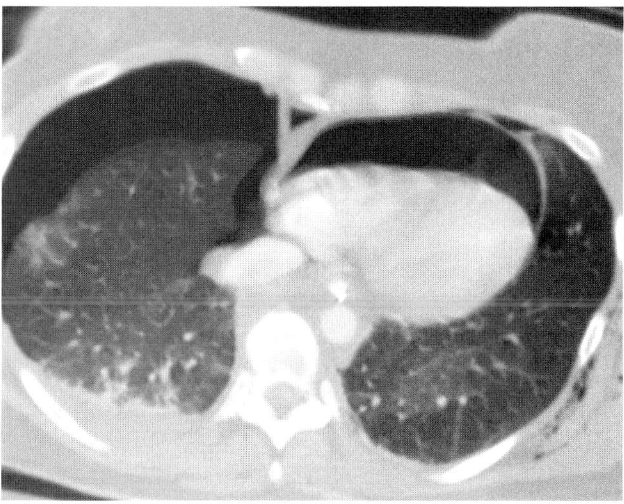

You are shown an image of a blunt trauma patient.

1. What is the pathologic process involving the heart?
2. What are some traumatic etiologies of this pathology?
3. What abnormalities might be present on physical examination?
4. What urgent treatment is indicated?

CASE 17

Tension Pneumopericardium

1. Tension pneumopericardium. (Mediastinal hematoma and right pneumothorax are also present.)
2. Air enters the pericardium through the pulmonary venous adventia (blunt); tracheopericardial communication (penetrating); esophagopericardial communication (penetrating); pleural to pericardial communication with tension pneumothorax (blunt or penetrating).
3. Tachycardia, distended neck veins, pulsus paradoxicus, muffled heart sounds.
4. Vent the pericardial space by needle insertion or pericardial window.

Reference

Mirvis SE: Diagnostic imaging of acute thoracic injury, *Semin Ultrasound CT MR* 25:156–179, 2004.

Cross-Reference

Emergency Radiology: THE REQUISITES, p 244.

Comment

Pneumopericardium is a relatively uncommon result of blunt chest trauma. Air can enter the pericardial space either through the pulmonary perivascular connective tissue or ostia of the pulmonary veins or through direct communication between the pericardial space and esophagus, trachea, or pleural space, either from blunt or, more commonly, penetrating trauma. If the air enters, but cannot exit the pericardial space (one-way valve effect) then positive pressure will increase leading to cardiac tamponade. In the setting of blunt trauma, it is usually the combination of positive airway pressure support and severe lung injury that leads to this life-threatening process. Tension pneumopericardium may develop in the acute trauma setting or may be seen hours to days after injury as patients with severe lung injury receive prolonged positive pressure ventilator assistance. Clinical evidence of tamponade may be subtle or may develop gradually, so imaging findings are often the first manifestation of the diagnosis.

Pneumopericardium is suspected by chest radiography with visualization of the pericardium as an opaque line surrounding the cardiac shadow. This line may be confused with the parietal pleura of the mediastinum seen with pneumomediastinum, which is often visualized tracking along the left mediastinal border. The parietal pleural line typically is thinner than the pericardium and descends below the left hemidiaphragm near the midclavicular line, rather than curving around the heart. Both entities can often co-exist after blunt chest trauma and may be difficult to distinguish. Also, if there is tension pneumopericardium, the heart may appear globally smaller than usual ("small heart" sign) due to uniform compression. The diagnosis is easier to recognize by computed tomography as the intrapericardial air can be followed around the heart, the flattened low-pressure right ventricle is displaced away from the anterior chest wall, and the pericardium is obviously stretched away from the heart.

Notes

CASE 18

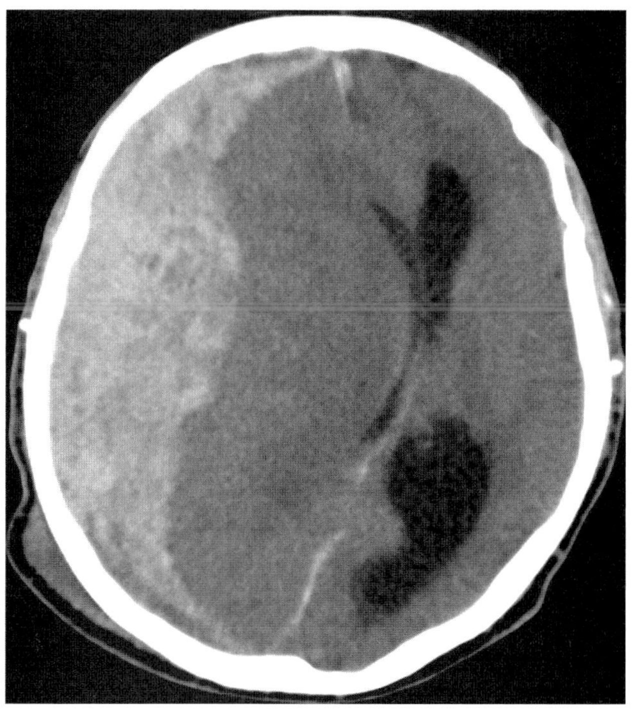

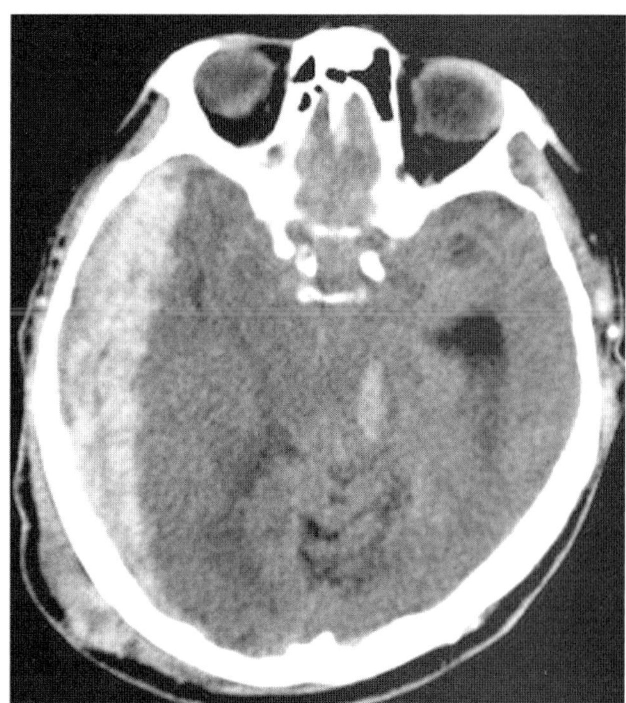

You are shown images of a blunt trauma patient.

1. Where is the extra-axial hematoma?
2. What types of cerebral herniation are demonstrated?
3. What major secondary injury can result from these herniations?
4. What is a Duret hemorrhage?

CASE 18

Acute Subdural Hematoma with Cerebral Herniation

1. Subdural space.
2. Trans-falcine and trans-tentorial or uncal.
3. Cerebral infarction due to compression of posterior cerebral artery and/or anterior cerebral artery along edge of tentorium or falx, respectively.
4. A hemorrhage seen in the brainstem (pons) in the setting of severe herniation. It is associated with essentially 100% mortality and is most likely due to occlusion of veins draining the brainstem.

Reference

Smirniotopoulus JG, Mirvis SE, Lefkowitz DM: Imaging of craniocerebral trauma. In Mirvis SE, Shanmuganathan K, eds: *Imaging in Trauma and Critical Care*, 2nd ed, Philadelphia, WB Saunders, 2003, pp 50–61.

Cross-Reference

Emergency Radiology: THE REQUISITES, pp 2–5.

Comment

Subdural hematomas (SDHs) are commonly seen in the acute post-trauma setting and usually are associated with concurrent underlying brain parenchymal injury. The subdural space lies between the inner (meningeal) layer of dura and the subarachnoid membrane. Classically, the subdural hematoma arises from a tear in one or more bridging cortical veins. When the head accelerates/decelerates, there is a lag between movement of the skull and brain. The lag produces a stretching of the bridging cortical veins that may tear if the strain is sufficient. The site of tearing is usually at the insertion of the flexible veins into the more rigid dural sinuses, allowing bleeding into the subdural compartment. The SDH occurs in from 10% to 30% of patients with severe head trauma and has a worse prognosis than epidural hematoma (EDH), with 30% to 90% mortality, in part related to commonly associated brain parenchymal injury including focal or diffuse cerebral edema, contusions, and diffuse axonal injury. Early surgical evacuation lowers mortality, emphasizing the need for rapid diagnosis. Factors that promote development of SDH from blunt trauma include cerebral atrophy, chronic renal disease, and a bleeding diathesis.

On computed tomography (CT), the SDH is usually a crescent-shaped collection of blood conforming to the cerebral contour. As with EDH the blood may appear uniformly clotted with a 60 to 90 Hounsfield units density, partially liquefied (incompletely clotted), or may manifest a "swirl" sign created by active extravasation of low-density blood into a hyperdense clot. Typically, there is no skull fracture associated with SDH as with EDH. Hemorrhage in the subdural space crosses sutures, but is limited by the dural sinuses. Often SDH extends from the cerebral convexity along the falx and tentorium. A SDH may appear isointense to cerebral cortex due to severe anemia (hemoglobin 8 to 10 g/dL), from admixing of cerebrospinal fluid from a torn arachnoid, or with digestion of hemoglobin gradually decreasing CT density over time. MRI and contrast-enhanced CT will detect isodense SDH. The mass effect due to the SDH will compress adjacent sulci and displace the grey-white interface medially, suggesting its presence even when isoattenuating with the cerebral cortex. Occasionally, SDH may exhibit a central convex bulge, as in the current case, and should not be confused with EDH.

Notes

CASE 19

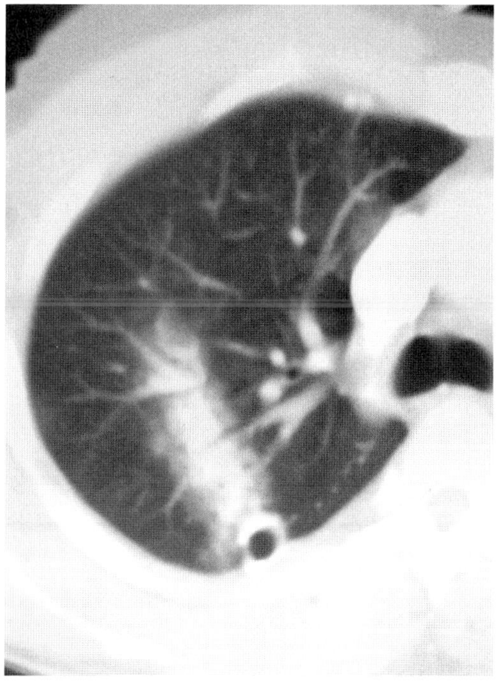

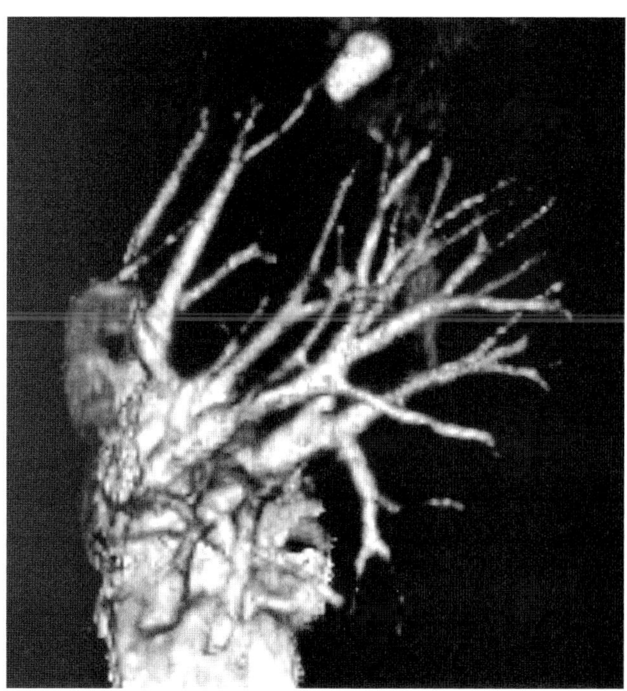

You are shown images of a patient with penetrating chest trauma.

1. What is the diagnosis?
2. What is the major complication?
3. What is the indicated treatment?
4. Name other types of nontrauma pathology that can cause the same lesion as a complication.

CASE 19

Pulmonary Artery Pseudoaneurysm

1. Pulmonary artery branch pseudoaneurysm.
2. Hemorrhage into airway.
3. Selective coil embolization.
4. Improper Swan-Ganz placement, infection (mycotic, tuberculosis), vascular abnormality (Marfan, Behçet's, cystic medial necrosis).

Reference

Hubler B, Earls JP, Stevens K: Traumatic pulmonary arterial and venous pseudoaneurysms, *AJR Am J Roentgenol* 69:1354, 1997.

Comment

Pulmonary artery pseudoaneurysm (PAP) is a rarely reported complication of blunt or penetrating trauma. A pseudoaneurysm results from a tear or disruption of all three layers of a vessel wall. Extravasated blood is contained by compressed extravascular tissue or a clot, which makes up the wall of the pseudoaneurysm. PAPs are most commonly encountered as a result of pulmonary artery perforation after improper Swan-Ganz catheter placement. Other causes include mycotic, syphilitic, or mycobacterial infection and vascular abnormalities such as cystic medial necrosis, Behcet's disease, and Marfan syndrome.

Hemoptysis is common and results from leakage of blood into the bronchial tree.

Findings of PAP on chest radiographs are nonspecific and include an area of consolidation or a mass that becomes more sharply defined as surrounding hemorrhage clears. Depending on the clinical history, a focal lung mass that remains stable or increases in size is suggestive of PAP. Diagnosis is made by computed tomography (CT) or angiography. On CT, and with an appropriately timed iodinated contrast bolus, PAP appears as an enhancing round lung mass that is isointense to the central pulmonary arteries.

Pulmonary arterial and venous pseudoaneurysms are rare after blunt or penetrating trauma but should be suspected in a trauma patient with hemoptysis and when a chest radiograph shows an area of parenchymal density that becomes mass-like on subsequent studies. The diagnosis can be confirmed by CT or angiography, and urgent treatment is necessary to avoid life-threatening hemorrhage.

Notes

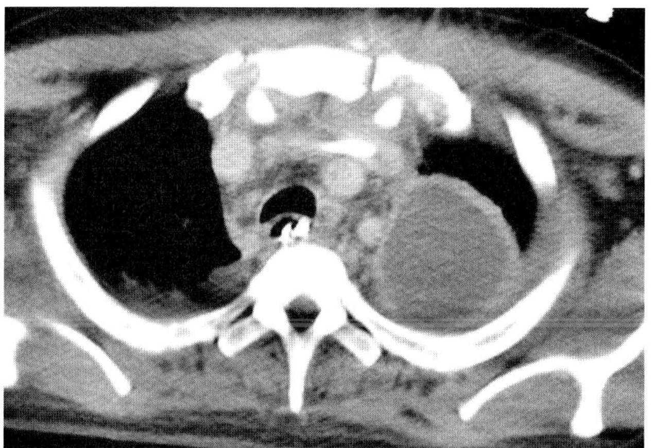

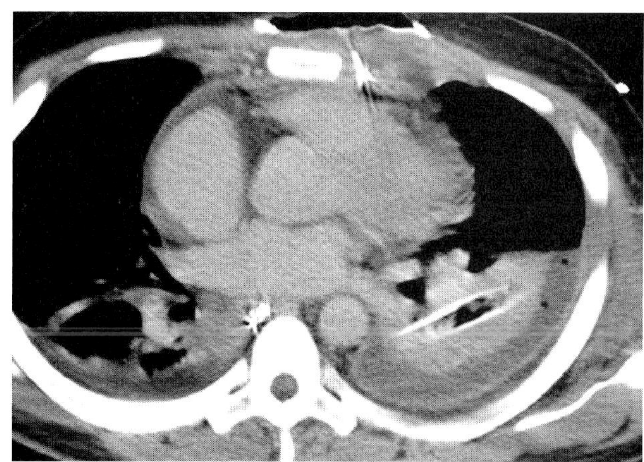

1. What is the diagnosis?
2. What is the most common etiology of this pathology?
3. What computed tomography findings indicate the diagnosis?
4. What is the primary method of management of this pathology?

CASE 20

Pleural Empyema

1. Pleural empyema.
2. Bacterial pneumonia.
3. Thickened and enhanced pleura ("split pleura" sign), increased density of extrapleural fat, smooth walls of collection, gas bubbles within fluid.
4. Percutaneous catheter drainage.

References

Kraus GJ: The split pleura sign, *Radiology* 243:297–298, 2007.

Waite RJ, Canbonneau RJ, Balikian JP, et al: Parietal pleural changes in empyema: appearances at CT, *Radiology* 175:145–150, 1990.

Cross-Reference

Emergency Radiology: THE REQUISITES, pp 243–244.

Comment

Thoracic empyema is defined as purulent content in the pleural cavity. Empyema most commonly occurs in the setting of bacterial pneumonia. Empyemas evolve over time, beginning with an exudative phase characterized by inflamed pleura that weeps proteinaceous fluid into the pleural space. Next is the fibrinopurulent phase, in which neutrophils accumulate and fibrin is deposited on the pleural surfaces. Finally, there is an organizing phase with formation of new granulation tissue and pleural fibrosis producing a pleural rind. Progression from the exudative phase to the organizing phase is unpredictable and may occur fairly rapidly (within 7 days). Abnormally high computed tomography (CT) attenuation in the extrapleural tissues (fat) can be expected to accompany the exudative pleural effusion, particularly with empyema, but not with transudative effusion. Pleural changes similar to those of empyema can be seen with malignant effusions (especially after talc pleurodesis), mesothelioma, hemothorax, and after lobectomy.

CT is typically utilized to diagnose empyema and to distinguish it from transudative pleural fluid collections and lung abscesses. Empyemas are typically ovoid in shape, make obtuse margins with the chest wall, compress and displace the surrounding lung, and have thin, smooth, and uniform walls. Lung abscesses are typically round, destroy adjacent lung, and have thick, nonuniform, and irregular walls. Inflammation of the visceral and parietal pleura leads to increased enhancement and thickening, creating the "split pleura" sign with the visceral and the parietal pleura separated by empyema fluid or an exudative effusion. This finding is seen in about 70% of cases. Also, abnormally high attenuation and thickening of the extrapleural tissues can be expected to accompany exudative pleural effusion, particularly empyema, but not transudative effusion. Although the mean attenuation of exudates is significantly higher than that of transudates, the clinical use of CT numbers to characterize pleural fluid is not recommended, as their accuracy is only moderate. It is important to distinguish empyema from abscess and to detect loculation in empyemas, which is a poor prognostic feature for successful drainage. Catheter drainage has been reported as a primary method of empyema management, with a cure rate of 80% to 90%.

Notes

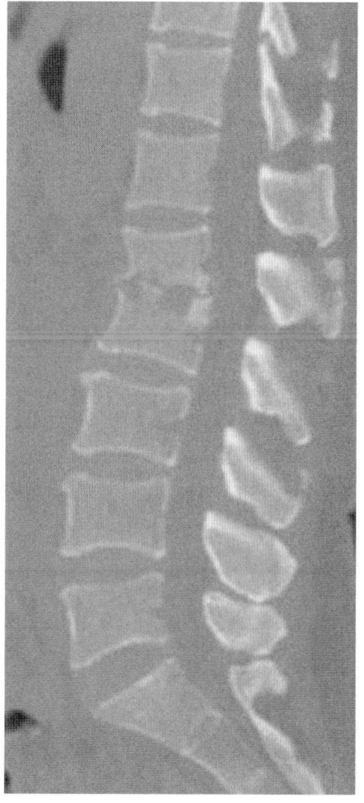

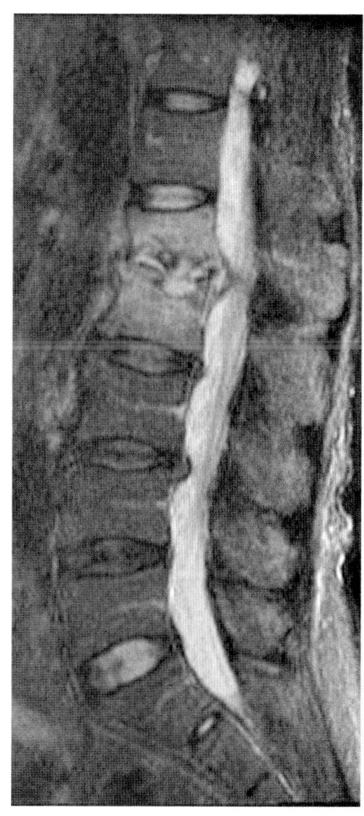

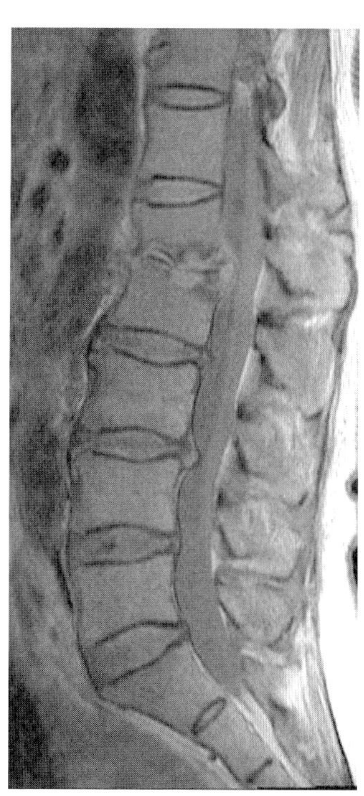

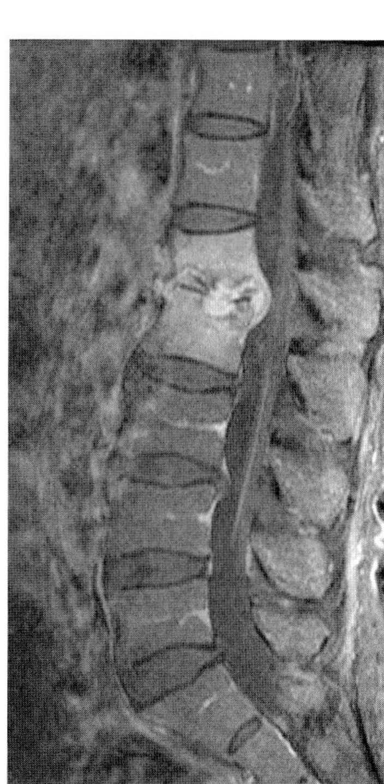

You are shown MDCT and MR images of a 56-year-old man with back pain.

1. What are the imaging findings?
2. What is the best diagnosis?
3. Name four predisposing conditions associated with this diagnosis.
4. What are the three MR findings that have a high sensitivity in diagnosing this condition?

CASE 21

Discitis and Vertebral Osteomyelitis

1. Destruction of the endplates with loss of intervertebral disc space height at the L1-L2 level, hypointense signal at the end plates of L1-L2 vertebra on noncontrast T1-weighted image with enhancement following administration of contrast material, and enhancing fluid collections within the L1-L2 disc space and the epidural space posterior to the disc.
2. Discitis and vertebral osteomyelitis L1-L2 levels.
3. Diabetes mellitus, intravenous drug abuse, postoperative nonspinal infection, and immunosuppression.
4. Paraspinal or epidural inflammatory changes, intervertebral disc enhancement, and hyperintense signal in the disc space on T2-weighted sequences.

References

Leddermann HP, Schwetizer ME, Carrino JA: MR imaging findings in spinal infections: rules or myths? *Radiology* 228:506–514, 2003.

Sharif HS: Role of MR imaging in the management of spinal infections, *AJR Am J Roentgenol* 158: 1333–1345, 1992.

Cross-Reference

Emergency Radiology: THE REQUISITES, pp 45–47, 231–232.

Comment

Symptoms and clinical findings in patients with infective spondylitis or discitis are often nonspecific. Clinically, it can be extremely difficult to differentiate infection from other major categories of spinal disorders such as degenerative, noninfectious inflammatory, and neoplastic processes. Back pain is an early symptom associated with localized tenderness, either with or without a neurological deficit. Imaging is often mandatory to confirm and localize the site of infection. Early diagnosis and prompt treatment are required to minimize permanent neurological deficits and spinal deformity.

Primary infection of the intervertebral disc may occur by hematogeneous spread in the pediatric age groups due to the preservation of the blood supply to the disc. In older age groups, the infection invariably results from extension from a contiguous site, typically the vertebral body or paraspinal soft tissues, or is implanted directly. Blood-borne spread results in the organism lodging in the bone marrow, with the resulting osteomyelitis leading to discitis. Diabetes mellitus in the elderly, intravenous drug abuse, immunosuppression, postoperative nonspinal infections, endocarditis, urosepsis, and septic phlebitis are underlying conditions associated with spinal infections. Common bacterial organisms causing pyogenic spondylitis include *Staphylococcus aureus*, *Escherichia coli*, *Salmonella*, *Pseudomonas aeruginosa*, and *Klebsiella pneumonia*.

MR findings with excellent sensitivity in demonstrating discitis and spinal osteomyelitis are anterior and lateral paraspinal or epidural extension of enhancing inflammatory tissue, enhancement seen within the intervertebral disc space, hyperintense or fluid equivalent signal within the intervertebral disc on T2-weighted images, and erosion or destruction of an adjacent vertebral body endplate. Other less sensitive MR findings include effacement of the nuclear cleft, loss of height of the intervertebral disc, disc hypointensity on T1-weighted sequences, and involvement of several spinal levels. Endplate signal abnormalities seen with spinal neoplasms, degenerative disease, noninfectious inflammatory disease, neuropathic spondyloarthropathy, and hemodialysis-associated spondyloarthropathy can be mistaken for infection. Large abscesses, subligamentous spread, skip lesions, epidural extension, and involvement of part of the vertebral body, especially the posterior elements, are suggestive of tuberculous spinal infections.

Notes

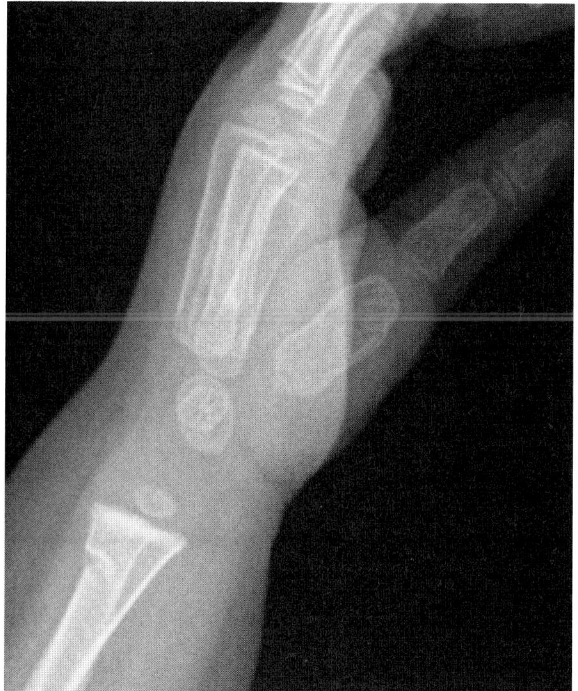

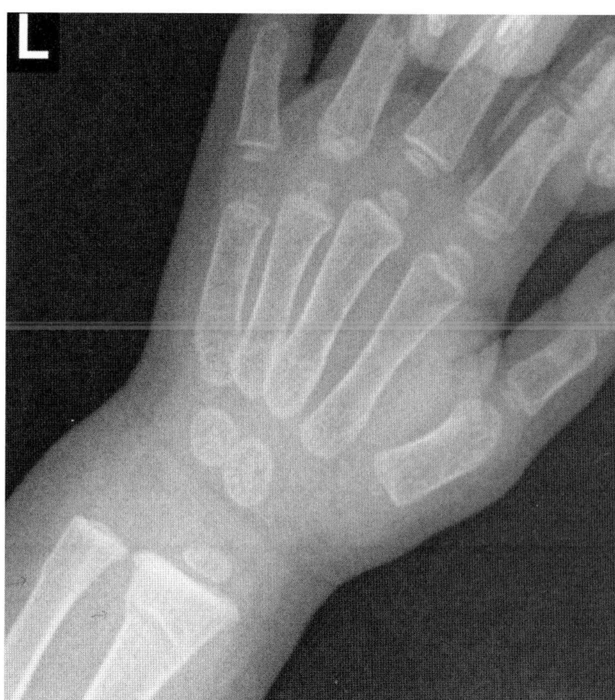

1. What osseous abnormalities are present in this patient?
2. These injuries are often sustained after what kind of trauma?
3. In what age group is this abnormality most often found?
4. Name the most common anatomical site of this type of fracture.

CASE 22

Torus Fracture of the Distal Radius and Ulna

1. Buckle (torus) fractures of the distal radius and ulna.
2. Fall on an outstretched hand.
3. Pediatric patients.
4. Distal forearm.

Reference

Irwin GJ: Fractures in children, *Imaging* 16:140–152, 2004.

Cross-Reference

Emergency Radiology: THE REQUISITES, pp 129, 209–210.

Comment

Torus or buckle fractures are almost always seen in children. They most commonly occur in metaphyseal regions due to greater bone porosity in that region. A torus fracture results from the more cortical diaphyseal bone being compressed into the more porous metaphyseal bone, resulting in a buckling of the cortex. These fractures most often occur as a result of an axial stress applied to the long axis of the bone. This is often due to a fall on an outstretched hand when occurring in the upper extremity.

Torus fractures can be quite subtle and difficult to detect on radiographs. The typical radiographic appearance is unilateral or bilateral bulging of the cortex with associated soft tissue swelling. Comparison views of the opposite limb may be useful in equivocal cases.

Buckle fractures are treated with casting or splint application. Little to no radiographic follow-up is needed after application of the cast since these fractures uniformly heal without sequelae.

Notes

CASE 23

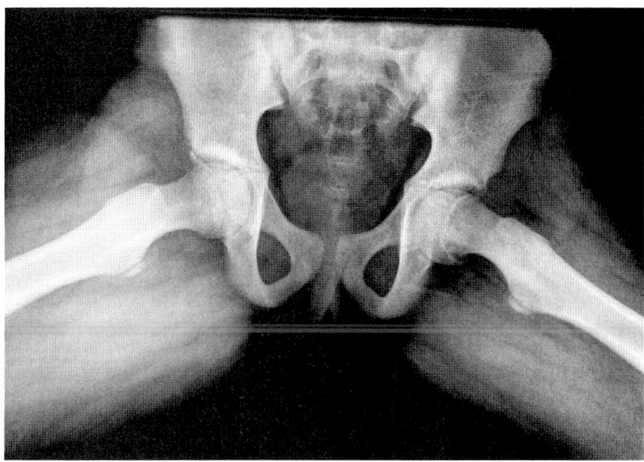

1. What is the abnormality in this 14-year-old male patient with hip pain?
2. How often is this condition bilateral?
3. What is the line of Klein?
4. Name two potential postsurgical complications.

CASE 23

Slipped Capital Femoral Epiphysis

1. Slipped capital femoral epiphysis.
2. The condition is bilateral in 20% to 37% of cases.
3. An imaginary line drawn through the superior margin of the femoral neck should always intersect a portion of the epiphysis. Failure of this line to intersect the epiphysis indicates medial femoral head displacement.
4. Potential postsurgical complications include progression of slip, osteoarthritis, hardware failure, chondrolysis, and avascular necrosis.

Reference

Boles CA, El-Khoury GY: Slipped capital femoral epiphysis, *Radiographics* 17:809–823, 1997.

Cross-Reference

Emergency Radiology: THE REQUISITES, pp 211–212.

Comment

Slipped capital femoral epiphysis (SCFE) is the most common hip abnormality seen in adolescence. The typical patient is an overweight 14-year-old male presenting with hip pain of one to two weeks duration. Additional symptoms include limp, vague groin discomfort, or pain in the thigh or knee. The condition is bilateral in 20% to 37% of cases.

SCFE originates from a fracture through the proximal femoral epiphysis that has usually occurred without significant trauma. SCFE is most commonly seen during the rapid growth period of adolescence. During that time, the epiphyseal plate orientation changes from horizontal to oblique, making it more prone to vertical shear forces.

SCFE can be categorized as mild, moderate, or severe and may be acute, acute-on-chronic, or chronic. The diagnosis is most often made with anteroposterior and frog leg lateral radiographs of the pelvis. Early findings can be subtle and include osteopenia and mild widening or irregularity of the physeal plate, with varying degrees of medial displacement of the femoral head from the metaphysis. The line of Klein refers to an imaginary line drawn along the superior margin of the femoral neck, which should always intersect a portion of the epiphysis. In SCFE, this line does not intersect the epiphysis due to medial femoral head displacement. Because early symptoms may be vague and radiographic findings subtle, there is a high rate of delay in diagnosis that may lead to progression of slip or increased risk of early onset osteoarthritis.

Treatment of SCFE is surgical, with stabilization across the physis with a pin or screw. Postsurgical follow-up radiographs are required to evaluate for physeal fusion and to exclude potential complications such as hardware failure, chondrolysis, avascular necrosis, or secondary osteoarthritis.

Notes

CASE 24

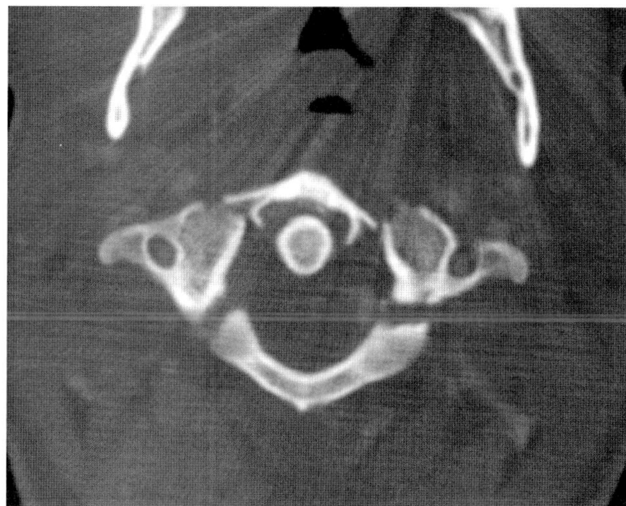

1. What is the mechanism of injury that has caused this fracture?
2. True or false: Neurological deficits are uncommon in this type of injury.
3. What lateral plain film finding may be seen with rupture of the transverse atlantal ligament, indicating an unstable injury?
4. In addition to motor vehicle collision and fall onto head from a significant height, what is a common cause of this fracture?

CASE 24

Jefferson Burst Fracture

1. Axial loading.
2. False. Neurological deficits are uncommon due to the lateral displacement of the fracture fragments and the width of the spinal canal at the C1 level, which both limit cord compression.
3. An atlantodental interval greater than 4 mm.
4. Diving accidents into shallow water. In this type of trauma, the head strikes the bottom of the pool and the force is transmitted to the cervical spine.

Reference

Harris JH, Mirvis SE: Vertical compression injuries. In Harris JH, Mirvis SE, eds: *The Radiology of Acute Cervical Spine Trauma*, 3rd ed, Baltimore, Williams and Wilkins, 1996, pp 340–345.

Cross-Reference

Emergency Radiology: THE REQUISITES, p 218.

Comment

A Jefferson fracture is a burst fracture of the C1 vertebra. The mechanism of injury involves an axial loading force that has been transmitted through the occipital condyles and into the lateral masses of C1, driving them laterally. Although a Jefferson fracture is classically described as bilateral fractures of the anterior and posterior rings, two- and three-part fractures of the C1 ring are common variants. This fracture is rarely seen in children.

Plain film findings on the lateral cervical spine radiograph include prevertebral soft tissue swelling and posterior C1 arch fractures. If the transverse antlantal ligament connecting the two lateral masses of C1 is ruptured, the atlantodental interval will be abnormally wide (greater than 4 mm). The open mouth odontoid view will show bilateral lateral displacement of the C1 lateral masses.

Cervical spine computed tomography (CT) demonstrates the anterior arch fracture(s), the degree of displacement, and any additional fractures within the cervical spine. Fifty percent of patients with a Jefferson fracture have an additional cervical spine injury, most commonly a C2 fracture. CT angiography of the neck is valuable to exclude a vertebral artery injury. A minimally displaced Jefferson fracture is treated by rigid cervicothoracic brace. An unstable fracture will require halo placement or C1-C2 surgical fusion.

Notes

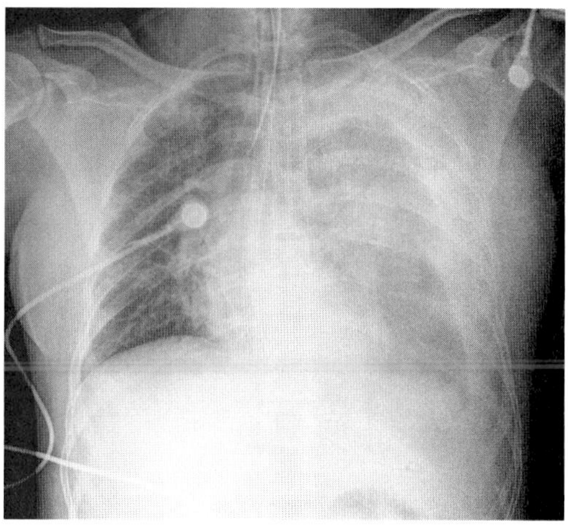

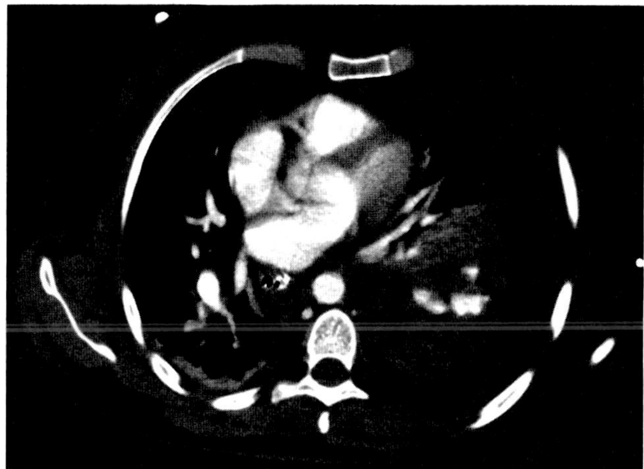

1. What are two potential causes of the foci of high density within the left lung on this contrast-enhanced computed tomography of a blunt trauma patient?
2. Name two ways in which you could differentiate between these two etiologies on computed tomography.
3. What are sources of bleeding into the pleural space in a trauma patient?
4. Name two indications for surgical treatment of an acute hemothorax.

CASE 25

Left Hemothorax with Active Bleeding

1. Active bleeding or retained contrast material from recent angiographic procedure.
2. Active bleeding would measure within 10 Hounsfield units of the nearest largest artery, typically the aorta. If delayed images were performed, the focus of high density may increase in size. Retained contrast material is typically much higher in density and would not change in size on delayed images.
3. Bleeding into the pleural space can originate from injury to the pleura, chest wall, lung, diaphragm, or mediastinum.
4. Chest tube output greater than 200 mL of blood per hour or hemothorax greater than 1 L upon chest tube insertion.

Reference

Sangster GP, Gonzales-Belcos A, Carbo AI, et al: Blunt traumatic injuries of the lung parenchyma, pleura, thoracic wall, and intrathoracic airways: multidetector computed tomography imaging findings, *Emerg Radiol* 14:297–310, 2007.

Cross-Reference

Emergency Radiology: THE REQUISITES, pp 60, 243–244.

Comment

Hemothorax is seen in approximately 30% to 50% of patients who sustain blunt chest trauma. Bleeding into the pleural space can originate from injury to the pleura, chest wall, lung, diaphragm, or mediastinum. When the size of a hemothorax reaches approximately 200 mL, an upright chest radiograph demonstrates blunting of the costophrenic angle, often with a "meniscus" sign: a concave upward sloping of fluid in the costophrenic angle. On a supine chest radiograph, a hemothorax layers in the dependent portion of the pleural space and causes increased density of the entire hemithorax or a rim of density surrounding the lateral aspect and apex of the lung. A large hemothorax can cause contralateral shift of the mediastinum due to mass effect.

Computed tomography (CT) is highly sensitive in detecting a small hemothorax. Blood in the pleural space measures 35 to 90 Hounsfield units (HUs), depending on the amount of clot present. A hemothorax due to a venous origin typically is self-limiting. Arterial bleeding may increase in size over time and often requires treatment. Active bleeding within a hemothorax is seen on CT as a focus of high density, typically within 10 HU of the nearest large artery. If delayed images are performed, the focus persists as a region of high density and may increase in size. If angiographic embolization has been performed for treatment of active bleeding in the pleural space, CT may show very high density residual contrast agent in the region where embolization was done, a finding that should not be confused with a site of new or recurrent bleeding.

Notes

CASE 26

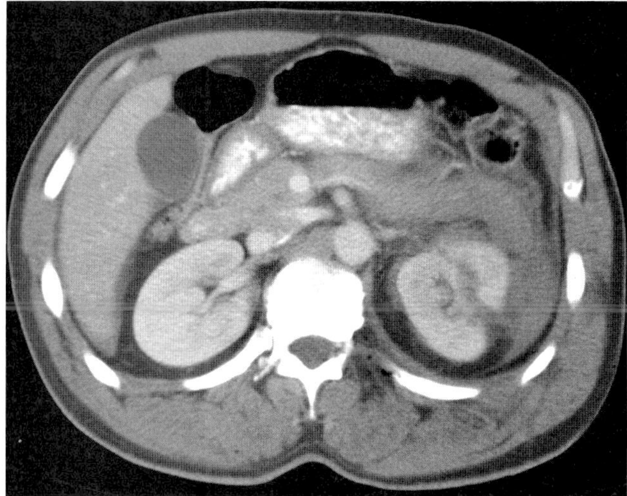

1. What is the diagnosis?
2. Does this injury involve the renal collecting system?
3. True or false: The absence of hematuria excludes a major renal injury.
4. Name three potential complications of renal trauma.

CASE 26

Left Renal Laceration

1. Left renal laceration with small amount of perinephric hematoma.
2. Extension into the collecting system is difficult to determine based on this initial computed tomography image. Delayed images of the kidneys done 1 to 2 minutes after the initial abdominal-pelvic computed tomography should be completed. These images may show contrast-enhanced urine leak from the kidney in a patient with a collecting system injury.
3. False. Hematuria is absent in up to 25% of patients with a major renal injury and is thus a poor predictor of renal trauma.
4. Urinoma, perinephric abscess, formation of arteriovenous fistula.

Reference

Lee VJ, Oh SV, Rha SE, et al: Renal trauma, *Radiol Clin North Am* 45:581–592, 2007.

Cross-Reference

Emergency Radiology: THE REQUISITES, pp 99–102.

Comment

Renal injury is seen in approximately 10% of all patients with blunt abdominal trauma. Patients with renal trauma may be asymptomatic, present with flank pain, or have hematuria.

The decision to image for evaluation of potential renal injury rests not only on the presence of hematuria but also on the mechanism of injury and clinical factors such as hemodynamic stability, the reliability of the clinical examination, a decreasing hematocrit, or evidence of major flank trauma.

Computed tomography (CT) is the test of choice for assessment of renal injury owing to its high diagnostic accuracy. An initial abdominal-pelvic CT is performed with the use of intravenous contrast, followed by 1- to 2-minute delayed images through the upper abdomen, including the kidneys. If a ureteral injury or bladder injury is suspected, delayed images through the pelvis should also be performed. Delayed images are useful in detection of a collecting system injury or presence of a renal vascular injury.

Renal lacerations appear on CT as a linear or branching hypodensity. Size and length of laceration, extension into the collecting system, and presence of a vascular injury—such as pseudoaneurysm, active extravasation of contrast, or involvement of the renal hilar vessels—are important predictors of outcome and will influence management. In general, renal injuries may be characterized as minor or major. Minor renal injuries include renal contusion, small subcapsular hematoma, lacerations less than 1 cm deep, or small perinephric hematoma. Minor injuries rarely require treatment. Major renal injuries include main renal artery or vein injury, laceration with involvement of the collecting system, shattered kidney, or devascularized kidney. Major renal injuries often require angiographic or surgical treatment.

Notes

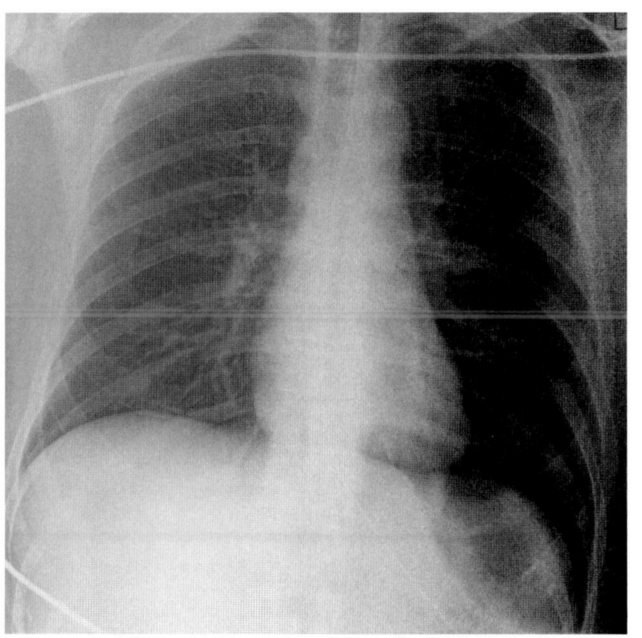

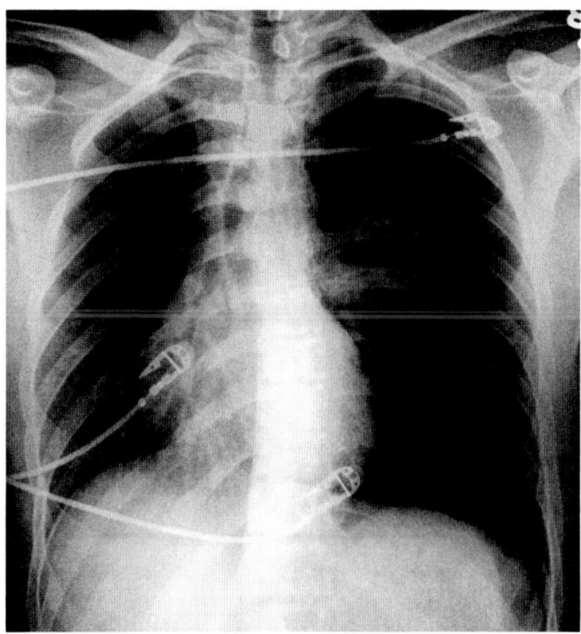

1. What is the diagnosis on the first image?
2. What are three findings that support that diagnosis?
3. Name four instances in which this condition would require urgent treatment.
4. What is the diagnosis on the second image of a different patient?

CASE 27

Left Pneumothorax and Tension Left Pneumothorax

1. Left pneumothorax.
2. Hyperlucent left upper quadrant, left "deep sulcus" sign, and sharply outlined left hemidiaphragm.
3. Pneumothorax greater than 20%, respiratory distress, or tension pneumothorax. Chest tube insertion also may be considered in a patient with a very small pneumothorax who will be placed on a mechanical ventilator or who will be undergoing a lengthy operative procedure.
4. Left tension pneumothorax.

References

Kuhlman JE, Pozniak MA, Collins J, et al: Radiographic and CT findings of blunt chest trauma: aortic injuries and looking beyond them, *Radiographics* 18:1085–1106, 1998.

Miller LA: Chest wall, lung and pleural space trauma, *Radiol Clin North Am* 44:213–224, 2006.

Cross-Reference

Emergency Radiology: THE REQUISITES, pp 60, 242–243.

Comment

Pneumothorax occurs in 30% to 40% of patients after blunt chest trauma. The most common cause is a rib fracture that lacerates the lung, but it may be caused by rupture of a preexisting bleb at time of impact. Clinical signs of pneumothorax can be difficult to elicit in a patient who has multisystem trauma. Detection of even a small, asymptomatic pneumothorax is important because up to one third can develop into a tension pneumothorax with potential cardiopulmonary decompensation.

Radiographic signs of a pneumothorax differ based on the patient's position. In the supine position, air collects within the anterior costophrenic sulcus. This appears radiographically as abnormal lucency in the lower chest or upper abdomen, an abnormally wide and deep costophrenic sulcus (the "deep sulcus" sign), a sharply outlined cardiac or diaphragmatic border, depression of the hemidiaphragm, or a "double diaphragm" sign that is seen when air outlines both the dome and the anterior insertion of the diaphragm.

On the upright chest radiograph, a pneumothorax is seen as a thin, sharply defined line that represents the visceral pleura. No lung markings are seen beyond this line. A small pneumothorax may not be detectable at all on a portable chest radiograph. An upright expiratory chest radiograph or computed tomography can assist in making the correct diagnosis in questionable cases.

Generally, patients who are asymptomatic or who demonstrate a greater than 20% pneumothorax are considered for chest tube placement. Chest tube insertion also may be considered in a patient with a small pneumothorax who will be placed on a mechanical ventilator or who will be undergoing a lengthy operative procedure.

Notes

CASE 28

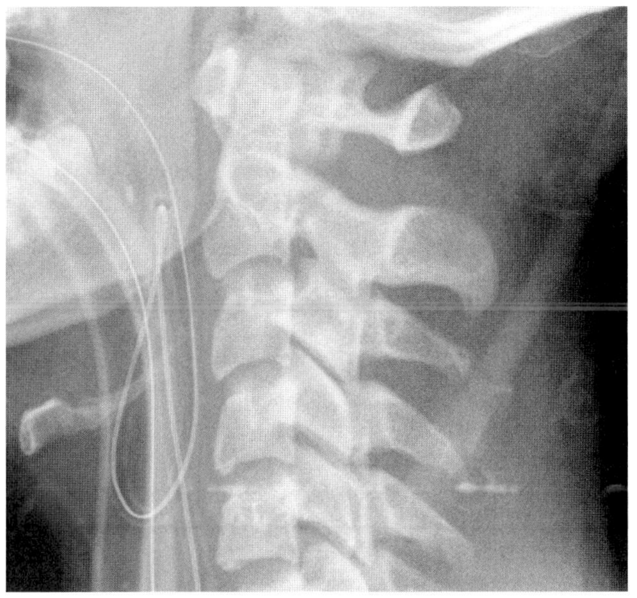

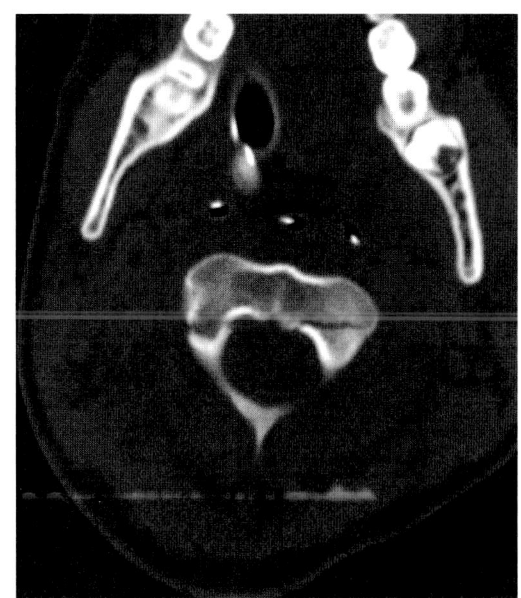

1. What anatomical part of C2 is involved in this fracture?
2. What is an atypical hangman fracture?
3. Why are neurologic deficits uncommon in this type of fracture?
4. True or false: This fracture is common in children.

CASE 28

C2 Hangman Fracture

1. Bilateral pars interarticularis.
2. A variant of the hangman fracture that involves vertical fractures through the posterior C2 body rather than through the pars interarticularis.
3. There is a low rate of spinal cord injury due to the width of the spinal canal at the C2 level and also the decompression of the spinal canal from the traumatic separation of the C2 body and posterior C2 arch.
4. False. This fracture is quite rare in children.

References

Levine AM, Edwards CC: The management of traumatic spondylolisthesis of the axis, *J Bone Joint Surg Am* 67:217–226, 1985.

Mirvis SE: Imaging of cervical spine trauma. In Mirvis SE, Shanmuganathan K, eds: *Imaging in Trauma and Critical Care*, 2nd ed, Philadelphia, WB Saunders, 2003, pp 185–293.

Cross-Reference

Emergency Radiology: THE REQUISITES, p 219.

Comment

A hangman fracture, also known as traumatic spondylolisthesis of the axis, consists of bilateral pars interarticularis fractures of the C2 vertebra. A hangman fracture is most commonly seen in motor vehicle collisions that involve rapid deceleration. This fracture is rare in children.

Cervical spine radiographs can diagnose up to 90% of hangman fractures. On radiographs the fracture line through the C2 pars interarticularis is often readily seen. Prevertebral soft tissue swelling may or may not be present. A variant of the fracture is a vertical fracture line through the posterior C2 body rather than through the pars and is known as an atypical hangman fracture. In this type of fracture, disruption through the posterior axis ring may be seen on the lateral cervical spine radiograph, reflecting involvement of the posterior C2 body cortex.

Cervical spine computed tomography (CT) may be used for evaluation of additional fractures, most commonly odontoid, posterior C1 arch, and C2 hyperextension teardrop fractures. CT can also determine if there is fracture involvement of the C2 vertebral foramina in atypical hangman fractures, a risk factor for vertebral artery injury.

Various classification schemes have been created in order to guide the management of hangman fractures. The classification of Effendi and colleagues, modified by Levine and Edwards, is used widely. This classification divides hangman fractures into four types based on the radiographic findings and likely mechanism of injury. Type I fractures are stable and include nondisplaced fractures and fractures with no angulation and less than 3 mm of anterior translation of the C2 vertebral body in relation to C3. These fractures likely result from a hyperextension-axial loading force. Type II fractures are unstable, with significant angulation and translation. The mechanism is thought to be a combination of hyperextension, axial loading, and hyperflexion. Type IIa fractures are a subset of type II fractures with minimal translation but severe angulation. A type III fracture will have a unilateral or bilateral facet dislocation in addition to being severely angulated and displaced.

Opinions vary regarding the optimal treatment of the different fracture types and may include traction and external immobilization with halo placement or open reduction and internal fixation.

Notes

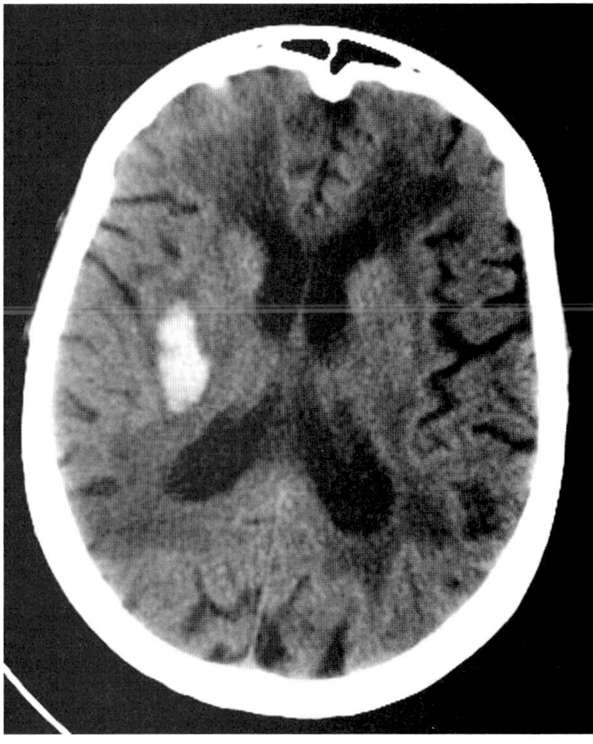

1. Name three potential etiologies of the intracranial bleed.
2. What causes the rim of hypodensity surrounding the lesion?
3. What are other common sites of hypertensive hemorrhage?
4. True or false: It is rare for a hypertensive hemorrhage to increase in size on a subsequent head computed tomography.

CASE 29

Hypertensive Hemorrhage in Right Basal Ganglia

1. Hypertensive hemorrhage, bleeding from tumor, arteriovenous malformation, amyloidosis, coagulopathy, cocaine use, trauma, or rupture of an aneurysm.
2. The hypodense rim is thought to represent edema or extruded plasma.
3. The basal ganglia, thalamus, pons, cerebellum, and centum semiovale.
4. False. Up to 40% will enlarge in the first hours after rupture. The increased size is often associated with clinical deterioration.

Reference

Panagos PD, Jauch EC, Broderick JP: Intracerebral hemorrhage, *Emerg Med Clin North Am* 20:631–655, 2002.

Cross-Reference

Emergency Radiology: THE REQUISITES, pp 1–2, 12.

Comment

Hypertensive hemorrhage is the second most common cause of intracranial hemorrhage after trauma. Additional causes of spontaneous intracranial hemorrhage include tumor, arteriovenous malformation, amyloidosis, coagulopathy, cocaine use, and rupture of an aneurysm.

The pathophysiology of hypertensive hemorrhage is incompletely understood. It is theorized that gradual damage of intracranial blood vessels in the hypertensive patient results from deposition of lipid-laden macrophages and cholesterol. Common sources of hypertensive hemorrhage are the perforator arteries that supply the basal ganglia, thalamus, and pons. Hypertensive hemorrhage may also occur in the cerebellum or centrum semiovale.

The typical patient with hypertensive hemorrhage is 50 to 70 years of age and has a history of hypertension. Presenting symptoms may include acute onset of severe headache and vomiting. The remaining neurological symptoms will depend on the exact site of cerebral hemorrhage.

The most common computed tomography (CT) finding in hypertensive hemorrhage is an intraparenchymal hematoma in the putamen or globus pallidus. Intraventricular hemorrhage with acute communicating hydrocephalus may result from decompression of the hematoma into the ventricular system. The CT appearance of the intraparenchymal hematoma will differ depending on the amount of time since the event. A CT performed immediately after and up to 4 hours after the event will show a hyperdense intraparenchymal hematoma measuring 40 to 90 Hounsfield units in density. The density will gradually decrease, starting from the periphery. At 1 to 6 weeks, there may be peripheral enhancement of the hematoma on contrast-enhanced CT. The hematoma will progressively become more hypodense until a focal area of encephalomalacia remains.

Notes

CASE 30

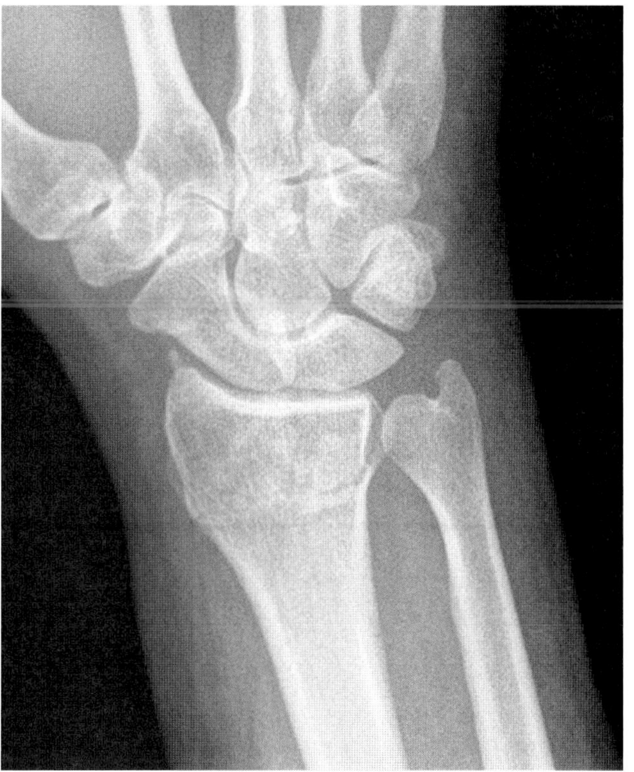

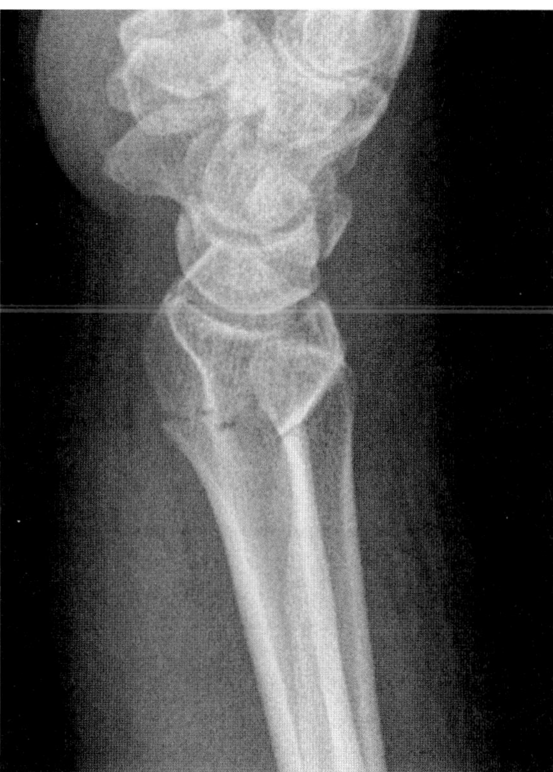

1. What is the eponym of this fracture?
2. What is the classic deformity seen on physical examination of a patient with this fracture?
3. In addition to degree of angulation and presence of intra-articular extension, name three other radiographic findings that should be included in the assessment.
4. What additional fracture is seen in the majority of patients with this injury?

ANSWERS

CASE 30

Colles' Fracture

1. Colles' fracture.
2. The "dinner fork" deformity. This finding is a result of the angulation of the distal radial fracture fragment.
3. The presence of radial shortening, distal radioulnar subluxation, or scapholunate dissociation.
4. An ulnar styloid fracture.

Reference

Goldfarb CA, Yin Y, Gilula LA, et al: Wrist fractures: what the clinician wants to know, *Radiology* 219: 11–28, 2001.

Cross-Reference

Emergency Radiology: THE REQUISITES, pp 126–128.

Comment

A Colles' fracture is a dorsally angulated transverse fracture of the distal radial metaphysis, usually 2 to 3 cm proximal to the wrist joint. The typical patient is an elderly female with osteoporosis who falls on an outstretched arm with the wrist in dorsiflexion.

Clinically, the patient will have pain and swelling at the fracture site. The dorsal angulation of the distal radial fracture fragment results in the classic "dinner fork" deformity on clinical examination.

Radiographic evaluation of the wrist in a patient with suspected Colles' fracture should include four projections: posteroanterior, lateral, external oblique, and posteroanterior with ulnar deviation. Assessment of intra-articular extension, comminution, and angulation are important to determine stability. The presence of radial shortening, distal radioulnar subluxation, or scapholunate dissociation should also be determined. A fracture of the ulnar styloid accompanies the Colles' fracture in 60% of cases. Computed tomography with coronal and sagittal reformatted images may be required if there is significant comminution. Magnetic resonance imaging can be performed if a ligamentous injury is suspected.

The initial management of a Colles' fracture includes closed reduction and splint or plaster immobilization. Repeat radiographs are obtained to evaluate the neutralization of angulation and restoration of radial length, articular congruity, volar tilt, and presence of radial inclination. Repeat films at 1 week follow-up are performed to ensure that fracture reduction has not been lost. Surgical open reduction and internal fixation may be required if there is significant osteopenia or fracture comminution.

Notes

CASE 31

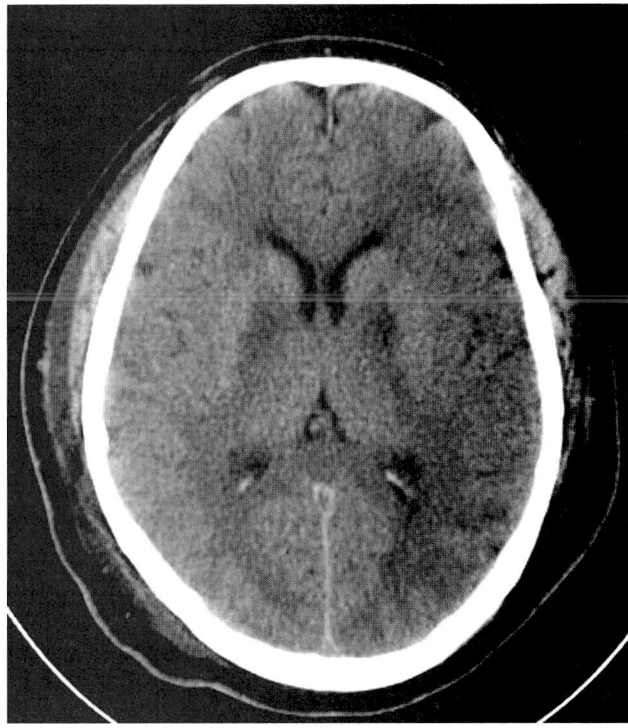

1. What is the best diagnosis? This patient was rescued from a house fire.
2. What other sites in the brain are involved by this entity?
3. Name three other acute processes that cause bilateral basal ganglia infarcts.
4. True or false: Clinical outcome is directly related to size of the globus pallidus lesions.

CASE 31

Bilateral Basal Ganglia Infarcts Due to Carbon Monoxide Poisoning

1. Bilateral basal ganglia infarcts due to carbon monoxide poisoning.
2. Within the white matter, especially the periventricular region and centrum semiovale, and the cerebral cortex. Acute demyelinization and cerebral atrophy may also be seen.
3. Global ischemia from cardiac arrest or strangulation, methanol intoxication, and acute cyanide poisoning.
4. False. Clinical outcome appears to depend on the severity of the white matter changes rather than the size of the globus pallidus lesions.

References

Hopkins RA, Fearing MA, Weaver LK, et al: Basal ganglia lesions following carbon monoxide poisoning, *Brain Inj* 20:273–281, 2006.

Silver DAT, Cross M, Fox B, et al: Computed tomography of the brain in acute carbon monoxide poisoning, *Clin Radiol* 51:480–483, 1996.

Cross-Reference

Emergency Radiology: THE REQUISITES, p 35.

Comment

Carbon monoxide poisoning is the most common cause of accidental poisoning in the United States, resulting in 800 deaths per year. The diagnosis is suspected by the appropriate clinical history such as a house fire or suicide attempt from inhalation of motor vehicle exhaust fumes. The diagnosis is confirmed by a measurement of the blood carboxyhemoglobin levels.

Noncontrast head computed tomography (CT) in carbon monoxide poisoning will frequently show low-density lesions involving part or all of the globus pallidus. While it is known that the basal ganglia are more metabolically active than white matter, and are thus more sensitive to ischemic insult, the precise pathology of cerebral abnormalities seen in carbon monoxide poisoning is poorly understood.

Magnetic resonance imaging is more sensitive than CT in detection of additional abnormalities, including white matter lesions (especially in the periventricular regions and centrum semiovale), the cerebral cortex, and the remainder of the basal ganglia. Affected areas often show increased signal intensity on T2-weighted and proton density sequences, but this pattern may vary in the presence of hemorrhage. Lesions can vary significantly in time of appearance, duration, and severity on imaging studies.

Other acute processes that preferentially cause basal ganglia infarcts include acute cyanide poisoning, global ischemia from cardiac arrest or strangulation (bilateral putamen, globus pallidus), and methanol intoxication (putamen). The prognosis often depends on the severity of the white matter changes and not on the size of the globus pallidus lesions.

Notes

CASE 32

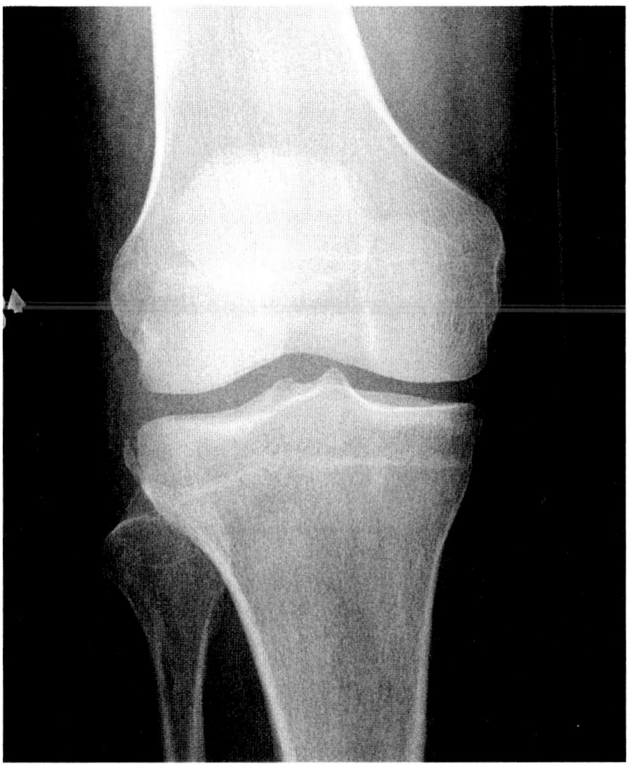

1. What is the finding?
2. What is the mechanism involved in this injury?
3. True or false: This injury is uncommon in children.
4. What is the "reverse" Segond fracture?

CASE 32

Segond Fracture

1. There is a vertical avulsion fracture of the lateral tibial plateau.
2. Internal rotation and varus stress.
3. True. When seen in this population it is usually the result of a sporting injury.
4. A small fracture of the medial tibial plateau representing avulsion of a portion of the medial collateral ligament. There may also be injuries to the posterior cruciate ligament or a medial meniscial tear.

Reference

Campos JC, Chung CB, Lektrakul N, et al: Pathogenesis of the Segond fracture: anatomic and MRI imaging evidence of an iliotibial tract of anterior oblique band avulsion, *Radiology* 219:381–386, 2001.

Cross-Reference

Emergency Radiology: THE REQUISITES, pp 144, 151.

Comment

A Segond fracture is a vertical avulsion fracture of the lateral tibial plateau at the site of attachment of the lateral capsular ligament, which is just distal to the articular surface of the tibial plateau. Recent research suggests that the insertion of the iliotibial tract and the anterior oblique band (the ligamentous attachment of the fibular collateral ligament to the mid-portion of the lateral tibia) may also play a role in the pathogenesis of this fracture. The mechanism of injury involves internal rotation and varus stress, leading to abnormal tension on the contralateral portion of the lateral collateral ligament.

Patients with a Segond fracture will present with acute pain, swelling, and tenderness of the lateral knee and a history of trauma to this region. Anteroposterior and lateral knee radiographs will demonstrate the characteristic small, vertically oriented fracture fragment adjacent to the lateral tibial plateau. A suprapatellar knee effusion is common. A fracture of the fibular head and/or intercondylar eminence of the tibia may be seen in association with this injury. Despite the small bony abnormality, there is a tear of the anterior cruciate ligament in 75% to 100% of cases and a medial or lateral meniscial tear in 66% to 75% of cases. Magnetic resonance imaging of the knee should be performed whenever this fracture is seen on radiograph in order to fully evaluate the meniscus and cruciate ligaments.

Notes

CASE 33

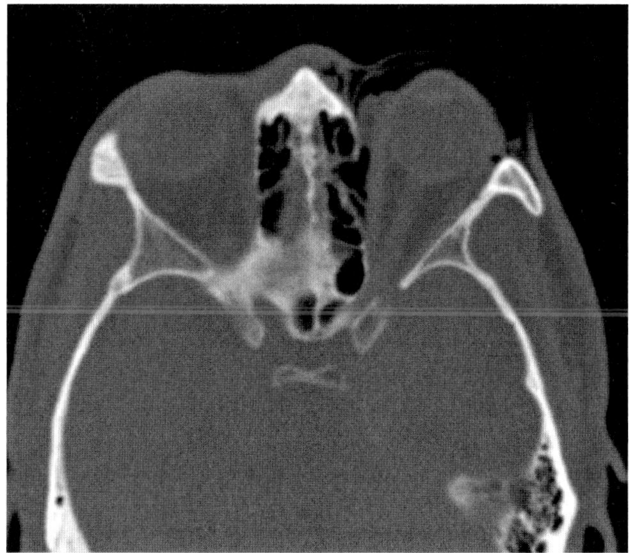

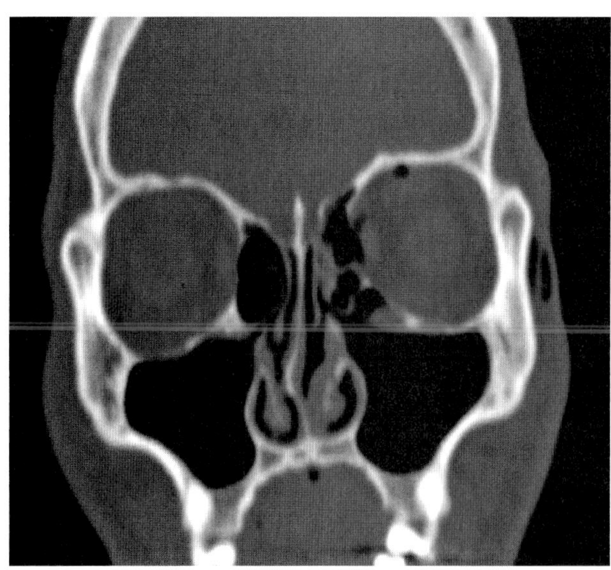

1. What is the diagnosis?
2. In what other orbital locations can this type of fracture occur?
3. Is this injury due to direct or indirect trauma?
4. What are the indications for surgical treatment of this fracture?

CASE 33

"Blow-out" Fracture of the Left Medial Orbital Wall

1. Blow-out fracture of the left medial orbital wall.
2. A blow-out fracture of the orbit may involve the medial wall, orbital floor, or, rarely, the orbital roof.
3. Indirect.
4. Surgery is reserved for those cases with impaired ocular mobility due to entrapment of the medial rectus muscle or cosmetically significant enophthalomos.

References

Hopper RA, Salemy S, Sze RW: Diagnosis of midface fractures with CT: what the surgeon needs to know, *Radiographics* 26:783–793, 2006.
Mauriello JA Jr, Lee HJ, Nguyen L: CT of soft tissue and orbital fractures, *Radiol Clin North Am* 37:241–252, 1999.

Cross-Reference

Emergency Radiology: THE REQUISITES, p 38.

Comment

"Blow-out" fractures occur as a result of indirect trauma when the eye is struck with an object that has a larger diameter than that of the bony orbit, such as a fist or a ball. The globe and intraorbital soft tissues are both retropulsed and compressed, causing an acute rise in the intraorbital pressure. This increased pressure gets transmitted to the thin medial orbital wall or to the orbital floor or roof, resulting in fracture. An orbital floor blow-out fracture is more common than one involving the medial wall. This is due to the added stability provided by the multiple bony septa arising from the ethmoid air cells which supports the medial orbital wall.

A patient with a medial orbital wall blow-out fracture will typically present with the expected history and periorbital soft tissue swelling. Orbital emphysema may be detected on examination, and there may be impaired oculomotor motility due to medial rectus muscle injury. Diagnosis is made with noncontrast orbital computed tomography. Coronal reformatted images are helpful in confirming the fracture site seen on standard axial images. A subtle medial wall fracture may be suspected by focal opacification of ethmoid air cells or a small focus of intraorbital air. Intraorbital hematoma and edema of the medial rectus muscle are commonly seen. Treatment is generally conservative.

Notes

CASE 34

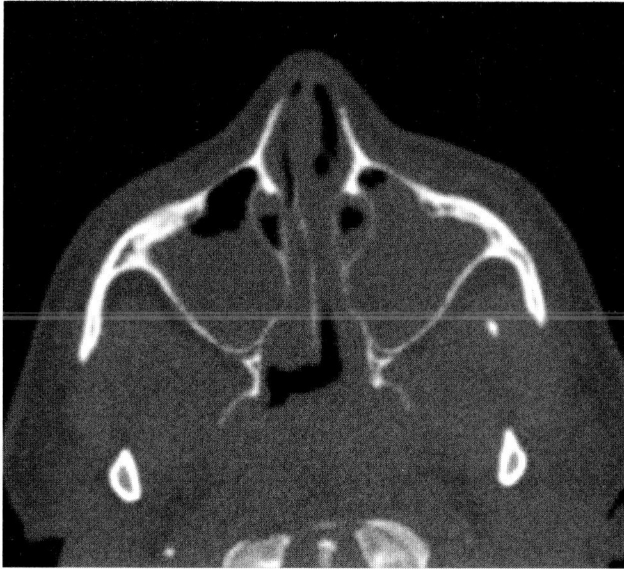

1. What is the diagnosis in this patient with a history of one week of facial pain and nasal congestion?
2. True or false: Bacterial infections are the most common cause of this condition.
3. Name three potential complications of this condition.
4. What are two findings that can be seen on contrast-enhanced head computed tomography in a patient with cavernous sinus thrombosis?

CASE 34

Acute Bilateral Maxillary Sinusitis

1. Acute bilateral maxillary sinusitis.
2. False. Viruses account for the majority of cases of acute sinusitis.
3. Orbital cellulitis, subperiosteal abscess, and cavernous sinus thrombosis.
4. A filling defect in the cavernous sinus and an enlarged ophthalmic vein.

Reference

Eustis HS, Mafee MF, Walton C, et al: MR imaging and CT of orbital infections and complications in acute rhinosinusitis, *Radiol Clin North Am* 36:1165–1183, 1998.

Cross-Reference

Emergency Radiology: THE REQUISITES, pp 50–54.

Comment

Acute sinusitis is a very common condition and refers to inflammation of the mucosa of the paranasal sinuses. Patients typically present with acute onset of nasal congestion and discharge, facial pain or pressure, and decreased sense of smell. The most common cause is a virus but superinfection with bacteria should be suspected if symptoms persist beyond 10 days.

Computed tomography (CT) is the primary imaging modality for evaluation of acute sinusitis. Findings on CT include sinus mucosal thickening, an air fluid level within the sinus lumen, complete opacification of the sinus, and an enhancing fluid collection within the sinus lumen with a central zone of nonenhancing pus. A significant limitation of CT is the high frequency of scans demonstrating similar abnormalities in asymptomatic patients. Clinical correlation with the presence and site of symptoms will increase the specificity. CT is most useful in evaluation of complications of acute sinusitis, including orbital cellulitis, subperiosteal abscess, and cavernous sinus thrombosis. Orbital cellulitis may be preseptal or postseptal. Postseptal cellulitis involves inflammation posterior to the orbital septum, with fat stranding in the orbital fat. Eyelid swelling and edema of the rectus muscles frequently accompany this process. A subperiosteal abscess is a medical and/or surgical emergency due to the potential for development of high intraorbital pressures and the resultant optic nerve ischemia. A subperiosteal abscess appears on contrast-enhanced CT as an extraconal mass with diffuse or ring-like enhancement. Significant proptosis, edema in the rectus muscles, or osteomyelitis of the orbital wall may be seen. Cavernous sinus thrombosis is due to septic thrombophlebitis in the ophthalmic vein. Patients are typically very ill. Filling defects within the cavernous sinus and an enlarged ophthalmic vein will be seen on contrast-enhanced CT.

Notes

CASE 35

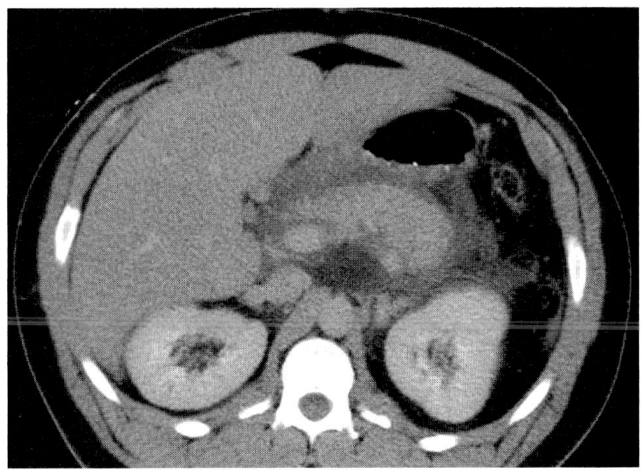

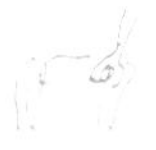

1. What are the findings in this 44-year-old female with acute upper abdominal pain?
2. What are the two most common causes of this condition?
3. What is the "colon cutoff" sign?
4. What are two other imaging modalities that may be used to diagnose this condition?

CASE 35

Acute Pancreatitis

1. There is diffuse pancreatic edema and peripancreatic fluid, consistent with acute pancreatitis.
2. Gallstones or alcohol abuse account for 60% to 80% of all cases of acute pancreatitis. Other causes include hypertriglyceridemia, drugs, infection such as mumps or cytomegalovirus, and cystic fibrosis. In 10% of cases no specific cause is found.
3. This sign has been described on abdominal radiographs in association with acute pancreatitis. It refers to distention of the colon to the level of the mid transverse colon with little gas seen distal to this level. It is thought to reflect alteration in peristalsis in the peripancreatic region.
4. Pancreatic ultrasound may be used, but is often limited by overlying bowel gas. Abdominal magnetic resonance imaging may be useful in the setting of iodine allergy.

Reference

Casas JD, Diaz R, Valeras G, et al: Prognostic value of CT in the early assessment of patients with acute pancreatitis, *AJR Am J Roentgenol* 82:569–574, 2004.

Cross-Reference

Emergency Radiology: THE REQUISITES, pp 291–293.

Comment

The majority of cases of acute pancreatitis are mild and respond to conservative treatment, but up to 25% of cases can result in a life-threatening illness due to development of sepsis and multisystem organ failure. Typical presenting symptoms include acute onset abdominal pain with radiation to the back, nausea, and vomiting. Chest radiograph findings are seen in about one half of patients, most commonly linear atelectasis in the left lung base or left pleural effusion. Abdominal radiographs may be completely normal or demonstrate pancreatic calcifications in the setting of chronic pancreatitis. The "sentinel loop" sign refers to a focal loop of dilated small bowel in the left upper quadrant, thought to reflect a focal ileus of the proximal jejunum adjacent to the nearby pancreatic inflammation. The "colon cutoff" sign describes distention of the colon to the level of the mid–transverse colon with little gas seen distal to this level. It is thought to reflect alteration in peristalsis in the peripancreatic region.

Computed tomography (CT) findings include focal or diffuse pancreatic edema, peripancreatic stranding, and heterogeneous pancreatic enhancement. The CT may be completely normal in up to 25% of patients. CT is most valuable in identifying complications such as pancreatic abscess or pseudocyst, splenic vein thrombosis, formation of a splenic artery pseudoaneurysm, or pancreatic necrosis.

Notes

CASE 36

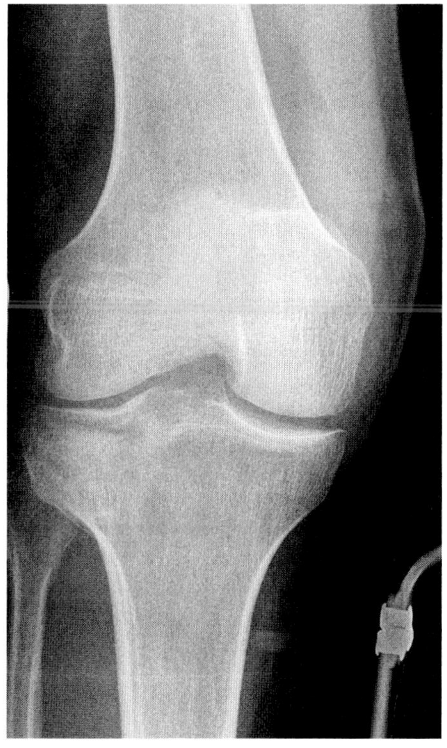

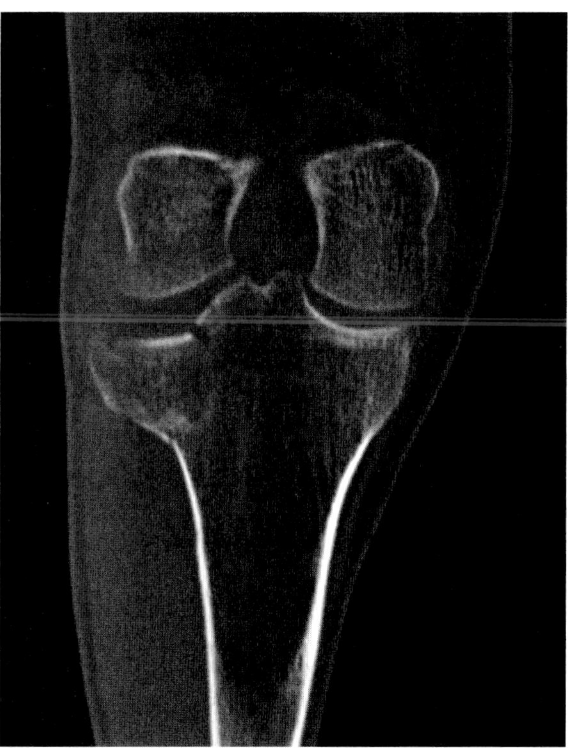

1. What are the findings on the frontal radiograph and the coronal reformatted computed tomography image of this patient with knee pain?
2. What is the mechanism responsible for this injury?
3. What does visualization of a fat-fluid level on a cross-table lateral knee radiograph indicate?
4. True or false: Medial tibial plateau involvement is seen in less than 1% of all tibial plateau fractures.

CASE 36

Tibial Plateau Fracture

1. Irregular lucency and a band of increased density along the lateral tibial plateau, consistent with tibial plateau fracture with mild bone compression.
2. Valgus stress.
3. Intra-articular involvement.
4. False. The medial tibial plateau is involved in up to 15% of all tibial plateau fractures.

References

Mulligan M: Extremity trauma. In Mirvis SE, Shanmuganathan K, eds: *Imaging in Trauma and Critical Care*, 2nd ed, Philadelphia, WB Saunders, 2003, pp 575–606.

Schatzker J, McBroom R, Bruce D: The tibial plateau fracture: the Toronto experience, *Clin Orthop* 138: 94–100, 1979.

Cross-Reference

Emergency Radiology: THE REQUISITES, pp 148–151.

Comment

Tibial plateau fractures are common in high-velocity trauma. Eighty-five percent of these fractures involve the lateral tibial plateau. Radiographic findings can be subtle; the fracture may be seen as a slight depression in the plateau with a line of increased density in the subplateau region indicating the fracture line. A cross-table lateral knee radiograph may show a fat-fluid level indicating a lipohemarthrosis from intra-articular involvement. Computed tomography may be used for more complete evaluation of the fracture. Greater than 3 mm of depression of the tibial plateau is considered clinically significant. Magnetic resonance imaging has the advantage of demonstrating potential associated soft tissue injuries such as a meniscial tear. The Schatzker classification of tibial plateau fractures is widely used and describes six types of fracture patterns. Type I is a simple split fracture of the lateral tibial plateau. Type II is a combination split-depression fracture. Type III is a simple depression fracture. Type IV is a fracture involving the medial rather than lateral tibial plateau. Type V fractures involve both the medial and lateral tibial plateaus. Type VI fractures describe a severe plateau fracture with separation of the plateau from the tibial shaft. Treatment of tibial plateau fractures may require open reduction and internal fixation with lateral tibial plate and screw placement.

Notes

CASE 37

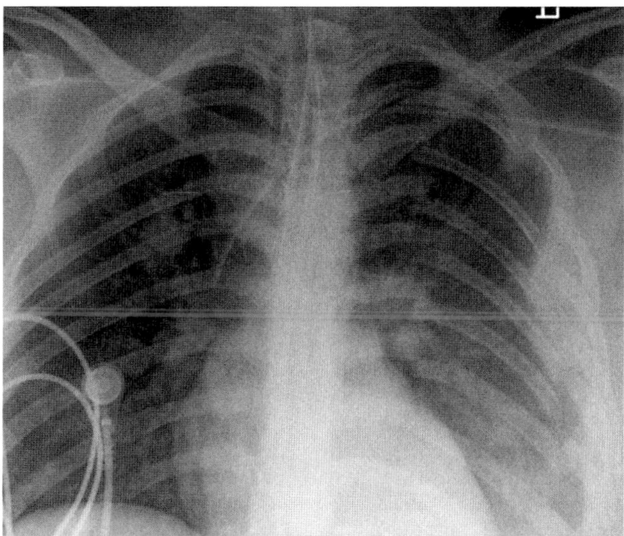

1. What is the diagnosis?
2. What may be seen on clinical examination of the chest in a patient with this condition?
3. What is the clinical significance of this condition?
4. True or false: Fractures of the first three ribs are associated with a higher incidence of traumatic aortic injury.

CASE 37

Left Flail Chest

1. Left flail chest. Left pulmonary contusion is also present.
2. Paradoxical motion of the flailed segment during respiration.
3. Patients will be at increased risk for developing pneumonia or requiring ventilatory support.
4. False.

Reference

Pettiford BL, Lukerich TD, Candreneau RJ: The management of flail chest, *Thorac Surg Clin* 17:25–33, 2007.

Cross-Reference

Emergency Radiology: THE REQUISITES, pp 74, 75.

Comment

Rib fractures are the most common musculoskeletal injury in blunt chest trauma. Fractures of the first three ribs indicate high velocity trauma, and 3% to 15% are associated with brachial plexus or subclavian vessel injury, although not with aortic injury. Fractures of the eighth through eleventh ribs should raise suspicion for splenic or hepatic injury. An extrapleural hematoma frequently accompanies rib fractures and is seen on chest radiographs and chest computed tomography as a focal, lobulated focus of soft-tissue density adjacent to the rib fracture usually with a margin convex to the lung. Any rib fracture can be complicated by laceration of an intercostal artery, potentially requiring angiographic embolization for control of bleeding. A flail chest refers to double or segmental fractures in three or more adjacent ribs. Patients with a flail chest may develop paradoxical motion of the flailed segment during respiration. This abnormal respiratory motion may lead to atelectasis, impaired pulmonary drainage, and pneumonia. Patients with a flail chest often have additional thoracic injuries such as hemothorax or pulmonary contusions or lacerations and are at a higher risk of requiring ventilatory support. Treatment options of flail chest range from aggressive pulmonary toilet with chest physiotherapy and pain management to mechanical ventilatory support and surgical fixation of the flail segment.

Notes

CASE 38

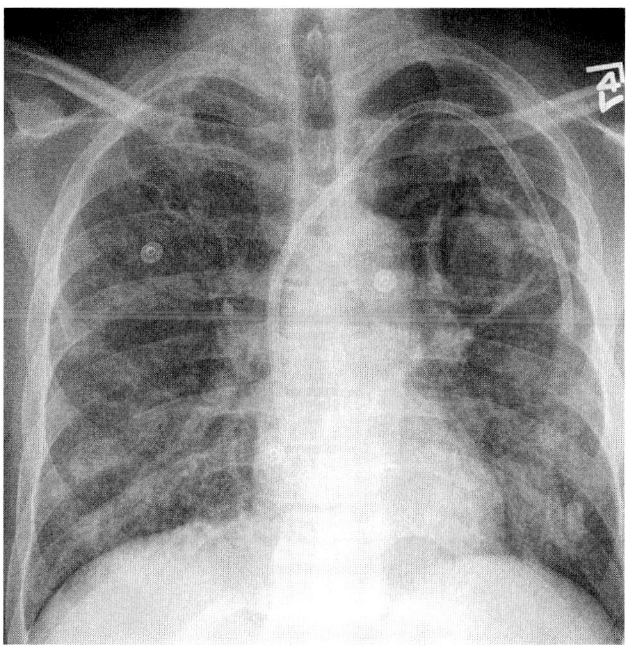

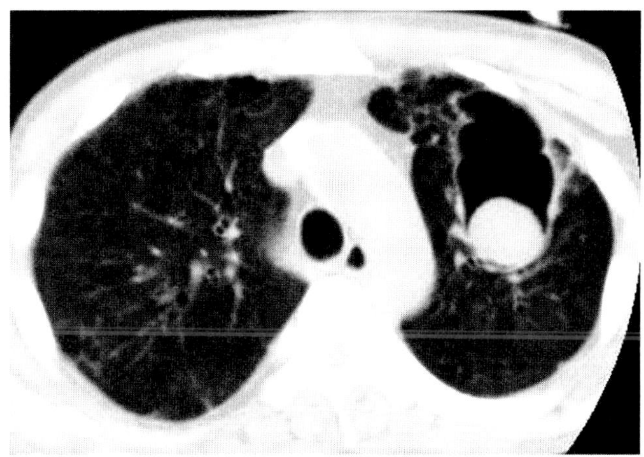

1. What are the findings?
2. What is the differential diagnosis?
3. What is the "air crescent" sign?
4. What is the most common symptom seen in patients with this condition?

CASE 38

Aspergilloma

1. The chest radiograph demonstrates a well-defined cavitary lesion containing a round opacity surrounded by a rim of air in the left upper lobe. Linear scarring is seen in both upper lobes. The chest computed tomography confirms these findings and also demonstrates changes of emphysema throughout the lungs.
2. Aspergilloma, necrotizing squamous cell carcinoma, intrapulmonary abscess, hematoma, hydatid cyst, and Wegener's granulomatosis.
3. This sign describes a thin rim of air that has dissected into a cavitary lung lesion containing an aspergilloma. The air is seen as a thin crescent between the top of the aspergilloma and the inner wall of the cavity.
4. The majority of patients are asymptomatic or may present with cough. Hemoptysis, ranging from mild to life-threatening, can also be seen in patients with an aspergilloma. The hemoptysis is typically due to erosion of nearby bronchial blood vessels.

References

Soubani AO, Chandrasekar PH: The clinical spectrum of pulmonary aspergillosis, *Chest* 121:1988–1999, 2002.

Zmeili OS, Soubani AO: Pulmonary aspergillosis: a clinical update, *QJM* 100:317–334, 2007.

Comment

Aspergillus is a common fungus found in water, soil, and decaying organic materials. Aspergillus infection can cause a spectrum of lung diseases, including invasive aspergillosis, chronic necrotizing aspergillosis, allergic bronchopulmonary aspergillosis, and aspergilloma.

Aspergillomas, also known as mycetomas or fungus balls, typically form in patients with underlying cavitary lung disease such as tuberculosis, sarcoidosis, cystic fibrosis, bronchiectasis, or bullae. Once inside the cavitary lesion, the fungus colonizes the cavity and grows to form a dense ball of aspergillus hyphae, cellular debris, and mucus.

The typical chest radiograph finding of an aspergilloma is a solid round or oval opacity within an upper lobe cavity. The cavity may be thick walled due to compression of surrounding lung tissue. An "air crescent" sign may or may not be present. The aspergilloma is often freely mobile within the cavity and will change position depending on the patient's body posture. There may be extensive ipsilateral apical pleural thickening. Computed tomography (CT) may be necessary for diagnosis if there is extensive lung disease or scarring.

No treatment is required if the patient is asymptomatic since the vast majority of cases remain stable. Treatment of mild hemoptysis includes CT-guided percutaneous placement of amphotericin B into the cavity. Severe hemoptysis may be treated with bronchial artery embolization. Surgical resection of the aspergilloma is reserved for those patients with severe recurrent hemoptysis.

Notes

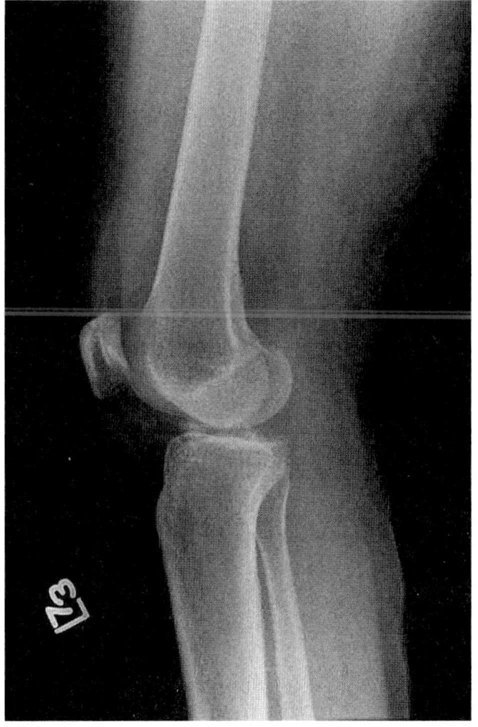

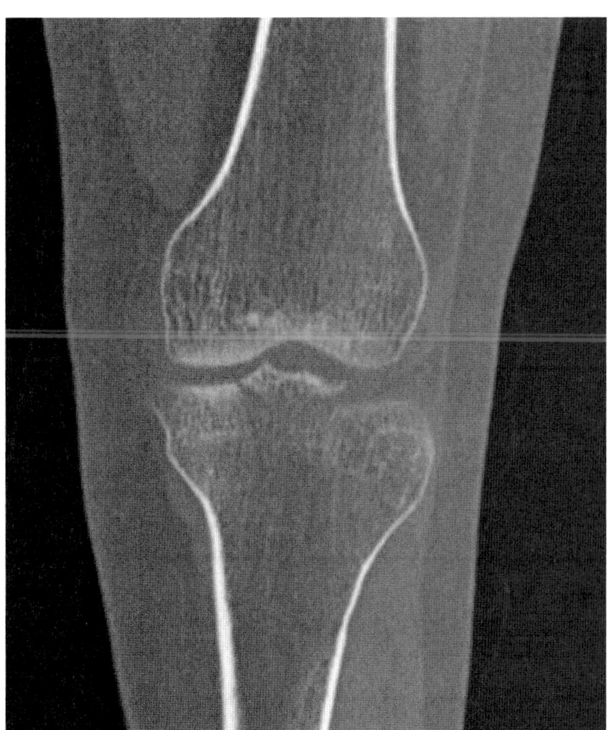

1. What are the findings on the cross-table lateral knee radiograph and coronal reformatted knee CT?
2. What is the diagnosis?
3. What causes the characteristic appearance of this condition?
4. In what other joint spaces can this condition be seen?

CASE 39

Lipohemarthrosis Due to Tibial Plateau Fracture

1. Cross-table lateral view of the left knee demonstrates a fat-fluid level in the suprapatellar bursa. There is irregularity of the superior margin of the tibial plateau. Coronal reformatted computed tomography image of the knee shows a central tibial plateau fracture.
2. Lipohemarthrosis of suprapatellar bursa due to tibial plateau fracture.
3. The differential densities of lower-density fat and higher-density blood released from the marrow of the joint involved with an intra-articular fracture.
4. Hip, elbow, and glenohumeral joints.

References

Costa DN, Cavalcanti CF, Sernik RA: Sonographic and CT findings in lipohemarthrosis, *AJR Am J Roentgenol* 188:W389, 2007.

Lee JH, Weissman BN, Nikpoor N, et al: Lipohemarthrosis of the knee: a review of recent experiences, *Radiology* 173:189–191, 1989.

Cross-Reference

Emergency Radiology: THE REQUISITES, pp 144, 148–151.

Comment

A lipohemarthrosis is formed by release of fat and blood from the bone marrow after an osseous injury. The presence of a lipohemarthrosis indicates an intra-articular fracture and is most commonly seen in tibial plateau fractures of the knee. Because of the differential densities of fat and blood, fat will float on the blood and a fat-fluid level will be seen in the joint space on a cross-table lateral view of the knee. A double fluid-fluid level may also be seen and consists of low-density fat floating on medium-density serum floating on high-density red blood cells.

Although most commonly associated with the knee joint, a lipohemarthrosis can also be seen in other joint spaces. Fractures of the humeral head or neck, or, less commonly, the glenoid, may cause a lipohemarthrosis of the glenohumeral joint. In this case, the fat-fluid level will only be seen on the frontal view of the shoulder with the patient upright. The humeral head may be slightly displaced inferiorly by the lipohemarthrosis. Intra-articular fractures of the elbow may rarely cause a lipohemarthrosis to be seen on the lateral view. A fracture of the femoral head or acetabulum may also rarely cause this condition to be seen in the hip joint.

Notes

CASE 40

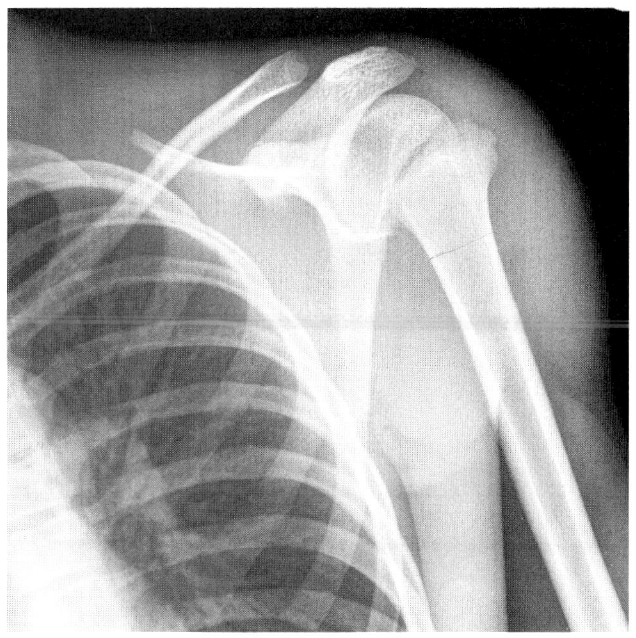

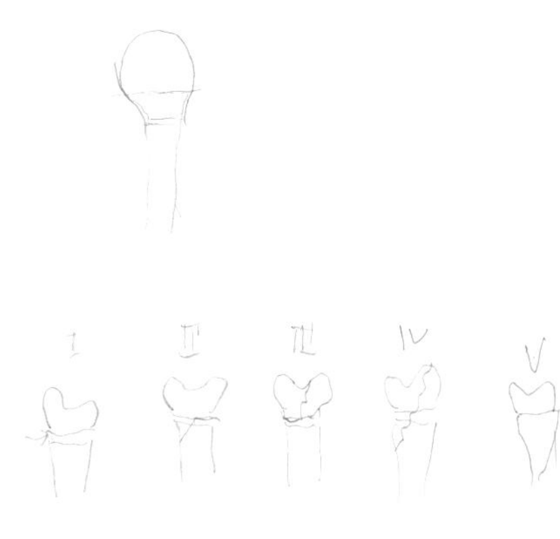

1. What is the finding?
2. What is the most common type of Salter-Harris fracture?
3. What is a Thurston-Holland fragment?
4. True or false: Computed tomography is the test of choice in the evaluation of Salter-Harris fractures.

CASE 40

Salter-Harris Fracture of the Left Humeral Head

1. Displaced Salter-Harris I fracture of the left humeral head.
2. Type II.
3. A metaphyseal corner fracture seen in type II Salter-Harris fractures.
4. False. Radiography is the test of choice. Computed tomography or magnetic resonance imaging is reserved for complex cases.

References

MacNealy GA, Rogers LF, Hernandez R, et al: Injuries of the distal tibial epiphysis: systematic radiographic evaluation, *AJR Am J Roentgenol* 138:683–689, 1982.

Rogers LF, Poznanski AK: Imaging of epiphyseal injuries, *Radiology* 191:297–308, 1994.

Cross-Reference

Emergency Radiology: THE REQUISITES, pp 208–211.

Comment

The Salter-Harris (SH) classification system categorizes epiphyseal plate fractures into types I through V and gives prognostic information.

A type I SH fracture occurs at the epiphyseal plate and is most commonly seen in the phalanges. This type can be difficult to diagnose if there is no displacement or widening of the epiphyseal plate. SH II fractures are the most common, accounting for 75% of all fractures involving the epiphyseal plate. This fracture involves the epiphyseal plate and metaphysis. Complications are rare in both type I and type II SH fractures.

Type III SH fractures involve the epiphyseal plate and the epiphysis. Growth disturbances manifested as limb length discrepancy or angular deformity are possible but rarely cause a significant function deficit. The epiphyseal plate, epiphysis, and metaphysis are all involved in SH IV fractures. These fractures have the worst prognosis due to higher risk of growth disturbance. SH V fractures are rare crush-type injuries of the epiphyseal plate via an axial loading injury. The diagnosis can be difficult and is often made retrospectively after growth disturbance is evident.

Radiographs are the test of choice in the evaluation of SH fractures. Radiographic findings include visualization of the fracture through the epiphysis or metaphysis, epiphyseal displacement, widening of the epiphyseal plate, or thin bone fragments within the physis.

Notes

CASE 41

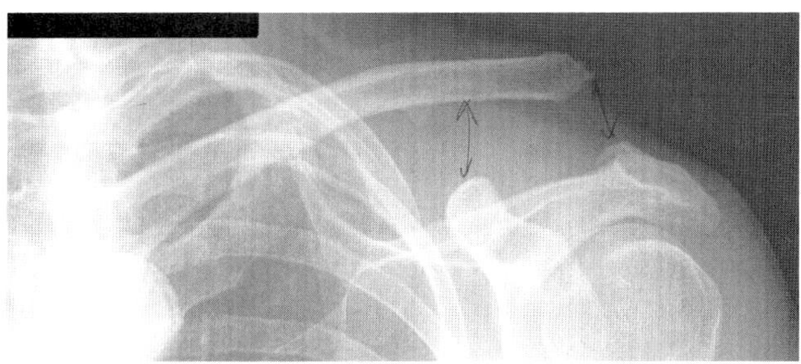

1. What is the usual mechanism of this injury?
2. What does the normal coracoclavicular interval usually measure?
3. Based on the classification system of Rockwood, what type (i.e., grade) of injury is this?
4. What radiographic projections constitute a complete radiographic assessment for this injury?

CASE 41

Acromioclavicular Joint Injury—Type III

1. Direct blow to the shoulder.
2. No more than 12 mm.
3. Type III.
4. Anteroposterior standing views with 15 degrees cephalad angulation obtained with and without weighted stress.

References

Ernberg LA, Potter HG: Radiographic evaluation of the acromioclavicular and sternoclavicular joints, *Clin Sports Med* 22:255–275, 2003.

Mulligan M: Extremity trauma. In Mirvis SE, Shanmuganathan K, eds: *Imaging in Trauma and Critical Care*, 2nd ed, Philadelphia, WB Saunders, 2003, p 575.

Cross-Reference

Emergency Radiology: THE REQUISITES, p 115.

Comment

The acromioclavicular (AC) joint is a small joint with a weak capsule reinforced superiorly and inferiorly by thickened areas referred to as the superior and inferior acromioclavicular ligaments, respectively. The acromioclavicular ligaments attach the clavicle to the acromion and blend into the trapezius and deltoid muscles. Vertical joint stability is maintained by the coracoclavicular ligament, which connects the coracoid process of the scapula to the undersurface of the clavicle.

Injuries to the AC joint usually result from a direct blow to the shoulder or, occasionally, a fall onto an outstretched hand. AC joint injuries are usually sprains, and they are unusual in children. All involve varying degrees of injury to the joint capsule. More severe injuries include disruption of the coracoclavicular ligament and insertions of the deltoid and trapezius muscles.

Anteroposterior standing views with 15 degrees cephalad angulation obtained with and without weighted (5 to 15 pounds suspended from each wrist) stress are standard radiographic projections of the AC joints. Frequently, both joints are evaluated to evaluate for symmetry. The normal AC joint is 3 to 4 mm wide, and there should be no more than 2 mm difference from side to side. The normal coracoclavicular interval should be no more than 12 mm. If the anteroposterior view without weighted stress demonstrates an obvious injury, the stress views can be deferred. However, a normal nonstress anteroposterior view does not preclude an injury.

AC joint injuries can be characterized (i.e., graded) as Rockwood type I to VI injuries. Type I injuries are mild AC capsule sprains that exhibit no radiographic abnormalities and are diagnosed by clinical examination. In type II injuries, there is disruption of the joint capsule, and radiographs demonstrate a wide AC joint. The coracoclavicular ligament and joint capsule are both disrupted in type III injuries, and radiographs demonstrate widening of both the AC joint and coracoclavicular interval with elevation of the clavicular head. Posterior displacement of the clavicular head seen with type IV injuries may be impossible to recognize on standard radiographic projections, although it is typically obvious clinically. In type V injuries, the clavicular head is markedly elevated into the lower neck soft tissues. Type VI injuries are characterized by inferior displacement of the clavicular head to a position inferior to the coracoid process.

Notes

CASE 42

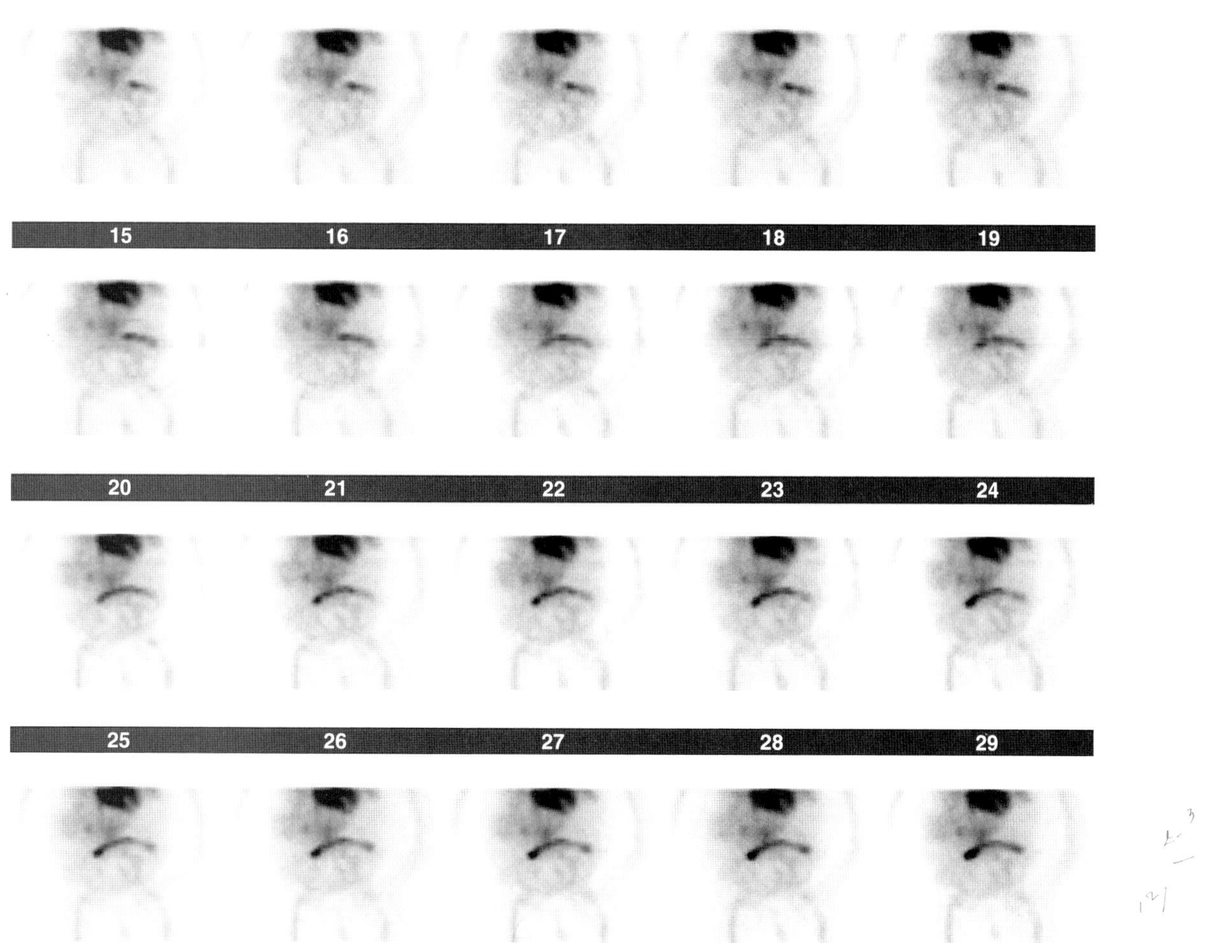

1. What are the criteria for active gastrointestinal hemorrhage on a ^{99m}Tc-labeled red blood cell scan?
2. What increases the likelihood of a positive ^{99m}Tc-labeled red blood cell scan during the assessment of acute lower gastrointestinal hemorrhage?
3. Approximately what percentage of patients with a normal ^{99m}Tc-labeled red blood cell scan experience recurrent lower gastrointestinal hemorrhage?
4. When the results of this study are positive, the odds of successful diagnosis and treatment with what other technique are increased?

CASE 42

Acute Lower Gastrointestinal Hemorrhage

1. Abnormal radiotracer localization with an appearance and configuration compatible with bowel lumen, increasing activity over the time course of the examination, and movement of activity (retrograde or antegrade) through bowel.
2. Transfusion with 2 units of red blood cells within 24 hours prior to the scan.
3. 15% to 27%.
4. Angiography.

Reference

Hammond KL, Beck DE, Hicks TC, et al: Implications of negative technetium 99m-labeled red blood cell scintigraphy in patients presenting with lower gastrointestinal bleeding, *Am J Surg* 193:404–407, 2007.

Cross-Reference

Emergency Radiology: THE REQUISITES, pp 289–291, 341–342, 378–379.

Comment

Acute lower gastrointestinal hemorrhage is a potentially life-threatening and common entity. Causes of lower gastrointestinal hemorrhage include diverticular disease, malignancy, and angiodysplasia, although the cause of hemorrhage is frequently undiagnosed. In most cases, hemorrhage spontaneously ceases without surgical or endovascular therapy, but in 15% to 27% of patients, gastrointestinal hemorrhage may recur. At times, colonoscopy can be used to both localize and treat the site of hemorrhage, yet in many instances, it fails to identify the source of bleeding. Angiography can also be used to identify and treat the site of hemorrhage, but if the patient is not actively bleeding at the time of examination, angiography may prove nondiagnostic.

^{99m}Tc-labeled red blood cell (RBC) scintigraphy can be used to detect active lower gastrointestinal hemorrhage occurring at a rate as low as 1 mL/min. If there is no clinical evidence of recent significant blood loss, the scan results will likely be negative. The greatest diagnostic yield of ^{99m}Tc-labeled RBC scintigraphy occurs when scanning is performed within 24 hours after the patient has been transfused with a minimum of 2 units of red blood cells. ^{99m}Tc-labeled RBC criteria for diagnosing active hemorrhage include abnormal radiotracer localization with an appearance and configuration compatible with bowel lumen, increasing activity over the time course of the examination, and movement of activity (retrograde or antegrade) through bowel by peristalsis.

Since up to 27% of patients without evidence of active bleeding on a ^{99m}Tc-labelled RBC scan may experience recurrent lower gastrointestinal hemorrhage, the value of scanning is somewhat controversial. However, scintigraphy can be used to predict successful angiographic diagnosis and intervention. In patients without clear clinical evidence of brisk ongoing hemorrhage, who may be best served by prompt angiographic assessment, a positive ^{99m}Tc-labelled RBC has been shown to significantly increase positive angiographic results compared to those with negative scintigraphic results. In this context, scintigraphy is particularly valuable when it reveals positive results within the first two minutes.

Notes

Case courtesy of Bruce Line, MD, Baltimore, MD.

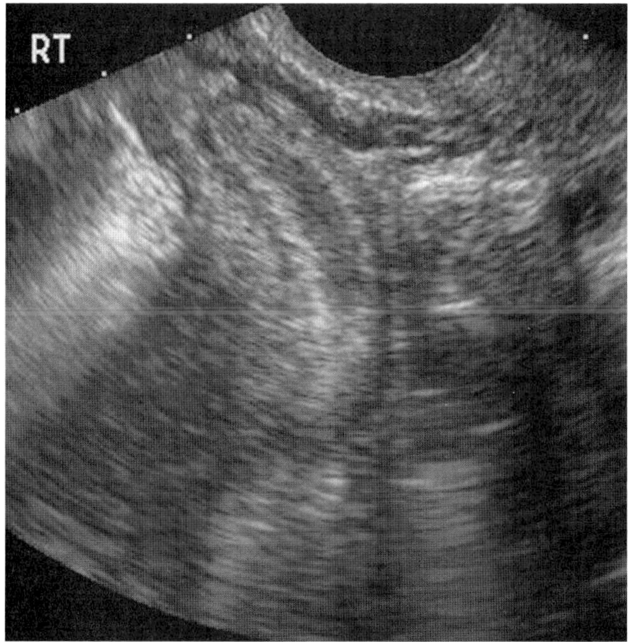

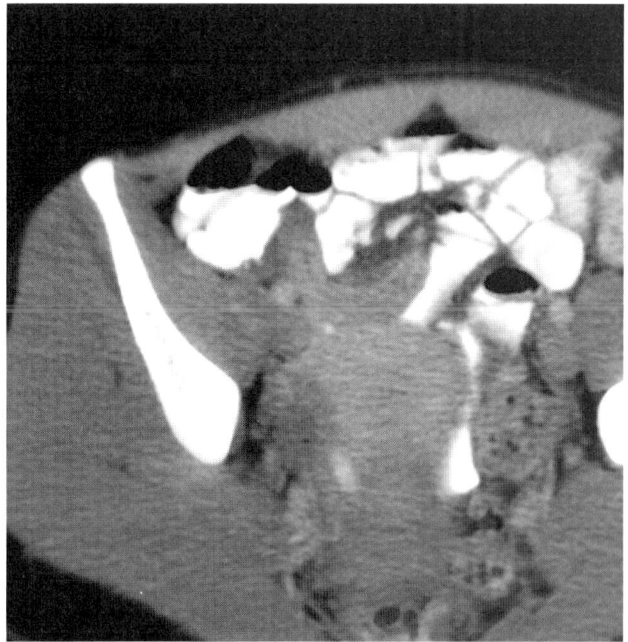

1. When acute appendicitis is suspected during transvaginal ultrasound examination, the appendix should be shown to be separate from what structures?
2. What are the gray-scale sonographic diagnostic criteria for acute appendicitis?
3. Why may women benefit most from the use of imaging in cases of suspected appendicitis?
4. What is the combined diagnostic accuracy of computed tomography and ultrasound for diagnosing acute appendicitis?

CASE 43

Acute Appendicitis

1. The ovary and fallopian tube.
2. Dilated (>6 mm diameter), blind-ending, noncompressible appendix.
3. The high frequency of gynecologic disorders and urinary tract infections that may mimic appendicitis.
4. 83% to 98%.

References

Bendeck SE, Nino-Murcia M, Berry GJ, Jeffrey RB Jr: Imaging for suspected appendicitis: negative appendectomy and perforation rates, *Radiology* 225: 131–136, 2002.

Molander P, Paavonen J, Sjoberg J, et al: Transvaginal sonography in the diagnosis of acute appendicitis, *Ultrasound Obstet Gynecol* 20:496–501, 2002.

Cross-Reference

Emergency Radiology: THE REQUISITES, pp 194, 283.

Comment

Utilizing clinical criteria, acute appendicitis can be diagnosed with a diagnostic accuracy of 80%. In women, in whom the symptoms of acute appendicitis overlap with urinary tract infections and gynecologic disease, the accuracy of clinical examination is only 60% to 68%. The use of computed tomography (CT) and ultrasonography (US) may increase diagnostic accuracy to 83% to 98%. Historically, based on clinical examination alone, negative appendectomy rates as high as 20% have been accepted. The use of imaging has lowered negative appendectomy rates, and the greatest impact has been demonstrated in women of reproductive age in whom negative appendectomy rates have been lowered from as high as 28% to 34% down to 7% to 8%.

In many centers, either CT or graded-compression US is used to evaluate patients in whom the clinical examination is suggestive, but not characteristic, of appendicitis. On the other hand, in those women in whom a gynecologic disorder, such as pelvic inflammatory disease, is suspected, a combination of transabdominal US and transvaginal pelvic US is generally utilized. Both CT and US demonstrate the appendix as a blind-ending tubular structure. On CT, the diagnosis of acute appendicitis can be rendered when the appendix is dilated greater than 6 mm diameter and there is adjacent inflammatory edema or fluid. Sonographic signs of acute appendicitis include a noncompressible dilated appendix (diameter > 6 mm). Occasionally, US may show echogenic inflammatory changes in the adjacent fat. Color Doppler interrogation may demonstrate increased appendiceal and periappendiceal flow related to hyperemia. With both CT and US, complicated appendicitis can be suspected if the appendix is replaced by an ill-defined inflammatory mass. During transvaginal pelvic US examination based on an initial suspicion for gynecologic disease, the appendix may be inferior to the right adnexa, and it should be shown to be separate from the ovary and fallopian tube.

Notes

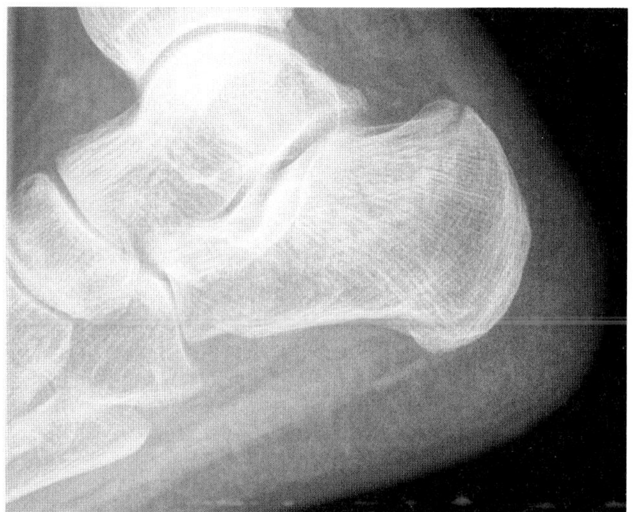

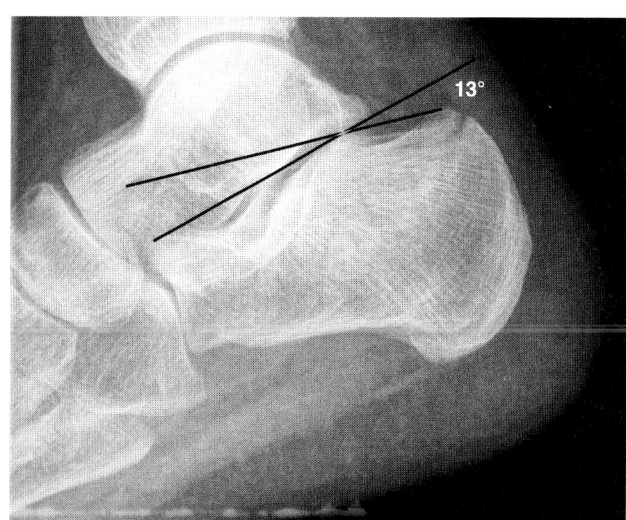

1. What is the usual mechanism of injury for calcaneal fractures?
2. How are calcaneal fractures characterized?
3. Are calcaneal fractures common in children?
4. What is the name of the angle measured in the above illustration?

CASE 44

Calcaneus Fracture

1. A direct blow to the calcaneus.
2. Intra-articular and extra-articular.
3. No.
4. Boehler's angle.

Reference

Daftary A, Haims AH, Baumgaertner MR: Fractures of the calcaneus: a review with emphasis on CT, *Radiographics* 25:1215–1226, 2005.

Cross-Reference

Emergency Radiology: THE REQUISITES, pp 156–158.

Comment

Calcaneal fractures account for 2% of all fractures in the body and 60% of tarsal fractures. They are more common in adults with only 5% occurring in children. Most calcaneal fractures occur as a result of axial loading. Usually, they result from a direct blow to the calcaneus. They are common in patients who fall from a height and land on their feet, and, in this setting, they are frequently associated with lumbar spine compression fractures. Due to altered mechanics through the foot, long-term outcomes have been historically poor.

Calcaneal fractures are characterized as intra-articular or extra-articular. Intra-articular fractures involve the posterior subtalar joint and account for 70% to 75% of calcaneal fractures. All fractures that spare the subtalar joint are extra-articular. Accurate characterization of subtalar joint involvement facilitates appropriate surgical care.

Although computed tomography is vital in the accurate assessment of calcaneal fractures, radiography remains the primary diagnostic tool of choice at most centers. Both axial and lateral views are used to evaluate the calcaneus, but the diagnosis can usually be made on the lateral projection. On the lateral projection, Boehler's angle is a measurement that may reveal subtle calcaneal fractures. Normally 20 to 40 degrees, Boehler's angle is formed by a line between the superior posterior margin of the tuberosity with the superior tip of the posterior facet and a second line between the superior tip of the posterior facet and the superior tip of the anterior calcaneal process. A depressed Boehler's angle indicates depression of the posterior facet that most likely results from fracture.

Notes

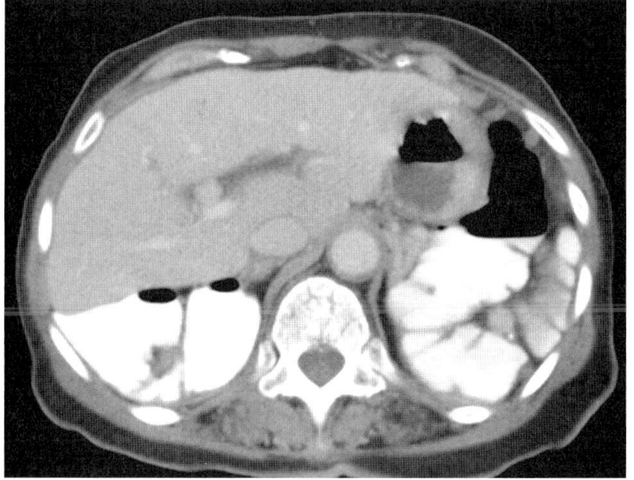

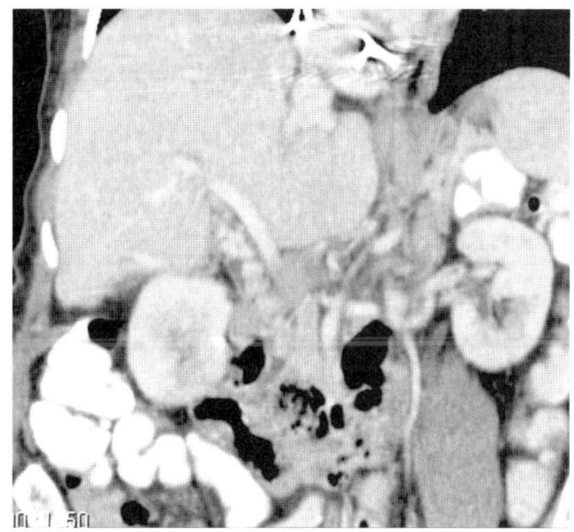

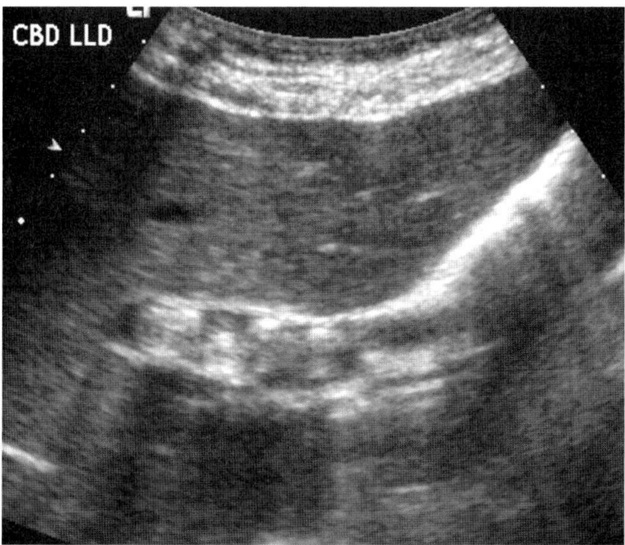

1. Where are the abnormalities located?
2. What is the sensitivity of ultrasound for detecting this abnormality?
3. What is the sensitivity of computed tomography for detecting this abnormality?
4. What is the most sensitive noninvasive means for detecting this abnormality or pathology?

CASE 45

Choledocholithiasis

1. The intrahepatic biliary ducts and both the proximal and distal common bile duct.
2. 70% to 75%.
3. 80% to 90%.
4. Magnetic resonance cholangiopancreatography.

Reference

Chung WS, Park MS, Yoon SW, et al: Diagnostic accuracy of multidetector-row computed tomography for common bile duct calculi: is it necessary to add non-contrast-enhanced images to contrast-enhanced images?, *J Comput Assist Tomogr* 31: 508–512, 2007

Cross-Reference

Emergency Radiology: THE REQUISITES, pp 294–296.

Comment

Choledocholithiasis can be the primary cause of acute right upper quadrant pain. Alternatively, it is detected as a cause of pancreatitis or ascending cholangitis. Occasionally, it is an incidental finding. The patient may be jaundiced, but liver function tests may also be normal.

Ultrasound (US) is a generally accepted means for diagnosing biliary duct stones when choledocholithiasis is the suspected cause of acute right upper quadrant pain. The sensitivity of US for identifying choledocholithiasis is somewhat low at 70% to 75%, although scanning the patient in various positions will maximize its sensitivity. In addition to calculi, scanning may demonstrate biliary duct dilation. While magnetic resonance cholangiopancreatography is the most accurate noninvasive means to diagnose choledocholithiasis, with sensitivity of 95% and specificity of 100%, its imaging times can be long and it may be difficult to obtain in an emergent fashion at many centers, whereas US is a quick examination that is widely available.

While its requirements for ionizing radiation and intravenous contrast make it a less desirable option than US for evaluating patients with suspected biliary stones, the sensitivity and specificity of computed tomography (CT) for detecting choledocholiths are both high at 80% to 90% and 90% to 100%, respectively. Thin-section (i.e., 3-mm-thick) images and coronal multiplanar reconstructed images maximize the accuracy of CT. Early studies had suggested that both unenhanced and intravenous contrast-enhanced images are necessary for CT to accurately detect biliary duct stones, although a recent study utilizing multidetector-row CT demonstrated no significant improvement in accuracy when unenhanced imaging was included with contrast-enhanced images reconstructed in axial and coronal planes.

Notes

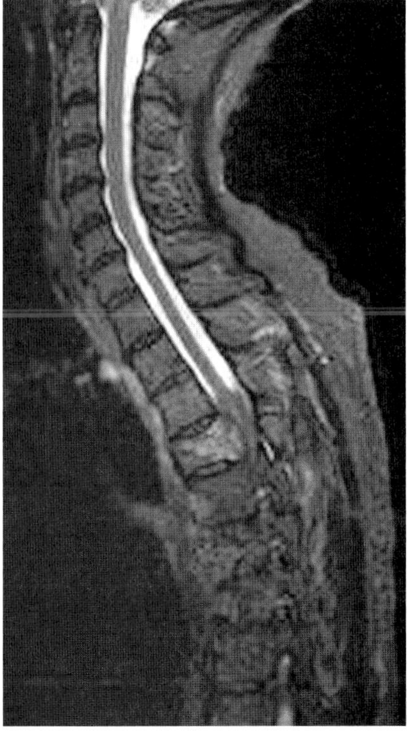

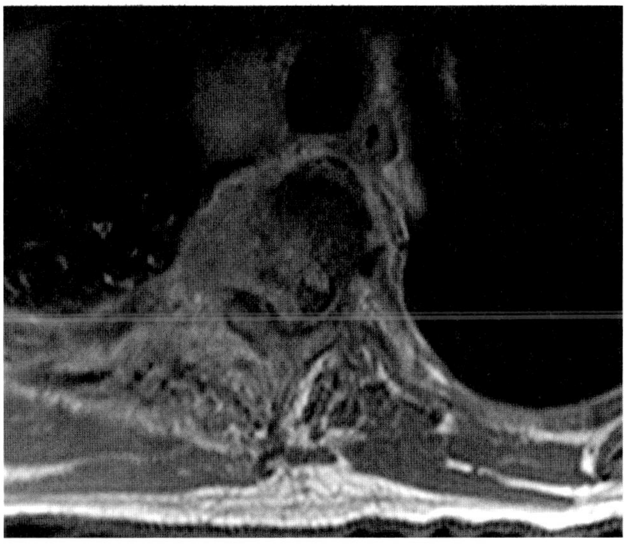

1. What is the diagnosis?
2. How frequently does this abnormality occur in cancer patients?
3. What is the probable outcome if this is not treated emergently and aggressively?
4. What is the utility of intravenous gadolinium when using magnetic resonance imaging to evaluate patients suspected of having this disorder?

CASE 46

Malignant Spinal Cord Compression

1. Malignant spinal cord compression.
2. 5% to 14% of cancer patients with metastatic disease.
3. Paraplegia.
4. Facilitate diagnosis of leptomeningeal or intrinsic spinal cord lesions that mimic cord compression.

References

Kwok Y, Tibbs PA, Patchell RA: Clinical approach to metastatic epidural spinal cord compression, *Hematol Oncol Clin North Am* 20:1297–1305, 2006.

Loughrey GJ, Collins CD, Todd SM, et al: Magnetic resonance imaging in the management of suspected spinal canal disease in patients with known malignancy, *Clin Radiol* 55:849–855, 2000.

Cross-Reference

Emergency Radiology: THE REQUISITES, pp 229–231.

Comment

Malignant cord compression is a relatively common complication of cancer with 5% to 14% of cancer patients developing metastatic spinal cord compression. In addition to metastatic disease, cord compression may result from multiple myeloma, lymphoma, and primary bone tumors. Patients typically present with back pain, and they may also exhibit weakness, sensory deficits, or incontinence. Untreated spinal cord compression causes paraplegia in nearly 100% of patients. Aggressive emergent treatment is required to limit neurologic damage and maintain quality of life, although long-term survival in these patients is limited.

Magnetic resonance imaging (MRI) is the most sensitive means to diagnose malignant cord compression. MRI may demonstrate cord compression by a mass extending from a vertebral body or through a neural foramen from the paraspinal region. Occasionally, MRI may reveal a pathologic compression fracture with compression of the spinal cord by displaced bone fragments. While the symptomatic lesion is usually detected at the thoracic level, multiple levels of metastatic disease are present in nearly 50% of patients, and approximately 25% exhibit more than one level of spinal cord compression. Consequently, imaging of the entire spine is recommended. Although contrast enhancement is not required to demonstrate cord compression, it facilitates diagnosis of significant alternative diagnoses that include leptomeningeal metastases and intrinsic spinal cord lesions.

Notes

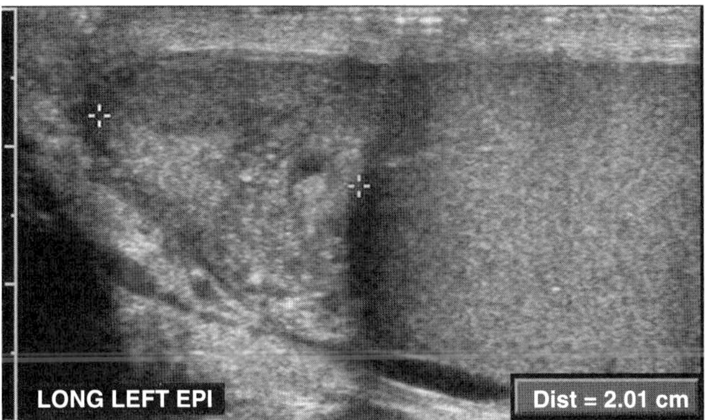

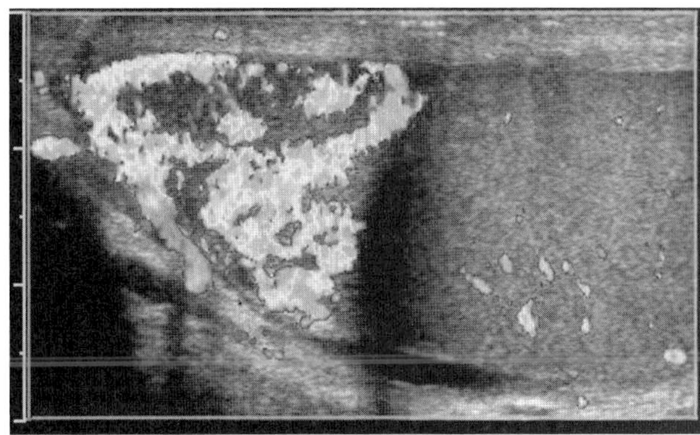
See also Color Plate

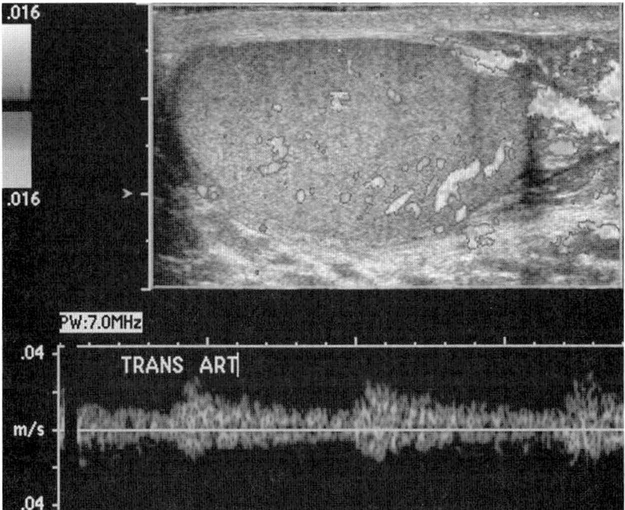

See also Color Plate

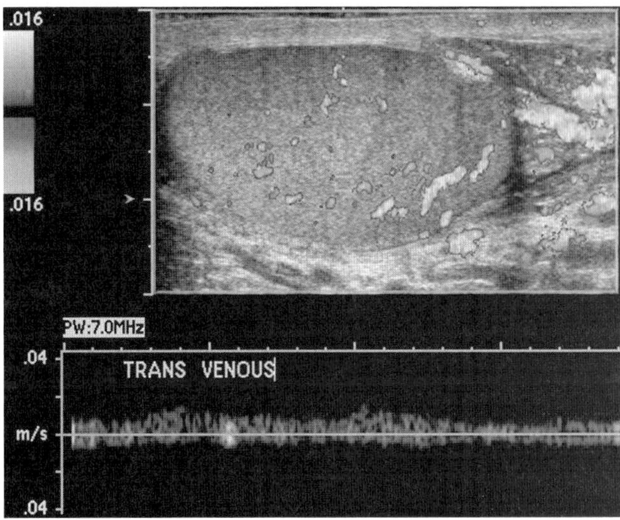

See also Color Plate

1. What are the primary epididymal abnormalities?
2. What is the primary differential diagnosis for sudden-onset acute scrotal pain?
3. Is isolated orchitis without associated epididymitis common?
4. What is the usual etiology of epididymitis in men older than 35 years of age?

CASE 47

Epididymitis

1. Enlarged and hypervascular epididymal head.
2. Epididymitis or epididymo-orchitis, testicular appendage torsion, and testicular torsion.
3. No.
4. A lower urinary tract infection.

Reference

Pearl MS, Hill MC: Ultrasound of the scrotum, *Semin Ultrasound CT MR* 28:225–248, 2007.

Cross-Reference

Emergency Radiology: THE REQUISITES, pp 198, 311, 383.

Comment

Epididymitis (or epididymo-orchitis) is a common cause of unilateral sudden-onset acute scrotal pain that is usually associated with scrotal erythema and swelling. Other entities in the differential diagnosis include testicular appendage torsion and testicular torsion. Additional signs that suggest epididymitis or epididymo-orchitis include fever, dysuria, and urethral discharge. When the clinical presentation does not clearly suggest epididymitis, Gray-scale and color Doppler ultrasound (US) can be used to reach the appropriate diagnosis.

Acute epididymitis is typically infectious. Commonly, the infection also involves the ipsilateral testis (i.e., epididymo-orchitis), and isolated infectious orchitis is rare. In young children and men older than 35 years, infection usually results from spread of a lower urinary tract infection from either the bladder or prostate. In adolescent and young adult men, epididymitis is usually caused by a sexually transmitted disease.

Gray-scale US usually demonstrates involvement of the epididymal head, although any part, or the entire epididymis, may be involved. The epididymis is usually enlarged (normal head diameter 5 to 12 mm, normal body and tail diameter 2 to 5 mm). Epididymal echotexture is typically hypoechoic, but it may be hyperechoic or heterogeneous if there is hemorrhage. Associated orchitis results in focal, multifocal, or diffuse reduced testicular echogenicity. The overlying skin is frequently thickened. There may be a hydrocele. Color Doppler US demonstrates increased flow due to hyperemia.

Notes

CASE 48

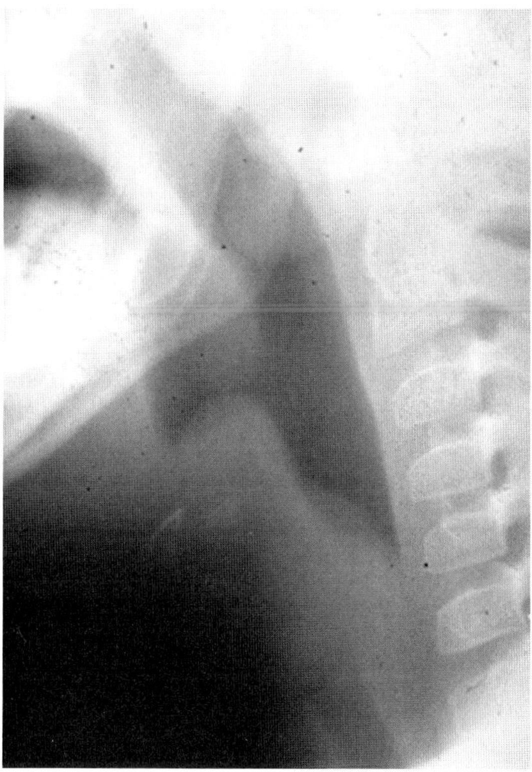

1. What is the diagnosis?
2. What is the major complication of this disease?
3. What are the radiographic diagnostic criteria on a lateral neck radiograph?
4. Is subglottic extension typical of this disease?

CASE 48

Acute Epiglottitis

1. Acute epiglottitis.
2. Sudden airway compromise.
3. Thickening of the epiglottis and aryepiglottic folds.
4. No.

References

John SD, Swischuk LE: Stridor and upper airway obstruction in infants and children, *Radiographics* 12:625–643, 1992.

John SD, Swischuk LE, Hayden CK Jr, Freeman DH Jr: Aryepiglottic fold width in patients with epiglottitis: where should measurements be obtained?, *Radiology* 190:123–125, 1994.

Cross-Reference

Emergency Radiology: THE REQUISITES, pp 48–50, 201.

Comment

Acute epiglottitis is a bacterial infection typically caused by *Haemophilus influenzae*. Due to the efficacy of the *H. influenzae* type B vaccine, acute epiglottitis is now an uncommon condition. Although it may affect adults, it is generally a disease of children. It may present without preceding upper airway infection with dysphagia, stridor, drooling, and high fever. Acute epiglottitis can lead to airway compromise which may be sudden and severe.

Radiographs are the initial means to diagnose epiglottitis. Given the risk for rapid severe airway compromise, it is advisable that portable examinations be performed in the emergency department with exceptional efforts made to limit manipulation of the neck and exciting the child. If a portable examination is not feasible, the patient should be accompanied by someone qualified to intubate the child should airway compromise develop.

The hallmark radiographic findings of acute epiglottitis are thickened epiglottis and aryepiglottic folds as demonstrated on the lateral neck radiograph. Aryepiglottic fold thickening is best appreciated and most predictive of epiglottitis at the upper half of the folds. Typically, the vocal cords and subglottic airway are spared, but, in severe cases, an anteroposterior neck radiograph may reveal subglottic airway narrowing caused by inferior extension of the inflammation.

Notes

Case courtesy of George Gross, MD, Baltimore, MD.

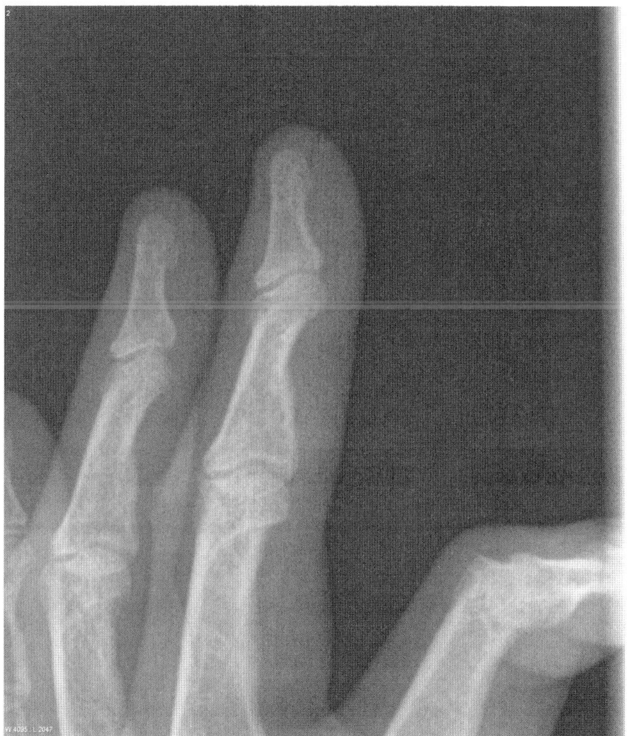

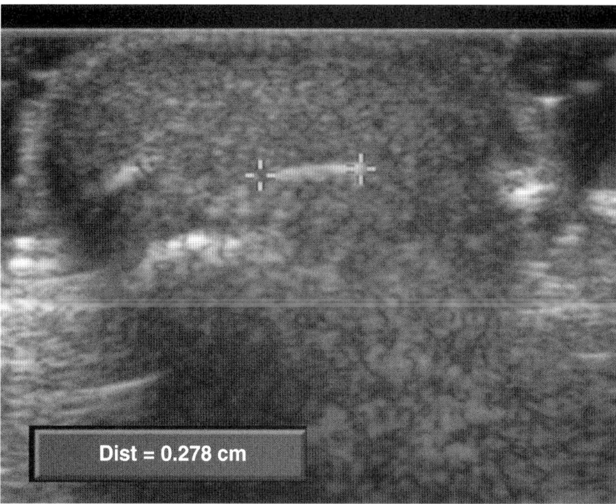

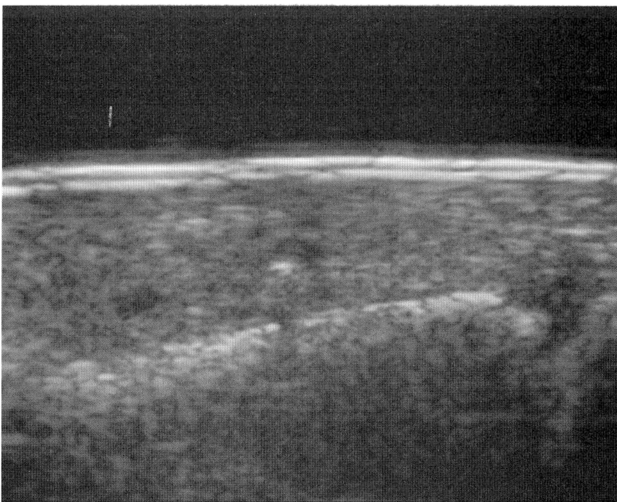

1. Are retained soft tissue foreign bodies commonly missed on initial clinical examination?
2. What is the significance of a missed retained foreign body?
3. What is the sensitivity of radiographs for detecting retained wood foreign bodies?
4. What is the size of the smallest superficial soft tissue foreign body detectable by ultrasound?

CASE 49

Retained Foreign Body

1. Yes. Up to 38% of retained foreign bodies may be missed in initial clinical examination.
2. Missed retained foreign bodies can lead to significant infection or inflammation. They are a common cause of litigation.
3. Less than 15%.
4. 2.5 mm in length and 1 mm in diameter.

References

Boyse TD, Fessell DP, Jacobson JA, et al: US of soft-tissue foreign bodies and associated complications with surgical correlation, *Radiographics* 21: 1251–1256, 2001.

Gibbs TS: The use of sonography in the identification, localization, and removal of soft tissue foreign bodies, *J Diag Med Sonogr* 22:5–21, 2006.

Cross-Reference

Emergency Radiology: THE REQUISITES, p 180.

Comment

Retained foreign bodies are a common occurrence in the emergency department. Most retained foreign bodies are wood, glass, or metal. Foreign body removal may seem a simple task, because of their typically small size, but up to 38% of retained foreign bodies are missed at initial clinical examination. Less than 15% of wooden foreign bodies are detected with radiographs, and many types of glass are radiolucent. Serious infection or inflammation may complicate untreated retained foreign bodies with nerve injury, tendon injury, allergic reaction, or other potential remote consequences. Missed foreign bodies have been reported to be the second most frequent source of litigation in emergency medicine.

Ultrasound (US) can be a valuable tool for identifying and localizing superficial soft tissue foreign bodies. When a high-resolution linear transducer is utilized, US can identify nonradiopaque foreign bodies with a sensitivity of 95% and a specificity of 89%. It allows detection of wood, glass, plastic, and metallic foreign bodies as small as 2.5 mm in length and 1 mm in diameter. Moreover, US can refine localization of foreign bodies detected radiographically, thereby facilitating rapid retrieval. Accuracy can be limited by gas introduced into the area of interest either through the wound itself or during pre-scanning attempts at retrieval. Due to the inherent limitations of the technique, deep foreign bodies may be difficult or impossible to localize sonographically.

Acutely, foreign bodies are typically echogenic, although in the subacute to chronic phases, wood can be isoechoic to soft tissues due to absorption of water. Foreign bodies may produce clean or dirty posterior acoustic shadowing. Flat or smooth objects, such as glass and metal, may produce posterior reverberation artifact. Sometimes, posterior shadowing is not apparent, although changing orientation of the transducer may produce shadowing and aid with object identification. If a foreign body is retained for more than 24 hours, it may elicit an inflammatory reaction that produces a hypoechoic rim surrounding the foreign body.

Notes

CASE 50

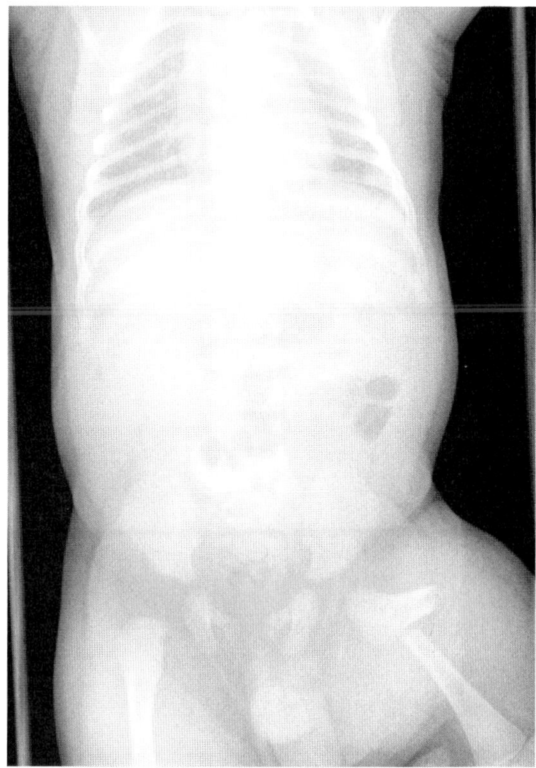

1. If this patient reportedly was dropped while his father was attempting to change his diaper, what diagnosis should be considered?
2. What age group suffers the greatest rate of child abuse?
3. In inflicted injury, in what bones are fractures most frequently identified?
4. In infants, what fractures are highly specific for inflicted injury?

CASE 50

Inflicted Injury (Child Physical Abuse)

1. Inflicted injury.
2. Children under 18 months of age.
3. Long bones, ribs, and skull.
4. Classic metaphyseal lesions (metaphyseal corner fractures) and posterior rib fractures.

References

Kleinman PK, Marks SC Jr, Richmond JM, Blackbourne BD: Inflicted skeletal injury: a postmortem radiologic-histopathologic study in 31 infants, *AJR Am J Roentgenol* 165:647–650, 1995.

Lonergan GJ, Baker AM, Morey MK, Boos SC: From the archives of the AFIP. Child abuse: radiologic-pathologic correlation, *Radiographics* 23:811–845, 2003.

Cross-Reference

Emergency Radiology: THE REQUISITES, pp 211–212, 377.

Comment

Child neglect and abuse are common. In the United States, approximately 1% of children are subjected to child abuse, with just over 75% suffering at the hands of their parents. Children under 18 months of age endure abuse or neglect at higher rates than other age groups, and they account for nearly half of all abuse-related fatalities. In all 50 states and the District of Columbia, all physicians are required by law to report suspected child abuse to appropriate authorities within 48 hours.

Musculoskeletal injuries are the most frequently encountered injuries in cases of child abuse. Most fractures affect the long bones, ribs, and skull. In the long bones, classic metaphyseal lesions (i.e., metaphyseal corner fractures or bucket handle fractures) are highly specific for abuse and rarely encountered in children other than infants. In infants, rib fractures are rarely caused by anything but abuse, and posterior rib fractures are highly specific for inflicted injury. Frequently, infants who die from inflicted injury have fractures at multiple sites. Fractures in various stages of healing are frequently encountered.

Special attention needs to be directed toward the circumstances of the injury. If the type of injury is incongruent with the reported history, inflicted skeletal injury should be suspected. Although household falls (e.g., changing tables, beds, counters, etc.) may cause injury, they rarely cause significant skeletal injury. Moreover, while a fall down stairs may result in head or extremity injuries, multifocal severe injuries are uncommon in falls unless there are unusual circumstances, such as a fall while in a walker. Inflicted injury should also be suspected when the injury is unusual for the child's developmental stage. For example, spiral long bone fractures are common in ambulatory children, but in nonambulatory children, they are uncommon and very suggestive of abuse.

Notes

Case courtesy of George Gross, MD, Baltimore, MD.

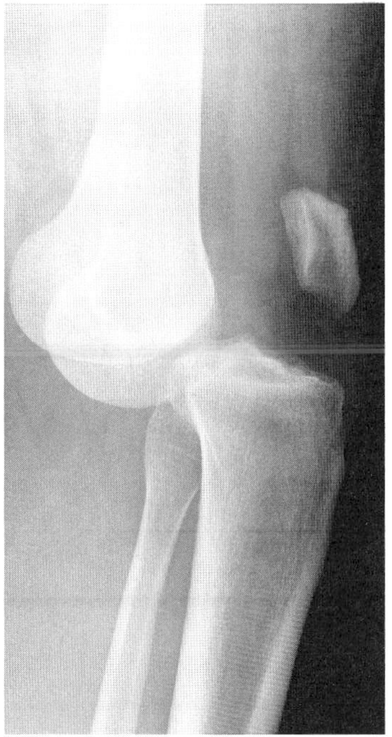

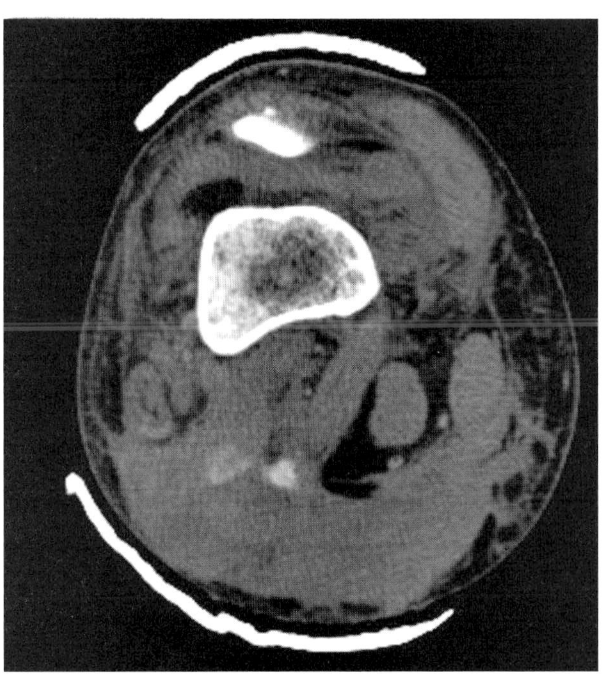

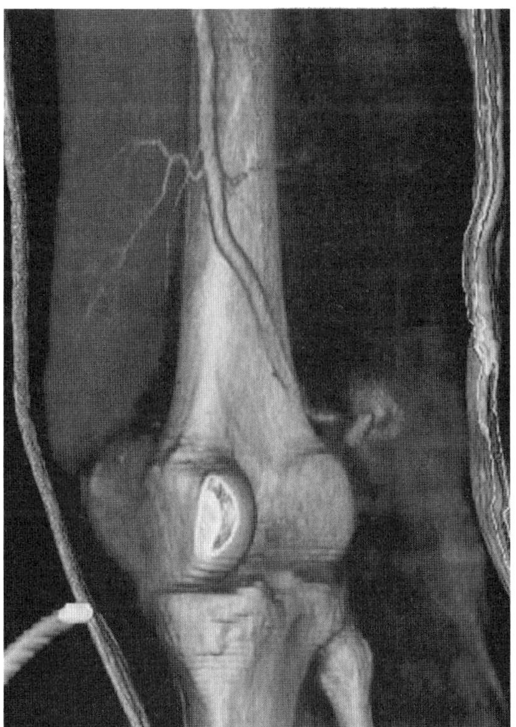

See also Color Plate

1. What type of knee dislocation is this?
2. What artery is injured?
3. What two types of knee dislocation are most frequently associated with arterial injury?
4. In the setting of knee dislocation, clinically significant arterial injuries are typically associated with what abnormality on physical examination?

CASE 51

Anterior Knee Dislocation with Popliteal Artery Transection

1. Anterior.
2. Popliteal artery.
3. Anterior and posterior.
4. Abnormal pedal pulses.

References

Inaba K, Potzman J, Munera F, et al: Multi-slice CT angiography for arterial evaluation in the injured lower extremity, *J Trauma* 60:502–506, 2006.

Rieger M, Mallouhi A, Tauscher T, et al: Traumatic arterial injuries of the extremities: initial evaluation with MD CT angiography, *AJR Am J Roentgenol* 186:656–664, 2006.

Cross-Reference

Emergency Radiology: THE REQUISITES, pp 145, 147.

Comment

Knee dislocations are rare injuries that result from major blunt trauma. The most common mechanisms include road traffic accidents and falls from a height, although crush injuries and violent sports mishaps may also cause dislocation. Dislocations are classified based on the displacement of the tibia relative to the femur. Anterior dislocations are most common. Posterior, medial, lateral, and posterolateral dislocations also occur. In addition to extensive soft tissue injuries with internal joint derangements, 29% to 50% of knee dislocations are associated with arterial injuries while 15% are associated with peroneal nerve injuries.

The popliteal artery is the most commonly injured artery. It is usually encountered with anterior and posterior dislocations. Clinically significant arterial injuries that occur with knee dislocation are typically associated with abnormal pedal pulses, although arterial injury can occur with normal pulses. Popliteal artery occlusions related to knee dislocation are frequently associated with lower leg ischemia that may necessitate amputation in up to 86% of cases in which prompt vascular repair is not undertaken. In contrast, prompt repair of popliteal occlusion is associated with amputation rates of 13% to 40%.

Angiography is the reference standard for diagnosing lower extremity arterial injuries. However, multidetector computed tomographic angiography (MD-CTA) is rapidly becoming a first-line tool for evaluating the acutely injured limb for arterial injury. When limited to those patients with clinical signs of arterial injury, the sensitivity of MD-CTA for clinically significant injuries approaches 100%. Generally, injuries are detected on axial MD-CTA images, although both multiplanar reconstructed images and volume-rendered images facilitate accurate injury characterization.

Notes

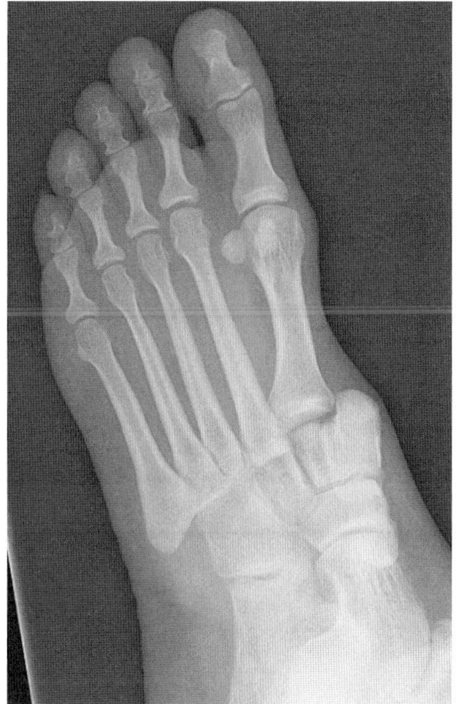

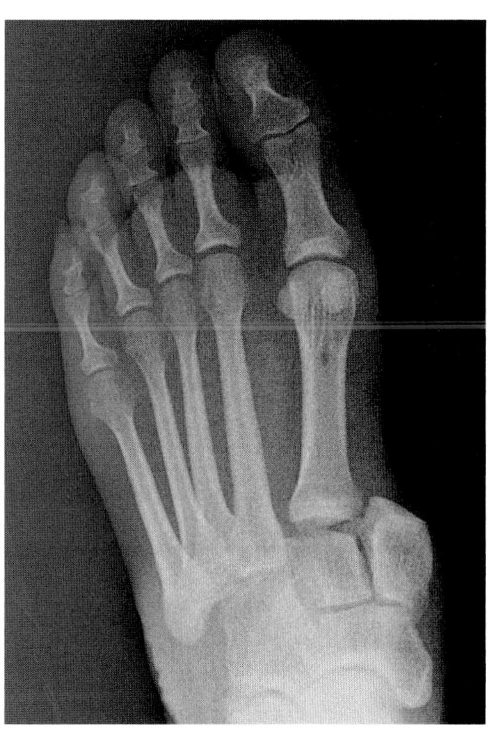

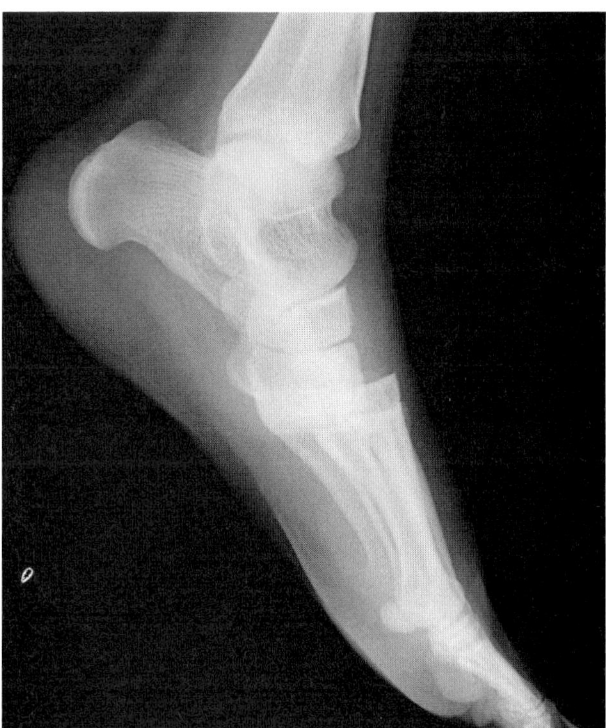

1. By what common eponym is this injury known?
2. What two mechanisms can cause this injury?
3. Is this the homolateral or divergent type of this injury?
4. How much offset in alignment between the medial margins of the fourth metatarsal and cuboid can be normal?

CASE 52

Lisfranc Fracture-Dislocation

1. Lisfranc injury.
2. Axial loading on a plantar flexed foot and twisting of the midfoot–hindfoot around the fixed forefoot.
3. Homolateral.
4. 2 to 3 mm.

Reference

Norfray JF, Geline RA, Steinberg RI, et al: Subtleties of Lisfranc fracture-dislocations, *AJR Am J Roentgenol* 137:1151–1156, 1981.

Cross-Reference

Emergency Radiology: THE REQUISITES, p 158.

Comment

Together, the five tarsometatarsal joints and associated interconnecting ligaments make up the Lisfranc joint. A Lisfranc injury represents dislocation of two or more tarsometatarsal joints with the second joint almost always involved. Injuries frequently occur from high-energy trauma, such as a fall from a height or motor vehicle collision, with axial loading on a plantar flexed foot, although they may occur from less severe trauma, such as secondary to stepping off a curb and sporting activities. Lisfranc injury may also be caused by twisting of the midfoot around the fixed forefoot. Typically, there are associated avulsion fractures at the Lisfranc joint. Other foot and ankle injuries are also common, especially transverse fractures at the proximal second metatarsal base and cuboid chip fractures. Although some injuries can be treated with closed reduction, results are frequently poor, and open reduction with internal fixation is generally required to preserve foot function.

Radiographic evidence of a Lisfranc injury may be very subtle. Occasionally, only one radiographic projection demonstrates the injury, so it is imperative to include all three standard projections (i.e., anteroposterior [AP], oblique, and lateral) in the radiographic examination of the acutely injured foot. On an AP projection of the normal foot, the lateral border of the first metatarsal aligns with the lateral margin of the medial cuneiform, while the medial margin of the second metatarsal aligns with the medial margin of the middle cuneiform. Normally, either oblique radiographs or AP radiographs demonstrate alignment between the lateral margins of the third metatarsal and lateral cuneiform, while the medial margins of the fourth metatarsal and cuboid are in alignment. Due to its bulbous configuration, the lateral margin of the fifth metatarsal base normally overlaps the lateral cuboid margin, although the majority of people demonstrate alignment of the cuboid with a small notch in the fifth metatarsal articulating surface. Although offset of 2 to 3 mm can be a normal finding at the fourth tarsometatarsal joint, this is usually a bilateral finding, and a comparison view of the other foot can help distinguish this normal variant from injury. On the lateral view, the dorsal borders of the first and second metatarsal should form an unbroken line with the medial and lateral cuneiforms, respectively. Incongruity of any of these relationships indicates a Lisfranc injury.

There are two subtypes of Lisfranc injury. A homolateral injury is associated with dislocation of all of the affected metatarsals in the same direction, usually lateral. In a divergent injury, the second through fifth metatarsals are displaced laterally while the first metatarsal is medially dislocated.

Notes

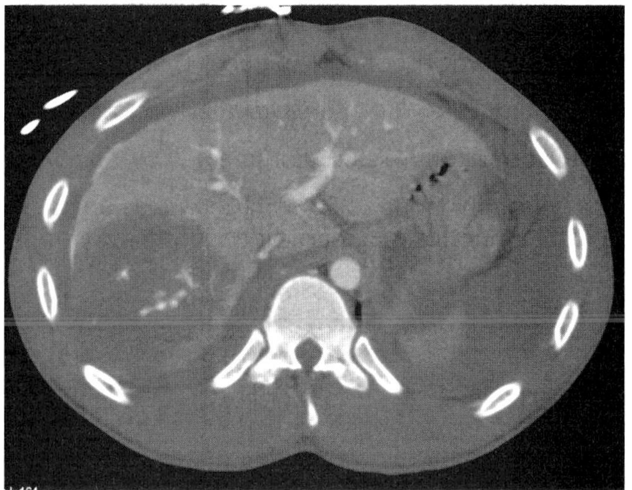

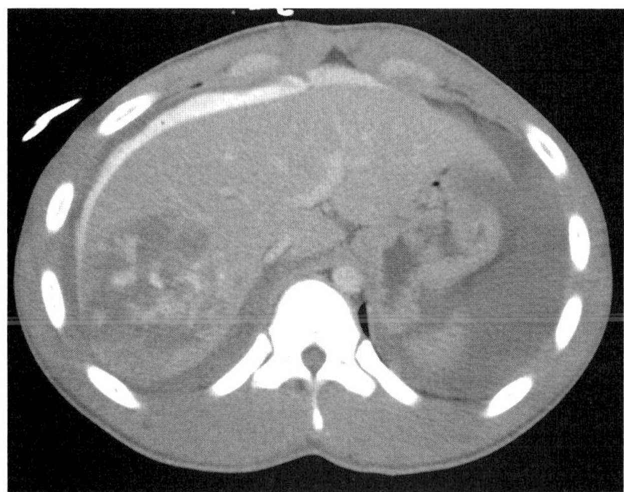

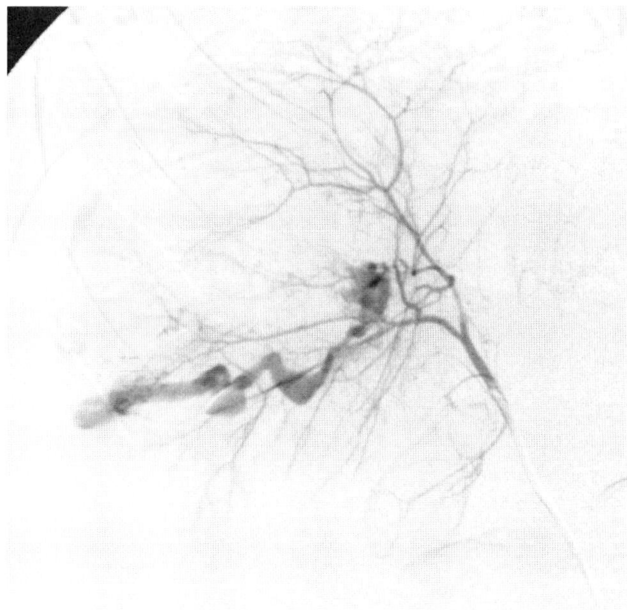

1. Which computed tomographic finding has the greatest immediate impact on management of this injury?
2. What is the role of interventional radiology in this setting?
3. What types of blunt hepatic injury are demonstrated by computed tomography?
4. On computed tomography, how can one differentiate pseudoaneurysms from active hemorrhage?

CASE 53

Liver Injury with Active Hemorrhage

1. Active arterial hemorrhage.
2. Endovascular control of the active arterial hemorrhage.
3. Contusion, intraparenchymal hematoma, subcapsular hematoma, vascular lesions, and active hemorrhage.
4. Pseudoaneurysms are focal collections of intravenous contrast seen on arterial-phase images with wash-out on later-phase imaging; active hemorrhage is an ill-defined contrast collection that enlarges on later-phase imaging.

Reference

Poletti PA, Mirvis SE, Shanmuganathan K, et al: CT criteria for management of blunt liver trauma: correlation with angiographic and surgical findings, *Radiology* 216:418–427, 2000.

Cross-Reference

Emergency Radiology: THE REQUISITES, pp 82–84.

Comment

The liver is the largest solid organ in the abdomen, and it is injured in 15% to 20% of patients who sustain blunt abdominal trauma. When appropriately selected, 50% to 96% of hemodynamically stable patients with blunt hepatic trauma can be successfully managed nonoperatively. Timely and accurate injury characterization with contrast-enhanced computed tomography (CT) is one key to successful nonoperative treatment. Abnormalities depicted by CT that can influence management of hepatic injury include extent of liver injury, associated nonhepatic injuries, active hemorrhage, and vascular injuries that predict an increased risk of hemorrhage. Coupled with the patient's hemodynamic status, abnormalities depicted by CT scan may indicate that surgery, imaging-based endovascular treatment, or a combination of the two may be more appropriate therapeutic options than nonoperative management.

Types of liver injury demonstrated by contrast-enhanced CT include contusions, hematomas (intraparenchymal or subcapsular), lacerations, vascular injuries, and active hemorrhage. Contusions are identified as low-attenuation areas of unclotted hemorrhage and/or bile. They can be associated with intraparenchymal high-attenuation hematomas. Subcapsular hematomas are hemorrhagic collections interposed between the liver capsule and enhancing liver parenchyma. Lacerations appear as nonenhancing linear or branching low-attenuation lesions. Vascular lesions are more common with lacerations extending to the central hepatic veins and/or retrohepatic inferior vena cava with frequently associated retrohepatic hematoma. Pseudoaneurysms are transient focal intravenous contrast collections with attenuation within 10 Hounsfield units of an adjacent artery seen in the arterial phase but not on portal venous or renal excretory phase imaging, while active hemorrhage is manifested by an ill-defined high-attenuation contrast collection on arterial phase images with subsequent enlargement on the later-phase images. The CT demonstration of major vascular injuries and/or active hemorrhage is of paramount importance to successful nonoperative management of hepatic injury since they indicate an increased likelihood of ongoing hemorrhage, and the combination of these two abnormalities is 85% sensitive for active arterial hemorrhage demonstrated at either angiography or surgery.

Notes

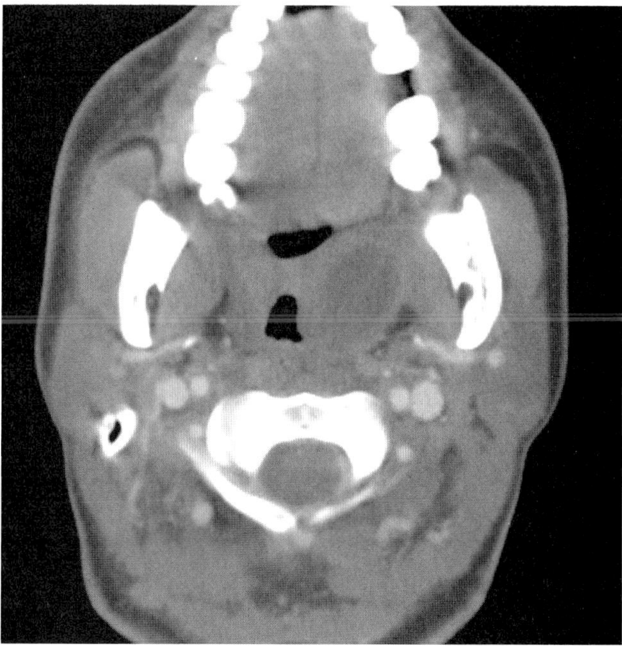

1. What is the role of computed tomography in the assessment of patients with peritonsillar cellulitis?
2. Why must peritonsillar abscess be differentiated from peritonsillar cellulitis?
3. Clinical diagnosis with needle aspiration or incision and drainage may lead to a false-negative diagnosis of peritonsillar abscess in what percentage of patients?
4. What is the reported sensitivity of computed tomography for peritonsillar abscess?

ANSWERS

CASE 54

Peritonsillar Abscess

1. To detect peritonsillar abscesses.
2. Peritonsillar abscesses are treated with drainage in addition to antibiotics, while peritonsillar cellulitis requires only antibiotic therapy.
3. 12% to 20%.
4. 100%.

Reference

Scott PM, Loftus WK, Kew J, et al: Diagnosis of peritonsillar infections: a prospective study of ultrasound, computerized tomography and clinical diagnosis, *J Laryngol Otol* 113:229–232, 1999.

Cross-Reference

Emergency Radiology: THE REQUISITES, pp 44–45.

Comment

Peritonsillar infection can be characterized by either peritonsillar cellulitis or peritonsillar abscess. Whereas treatment of peritonsillar cellulitis with antibiotics is usually adequate, a peritonsillar abscess usually requires drainage, in addition to antibiotics, in order for therapy to prove successful. Untreated or inadequately treated peritonsillar abscess can be complicated by airway compromise or abscess extension into the deeper neck soft tissues with subsequent spread to the skull base or mediastinum. Attempted incision and drainage or aspiration of a clinically suspected abscess, in order to confirm the diagnosis, can be difficult, painful to the patient, and potentially risky due to the proximity of the internal carotid artery in many patients. Moreover, attempted needle aspiration or incision and drainage may lead to a false-negative diagnosis of peritonsillar abscess, with potential for inadequate treatment, in 12% to 20% of cases due to sampling error.

Diagnostic imaging can be used to differentiate between peritonsillar cellulitis and peritonsillar abscess, thereby sparing unnecessary attempts at drainage. Both computed tomography (CT) and intraoral ultrasound (US) can be used to differentiate peritonsillar abscess from uncomplicated cellulitis, although there are few data in the literature regarding their accuracy for detecting peritonsillar abscess. In one study, the sensitivity and specificity of CT for abscess are 100% and 75%, respectively, and the respective values for US are 89% and 100%, respectively.

Notes

CASE 55

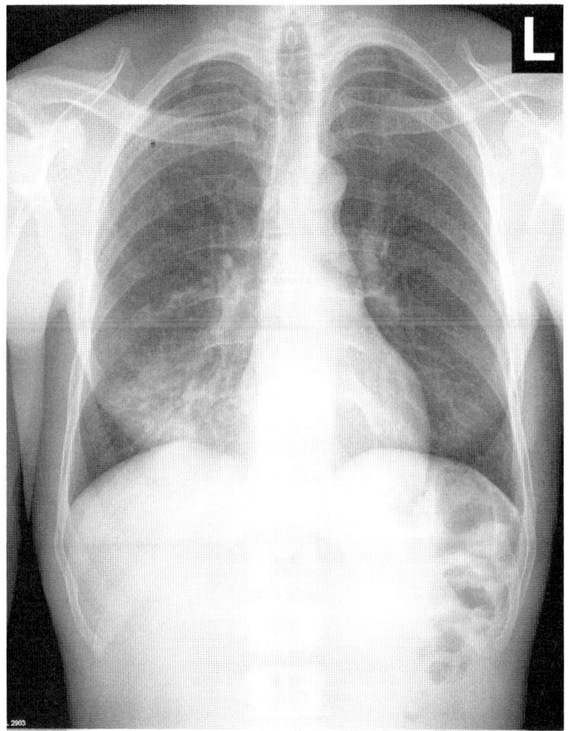

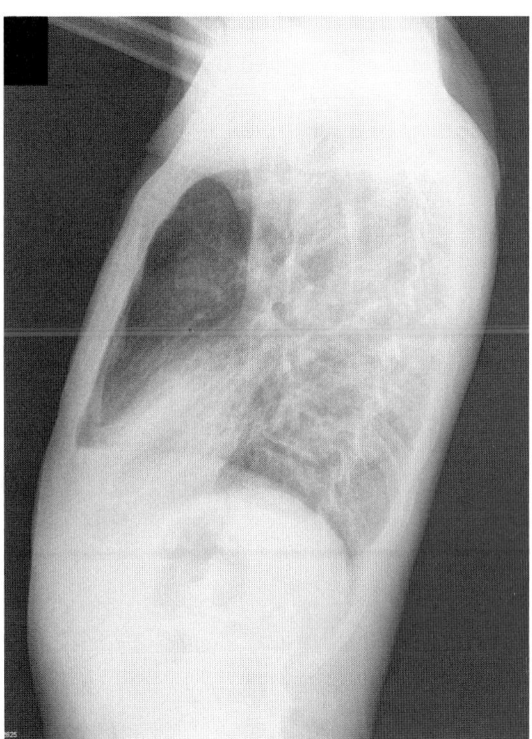

1. What is the most likely infectious etiology for this diagnosis?
2. In what patient population can community-acquired pneumonia present with confusion rather than fever and cough?
3. What radiographic features of pneumonia suggest a bacterial etiology?
4. What is the most common type of pneumonia in HIV-infected patients?

CASE 55

Community-acquired Lobar Pneumonia

1. *Streptococcus pneumoniae,* although the pathologic organism often is not isolated.
2. The elderly.
3. Lobar consolidation, air bronchograms, and parapneumonic pleural effusions.
4. Community-acquired.

References

Tarver RD, Teague SD, Heitkamp DE, et al: Radiology of community-acquired pneumonia, *Radiol Clin North Am* 43:497–512, 2005.

Waite S, Jeudy J, White CS: Acute lung infections in normal and immunocompromised hosts, *Radiol Clin North Am* 44:295–315, 2006.

Cross-Reference

Emergency Radiology: THE REQUISITES, pp 235–236.

Comment

Up to 5 million cases of community-acquired pneumonia (CAP) are diagnosed in the United States annually, and it was the eighth leading cause of death as recently as 2004. In the 80% of patients treated as outpatients, mortality is low at 1%. However, in the 20% treated as inpatients, the mortality is 12%. Outcome is negatively influenced by predisposing co-morbidities that include advanced age, diabetes mellitus, chronic obstructive pulmonary disease, immunocompromise, congestive heart failure, and renal failure.

While those infected with human immunodeficiency virus (HIV) are susceptible to atypical infections, CAP occurs frequently over the course of HIV disease. Bacterial pneumonia is more prevalent than in the general population, and it occurs with greater frequency at lower CD4 counts. Similar to immunocompetent patients, bacterial pneumonia is still typically community acquired with *S. pneumoniae* the most common infectious agent.

Typical clinical manifestations of CAP in both immunocompetent and immunocompromised patients include cough, fever, chills, and malaise, although the clinical course is more fulminant with immunocompromise. The elderly may present with confusion or decreased physical ability to function rather than the usual clinical findings.

The responsible organism remains unidentified in up to 50% of patients with CAP. In those cases in which an organism is isolated, *S. pneumoniae* is the causative agent in 40%. Other common causes of CAP include *Mycoplasma pneumoniae,* viruses, most typically influenza, and *Chlamydia pneumoniae.* Less frequent, yet important, causes of CAP include *Staphylococcus aureus, Klebsiella pneumoniae,* and *Legionella pneumophila.* Although the responsible organism can be difficult to suggest radiographically due to overlapping radiographic manifestations, lobar consolidation implies a bacterial source. In the case of *S. pneumoniae,* lobar consolidation is typical with multifocal disease encountered in 33%. Pleural effusions are not uncommon in bacterial pneumonia.

Notes

CASE 56

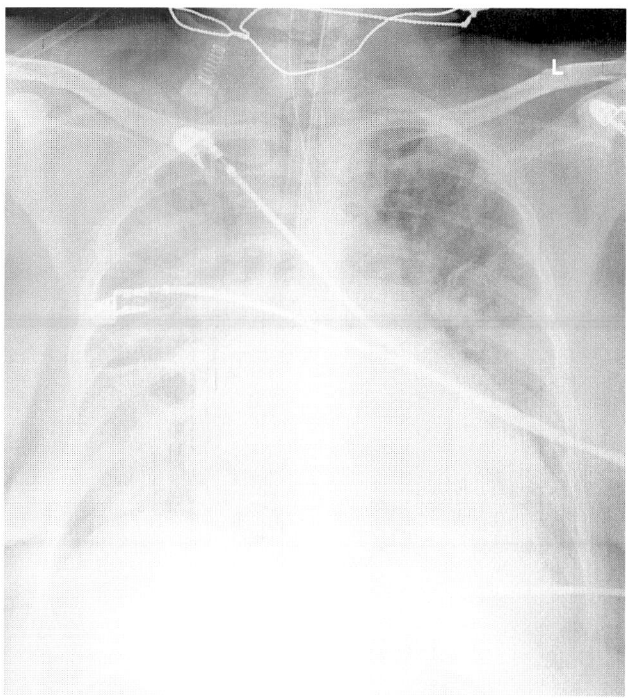

This is an anteroposterior chest radiograph of a 65-year-old woman with a history of chronic renal failure.

1. What is the diagnosis?
2. What are the two most common etiologies of this process?
3. What clinical symptom and sign are most frequently encountered in patients who are diagnosed with this process?
4. What are the three stages of this process? In which stage is this patient?

CASE 56

Alveolar Pulmonary Edema

1. Pulmonary edema.
2. Left heart failure and fluid overload.
3. Dyspnea and tachypnea.
4. Pulmonary venous hypertension, pulmonary interstitial edema, and alveolar edema. This patient has alveolar edema.

References

Gluecker T, Capasso P, Schnyder P, et al: Clinical and radiologic features of pulmonary edema, *Radiographics* 19:1507–1531, 1999.

Hansell DM, Armstrong P, Lynch DA, McAdams HP: Pulmonary vascular diseases and pulmonary edema. In *Imaging of Diseases of the Chest*, 4th ed, Philadelphia, Elsevier Mosby, 2000, pp 401–406.

Cross-Reference

Emergency Radiology: THE REQUISITES, p 236.

Comment

Pulmonary edema occurs when fluid accumulates in the extravascular spaces of the lung. Generally, it is the result of elevated pulmonary venous pressure (i.e., hydrostatic edema) or increased alveolar-capillary permeability, although the two mechanisms frequently work together. Hydrostatic edema is most commonly the result of cardiac disease with left heart failure or fluid overload from renal failure.

Clinical manifestations invariably include dyspnea and tachypnea which may require the patient to maintain erect positioning. Patients may be hypoxic. Clinical examination may reveal wheezing and diaphoresis. In severe cases, blood-tinged frothy sputum may be produced.

Hydrostatic edema typically evolves through three stages: pulmonary venous hypertension, interstitial pulmonary edema, and alveolar edema. On erect chest radiographs, pulmonary venous hypertension manifests as enlargement of the vessels in the upper lung zones (i.e., cephalization) relative to those in the lower zones. As hydrostatic pressure increases, fluid accumulates in the pulmonary interstitium, with interstitial pulmonary edema manifesting as pulmonary septal lines, bronchial wall thickening, and/or indistinct hilar and central pulmonary vessels. Pleural effusions may also develop. With continued fluid accumulation, lung attenuation generally increases. As the process progresses, fluid spilling into the air spaces causes alveolar edema with radiographs demonstrating areas of nodular or ill-defined density. The air space densities are frequently diffuse and patchy, although they may consolidate. One pattern of alveolar edema, "bat wing" edema, refers predominantly to central perihilar alveolar edema with relative sparing of the lung periphery. Although uncommon, the "bat wing" pattern of edema suggests acute rapid cardiac decompensation, such as that seen with a massive myocardial infarction, or fluid overload secondary to renal failure. When alveolar edema is present, it frequently masks the radiographic signs of pulmonary venous hypertension and interstitial edema.

Notes

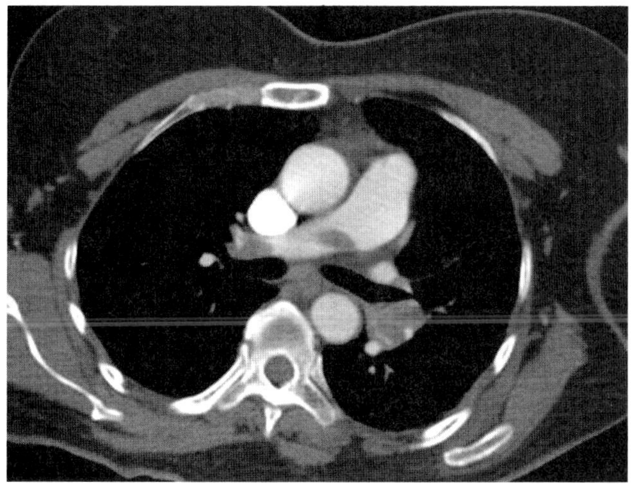

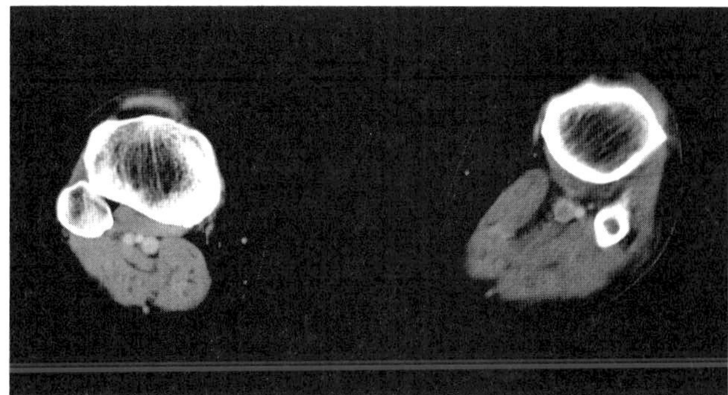

1. What are risk factors for venous thromboembolic disease?
2. Where do most pulmonary emboli lodge?
3. What are the common sites of deep venous thrombosis that lead to pulmonary embolism?
4. What is the negative predictive value of computed tomography for the detection of venous thromboembolic disease?

CASE 57

Pulmonary Embolism and Lower-extremity Deep Venous Thrombosis

1. Hypercoagulability, venous stasis, malignancy, orthopedic surgery, trauma, oral contraceptive pills, and pregnancy, among others.
2. Segmental or subsegmental pulmonary artery branches.
3. The deep veins of the legs.
4. 95% to 99%.

References

Quiroz R, Kucher N, Zou KH, et al: Clinical validity of a negative computed tomography scan in patients with suspected pulmonary embolism: a systematic review, *JAMA* 293:2012–2017, 2005.

Stein PD, Fowler SE, Goodman LR, et al: Multidetector computed tomography for acute pulmonary embolism, *N Engl J Med* 354:2317–2327, 2006.

Cross-Reference

Emergency Radiology: THE REQUISITES, pp 253–260.

Comment

Deep venous thrombosis (DVT) and pulmonary embolism (PE) constitute different manifestations of the same disease: venous thromboembolic disease. The incidence of PE is difficult to accurately determine, but its annual incidence in the United States is estimated to range from 0.65 to 1 per 1000 population. Venous thromboembolic disease is particularly common in hospitalized patients with an estimated 170,000 cases per year. PE may account for 10% to 15% of hospital deaths, and it is associated with an all-cause mortality of up to 17%. However, anticoagulation may reduce the mortality related to pulmonary embolism to approximately 1.0%. Risk factors for venous thromboembolic disease include hypercoagulability, venous stasis, malignancy, orthopedic surgery, trauma, oral contraceptive pills, and pregnancy.

Pulmonary emboli usually lodge in segmental or subsegmental branches, although large emboli may lodge in the central pulmonary arteries. Most emboli originate as thrombi within the deep veins of the legs, although some may originate in the pelvis. Upper-extremity DVT leading to PE is uncommon but may be seen with relatively greater frequency in those with indwelling venous catheters. Since PE and DVT constitute a disease continuum, in instances when evaluation for PE yields negative results, investigation for DVT frequently follows.

Given the positive impact of anticoagulation on patient outcome, coupled with its risks of hemorrhagic complications, accurate diagnosis is vital. With the advent and widespread availability of spiral, and then multidetector-row, computed tomography (CT) scanners, pulmonary artery CT angiography (CTA) has become the initial imaging test of choice in most instances of suspected pulmonary embolism. When CT scanning of the pelvis and legs, CT venography (CTV) is added to the scanning protocol, and the sensitivity for venous thromboembolic disease improves. For example, in the PIOPED II study (Stein et al, 2006), the sensitivity of CTA for thromboembolic disease was 83% while the sensitivity of combined CTA and CTV was 90%. Importantly, CTA has a negative predictive value of 95% to 99% for PE, either with or without CTV. If diagnostic quality of lower-extremity CTV is adequate, the addition of lower ultrasound examination for DVT has little proven value.

Notes

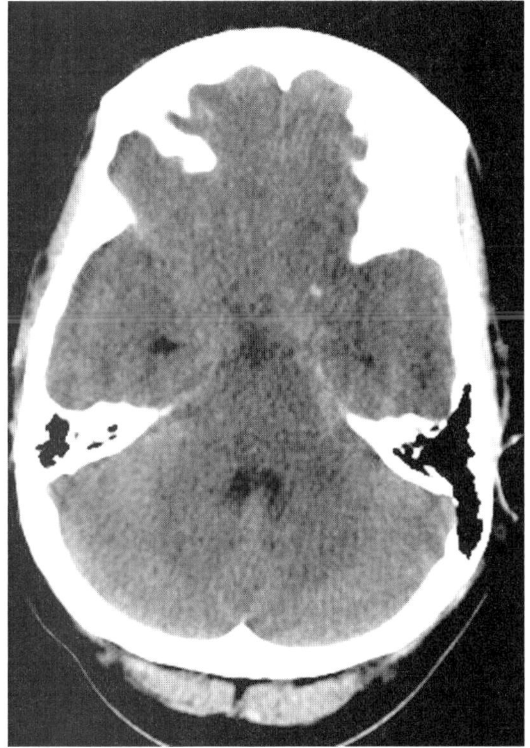

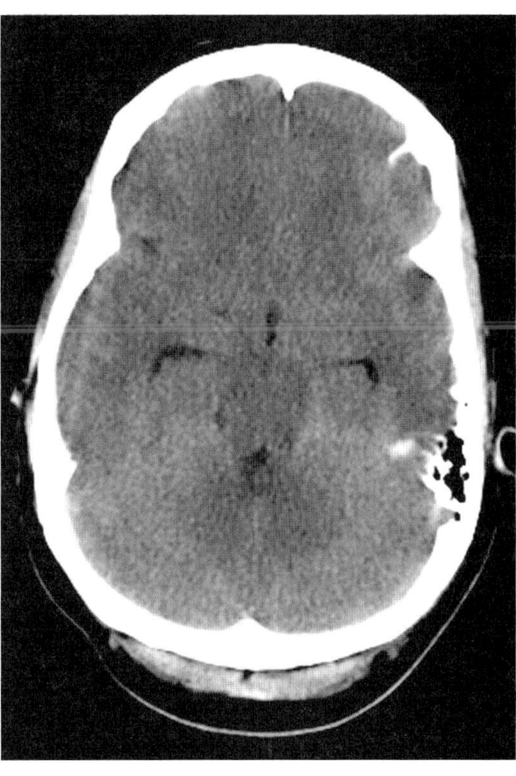

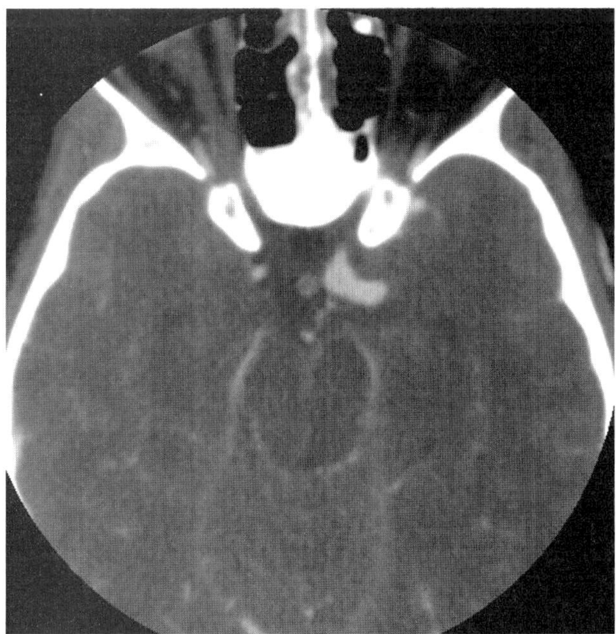

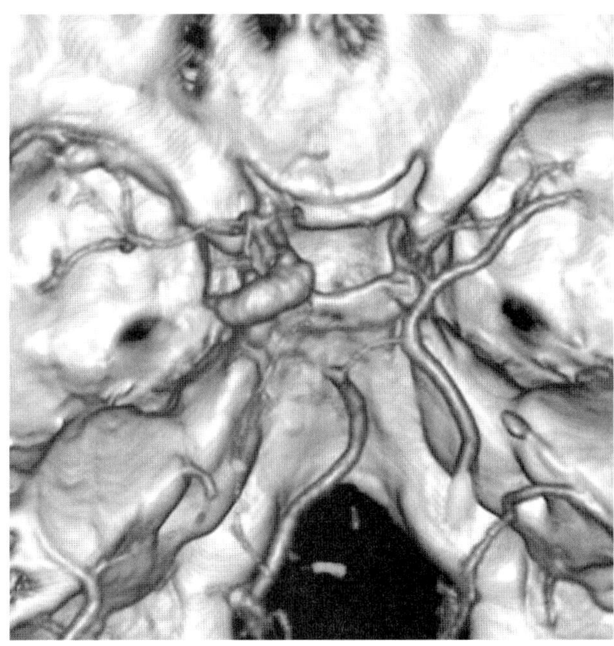

See also Color Plate

1. What is the likely source of subarachnoid hemorrhage (SAH) in this patient?
2. What is the typical clinical presentation of patients with acute nontraumatic SAH?
3. What is the current standard for diagnosing acute nontraumatic SAH in the emergency department?
4. What is the specificity of multidetector-row computed tomographic angiography for detecting cerebral aneurysms?

CASE 58

Ruptured Cerebral Aneurysm

1. Ruptured cerebral aneurysm.
2. "Thunderclap" headache.
3. Unenhanced head computed tomography followed by lumbar puncture if computed tomography does not demonstrate subarachnoid hemorrhage.
4. 93% to 100%.

References

Carstairs SD, Tanen DA, Duncan TD, et al: Computed tomographic angiography for the evaluation of aneurysmal subarachnoid hemorrhage, *Acad Emerg Med* 13:486–492, 2006.

Papke K, Kuhl CK, Fruth M, et al: Intracranial aneurysms: role of multidetector CT angiography in diagnosis and endovascular therapy planning, *Radiology* 244:532–540, 2007.

Cross-Reference

Emergency Radiology: THE REQUISITES, p 20.

Comment

Cerebral aneurysms may have a prevalence of up to 3% to 6% in the general population. Nontraumatic subarachnoid hemorrhage (SAH), which most frequently results from cerebral aneurysm rupture, has an incidence of 11 to 25 per 100,000. Untreated acute nontraumatic SAH is associated with high mortality; up to 25% of patients die in the first 24 hours, while the mortality rate at 3 months is 50%.

Patients with acute SAH usually present with a severe, sudden onset headache (i.e., "thunderclap" headache). The standard for diagnosing acute SAH in the emergency department is unenhanced head computed tomography (CT) followed by lumbar puncture when CT fails to reveal SAH, although the sensitivity of recent-generation multidetector-row CT (MDCT) scanners for detecting acute SAH may be as high as 100%. This approach may demonstrate the SAH, but it will not demonstrate the source of the hemorrhage. The diagnostic standard for diagnosing cerebral aneurysms and other vascular lesions that result in SAH has long been digital subtraction angiography (DSA). However, with the advent of MDCT, MDCT-angiography has taken its place as a powerful diagnostic tool with high sensitivity for cerebral aneurysms. The sensitivity of 4-channel MDCT-angiography for detecting cerebral aneurysms is 81% to 90%, while 16-channel MDCT-angiography has a sensitivity of 98%. Specificities range from 93% to 100%. Not only is MDCT-angiography generally obtainable more rapidly than DSA, but it also allows for reliable treatment planning.

Notes

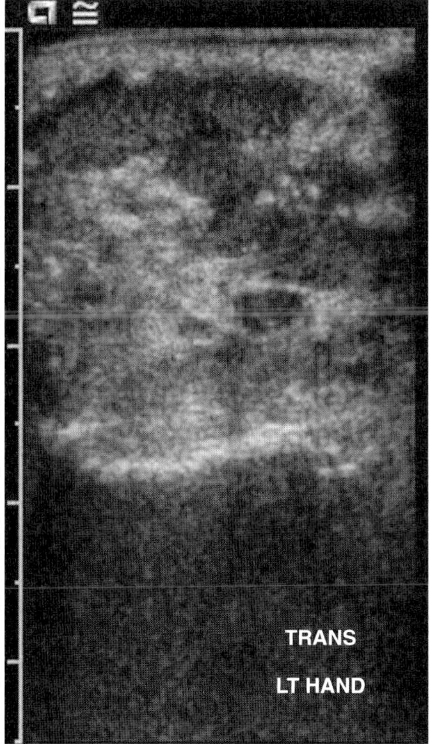

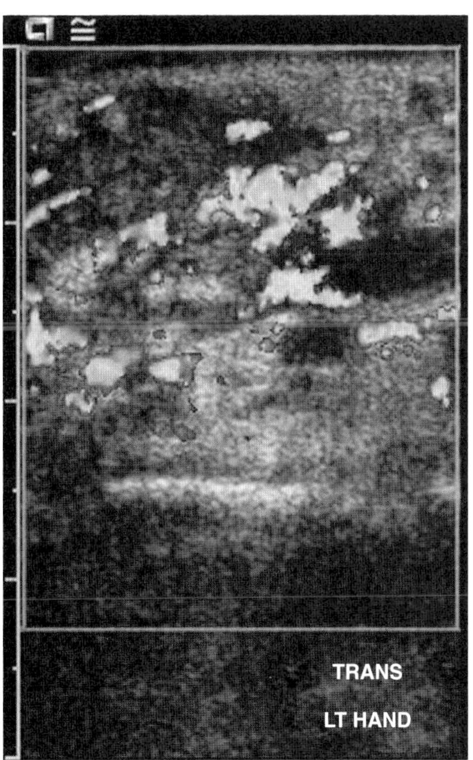

See also Color Plate

1. What ultrasound equipment is required to evaluate a patient with cellulitis for a superficial abscess?
2. What is the impact of ultrasound on the management of patients who present to the emergency department with cellulitis?
3. What is the typical ultrasound appearance of a superficial soft tissue abscess on ultrasound?
4. What can help diagnose a superficial soft tissue abscess with atypical sonographic features?

CASE 59

Superficial Soft Tissue Abscess

1. A linear high resolution transducer.
2. Ultrasound can alter clinical management in nearly half of patients.
3. A hypoechoic mass with posterior acoustic enhancement and internal debris.
4. Color Doppler interrogation may show areas of hypervascularity surrounding avascular regions. Palpation while scanning may show mobile debris within the abscess fluid.

References

Loyer EM, DuBrow RA, David CL, et al: Imaging of superficial soft-tissue infections: sonographic findings in cases of cellulitis and abscess, *AJR Am J Roentgenol* 166:149–152, 1996.

Tayal VS, Hasan N, Norton HJ, et al: The effect of soft-tissue ultrasound on the management of cellulitis in the emergency department, *Acad Emerg Med* 13: 384–388, 2006.

Cross-Reference

Emergency Radiology: THE REQUISITES, p 48.

Comment

Cellulitis is a soft tissue infection of the skin and subcutaneous tissues. Patients frequently present with a swollen, painful, and erythematous extremity and fever. Uncomplicated cellulitis is treated with antibiotics, but abscesses generally require drainage. The presence of focal swelling with fluctuance makes the clinical diagnosis of an abscess straightforward. However, in many cases, clinical diagnosis of an abscess in the setting of cellulitis can be challenging and inaccurate. In many instances, ultrasound (US) can significantly alter management decisions. For example, a recent study conducted by Tayal and colleagues (2006) demonstrated that the use of US can alter management decisions in approximately half of patients who present to the emergency department with cellulitis. In many cases, a clinically unsuspected abscess was identified, while in many others unnecessary attempts at drainage were avoided. If a deep soft tissue infection, such as one occurring in the buttocks, is suspected, either computed tomography or magnetic resonance imaging may be a more appropriate imaging choice than US and/or radiography.

US evaluation of superficial cellulitis and abscesses requires a high-resolution linear transducer. US manifestations of cellulitis include skin thickening, increased echogenicity of the subcutaneous tissues, and anechoic subcutaneous septations that result in a "cobblestone" appearance. An abscess typically appears as an anechoic mass with margins that may be poorly defined. Posterior acoustic enhancement, internal echogenic debris, and septations are also frequent findings. Color Doppler imaging may demonstrate abscess wall hyperemia outlining areas of absent flow within the fluid collection itself. Mobile debris within the collected fluid can be demonstrated by gently probing the area of interest with either the US transducer or a finger. The latter features may help identify atypical abscesses that are either hyperechoic or isoechoic to the subcutaneous tissues. Gas, although infrequently encountered, is virtually diagnostic of abscess if there is no history of open wound or attempted aspiration at the area of interest.

Notes

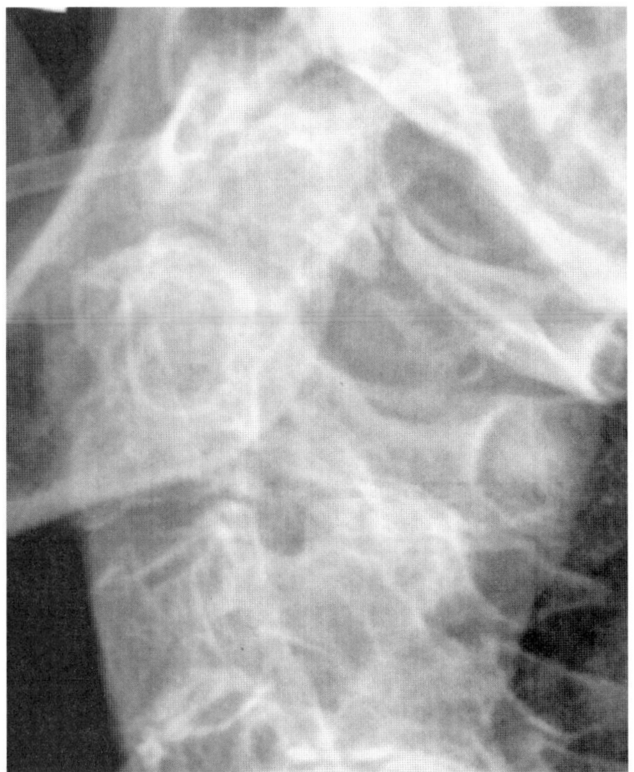

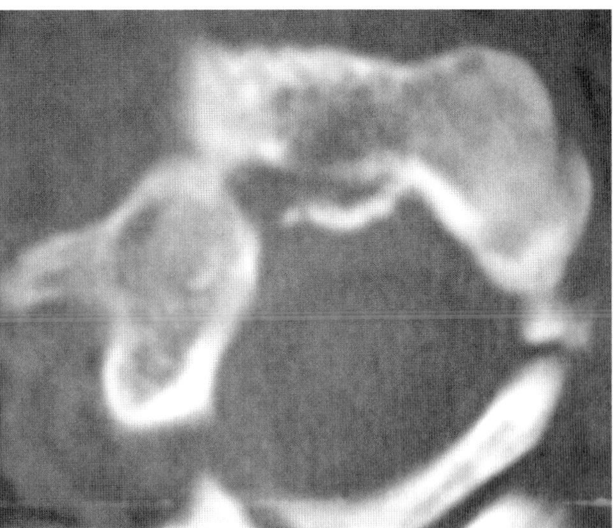

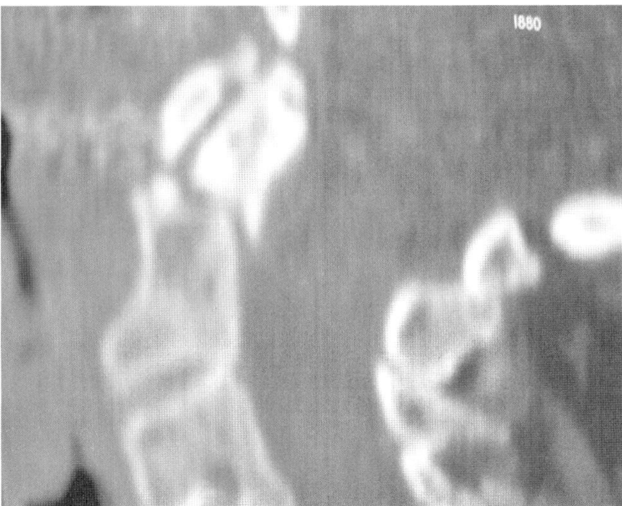

This patient complained of neck pain following a fall from the standing position.

1. What are the radiographic findings?
2. What is the diagnosis?
3. What classification is this fracture based on?
4. Which type of this fracture is prone to nonunion?

CASE 60

Type II Dens Fracture (Anderson-D'Alonzo Classification)

1. A subtle fracture line is seen at the lower dens. The posterior arch of the C1 vertebral body and the dens are posteriorly displaced. A step-off is seen in the spinolaminar line at the C1-C2 level.
2. Type II dens fracture (Anderson-D'Alonzo classification).
3. The type I, II, and III dens fractures are classified according to the anatomic location of the fracture site.
4. Type II dens fracture.

References

Anderson LD, D'Alonzo RT: Fractures of the odontoid process of the axis, *J Bone Joint Surg Am* 56: 1663–1674, 1974.

Lomoschitz FM, Blackmore CC, Mirza SK, Mann FA: Cervical spine fractures in patients 65 years and older: epidemiologic analysis regarding the effects of age and mechanism of injury on distribution, type, and stability of injury, *AJR Am J Roentgenol* 178: 573–577, 2002.

Cross-Reference

Emergency Radiology: THE REQUISITES, p 219.

Comment

Dens fractures are the most common type of fracture occurring in the body of the axis. This fracture may be caused by hyperflexion, hyperextension, lateral flexion, or a combination of these vector forces. Upper cervical spine (C1-C2) fractures are commonly seen in patients 65 years and older. Up to 40% of these fractures involve the C2 vertebra and 36% of these injuries are type II dens fractures. Low-energy injuries from a fall from the standing position or seated height are a common mechanism in this age group.

Anderson and D'Alonzo classified dens fractures into three types based on the anatomical location of the fracture. Type I fractures, rarely seen in clinical practice, are oblique fractures of the superolateral aspect of the dens. The alar ligament avulses a bone fragment from its site of attachment to the odontoid process. Type II fractures occur at the base of the odontoid process and do not extend into the body of C2. Type III fractures involve the body of the C2 vertebra. Associate fractures of the atlas are seen in 56% of patients with type II dens fractures.

On radiographs type II dens fractures may be extremely subtle to visualize. Mach effect mimicking a type II dens fracture is a well-known pitfall on the open-mouth radiograph. The Mach effect results from the posterior-inferior arch of the C1 vertebra. Demonstrating this line extending beyond the dens or repeating the radiograph in a slightly different position helps to exclude a dens fracture. The transverse or oblique orientation of the fracture line makes it difficult to visualize these injuries even on high-resolution axial computed tomography (CT). Isotropic high-resolution sagittal and coronal reformatted multi-detector CT images should be performed routinely to demonstrate dens fractures.

Nonunion is commonly seen following type II dens fractures if optimal alignment (displacement > 2 mm) is not maintained between the odontoid process and body of the C2 vertebra. Nonunion results in instability at the atlantoaxial joint.

Notes

CASE 61

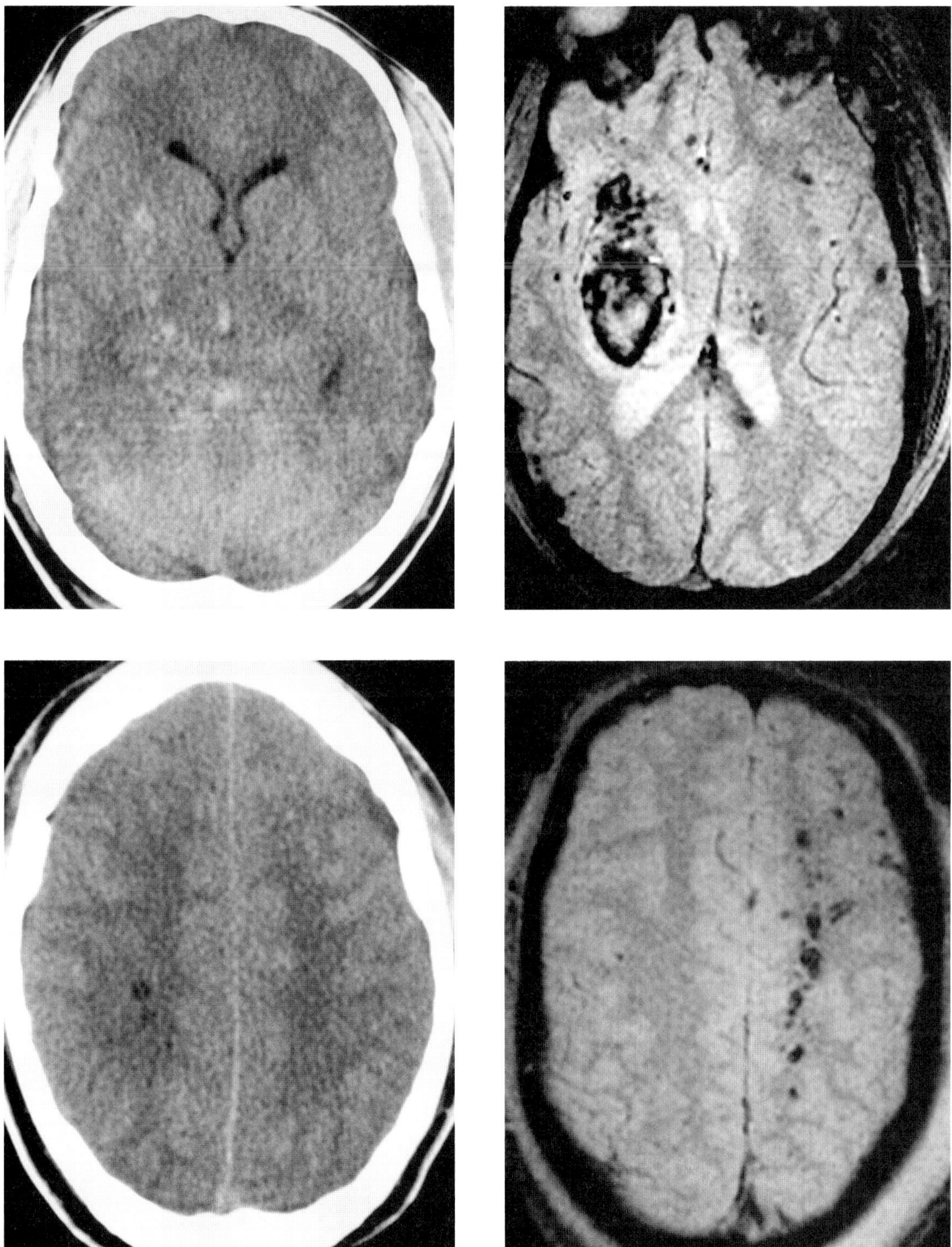

You are shown images of a patient with blunt trauma to the head and altered level of consciousness.

1. What are the computed tomographic and magnetic resonance imaging findings?
2. What is the diagnosis?
3. Name other anatomical sites that are involved in this injury?
4. What is the most sensitive magnetic resonance sequence to demonstrate this injury?

CASE 61

Diffuse Axonal Shear Injury

1. Hemorrhagic lesions are seen in the gray–white junction in both hemispheres, posterior left corpus callosum, right deep nucleus, and external capsule. Magnetic resonance imaging shows more lesions than noted on computed tomography.
2. Diffuse axonal shear injury.
3. Body and genu of corpus callosum, brain stem, cerebellum.
4. Gradient-echo sequence.

References

Hammoud DA, Wasserman BA: Diffuse axonal injuries: pathophysiology and imaging, *Neuroimaging Clin North Am* 12:205–216, 2002.

Kinoshita T, Moritani T, Hiwatashi A, et al: Conspicuity of diffuse axonal injury lesions on diffusion-weighted MR imaging, *Eur J Radiol* 56:5–11, 2005.

Cross-Reference

Emergency Radiology: THE REQUISITES, pp 8, 9.

Comment

Diffuse axonal shear injury (DAI) is seen most commonly following motor vehicle collisions. The rotational acceleration force typically produces injuries at the interfaces between two adjacent tissues and is unrelated to the site of impact. The extent and distribution of injury is clearly related to the magnitude of the rotational acceleration. The axonal damage seen on microscopy is usually underestimated on macroscopic inspection of the brain.

The lesions are small and often not well demonstrated by computed tomography (CT). The CT may be unremarkable if the injuries occur without hemorrhage. Multiple small punctate hemorrhagic lesions are seen at the gray–white junction of both hemispheres in patients with lobar white matter shearing injury. This is the most common location to see DAI. The splenium is the second most common location to be involved by DAI. Shearing occurs at the posterior white matter tracts connecting the two relatively more mobile cerebral hemispheres and the less mobile corpus callosum. Lesion may also be seen within the body and genu of the corpus callosum. These lesions are usually seen in conjunction with lesions in the splenium. Brain stem lesions are usually seen in patients with severe brain injury. The shearing lesions are characteristically seen in the dorsolateral aspect of the brain stem with sparing of a small rim of brain parenchyma peripheral to the lesion. Associated shearing injury will be seen in more peripheral areas including the hemispheres and corpus callosum. A small amount of intraventricular hemorrhage or a small subdural hematoma may also be seen in patients with DAI. Uncommon locations for shearing injury include the pituitary stalk, optic chiasm, and hippocampus.

Magnetic resonance imaging (MRI) is the imaging modality of choice to diagnose and demonstrate the extent of lesions seen in patients with DAI. Hemorrhagic and nonhemorrhagic shearing lesions are optimally demonstrated on gradient echo sequences. Magnetic field inhomogeneities caused by the paramagnetic blood breakdown products help to visualize the lesions on gradient echo sequences. Other MR sequences that are sensitive in demonstrating shear injury include fluid attenuated inversion recovery and diffusion or T2-weighted sequences. Preliminary studies suggest more advanced techniques like susceptibility weighted images and peak apparent diffusion coefficient values are more sensitive in diagnosing parenchymal hemorrhage and predicting outcome in DAI compared with conventional MRI.

Notes

CASE 62

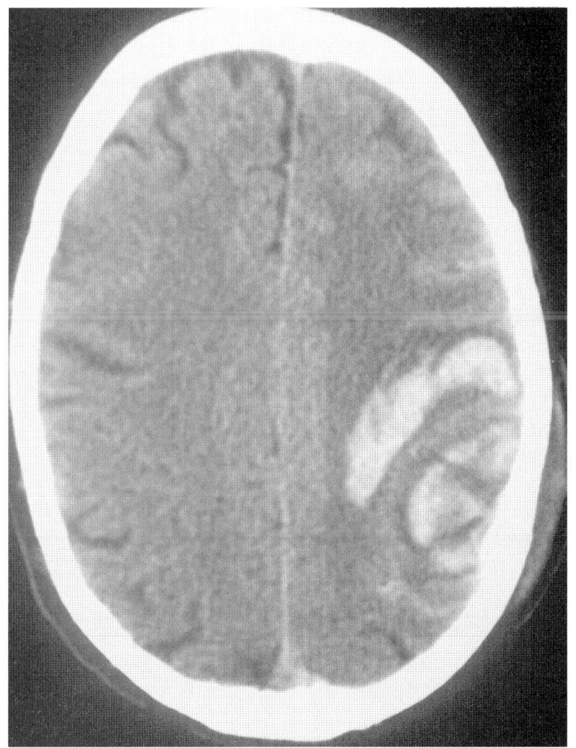

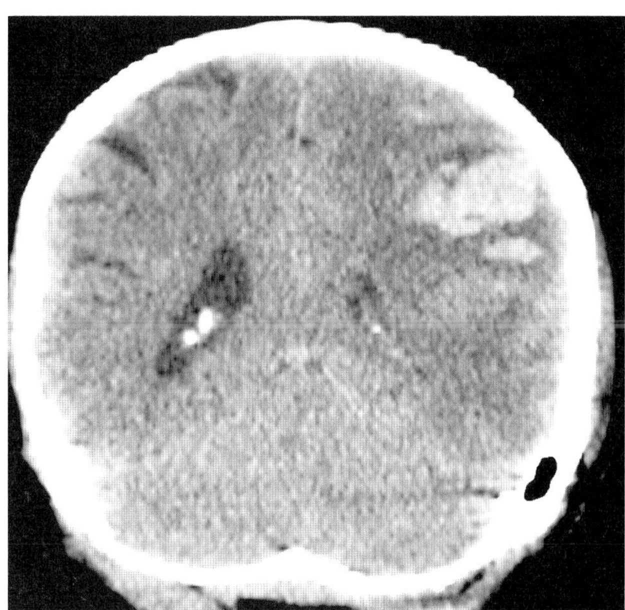

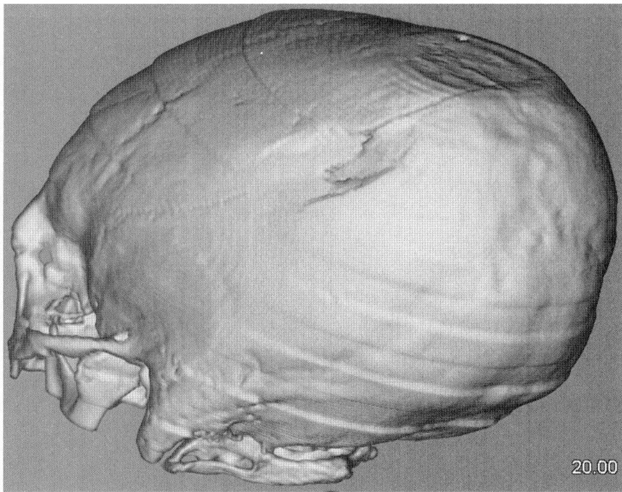

See also Color Plate

You are shown images of a patient assaulted with a lead pipe.

1. What are the computed tomography findings?
2. What is the diagnosis?
3. What are the common sites of injury to the brain following a fall with an impact site at the occiput?
4. What are the indications for treatment of depressed skull fracture?

CASE 62

Depressed Comminuted Skull Fracture with Underlying Parenchymal Contusion

1. There is a depressed comminuted fracture of the left temporoparietal bone with a large temporoparietal contusion and subarachnoid blood. Left-sided cerebral edema with local mass effect on the left lateral ventricle is seen.
2. Depressed comminuted skull fracture with underlying parenchymal contusion.
3. Contrecoup contusions are typically seen at the anterior–inferior frontal lobes (over the floor of the anterior cranial fossa) and bilateral anterior temporal lobes.
4. To improve neurological deficits, correct cosmetic deformities, and prevent infections.

References

Gentry LR, Godersky JC, Thompson B: MR imaging of head trauma: review of the distribution and radiopathologic features of traumatic lesions, *AJR Am J Roentgenol* 150:663–672, 1988.

Klufas RA, Hsu L, Patel MR, et al: Unusual manifestations of head trauma, *AJR Am J Roentgenol* 166: 675–681, 1996.

Cross-Reference

Emergency Radiology: THE REQUISITES, pp 6, 7.

Comment

Cerebral contusions are surface lesions often confined to the gray matter with sparing of the white matter. A contusion consists of a focal area of edema and hemorrhage. Severe contusions may extend and involve the underlying white matter. Contusion may be seen as a coup or contrecoup injury. Coup injuries occur when a force is directly transmitted through the skull to the underlying brain parenchyma by a direct blow to the calvarium, penetrating foreign body, or depressed bone fragment. Contrecoup injuries are characteristically seen contralateral to the impact site, for example, a backward fall on the occiput. This results in an area of contusions in the anterior and inferior aspects of the frontal lobes over the orbital roofs bilaterally. These patients may also have contusions over the anterior temporal lobes. These contusions result from the rubbing of the cortex over the irregular surface of the floor of the anterior cranial fossa and from direct impact on the anterior middle cranial fossa. An occipital fracture is not an uncommon finding in these patients.

Cerebral contusions are demonstrated on computed tomography (CT) as an ill-defined high-attenuation area seen superficially within the brain parenchyma. Areas of low attenuation may be seen within and surrounding the lesion, representing edema and tissue necrosis. Depending on the size of the lesion and edema, mass effect may be seen on the adjacent parenchyma and ventricles. The amount of edema may increase up to 3 to 5 days following injury. Surgical evacuation of large hematomas (cerebral bleed > 5 cm diameter) in the temporal lobes or the posterior cranial fossa may be required due to life-threatening herniation, brain stem compression, or obstructive hydrocephalus.

With time uncomplicated cerebral contusions decrease in size and attenuation values. These changes are usually evident in a week. Ring enhancement following administration of intravenous contrast material may be seen in hemorrhagic contusions on follow-up CT and mimic a neoplasm, infection, or infarction.

Magnetic resonance imaging (MRI) is more sensitive than CT in demonstrating cerebral contusions but is not required routinely in the acute trauma setting. MRI should be limited to those patients in whom CT fails to explain the objective neurologic deficits.

Notes

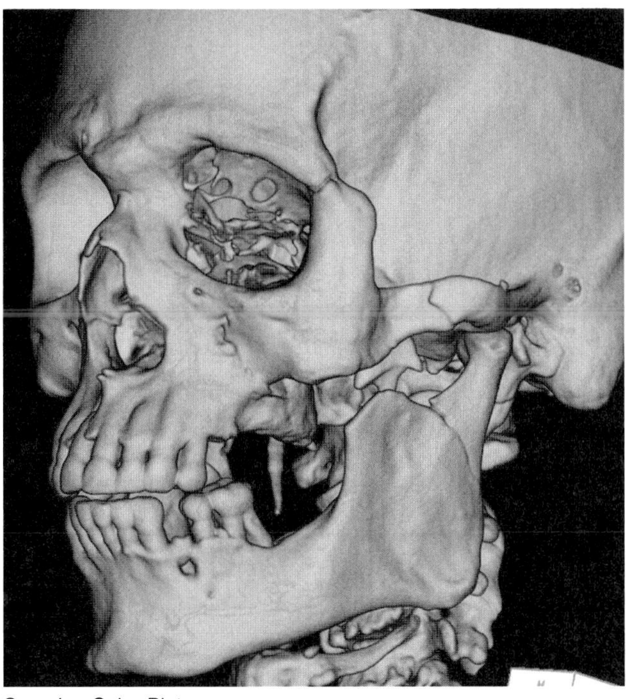

See also Color Plate

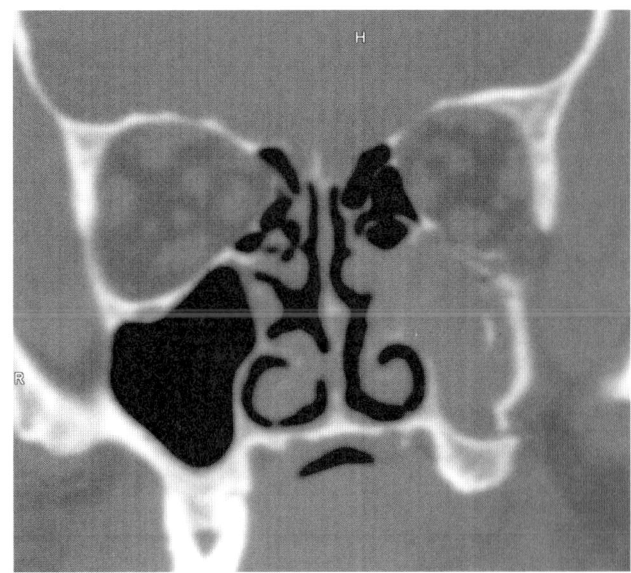

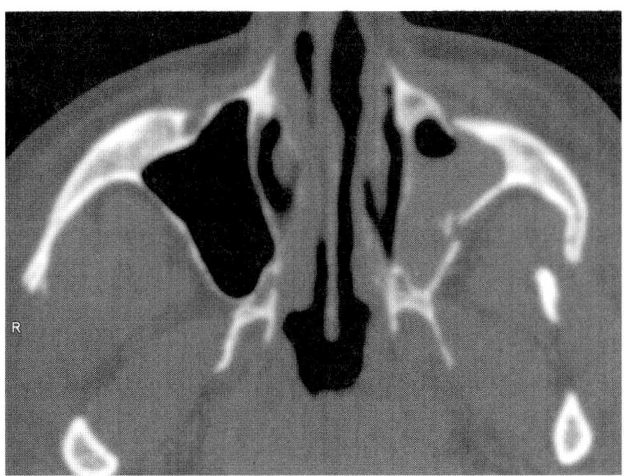

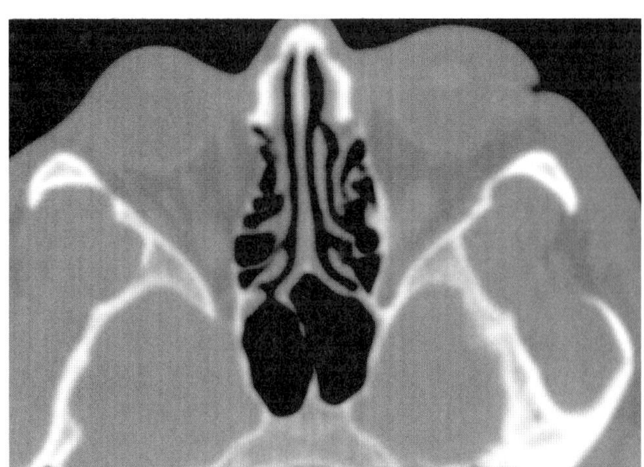

You are shown images of a patient with assault to the left side of face with pain and swelling.

1. What is the diagnosis?
2. What are the five fractures seen in this injury?
3. What are the four articulations of the zygoma to the skull and face?
4. Give four objective clinical findings seen in patients with this injury.

CASE 63

Zygomaticomaxillary Complex Fracture

1. Zygomaticomaxillary complex (ZMC) fracture.
2. Lateral wall of orbit, orbital rim and adjacent floor, zygomatic arch, anterior and lateral walls of the maxillary antrum. (The fracture of the mandibular neck seen on the three-dimensional volume rendered image is not part of the ZMC fracture.)
3. Frontozygomatic suture, zygomatico-maxillary suture, sphenozygomatic suture, and zygomatico-temporal suture.
4. Diplopia on upward gaze, sensory loss over the infraorbital nerve, soft tissue emphysema, and a step off at the inferior orbital rim.

References

Hopper RA, Salemy S, Sze RW: Diagnosis of midface fractures with CT: what the surgeon needs to know, *Radiographics* 26:783–793, 2006.

Strong EB, Sykes JM: Zygoma complex fractures, *Facial Plast Surg* 14:105–115, 1998.

Cross-Reference

Emergency Radiology: THE REQUISITES, p 39.

Comment

The zygoma is the second most commonly fractured facial bone. The prominent convex shape of the malar eminence makes it vulnerable to injury. Assault accounts for the majority of the fractures. About 25% of patients with a ZMC fracture will have other associated facial fractures. Minimally displaced ZMC fractures may result in significant functional and cosmetic deformity. The majority (70% to 90%) of ZMC fractures require surgical fixation.

Clinical findings associated with ZMC fractures include a step off on palpation of the inferior orbital rim or zygoma, soft tissue emphysema from disruption of the anterior wall of the maxillary sinus, and anesthesia over the infraorbital nerve distribution. The nerve is often injured due to the orbital floor fracture. Diplopia, especially on upward gaze, commonly occurs from edema or impingement of the inferior rectus muscle by a bone fragment from the orbital floor fracture. Trismus results from impingement by the zygomatic arch on the coronoid process and temporalis muscle. Other findings include enophthalmus or exophthalmus depending on whether the orbital volume is increased or decreased by the injury.

The body of the zygoma can be considered the central convex prominence with four processes extending to attach with the frontal, temporal, sphenoid, and maxillary bones at the frontozygomatic, zygomatico-temporal, sphenozygomatic, and zygomaticomaxillary sutures, respectively. The weakest bone of the ZMC complex is the orbital floor. The strongest is the frontozygomatic buttress.

A significant direct blow to the malar eminence commonly disrupts all four buttresses mentioned above. Hence this injury is called a tetrapod or quadripod fracture. The term "tripod fracture" is used commonly in the old literature to describe this injury. This term fails to recognize the posterior relationship of the zygoma to the sphenoid bone at the skull base. Maxillofacial surgeons prefer the term ZMC fracture. The following injuries are seen in a classical ZMC fracture: (1) fracture of the zygomatic arch, (2) anterior inferior orbital rim and orbital floor, (3) anterior and lateral wall of the maxillary antrum, and (4) lateral wall of the orbit or diastasis of the zygomaticofrontal suture. A comminuted fracture may often be seen at the zygomaticomaxillary and zygomaticotemporal buttresses. Typically, posterior, inferior, and medial displacement of the zygoma results from the external force and pull of the masseter muscle. Multidetector computed tomography is the imaging modality of choice to diagnose this injury.

Notes

CASE 64

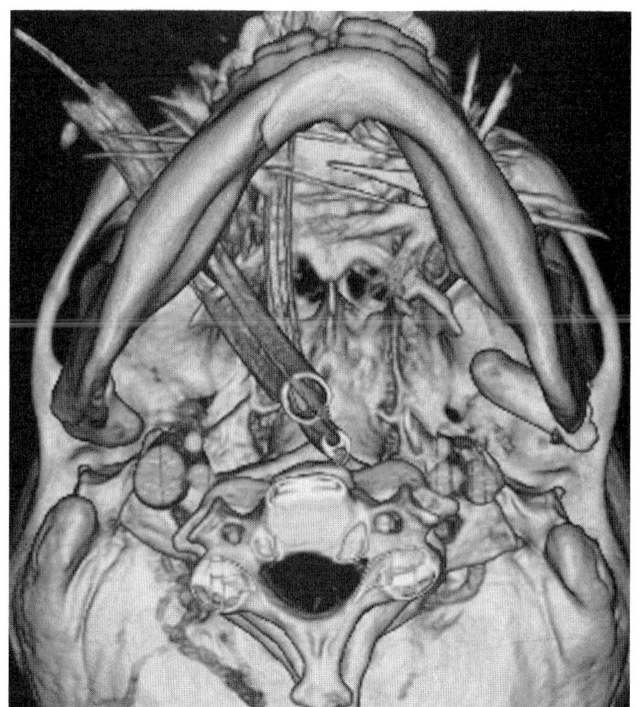

See also Color Plate

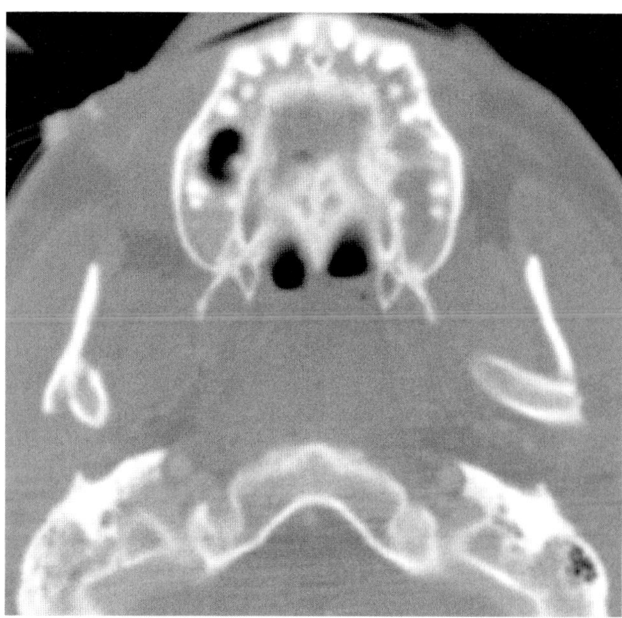

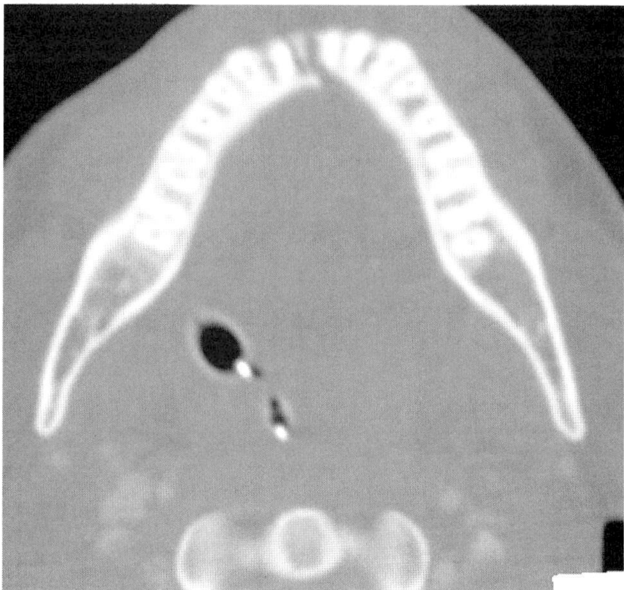

You are shown images of an assaulted patient with bilateral facial pain.

1. What injuries are seen?
2. What is the most common location for mandibular facture?
3. What fractures are better seen on a panorex study when compared with routine radiographs of the mandible?
4. What is the mechanism of this injury?

CASE 64

Flail Mandible

1. Fracture of both mandibular necks and the symphysis mentus. Bilateral dislocations are seen at the temporomandibular joints.
2. The body of the mandible.
3. Fractures occurring in the posterior third of the mandible are better seen on the panorex study compared with radiographs.
4. Direct blow to the chin.

References

Ceallaigh PO, Ekanaykaee K, Beirne CJ, et al: Diagnosis and management of common maxillofacial injuries in the emergency department. Part 2: mandibular fractures, *J Emerg Med* 23:927–928, 2006.

Turner BG, Rhea JT, Thrall JH, et al: Trends in the use of CT and radiography in the evaluation of facial trauma, 1992–2002: implications for current costs, *AJR Am J Roentgenol* 183:751–754, 2004.

Cross-Reference

Emergency Radiology: THE REQUISITES, pp 40, 41.

Comment

Like the nose and zygoma, the mandible is vulnerable to fracture because of its prominent contour. Its U-like shape makes it likely to fracture at two sites, or there may be a second injury involving the temporomandibular joints. The mandible can be divided into six anatomical regions: the symphysis, body, angle, ramus, condyle, and coronoid process. Fractures are classified into six different types based on the anatomical location of the injury. The anatomical location of the fracture and the percentages of the area involved may vary in the literature. The most common location for a fracture is the body (30%), followed by the angle (28%), neck (26%), symphysis (10%), ramus, and coronoid process.

Radiographic series including posterior anterior, bilateral oblique, Towne, and true lateral views will demonstrate most fractures of the mandible. A horizontal panorex study helps in visualization of the entire mandible on a single radiograph, especially so with the posterior third of the mandible. Both these radiographic studies are time intensive (average time 28 minutes; range, 10 to 60 minutes) and require the patient's cooperation to obtain adequate views. Multidetector computed tomography (MDCT) is much faster, accurate, less expensive, and more comfortable for the patient compared with radiographs. Axial, coronal, and curved multiplanar reformatted, and volume-rendered three-dimensional MDCT images are helpful to accurately diagnose all fractures and to plan treatment.

A flail mandibular fracture involves the symphysis mentus with associated bilateral fractures of condyle, ramus, or angle of the mandible. Injuries to the temporomandibular joints are also common. Clinical findings include malocclusion, trismus, limitation of mandibular motion, and intraoral bleeding. The airway may be occluded because of a large bilateral pharyngeal hematoma, or because of an inability to maintain the tongue in an anterior position when the patient is lying in the supine position.

The majority of mandibular fractures are considered compound fractures (all fractures posterior to the second molar tooth). Patients with open mandibular fractures will require antibiotics.

Notes

CASE 65

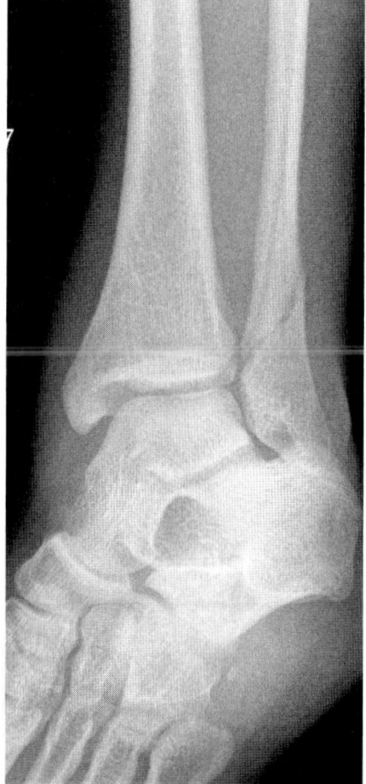

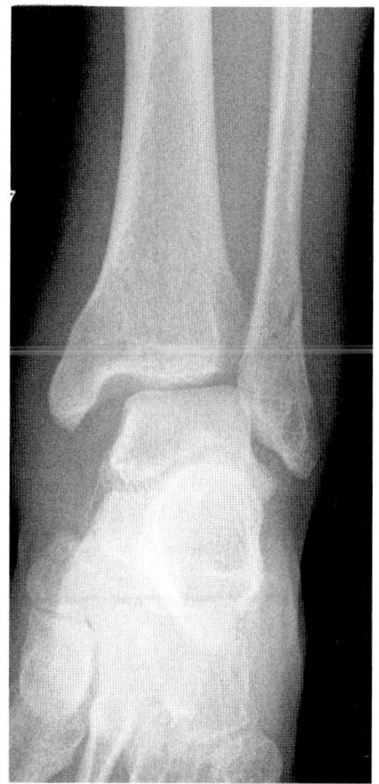

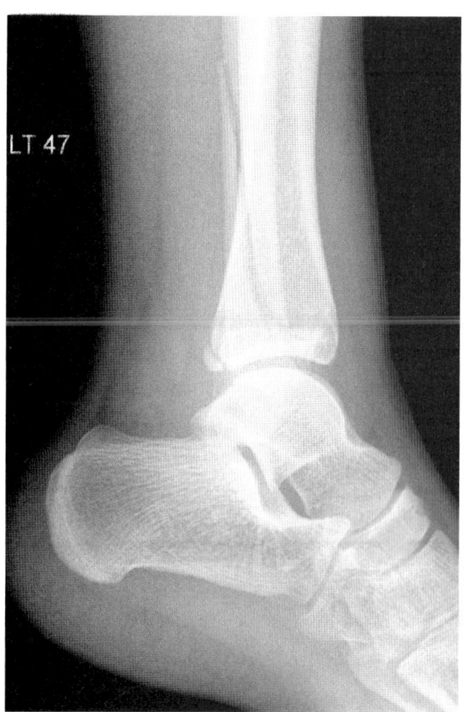

You are shown images of a patient with pain and swelling over the ankle following a fall.

1. What is the mechanism of this injury?
2. Describe the typical radiographic appearance of the fibula fracture seen with this injury.
3. Which ligament fails initially with this mechanism?
4. What are the radiographic features of stages III and IV of this injury?

CASE 65

Supination External Rotation Injury of the Ankle

1. Supination external rotation.
2. The fibula fracture typically begins at the level of the tibial plafond and extends a variable distance proximally.
3. The initial failure occurs at the anterior inferior tibiofibular ligament.
4. A "posterior malleolar" fragment indicates a stage III injury. A medial joint space greater than 4 mm and significant displacement at the fibula fracture indicate a stage IV injury.

Reference

Wilson AJ: The ankle. In Rogers LF, ed: *Radiology of Skeletal Trauma*, New York, Churchill Livingstone, 2002, pp 1222–1318.

Cross-Reference

Emergency Radiology: THE REQUISITES, pp 151–155.

Comment

Supination external rotation is the most common mechanism for malleolar fracture. This fracture pattern is seen in 40% to 70% of patients with ankle injury. Other mechanisms of malleolar fracture include supination adduction, pronation external rotation, and pronation adduction. The anatomical location and the orientation of the fibula fractures vary with the four mechanisms. The typical spiral fibula fracture seen with supination external rotation injuries is usually the most obvious component of the injury. This fracture is best demonstrated on the lateral radiograph of the ankle.

The failure of structures around the ankle occurs in a very characteristic pattern with supination external rotation injuries. The initial structure to fail is the anterior inferior tibiofibular ligament, followed by the fibula. In the third stage the posterior inferior tibiofibular ligament fails. Stage IV injuries involve the medial aspect of the ankle mortis. This results in either a rupture of the deltoid ligament or a transverse fracture of the medial malleolus. Avulsion bone fragments may also be seen arising from either the tibial or fibula attachment with an injury to the anterior inferior tibiofibular ligament.

Stage III involves the posterior inferior tibiofibular ligament. The injury may be a purely soft tissue injury or avulse a bone fragment from its attachment to the posterior lip of the tibia. This fracture may be referred to as Volkmann's fragment or posterior malleolar fracture. Often the fragment is small and extra-articular, but a large fragment may extend intra-articularly into the ankle joint. The bone fragment is usually demonstrated on the lateral radiograph of the ankle.

It is important to try and differentiate a stable stage II injury from a completely unstable stage IV injury, with rupture of the deltoid ligament. Radiographic findings that indicate more than a stage II injury include a lateral talar shift seen as an increase in the medial joint space (> 4 mm), a posterior malleolar fracture, and a significantly displaced fibula fracture. The majority of stage IV injuries demonstrate a transverse fracture of the medial malleolus. Magnetic resonance imaging of the ankle can be used to demonstrate the soft tissue injury in atypical malleolar fractures.

The treatment depends more on the ligament and bony injury than on the actual stage of injury by any classification system. The basis of treatment is to restore normal tibiotalar alignment. Undisplaced malleolar fractures do not require surgical reduction. Reversal of the injuring force is the principle of reduction of ankle fractures.

Notes

CASE 66

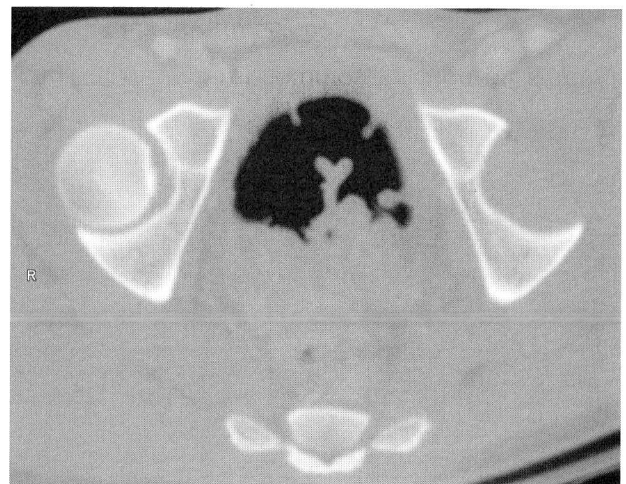

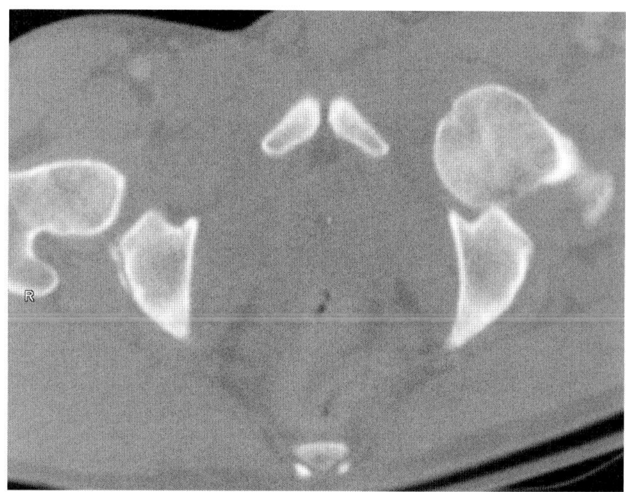

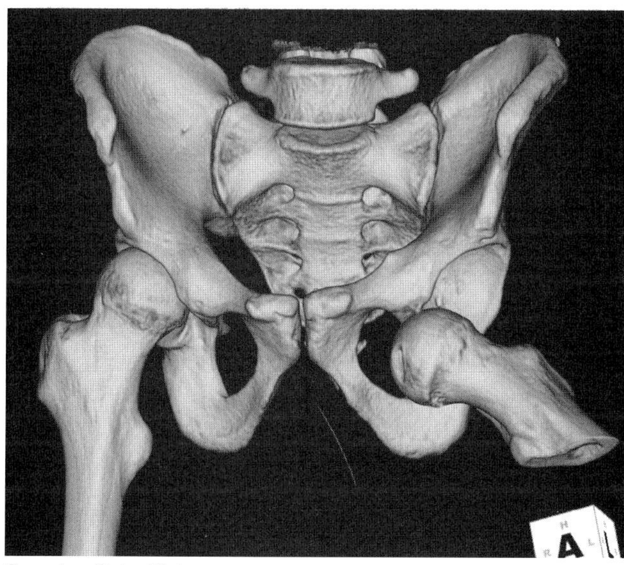

See also Color Plate

You are shown images of a patient with pelvic pain caused by a motor vehicle collision.

1. What is the diagnosis?
2. What position was the femur in at the time of injury?
3. Name three common fractures seen with hip dislocations.
4. Name two complications of hip dislocation.

CASE 66

Anterior Dislocation of the Left Hip

1. Anterior dislocation of the left hip joint with no fractures.
2. An unsuspecting driver with a flexed, externally rotated, and abducted femur at the hip.
3. Acetabular fracture, femoral head, and neck fractures.
4. Post-traumatic arthritis and avascular necrosis of the femoral head.

Reference

Levin P: Hip dislocation. In Browner BD, Jupiter JB, Levine A, Trafton PG, eds: *Skeletal Trauma*, Philadelphia, WB Saunders, 1998, pp 1713–1750.

Cross-Reference

Emergency Radiology: THE REQUISITES, p 142.

Comment

The hip joint is an extraordinarily stable ball and socket joint. The stability results from the bony relationship between the femoral head and the acetabular socket which has been further deepened by the labrum. The tough thick fibrous capsule with its ligamentous condensations and surrounding muscular anatomy also helps to increase the stability of the joint.

Hip dislocations are almost always due to high-energy trauma. The type of hip injury that occurs depends on multiple factors, including the position of the femur at the time of impact, the amount and direction of the predominant force, the amount of anteversion at the acetabulum, and the bony mineralization of both the femur and acetabulum. Posterior dislocation is the most common type of dislocation seen. Anterior dislocations are seen much less frequently compared with posterior dislocations. Anterior inferior dislocations usually occur if the inner aspect of the knee strikes the dashboard with a relaxed hip in a flexed position with abduction and external rotation. Anterior and superior dislocation of the hip occurs when forces act on a hip that is in an extended position. Modern classifications of hip dislocation have abandoned the term "central dislocation" where there is medial displacement of the femoral head associated with a medial wall fracture of the acetabulum.

An anteroposterior radiograph is the commonest imaging modality performed to evaluate hip dislocations. It is important to obtain 450 internal and external oblique views (Judets views) centered on the affected hip. A minor discrepancy in the size of the femoral heads may indicate a hip dislocation. With anterior dislocation the dislocated femoral head appears larger on an anteroposterior radiograph. Shenton's line will be abnormal. The iliac oblique radiograph is useful for evaluating the posterior column and anterior wall of the acetabulum. The obturator oblique radiograph is useful for evaluating the anterior column and posterior wall of the acetabulum. The different profiles of the femoral head should be carefully evaluated on all three radiographs for fractures. Demonstration of intra-articular bone fragments, femoral neck, and acetabular fractures are important to plan reduction and surgical approach.

Multidetector computed tomography (CT) is usually obtained following successful reduction of the dislocated hip. Intra-articular bony fragments, the anatomy, size, and the amount of displacement of acetabular and femoral head fractures are well demonstrated by CT. The amount of soft tissue injury and joint effusions are better demonstrated on CT. Presence of an air bubble within the hip joint on CT may reflect a hip that was forcibly distracted with traumatic hip dislocation.

Recognized complications of hip dislocation include post-traumatic arthritis and avascular necrosis of the femoral head. Loss of articular cartilage and congruence between the femoral head and the articular surface of the acetabulum predisposes to development of early post-traumatic osteoarthritis. A strong correlation has been demonstrated between the development of avascular necrosis and the time the hip remained dislocated.

Notes

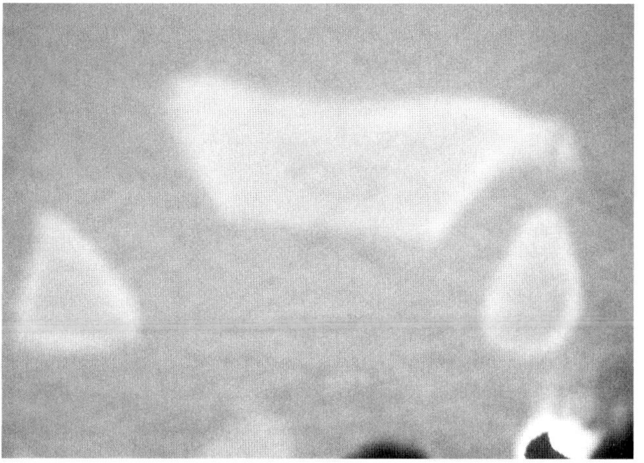

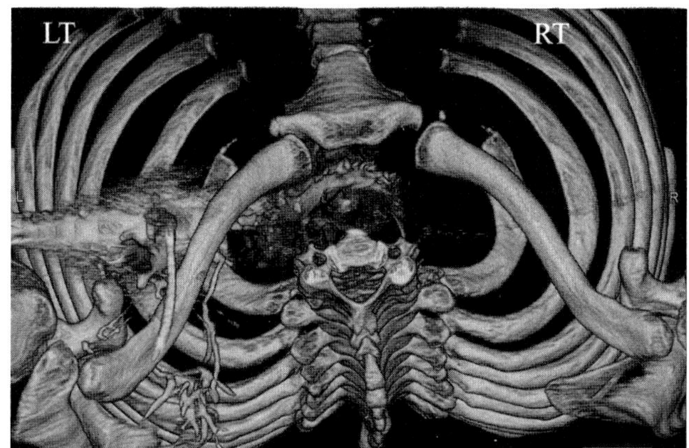

See also Color Plate

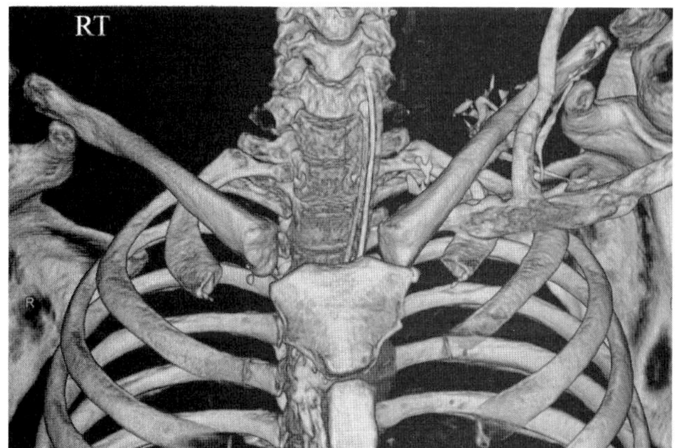

See also Color Plate

You are shown images of a blunt trauma patient with anterior chest pain.

1. What is the diagnosis?
2. What are the different types of this injury?
3. What is the mechanism of this injury?
4. What associated mediastinal injuries might occur with this injury?

CASE 67

Posterior Dislocation of the Right Sternoclavicular Joint

1. Posterosuperior dislocation of the right sternoclavicular joint.
2. Either anterosuperior or posterosuperior dislocation.
3. A blow to the posterior aspect of the shoulder or a direct blow to the anteromedial aspect of the clavicle.
4. Injuries to the common carotid or subclavian arteries, brachiocephalic vein, trachea, esophagus, superior vena cava, and recurrent laryngeal nerve might be seen following a posterior dislocation.

Reference

Wilson AJ: The shoulder and humeral shaft. In Rogers LF, ed: *Radiology of Skeletal Trauma*, New York, Churchill Livingstone, 2002, pp 607–618.

Cross-Reference

Emergency Radiology: THE REQUISITES, p 115.

Comment

Dislocations of the sternoclavicular joint are uncommon and may be classified as anterior or posterior. Usually there is also superior displacement of the medial aspect of the clavicle. The rarity of this injury and the difficulty in optimally visualizing the sternoclavicular joint on radiographs can often lead to missing this condition.

Anterior dislocations are more common compared with posterior dislocations. An indirect blow to the posterior or the anterior aspect of the shoulder could result in an anterior or posterior dislocation, respectively. The clavicle acts as a lever, and the costosternal joint forms the fulcrum. A direct blow to the medial aspect of the clavicle may also result in a posterior dislocation. Rarely, spontaneous sternoclavicular dislocations may occur without a history of trauma due to developmental anomalies or degenerative arthritis of the sternoclavicular joint.

Associated injuries may occur following posterior dislocation because of the close posterior relationship of the great vessels of the mediastinum, trachea, esophagus, recurrent laryngeal nerve, superior vena cava, and brachiocephalic veins to the sternoclavicular joint. Any one or more of these structures could be injured by the posterior displacement of the clavicle or during surgical manipulation of the sternoclavicular joint.

Radiographs, including the anteroposterior, oblique, and special projections, poorly demonstrate the anatomical relationship between the clavicle and manubrium. Overlap of mediastinal structures and the thoracic spine makes interpretation of these radiographs difficult. The medial end of the affected clavicle will be displaced and seen at a different level. It may be impossible to determine if the displacement is anterior or posterior on radiographs.

Multidetector computed tomography (MDCT) is the imaging modality of choice to diagnose sternoclavicular dislocations. CT demonstrates the precise relationship between the medial end of the clavicle and manubrium. Soft tissue injuries that may result from posterior dislocation can also be seen on MDCT. Ability to perform high-resolution reformatted and volume-rendered three-dimensional images helps to accurately determine the amount of displacement and the relationship between the medial clavicle and adjacent vital mediastinal structures.

Closed reduction is usually the treatment of choice unless there is impingement of vital mediastinal structures from posterior displacement of the clavicle, in which case open reduction is advocated.

Notes

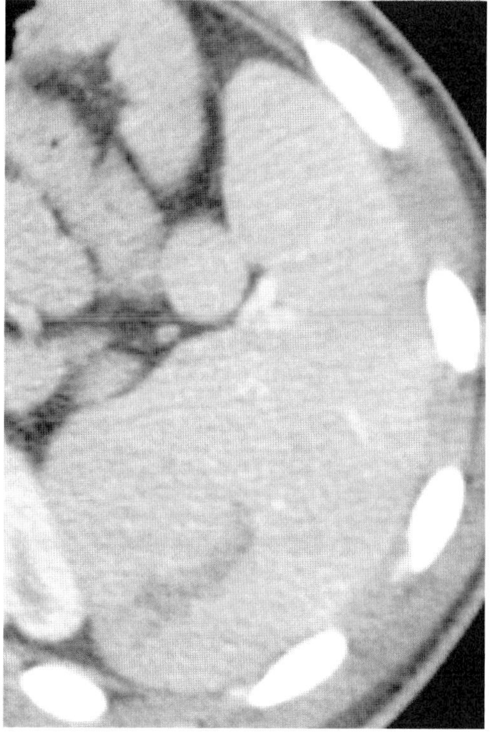

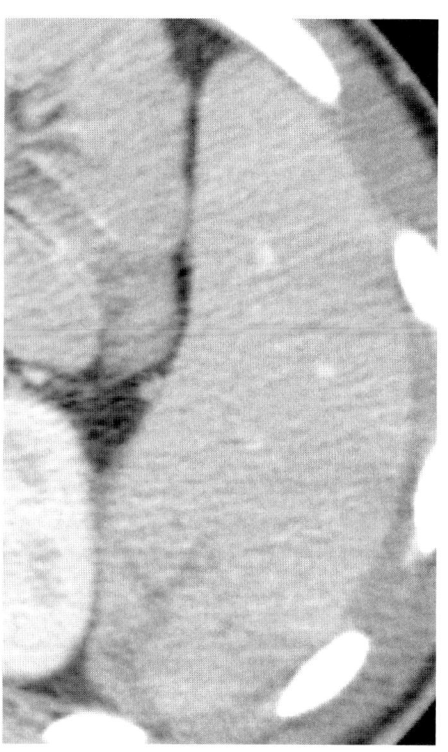

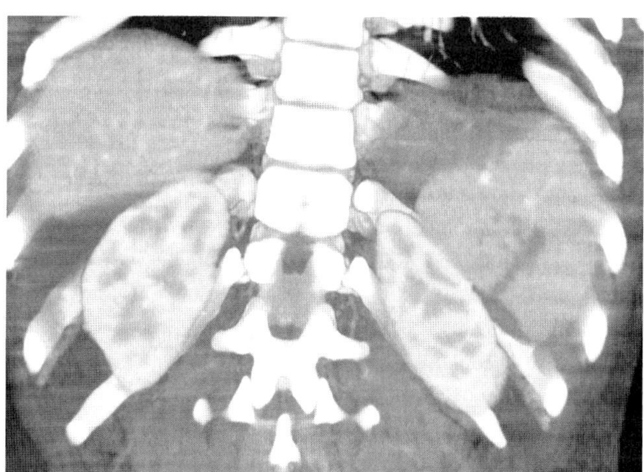

You are shown images of patient with abdominal pain following a motor vehicle collision.

1. What is the best diagnosis?
2. What is the appearance of this injury on excretory phase computed tomography (3 minutes after injection of intravenous contrast material)?
3. What imaging findings are used in grading splenic injury?
4. What splenic injuries require aggressive surgical or transcatheter embolization?

CASE 68

Splenic Laceration

1. Splenic lacerations.
2. Lacerations appear smaller or may become invisible on excretory phase images. This is because lacerations fill in with contrast material and become similar in attenuation to normal splenic parenchyma.
3. The length and number of lacerations, surface area of hematomas, splenic active bleeding, and vascular injury.
4. Splenic active bleeding and vascular injury.

References

Marmery H, Shanmuganathan K: Multidetector-row computed tomography imaging of splenic trauma, *Ultrasound CT MR* 27:404–419, 2006.

Marmery H, Shanmuganathan K, Alexander MT, et al: Optimization of selection for nonoperative management of blunt splenic injury: Comparison of MDCT grading systems, *AJR Am J Roentgenol* 189:1421–1427, 2007.

Cross-Reference

Emergency Radiology: THE REQUISITES, p 88.

Comment

Five principal types of splenic injuries are seen on contrast-enhanced computed tomography (CT) in patients admitted following blunt abdominal trauma. These injuries include hematomas, lacerations, active bleeding, vascular injury, and infarcts. Acute splenic lacerations are seen on contrast-enhanced CT as low-attenuation linear or branching areas with jagged or irregular margins. On excretory phase images obtained at about 3 minutes administration of contrast material, lacerations fill in with contrast material and appear smaller or become similar in attenuation to the adjacent, normal splenic parenchyma. It is important to image the spleen during the portal venous phase following administration of contrast to accurately determine the extent of lacerations.

The American Association for the Surgery of Trauma (AAST) injury scale and multidetector-computed tomography (MDCT)-based grading system use the number and length of lacerations, surface area or thickness of splenic hematomas (subcapsular or intraparenchymal), presence of splenic active bleeding, or vascular injuries to grade splenic injury. With healing, the margins of lacerations become less evident, rounded, and decrease in size until they become similar in attenuation to normal splenic parenchyma. A peripheral scar or a contour abnormality may form in the spleen at the site of injury. Development of a post-traumatic cyst is extremely uncommon in the normal healing process. Uncomplicated lacerations usually heal within 4 to 6 weeks.

Splenic clefts, lobulations, or streak artifact may mimic splenic lacerations. Splenic clefts have a smooth rounded margin and may contain fat or fibrous tissues within them, and on excretory phase images they typically do not become similar in attenuation to normal splenic parenchyma. Careful review of delayed-phase images may help to differentiate a splenic cleft from a laceration.

Notes

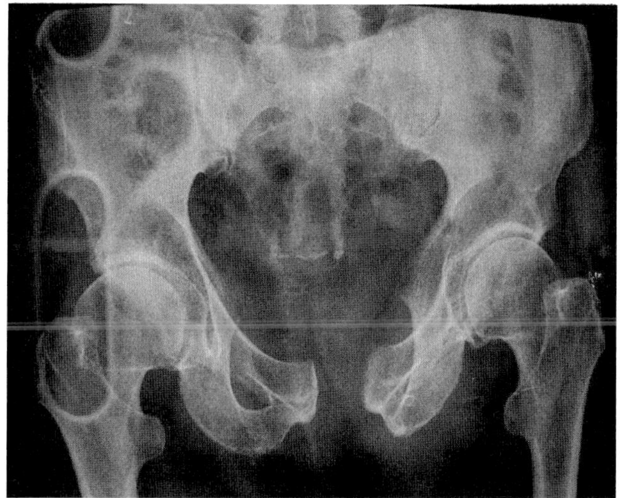

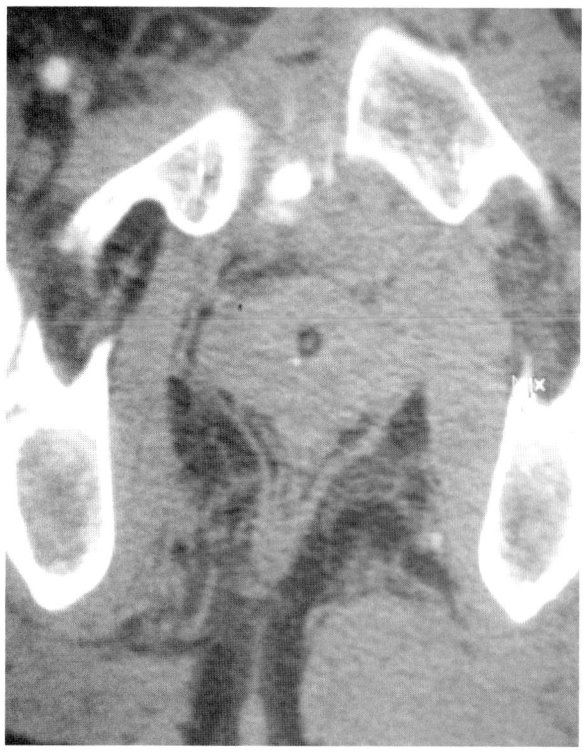

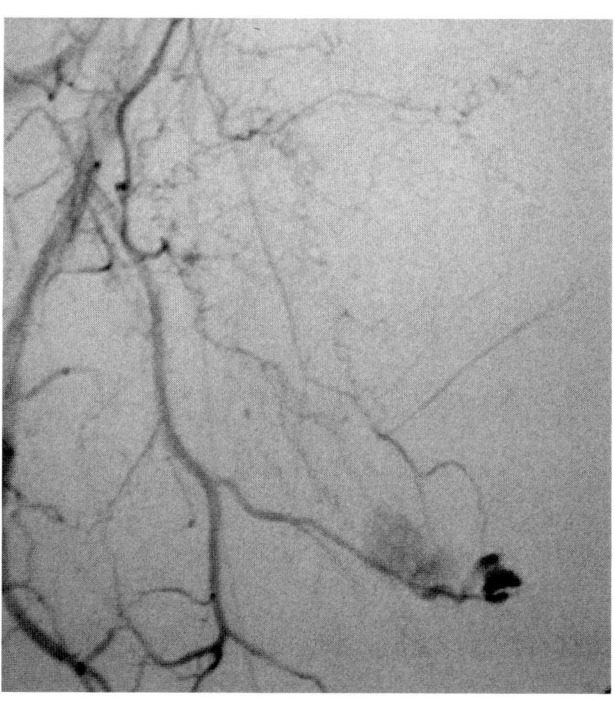

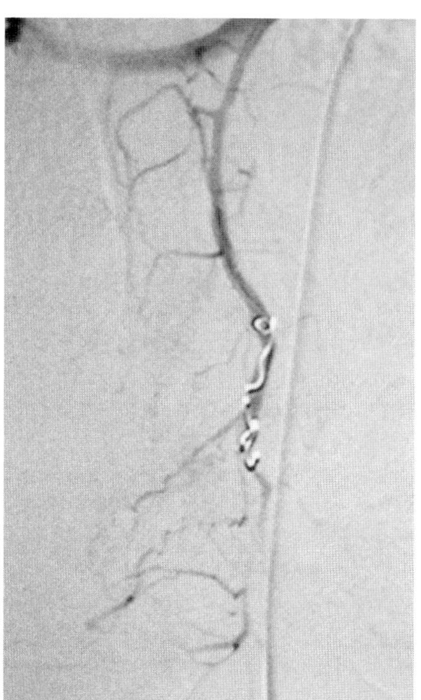

You are shown images of a patient with pelvic pain due to a motor vehicle collision.

1. What are the radiographic findings?
2. What are the computed tomographic findings?
3. What are the arteriographic findings seen in the first image?
4. What types of pelvic fractures are associated with significant pelvic hemorrhage?

CASE 69

Type II Anteroposterior Compression Pelvic Fracture

1. There is diastasis of the symphysis pubis and anterior right sacroiliac joints. This represents a type II anteroposterior compression fracture (Young-Burgess pelvic fracture classification).
2. Diastasis of the symphysis pubis, pelvic floor hematoma, and an irregular area of active bleeding within the hematoma.
3. Selective internal iliac arteriogram shows bleeding from a branch of the internal pudendal artery.
4. Type III lateral compression, vertical shear, combined mechanism, types II and III anteroposterior compression pelvic fractures (Young-Burgess pelvic fracture classification).

References

Ben-Menachem Y, Coldwell DM, Young JWR, et al: Hemorrhage associated with pelvic fractures: causes, diagnosis, and emergent management, *AJR Am J Roentgenol* 57:1005–1014, 1991.

Eastridge BJ, Starr A, Minei JP, et al: The importance of fracture pattern in guiding therapeutic decision-making in patients with hemorrhagic shock and pelvic ring disruptions, *J Trauma* 53:446–450, 2002.

Cross-Reference

Emergency Radiology: THE REQUISITES, p 138.

Comment

Pelvic hemorrhage is a well recognized complication seen in patients with pelvic ring disruption after blunt force trauma. Patients admitted with significant hemorrhage related to pelvic fractures have a greater than 50% mortality rate. The high morbidity and mortality rates associated with pelvic fractures are directly and primarily related to the amount of associated hemorrhage. Patients, especially those with posterior pelvic ring disruption or fractures, are likely to bleed. The hemorrhage may be from injury to the branches of the iliac arteries, the rich pelvic venous plexus, or cancellous bone fragments. Associated injuries, including long bone fractures and intraperitoneal injuries, are seen in up to 55% of patients. These injuries may also produce additional substantial blood loss. A balanced multidisciplinary approach is necessary to prioritize the treatment depending on the source of hemorrhage.

Multiple different classification systems are available to classify pelvic fractures. The Young-Burgess method classifies pelvic fractures according to the major direction of the disrupting force. The forces described include lateral compression (LC), anteroposterior compression (APC), vertical shear, and a complex mechanism. The LC and APC pelvic fractures each have three subgroups. LC fractures are by far the most common type of injury seen. Identifying the orientation of pubic rami fractures and displacement of the major fragments on radiographs or computed tomography are helpful to establish classification. Determining the pelvic fracture pattern may help to identify patients at greater risk of hemorrhage and guide appropriate therapy. For example, the highest prevalence of arterial injuries is seen involving the superior gluteal and internal pudendal arteries in patients with APC II and APC III fractures. The superior gluteal artery is in close proximity to the sacrospinous ligament and pyriformis fascia and the internal pudendal artery to the sacrotuberous ligament. These arteries are usually injured when these ligaments are torn.

Application of a pelvic binder helps to reduce the amount of space in the true pelvis into which hemorrhage could occur. This also stabilizes the bone fragments and the pelvic ring and helps injured vessels to form a stable clot. Pelvic angiography helps to localize the site of arterial hemorrhage and control the bleeding by performing selective distal embolization.

Notes

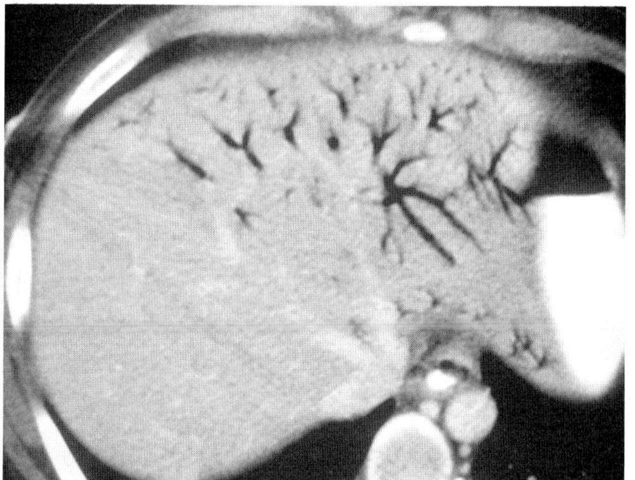

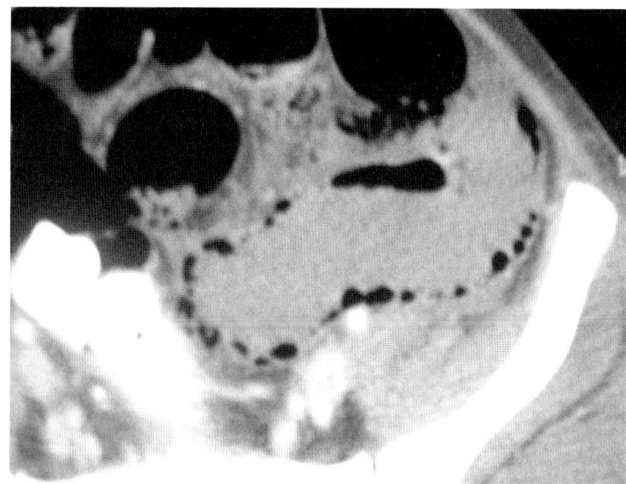

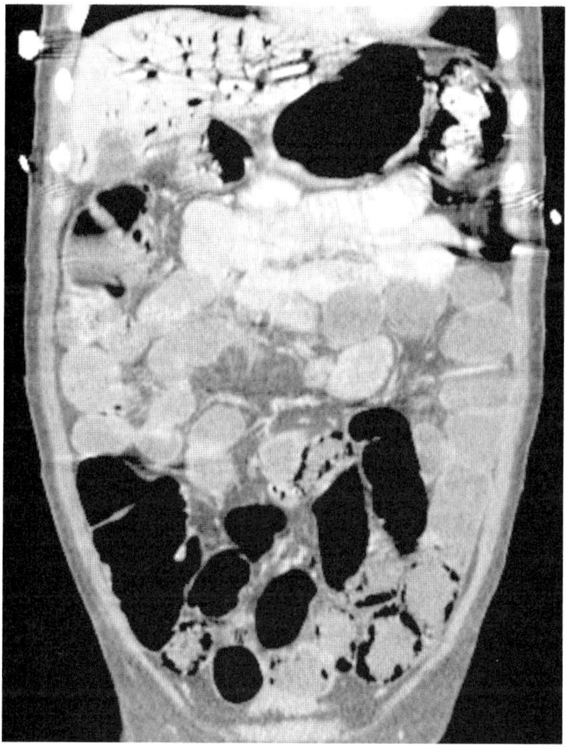

You are shown contrast-enhanced multidetector computed tomographic (MDCT) images in a patient with severe abdominal pain.

1. Describe the abnormal computed tomographic (CT) findings.
2. What is the best diagnosis?
3. Name three common contrast-enhanced CT findings seen in this entity.
4. What is the most specific contrast-enhanced CT finding seen in this entity?

CASE 70

Infarction of Small Bowel

1. Diffuse dilatation of loops of small bowel, pneumatosis intetinalis, portal venous gas, and lack of enhancement of dilated ileal loops (with pneumatosis on multiplanar reconstruction [MPR] image).
2. Transmural infarction of small bowel.
3. Bowel wall thickening, dilatation of bowel loops, and abnormal enhancement of bowel wall.
4. Lack of contrast enhancement of bowel wall is the most specific computed tomographic finding of bowel infarction.

References

Rha SE, Ha HK, Lee SH, et al: CT and MR imaging findings of bowel ischemia from various primary causes, *Radiographics* 20:29–42, 2000.

Wiesner W, Khurana B, Hoon J, et al: CT of acute bowel ischemia, *Radiology* 226:635–650, 2003.

Cross-Reference

Emergency Radiology: THE REQUISITES, pp 290–291.

Comment

Bowel ischemia may involve the small or large bowel, be segmental or diffuse, and involve part or the entire wall of the bowel. Partial ischemic colitis is the commonest type of colitis seen in patients older than 50 years of age. This is usually a self-limiting disease. Transmural bowel infarction is typically associated with a high mortality rate (50% to 90%). Primary causes of insufficient blood flow to the bowel may result from occlusive or nonocclusive causes, including arterial or venous thromboembolism, low flow or vasospasm, intestinal obstruction, neoplasms, vasculitis, radiation, drugs, and trauma. Up to 60% to 70% of all cases of bowel ischemia are due to arterial thrombosis or embolism of the superior mesenteric artery.

Multidetector computed tomography (MDCT) and magnetic resonance imaging currently play an important role in demonstrating the primary cause and bowel wall changes seen with intestinal ischemia. The sensitivity of diagnosing bowel ischemia by computed tomography (CT) is currently as high as 82% and is comparable to angiography. CT evaluation of bowel ischemia requires both oral and rectal administration of contrast material or water. Administration of intravenous contrast material helps to demonstrate thrombi in the mesenteric artery or veins. Unenhanced and enhanced CT images are essential to diagnose bowel wall hemorrhage and differentiate the various patterns of bowel wall enhancement.

The radiological manifestations of bowel ischemia are similar regardless of the primary cause. The most common CT finding seen is focal or diffuse bowel wall thickening (26% to 96%). The amount of thickening does not reflect the severity of ischemia. The normal bowel wall may vary in thickness (3 to 5 mm) depending on the amount of distention. Abnormal attenuation within the thickened bowel wall may be seen due to edema (homogeneous hypoattenuation) or hemorrhage (hyperattenuation areas) on unenhanced CT. The target sign, alternating high and low attenuation associated with bowel wall thickening, may be seen with submucosal edema or hemorrhage on enhanced CT. Lack of enhancement of bowel wall on enhanced CT is the most specific CT finding of bowel ischemia.

Luminal dilatation and air fluid levels are more commonly (56% to 91%) seen following bowel infarction compared with bowel ischemia. This results from interruption of normal intestinal peristalsis by ischemia. Other CT findings suggestive of transmural infarction include destruction of intramural nerves and muscle leading to extreme thinning of the bowel wall (especially the small bowel), pneumatosis, and portal venous gas. Both pneumatosis and portal venous gas are more specific but less frequently (3% to 28%) seen CT findings. Presence of free intraperitoneal air is an ominous CT finding that indicates perforation of infarcted bowel. Mesenteric fat stranding, mesenteric fluid, and ascites are other nonspecific CT findings seen in patients with acute ischemic bowel.

Notes

CASE 71

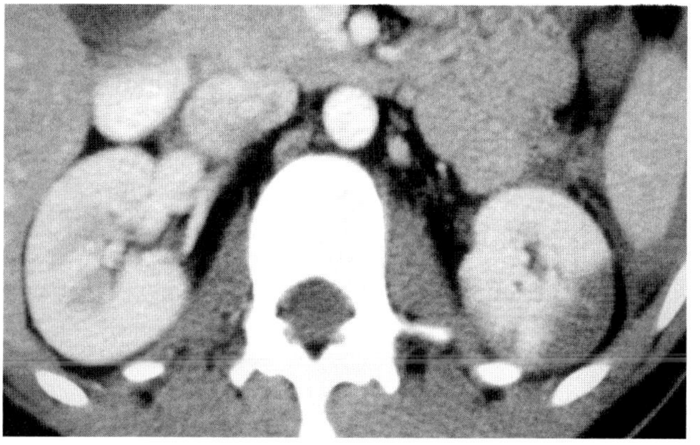

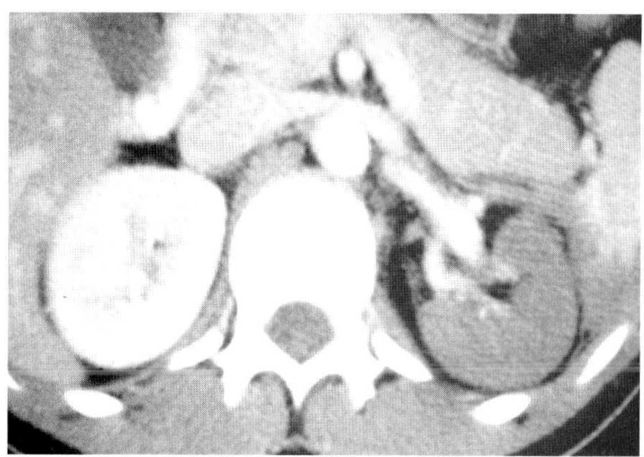

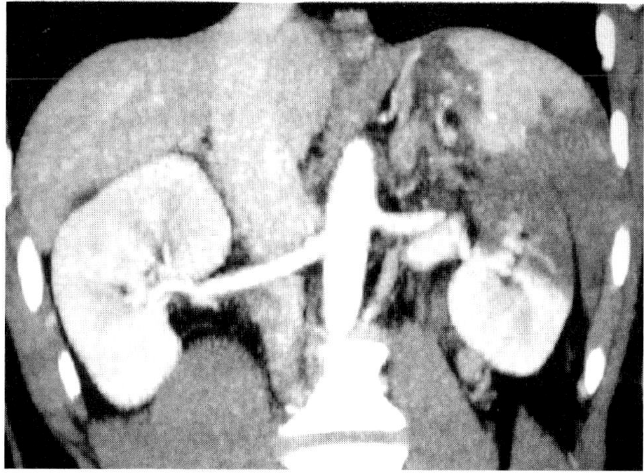

You are shown images of a patient with abdominal pain following blunt trauma.

1. What is the best diagnosis?
2. What is the most common site for this injury?
3. Describe the role of arteriography in the diagnosis and treatment of this injury.
4. What is the mechanism of this injury?

CASE 71

Segmental Renal Infarct

1. Left upper pole renal segmental infarction and perisplenic blood.
2. Upper poles of the kidney.
3. Multidetector computed tomography can accurately diagnose segmental renal infarcts. Renal arteriography is not indicated for diagnosis or treatment.
4. An intimal injury with subsequent thrombosis or avulsion of the capsular, accessory, or intrarenal segmental artery causes parenchymal infarction.

References

Kawashima A, Sandler CM, Corl FM, et al: Imaging of renal trauma: a comprehensive review, *Radiographics* 21:557–574, 2001.

Lewis DR, Mirvis SE, Shanmuganathan K: Segmental renal infarction after blunt abdominal trauma: clinical significance and appropriate management, *Emerg Radiol* 3:236–240, 1996.

Cross-Reference

Emergency Radiology: THE REQUISITES, p 100.

Comment

Blunt trauma is a potential cause of segmental renal infarction. The majority of the cases reported in the literature are due to embolic events from valvular heart disease. Other well-known etiologies includes emboli from sites of atherosclerotic plaques in the abdominal aorta or renal artery, renal artery aneurysms, angiography catheter manipulation, and vasculitis.

Stretching of the accessory renal artery, extra- or intrarenal artery branch, or a capsular artery during blunt impact produces either an intimal injury, with subsequent thrombosis, or an avulsion of the vessel. Prolonged interruption of the arterial flow will ultimately result in an infarct. There are a total of five renal segments each supplied by its own segmental renal artery. Each segmental artery is an end vessel to the parenchymal segment it supplies. The commonest location is the upper pole of the kidney, but other locations include the lower pole and the anterior and posterior interpolar region.

A segmental renal artery infarction is seen on contrast-enhanced multidetector computed tomography (MDCT) as a well-defined, well-demarcated, wedge-shaped non-enhancing region. The base of the infarct is typically seen at the periphery and the apex at the hilum of the kidney. The presence of other associated, minor renal parenchymal injuries or a small perinephric hematoma should not preclude the diagnosis of segmental renal artery infarct by enhanced MDCT.

Up to 71% of renal infarcts are the only form of renal injury seen following blunt trauma. The radiological and urological literature suggests that delayed renal hemorrhage or significant renal function loss does not occur on follow-up and renal infarcts should be managed non-operatively. The MDCT appearance of segmental renal artery infarct is characteristic, and renal arteriography should not be performed unless required for concurrent injuries.

Notes

CASE 72

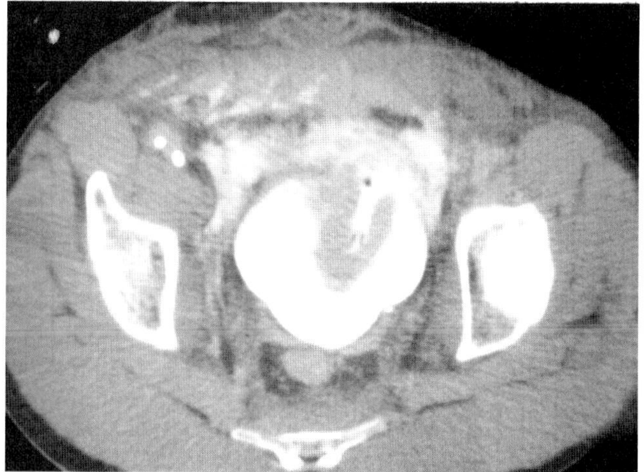

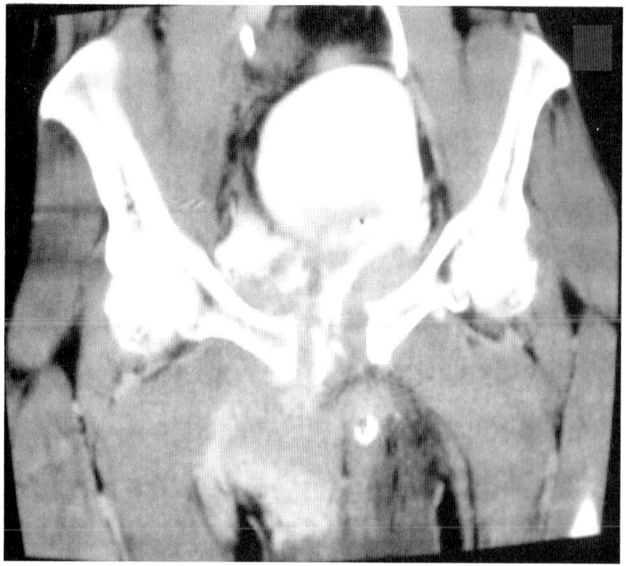

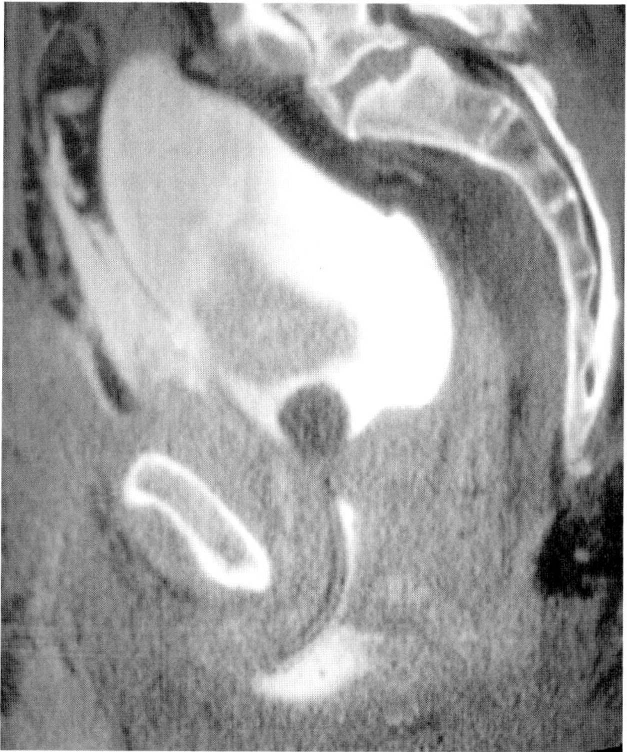

You are shown transverse, coronal, and sagittal multidetector computed tomography images in the region of the pelvis. This patient was admitted after a motor vehicle collision.

1. What is the best diagnosis?
2. What are the different types of this injury?
3. Name the anatomical space where the extravasated urinary contrast material is seen anterior to the bladder on the axial and coronal images.
4. Is the urogenital diaphragm intact in this patient?

CASE 72

Extraperitoneal Bladder Rupture

1. Extraperitoneal bladder rupture.
2. There are five different injury types including bladder wall contusion, interstitial, extraperitoneal, intraperitoneal, and combined intra- and extraperitoneal bladder rupture.
3. Space of Retzius.
4. No. Contrast material is seen in the perineum and right thigh, indicating that the urogenital diaphragm is ruptured.

References

Chan DPN, Abujudeh HH, Cushing GL Jr, et al: CT cystography with multiplanar reformation for suspected bladder rupture: experience in 234 cases, *AJR Am J Roentgenol* 187:1296–1302, 2006.

Vaccaro JP, Brody JM: CT cystography in the evaluation of major bladder trauma, *Radiographics* 20: 1373–1381, 2000.

Cross-Reference

Emergency Radiology: THE REQUISITES, pp 103–105.

Comment

Bladder ruptures are seen in 5% to 10% of patients with pelvic fractures. Up to 83% of patients with bladder rupture have a pelvic fracture. The most common mechanism of bladder rupture is motor vehicle collision. Gross hematuria invariably accompanies significant bladder injury. Either a conventional or a computed tomographic (CT) cystogram should be performed in all patients with gross hematuria and pelvic fractures.

Both conventional and CT cystogram require sufficient bladder distention to avoid false negative studies. Adequate bladder distention is achieved by instilling 350 to 400 mL of contrast material (30% contrast material for conventional and 4.4% contrast material for CT cystography). If pelvic angiography is contemplated, conventional cystography should be performed following completion of that procedure.

Based on the type of wall injury and location, five patterns of bladder injury are seen following blunt trauma. No reliable data are available as to the prevalence of bladder contusions. Bladder contusions result in partial or incomplete tear of the mucosa. Although hematuria is present, the cystogram is typically normal. No specific treatment is required. Bladder wall irregularities with no frank extravasation of contrast material are seen on cystography in patients with interstitial bladder rupture. Interstitial bladder ruptures are rarely seen following blunt trauma.

Extraperitoneal bladder ruptures are the most common type of bladder injury (80% to 90%). Urinary contrast material typically extravasates into the extravesicle spaces due to a transmural bladder wall injury. The wall injury results from shearing of the ligamentous attachment of the bladder or from direct laceration by bone fragments. Extravasated contrast material may track into the adjacent anterior perivesicle space of Retzius, the pelvic floor, or posteriorly and superiorly into the retroperitoneum. Extravasated contrast material into the space of Retzius may extend along the anterior abdominal wall up to the umbilicus. Injury to the superior fascia of the urogenital diaphragm will permit contrast material to track into the scrotum. Extravasation of contrast material into the thigh and penis implies an injury to the inferior fascia of the urogenital diaphragm. The majority of extraperitoneal bladder ruptures are treated conservatively with either transurethral or supra pubic bladder drainage. Large tears may require surgical repair.

Intraperitoneal bladder ruptures account for 10% to 20% of all ruptures. Contrast extravasates into the peritoneal recesses and outlines bowel loops. The site of rupture is at the bladder dome. This injury typically occurs from direct impact to a full bladder. Surgical repair is the treatment of choice. Combined intraperitoneal and extraperitoneal ruptures are seen in 5% to 12% of all cases.

Notes

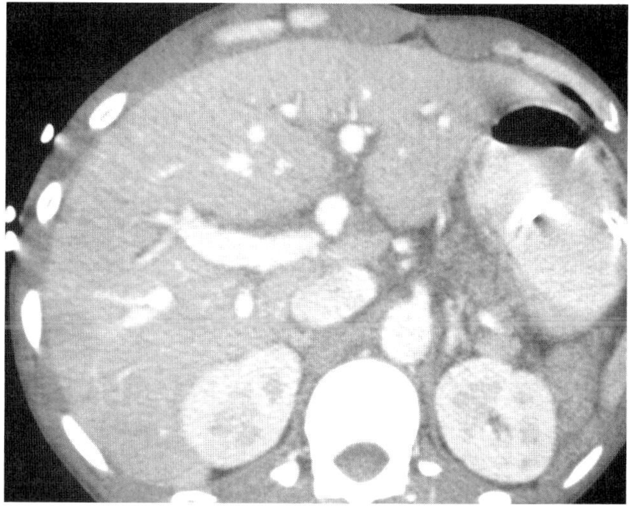

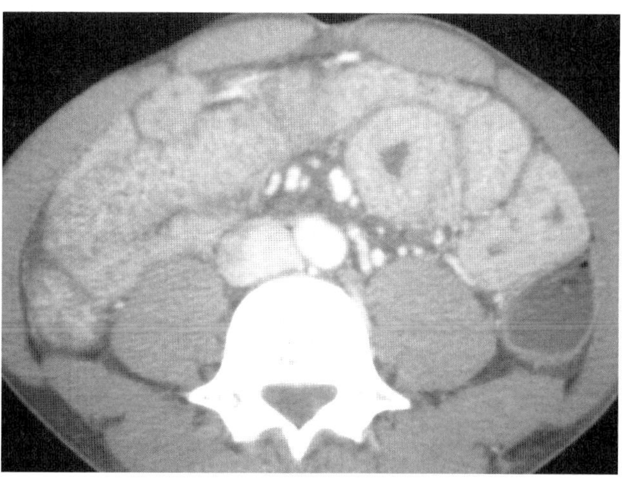

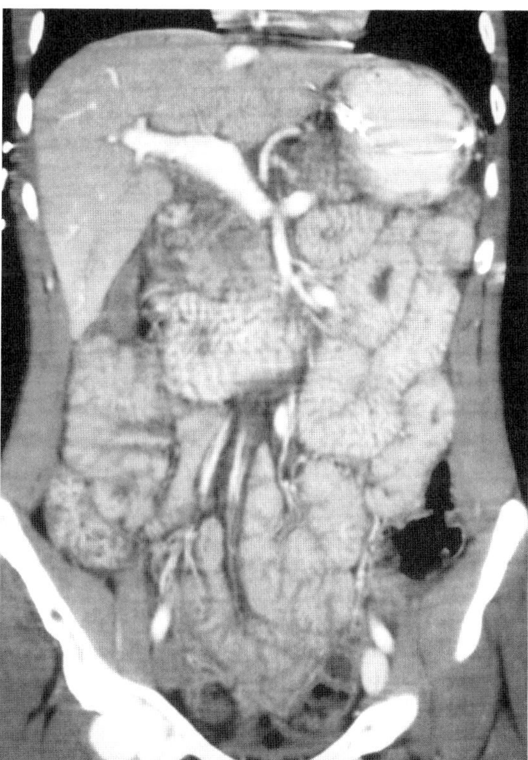

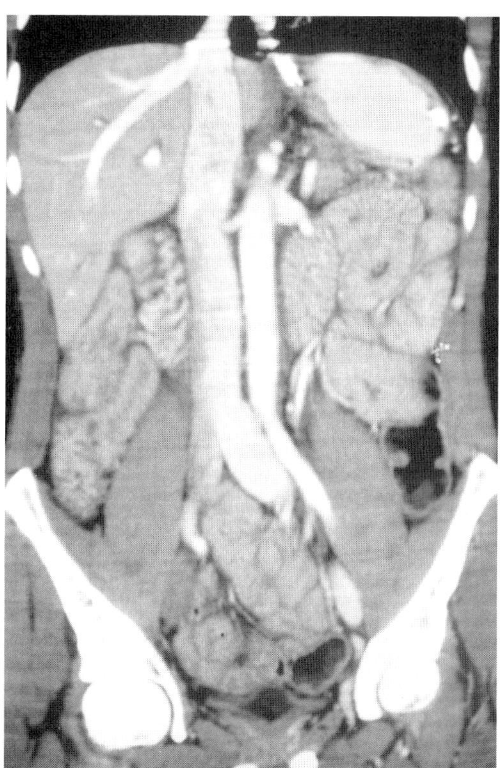

You are shown transverse and coronal reformatted images obtained in a patient admitted following blunt abdominal trauma.

1. What is the diagnosis?
2. What do the low attenuation areas around the portal vein and branches represent?
3. What other trauma-related conditions could give similar computed tomography (CT) findings?
4. What CT findings help to differentiate periportal lymphedema from intrahepatic biliary dilatation?

CASE 73

Periportal Lymphedema from Volume Overload

1. Diffuse periportal low attenuation, small bowel wall thickening, and marked distention of the inferior vena cava indicate volume overload from rapid vigorous intravenous fluid resuscitation.
2. The low attenuation areas represent distended periportal lymphatics.
3. Tension pneumothorax and pericardial tamponade may cause diffuse periportal lymphedema. Focal periportal lymphedema may be seen adjacent to liver lacerations.
4. Periportal lymphedema typically is seen as a low-attenuation area surrounding the portal vein and its branches. Biliary dilatation is usually seen only anterior to the portal vein and its branches.

References

Chapman VM, Rhea JT, Sacknoff R, et al: CT of non-traumatic abdominal fluid collections after initial fluid resuscitation of patients with major burns, *AJR Am J Roentgenol* 182:1493–1496, 2004.

Shanmuganathan K, Ameroso M, Mirvis SE: Periportal low density on CT in patients with blunt trauma: association with elevated venous pressure, *AJR Am J Roentgenol* 160:279–283, 1993.

Comment

Low-attenuation areas seen around the portal vein and branches secondary to many conditions have been well described in the medical literature. Nontraumatic causes include acute liver transplant rejection, congestive cardiac failure, malignant periportal or retroperitoneal lymph adenopathy, and hepatitis. Periportal edema after trauma usually indicates an acute elevation of the central venous pressure, which may be due to vigorous, rapid intravenous fluid resuscitation, cardiac tamponade, or tension pneumothorax.

The intrahepatic lymphatic system, unlike the intrahepatic bile ducts which are anterior to the portal vein, surrounds the portal vein, hepatic arteries, and bile ducts within the interlobar connective tissue. Intrahepatic lymphatics become visible when fluid accumulates due to lymphatic obstruction or increased flow. Elevated central venous pressure caused by rapid expansion of the intravascular volume during intravenous resuscitation is the most common cause of periportal low density seen following trauma, although tension pneumothorax and cardiac tamponade are other important causes.

Other computed tomographic (CT) findings related to elevated central venous pressure include a distended inferior vena cava, which may demonstrate a diameter greater than the adjacent aorta without respiration-related variations on subsequent images. Diffuse bowel edema with small bowel wall thickening is a second CT sign of elevated central venous pressure. In patients with prolonged, severely elevated central venous pressure, edema may also develop in walls of the large bowel and stomach, as well as throughout the retroperitoneum. Characteristically, these abnormalities resolve with restoration of euvolemia.

Focal periportal low attenuation seen adjacent to liver lacerations represents hemorrhage extending into the periportal space. Diffuse small bowel wall edema is also seen in trauma patients with hypoperfusion syndrome (shock bowel) secondary to hypovolemia, and it is important to distinguish this pattern from patients with raised central venous pressure. The CT signs of hypovolemia include a flattened inferior vena cava, a small abdominal aorta, and hyperattenuation of renal parenchyma due to slow perfusion. The bowel is typically distended, and the fluid is filled with abnormally increased mural enhancement. A follow-up CT in 4 to 6 hours' time may be required in patients with abdominal pain to diagnose concurrent partial or full thickness small bowel injury, which may be masked by the diffuse bowel wall edema due to the volume overload.

Notes

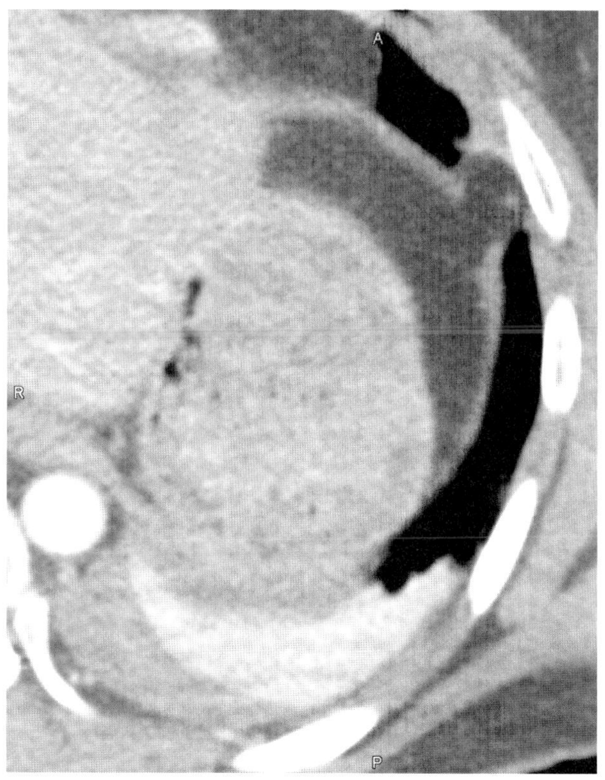

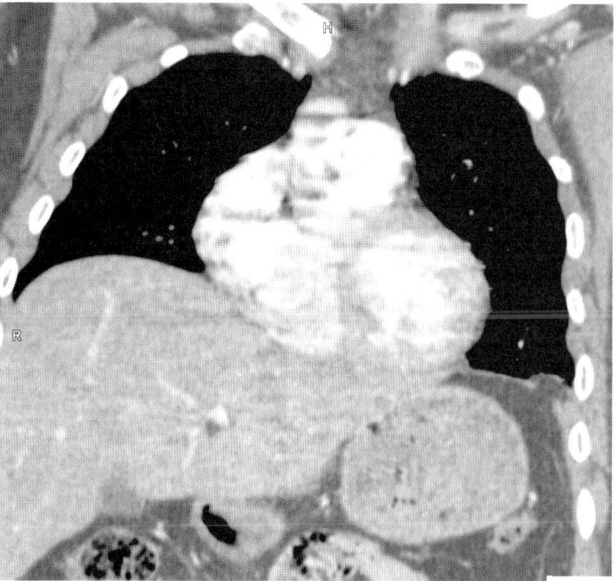

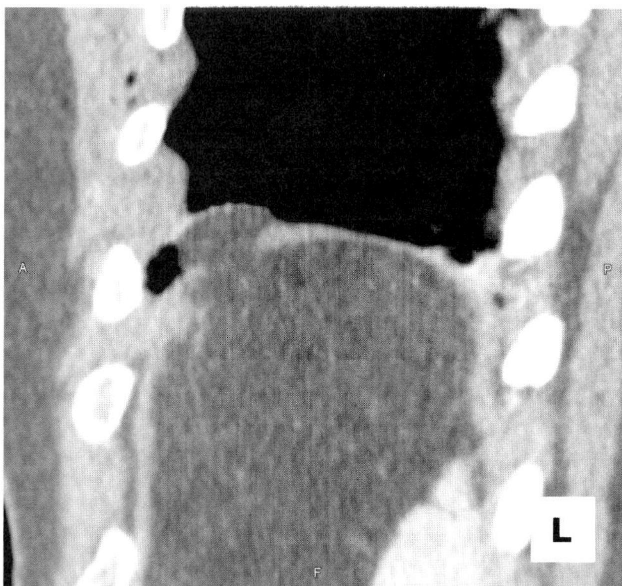

You are shown images of a patient who was stabbed in the left thoracoabdominal region.

1. What are the abnormalities associated with the correct diagnosis?
2. What penetrating wound entry sites are likely to be associated with a diaphragm injury?
3. What delayed complication can result from an occult diaphragm injury?
4. Name three minimally invasive surgical techniques used to diagnose penetrating diaphragm injuries.

CASE 74

Left Hemidiaphragm Injury

1. Left hemidiaphragm injury with herniation of abdominal fat into the thoracic cavity through a small diaphragm defect.
2. Entry sites at the throracoabdominal region, lower chest, upper abdomen, and flanks.
3. Incarceration or strangulation of the abdominal structure herniating through the diaphragmatic defect.
4. Diagnostic peritoneal lavage (DPL), video-assisted thoracoscopic surgery (VATS), and laparoscopy.

References

Freeman RK, Al-Dossari G, Hutcheson KA, et al: Indications for using video-assisted thoracoscopic surgery to diagnose diaphragmatic injuries after penetrating chest trauma, *Ann Thorac Surg* 72:342–347, 2001.

Murray JA, Demetriades D, Cornwell EE 3rd, et al: Penetrating left thoracoabdominal trauma: the incidence and clinical presentation of diaphragm injuries, *J Trauma* 43:624–626, 1997.

Comment

The incidence of diaphragmatic injury following penetrating torso trauma varies based on the location of the entry site of the stab or gunshot wound. The incidence is highest, 26% to 45%, for patients with entry wounds at the lower chest or thoracoabdominal region, which is typically defined as the area between the nipple lines both anteriorly and posteriorly in the chest and costal margins inferiorly. Other entry sites commonly associated with a diaphragm injury include the upper abdomen and flanks.

The emergence of selective nonoperative management of hemodynamically stable patients without obvious clinical or computed tomographic (CT) evidence of organ injury as the treatment of choice for torso trauma increases the risk of missing asymptomatic but significant diaphragm injuries.

Although the majority of patients with a diaphragm injury are likely to have an associated injury to organs in the upper abdomen or lower chest, up to 26% of patients with left thoracoabdominal wounds may be clinically asymptomatic. The admission chest radiographs may be normal in 32% of patients due to the typically small size of the rent, in contrast to the characteristically large diaphragmatic tears caused by blunt trauma, with the average penetrating diaphragm injury measuring from 1 to 4 cm in length.

The commonly used minimally invasive surgical techniques to diagnose penetrating diaphragm injury include diagnostic peritoneal lavage (DPL), video-assisted thoracoscopic surgery (VATS), and laparoscopy. DPL had been considered the diagnostic standard for diagnosing diaphragm injury. However, the use of DPL to suggest diaphragm injury relies on an abnormal peritoneal lavage fluid red blood cell count, which is not a standardized measurement. Minimally invasive surgical techniques, such as VATS and laparoscopy, have proved to be safe methods for diagnosing and repairing asymptomatic or radiographically occult diaphragm injuries.

An ipsilateral pneumothorax or a hemothorax is a common finding seen on admission chest radiographs in patients with penetrating diaphragm injury. Other radiographic findings include elevation of the hemidiaphragm and obliteration of the diaphragmatic outline by either hemorrhage or herniated abdominal structures. Notably, admission chest radiographs are normal in up to 32% of patients with a left thoracoabdominal penetrating wound and a diaphragm injury.

High-resolution axial and multiplanar reformatted multidetector computed tomography (MDCT) images can demonstrate small diaphragm injuries. No studies have reported the sensitivity of MDCT in diagnosing diaphragm injury. Specific CT findings diagnostic of a penetrating diaphragm injury include the "CT collar" sign (constriction of a herniating viscus seen at the site of the diaphragmatic rent), herniation of abdominal viscera through a diaphragmatic defect into the thoracic cavity, and, in patients with a single stab wound, adjacent injuries on either side of the diaphragm. Nonspecific CT findings of diaphragm injury include wound tract extending up to the diaphragm, thickening of the diaphragm, and an isolated focal defect in the diaphragm without adjacent hematoma. Patients with nonspecific CT findings require further investigation with follow-up CT, laparoscopy, or VATS.

Notes

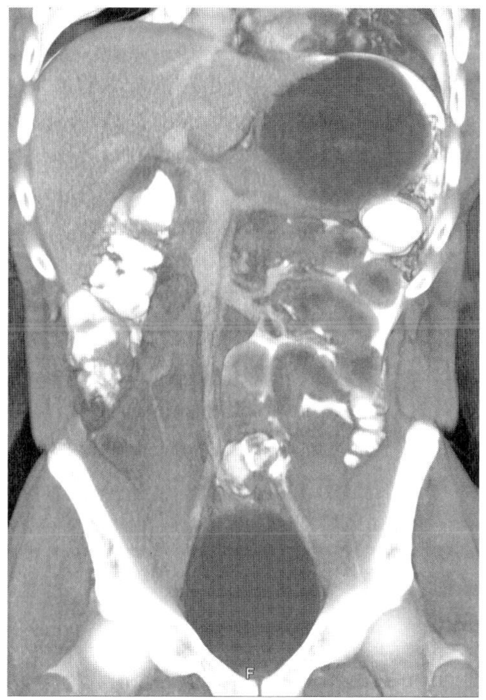

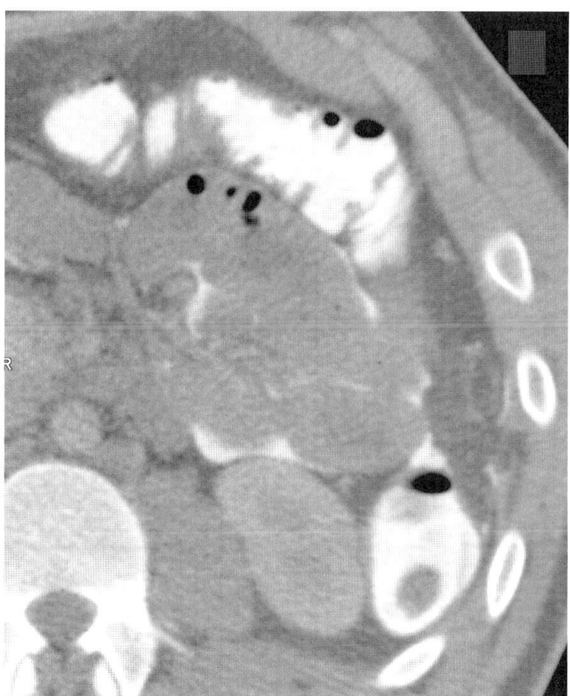

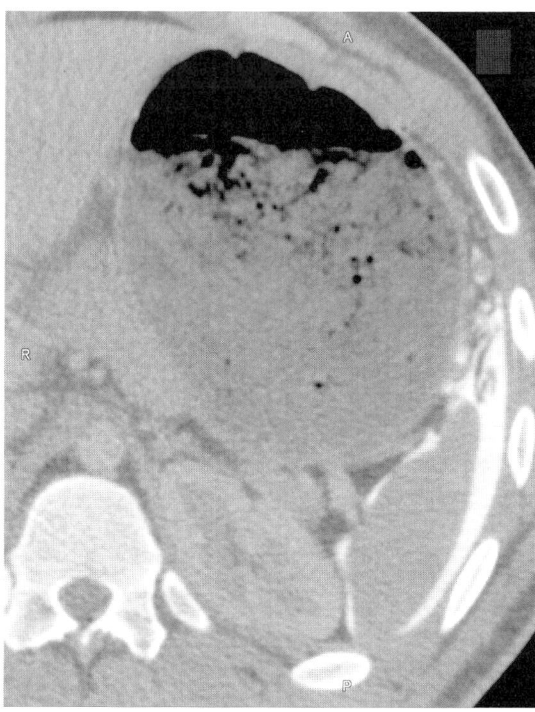

You are shown images of a patient who was stabbed in the upper left flank.

1. What are the computed tomographic (CT) findings of a full-thickness bowel injury caused by penetrating trauma?
2. In this patient, what CT finding indicates a full-thickness colonic injury?
3. The CT demonstrates what other injury that requires surgical repair?
4. What is the significance of free intraperitoneal air demonstrated by CT following penetrating trauma?

CASE 75

Penetrating Colon and Diaphragm Injury

1. Bowel wall thickening, discontinuity of bowel wall, and oral or rectal contrast material extravasation outside the lumen of bowel.
2. Colonic contrast material extravasation into the peritoneal cavity.
3. A small left hemidiaphragm injury is seen in the right image.
4. Free intraperitoneal air represents peritoneal violation. It is not a specific CT finding of bowel injury since it can be introduced by the missile or knife when the peritoneum is violated.

References

Múnera F, Morales C, Soto JA, et al: Gunshot wounds of abdomen: evaluation of stable patients with triple-contrast helical CT, *Radiology* 231:399–405, 2004.

Shanmuganathan K, Mirvis SE, Chiu WC, et al: Penetrating torso trauma: triple-contrast helical CT in peritoneal violation and organ injury—A prospective study in 200 patients, *Radiology* 231:775–784, 2004.

Comment

Bowel injury is common in patients admitted following penetrating injury to the torso. The incidence may be as high as 35% in patients with entry site in the abdomen. These injuries may remain occult for several hours. Multidetector computed tomography (MDCT) has been shown to be accurate and reliable in detecting peritoneal violation and intraperitoneal injuries, including injuries to the mesentery and bowel.

Contraindications for MDCT in penetrating trauma include hemodynamic instability, peritonitis, evidence of free intraperitoneal fluid on ultrasound examination, demonstration of free intraperitoneal air on abdominal or chest radiographs, bright red blood per rectum, and aspiration of blood through a nasogastric tube.

A triple contrast MDCT should be routinely performed to evaluate for peritoneal violation and to demonstrate the extent of intraperitoneal and retroperitoneal injury. Routine administration of intravenous, oral, and rectal contrast material is essential to diagnose intraperitoneal injuries. Administration of positive oral and rectal contrast material to opacity and to distend the bowel helps to increase the ability to detect bowel and mesenteric injuries. Delayed images should also be obtained during the renal excretory phase to evaluate the renal collecting systems for signs of urine leak.

MDCT findings of bowel injury include extravasation of gastrointestinal contrast material, bowel wall thickening, discontinuity or a defect in the bowel wall, and a wound tract extending up to the wall of the hollow viscus. Free intraperitoneal blood may result from an injury to the peritoneal lining itself or to the abdominal wall, or extra peritoneal injuries may also bleed into the peritoneum through the wound tract. Intraperitoneal air may be introduced into the peritoneal cavity by the bullet or knife during violation of the peritoneum. Consequently, free intraperitoneal blood and intraperitoneal air are not considered. CT signs are strongly suggestive of bowel injury in the setting of penetrating trauma. Conversely, CT findings of bowel wall thickening are considered a nonspecific sign of significant bowel injury in blunt trauma. The majority of patients with penetrating abdominal injury in whom CT demonstrates bowel wall thickening have a full-thickness bowel injury that requires surgical repair.

Notes

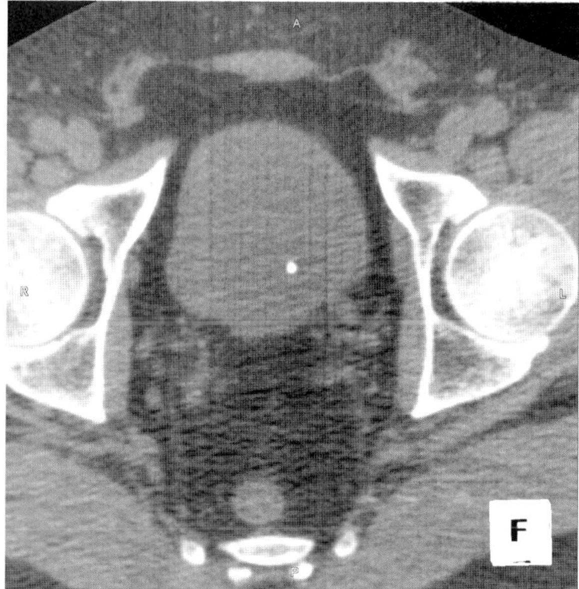

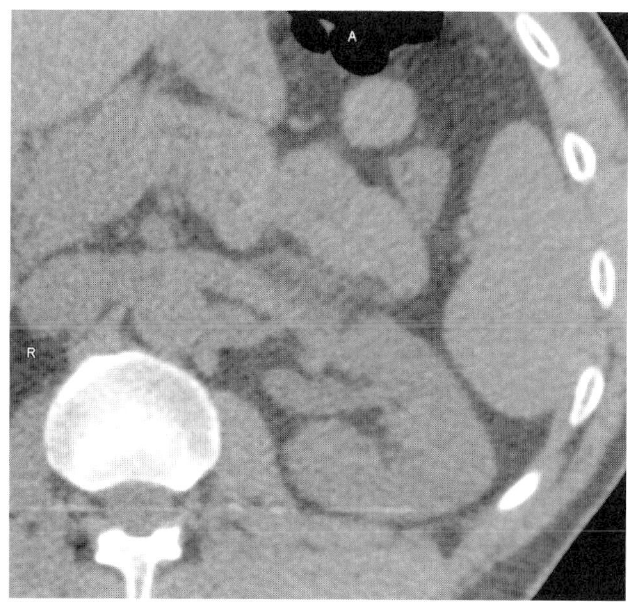

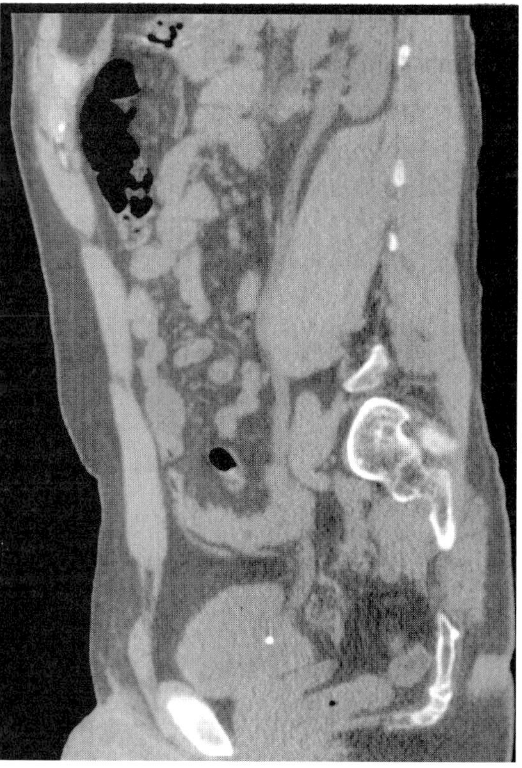

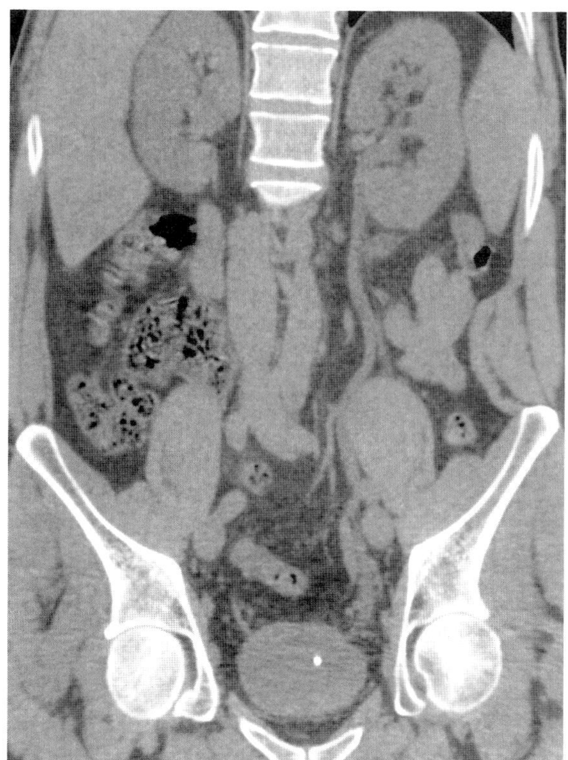

You are shown images of a patient who presented with left flank pain.

1. What is the best diagnosis?
2. Why does the patient have left hydronephrosis and hydroureter?
3. What are the causes of urinary tract obstruction when stones are not seen?
4. What are the three most common sites at which a stone may cause ureteral obstruction?

CASE 76

Recent Passage of a Ureteral Stone into the Bladder

1. Recent passage of a left ureteral stone into bladder with left hydroureter and hydronephrosis.
2. Obstruction secondary to ureterovesical junction mucosal edema caused by recently impacted stone.
3. Mucosal edema from recent passing of a stone, blood clot, sloughed renal papilla in patients with papillary necrosis, transitional cell carcinoma, and ureteral strictures.
4. Ureteropelvic junction, the pelvic brim, and ureterovesical junction.

References

Rucker CM, Menias CM, Bhalla S: Mimics of renal colic: alternative diagnoses at unenhanced helical CT, *Radiographics* 24(Suppl):S11–S28, 2004.

Tamm EP, Silverman PM, Shuman WP: Evaluation of the patient with flank pain and possible ureteral calculus, *Radiology* 228:319–329, 2003.

Cross-Reference

Emergency Radiology: THE REQUISITES, p 299.

Comment

Unenhanced multidetector computed tomography (MDCT) is the imaging modality of choice to evaluate patients with flank pain. It has a very high sensitivity of 95% to 98% and specificity of 98% to 99% for detecting renal calculi. About 33% to 55% of patients presenting with flank pain will have a renal or ureteral stone. On unenhanced CT, an alternate diagnosis may be seen in 9% to 30% of patients. In contrast to the accuracy of CT, abdominal radiographs are only 45% sensitive and 77% specific for demonstrating renal stones.

Ninety percent of the urinary calculi are calcified. The majority (67%) of renal stones have a chemical composition containing calcium oxalate (mixed or pure). Other stones may contain a chemical composition of calcium phosphate (6%), mixed struvite and apatite (15%), uric acid (8%), and cystine (3%). In patients undergoing treatment of AIDS with protease inhibitors, the medication may crystallize in the urine and result in the so-called indinavire stones that may not be demonstrated with CT. Regardless of their chemical composition, the majority of the renal stones seen with CT are visualized because the inherent attenuation of the stone is higher than the surrounding soft tissues.

Natural anatomical narrowing of the ureteral lumen at the ureteropelvic junction, pelvic brim, and ureterovesical junction makes it more likely for stones to lodge at one of these locations and cause obstruction. Demonstration of a calculus within the lumen of the ureter is the most direct sign of ureteral calculus. Secondary signs of asymmetric perinephric inflammatory changes, enlargement of the ipsilateral kidney, hydronephrosis, hydroureter, thickening of the ureteral wall, and periureteral fat stranding are useful in increasing diagnostic certainty.

At times it may be difficult to differentiate a ureteral calculus from extraureteral calcification (e.g., phlebolith). One sign that helps identify a stone, the soft tissue rim sign, occurs when the edematous wall of the ureter surrounds the calculus. The soft tissue rim sign can be seen in 50% to 77% of patients with ureteral calculi. The comet-tail sign, representing a vein that extends to the hilum of the phlebolith, is another sign that can help differentiate a phlebolith from ureteral calculus.

Hydronephrosis and hydroureter without an obstructing calculus may be due to mucosal edema induced by a recently passed calculus that had been impacted at the ureterovesical junction. Other causes include blood clot, transitional cell carcinoma, or a sloughed renal papilla in patients with papillary necrosis obstructing the ureter. If the latter causes are suspected, follow-up CT imaging with intravenous contrast may be useful for further evaluation.

Eighty percent of stones 4 mm or smaller initially seen at the ureterovesical junction will pass spontaneously. In patients with 4 mm or larger obstructing calculi seen in the vicinity of the ureterovesical junction, both supine and prone imaging may be required to determine if the stone is within the ureter or the bladder. With the patient positioned prone, stones within the bladder will fall to the most dependant (i.e., anterior) aspect of the bladder.

Notes

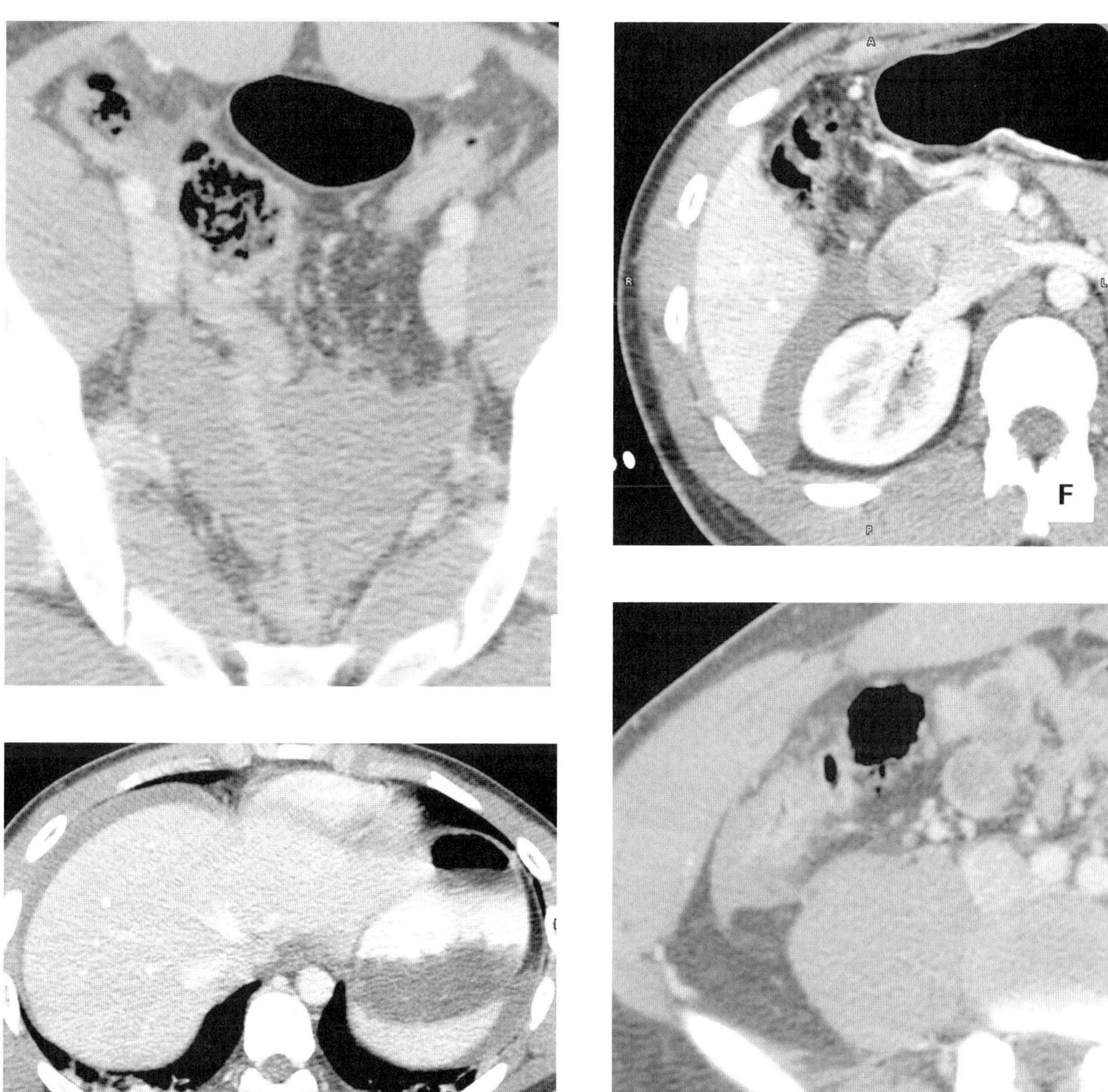

You are shown images of a patient who complained of abdominal pain after blunt force trauma. Computed tomography demonstrated normal abdominal and pelvic organs.

1. In what anatomic locations is the free fluid seen?
2. What is the best diagnosis?
3. What are causes for isolated free intraperitoneal fluid in blunt trauma?
4. What is the best management option in this situation?

CASE 77

Isolated Post-traumatic Free Fluid Without a Source

1. Perihepatic, perisplenic, hepatorenal fossa (Morison's pouch), right paracolic gutter, and pelvis.
2. Isolated free intraperitoneal fluid without solid organ injury.
3. Bowel or mesenteric injuries, subtle liver or spleen surface lacerations, intraperitoneal bladder injury, diapedesis of red blood cells from an extraperitoneal hematoma, and ascites unrelated to trauma. In women, small quantities of free fluid can be physiologic.
4. The radiologist and trauma surgeon should discuss the radiologic and clinical findings to plan optimal management.

References

Lubner M, Menias M, Rucker C, et al: Blood in the belly: CT findings of hemoperitoneum, *Radiographics* 27: 109–125, 2007.

Sirlin CB, Casola G, Brown MA, et al: US of blunt abdominal trauma: importance of free pelvic fluid in women of reproductive age, *Radiology* 219:229–235, 2001.

Cross-Reference

Emergency Radiology: THE REQUISITES, p 95.

Comment

Free intraperitoneal fluid identified as the sole computed tomographic (CT) finding in blunt abdominal trauma may indicate a significant occult injury. There is no clear consensus among the various trauma centers on how these patients should be managed to identify the occult injury. Important factors that should be taken into consideration when planning the management of patients with isolated free intraperitoneal fluid demonstrated with CT include the quantity and location of the free intraperitoneal fluid, the sex of the patient, the result of physical examination, and the presence of fever and leukocytosis. Some consider isolated intraperitoneal fluid a marker of bowel or mesenteric injury and a strong indication for laparotomies. Other etiologies for free fluid include preexisting ascites, occult surface lacerations to solid organs, intraperitoneal bladder injury, and decompression or diapedesis of red blood cells from the extraperitoneal hematoma into the peritoneal cavity. Female patients of reproductive age may have a small amount of "physiologic" free fluid in the cul-de-sac related to menstruation.

Routine follow-up CT is not required in asymptomatic female patients with small amounts of isolated free fluid in the pelvis. Male patients without pelvic fractures and with isolated free intraperitoneal fluid (irrespective of magnitude), female patients with moderate or large amounts of pelvic fluid, and free fluid in multiple locations or between the mesenteric leaves all require further careful observation with serial physical examinations, follow-up CT in 4 to 6 hours, diagnostic peritoneal lavage, or laparoscopy to determine the etiology of the fluid. Patients with moderate to large amounts of isolated free fluid, small amounts of fluid in multiple locations, or intermesenteric fluid require an aggressive management with laparotomies. It is important for the trauma surgeon and trauma radiologist to discuss the radiologic and clinical findings in these patients on an individual patient basis to better plan management.

Notes

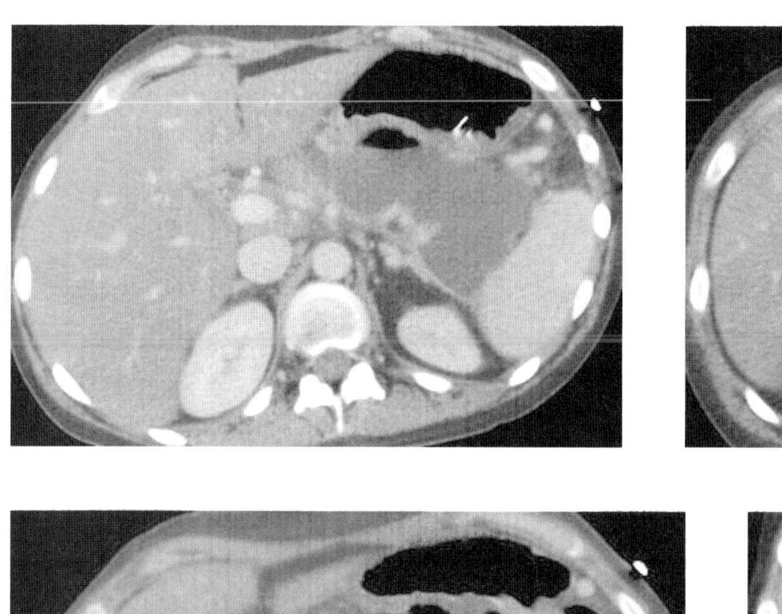

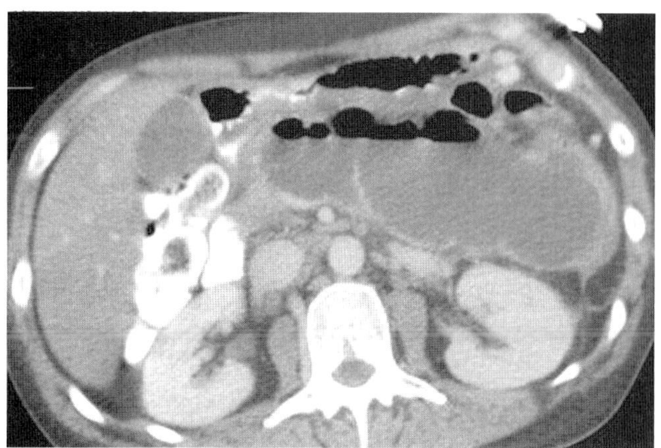

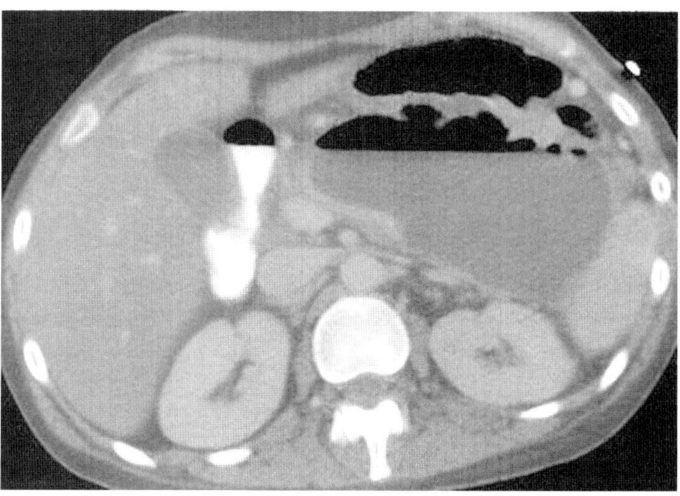

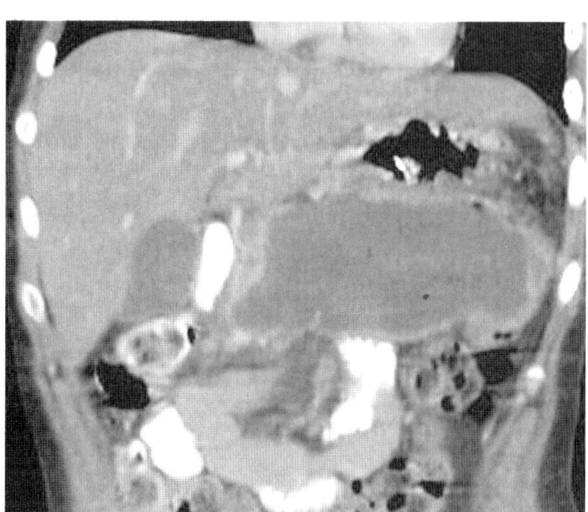

You are shown MDCT images of a 37-year-old woman presenting with abdominal pain and diabetic ketoacidosis.

1. In which anatomic space is the lesion located?
2. What is the best diagnosis?
3. What is the optimal technique to establish the diagnosis?
4. What are potential etiologies for the gas seen in the lesion?

CASE 78

Pancreatic Abscess

1. Anterior pararenal space
2. Pancreatic abscess.
3. Image-guided fine needle aspiration of the collection.
4. Infection due to a gas-forming organism, gastrointestinal fistula, iatrogenic intervention (placement of a drain or catheter), and infected necrosis of the pancreas.

References

Messiou C, Charmers AG: Imaging in acute pancreatitis, *Imaging* 16:314–322, 2004.

VanSonnenberg E, Wittich GR, Chon KS, et al: Percutaneous radiologic drainage of pancreatic abscesses, *AJR Am J Roentgenol* 168:979–984, 1997.

Comment

Pancreatic abscesses have mortality rates varying from 14% to 54%. The presentation can be either indolent or fulminant. The abscess tends to develop more than 4 weeks following pancreatitis or pancreatic injury. To optimally select management strategies and treatment, it is important not to confuse this entity with a bland peripancreatic fluid collection, pancreatic phlegmon, pseudocyst, pancreatic necrosis, or infected pancreatic necrosis.

MDCT demonstrates a pancreatic abscess as a well-defined circumscribed low- or mixed-attenuation collection within either the peripancreatic region or the pancreas. Margins may be either smooth or ill-defined. Peripheral enhancement, complex loculations and septations can be seen. It may contain little or no necrotic tissue. Typically, pus is obtained on percutaneous image-guided aspiration of the collection.

The infection usually occurs from gram-negative organisms originating from the gastrointestinal tract such as *Escherichia coli, Klebsiella, Proteus, Pseudomonas,* and *Enterobacter.* Spontaneous fistula with the gastrointestinal tract can occur in about 17% of patients. The air seen within the collection may result from infection due to gas-forming organisms, from gastrointestinal fistula, or from iatrogenic intervention. Unless there is a history of recent intervention, presence of gas within the collection should raise the suspicion of an abscess.

To plan optimal treatment, attempts should be made to differentiate pancreatic abscess from other recognized complications of pancreatitis such as intra- and peripancreatic fluid collections, pseudocyst, necrosis, and infected necrosis. Acute fluid collections occur in or adjacent to the pancreas, and about half resolve spontaneously. Pancreatic necrosis is seen on contrast-enhanced CT as a diffuse or focal area of solid attenuation (tissue) that lacks enhancement. Necrosis occurs in about 20% of patients with severe pancreatitis and is seen 48 to 72 hours after onset of clinical symptoms. Infected necrosis is associated with multiorgan failure, is seen in about 40% to 70% of patients with pancreatic necrosis, and can be suspected when areas of absent pancreatic enhancement are intermixed with locules of gas. Pseudocysts typically take at least 4 weeks to develop and have well-defined walls.

Percutaneous drainage and antibiotic therapy can cure the majority of the pancreatic abscesses. Patients in whom percutaneous drainage fails are candidates for surgery.

Notes

Fair Game

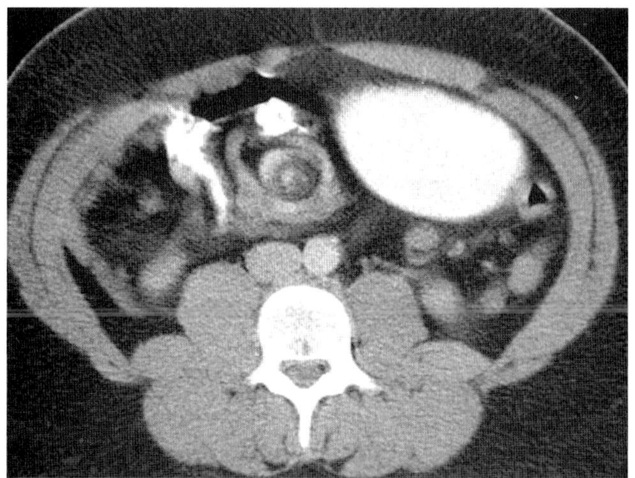

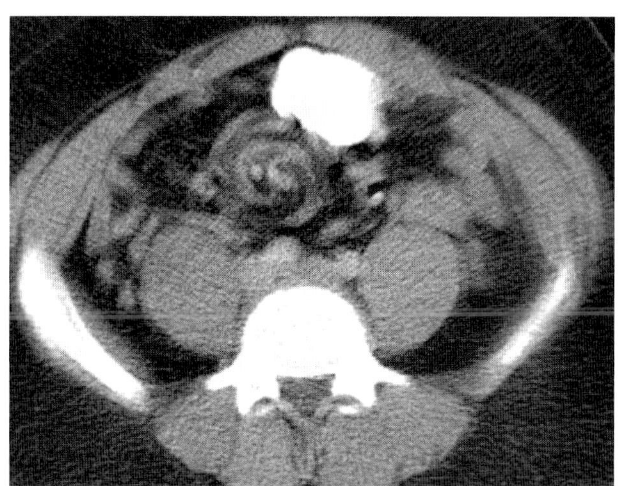

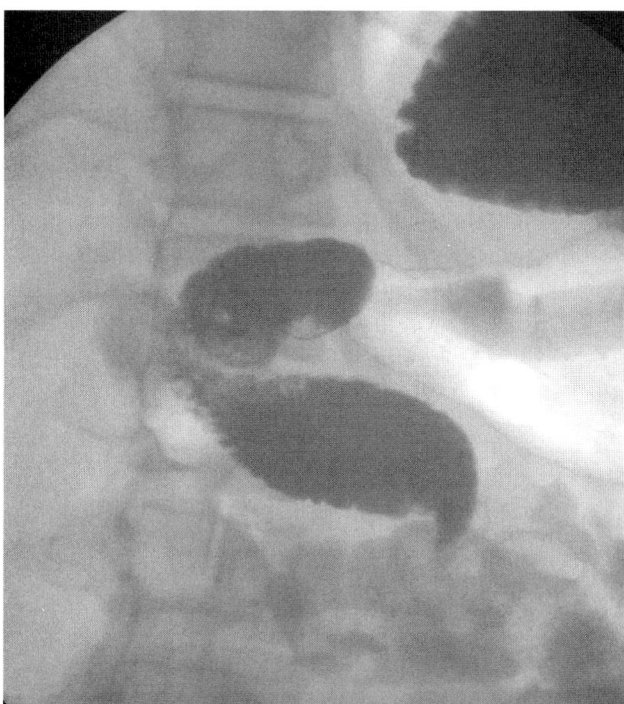

You are shown images of a patient with mid-abdominal pain.

1. What is the diagnosis?
2. What classic CT finding establishes the diagnosis?
3. What is the cause of this pathology?
4. What are two major complications?

CASE 79

Midgut Volvulus

1. Midgut volvulus.
2. The "swirl" or "whirlpool" sign.
3. Clockwise twisting of the bowel around the superior mesenteric artery axis due to a narrowed mesenteric attachment.
4. Bowel ischemia and perforation.

References

Magu S, Ratan KN, Agrawal K: Images: CT whirl sign—midgut volvulus, *Indian J Radiol Imaging* 16:83–84, 2006.

Pickhardt PJ, Bhalla S: Intestinal malrotation in adolescents and adults: spectrum of clinical and imaging features, *AJR Am J Roentgenol* 179:1429–1435, 2002.

Cross-Reference

Emergency Radiology: THE REQUISITES, pp 191, 278.

Comment

Midgut malrotation is estimated to occur in 1 in 500 live births. Reportedly 64% to 80% of patients present during the first month of life, but some remain undiagnosed beyond childhood. Midgut volvulus is a complication of malrotation in which clockwise twisting of the bowel around the superior mesenteric artery (SMA) axis occurs due to a narrowed mesenteric attachment. Recurrent episodes of colicky abdominal pain with vomiting over a period of months or years are typical and may eventually lead to imaging. The radiologist may encounter this entity in several different clinical settings such as an incidental imaging finding, the cause of acute abdominal symptoms, or a condition associated with abdominal situs abnormalities.

Computed tomography (CT) is usually the imaging technique of choice for patients presenting with acute abdominal pain. The CT "swirl" or "whirlpool" sign describes the swirling appearance of bowel and mesentery twisted around the SMA axis. Low attenuating fatty mesentery with enhancing engorged vessels radiate from the twisted bowel. In the central eye of the whirl, a soft tissue density pinpoints the source of the twist. Additional CT findings include duodenal obstruction, congestion of the mesenteric vasculature, and evidence of underlying malrotation. Accompanying superior mesenteric vascular compromise (first venous, followed by arterial) can lead to life-threatening ischemia of the small bowel and gangrenous necrosis. Mortality associated with midgut volvulus is at least 15%. CT reveals the presence and location of the volvulus and gives the added benefit of allowing early identification of potentially fatal complications, such as ischemia and perforation. On an upper GI series, the findings of malrotation with midgut volvulus include a dilated, fluid-filled duodenum, proximal small bowel obstruction, "corkscrew" pattern (proximal jejunum spiraling downward in the right- or mid-upper abdomen), and mural edema with thick folds.

Notes

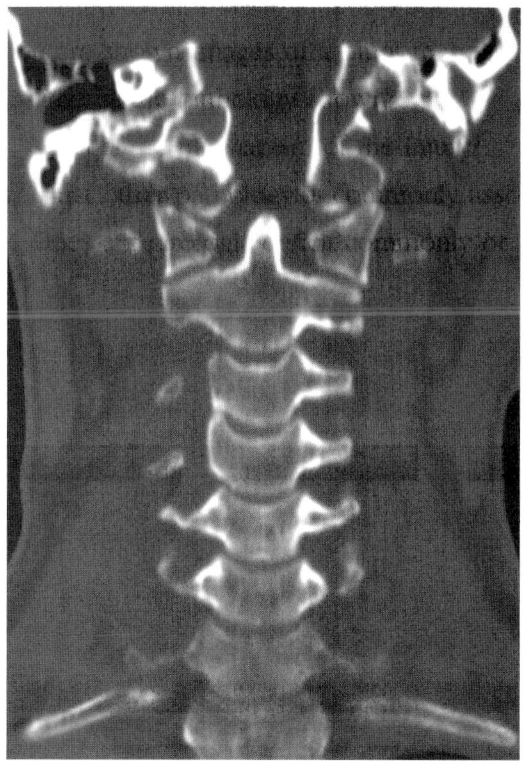

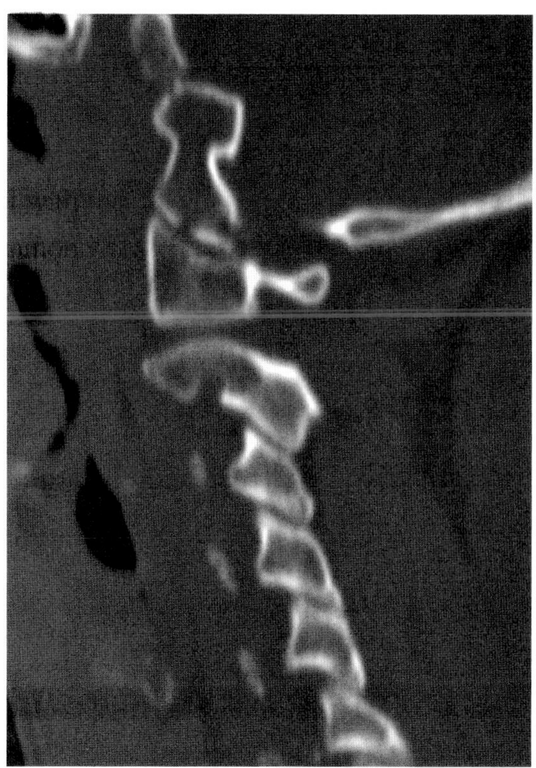

You are shown images of a blunt trauma patient.

1. What injury is shown?
2. Is it mechanically stable?
3. What is the mechanism of the injury?
4. What clinical signs, besides neck pain, may occur with this injury?

CASE 80

Type III Occipital Condyle Fracture

1. Type III occipital condyle fracture.
2. Considered unstable.
3. Distraction force.
4. Limited skull mobility, torticollis, dysphagia, brainstem and lower cranial nerve deficits.

Reference

Aulino JM, Tutt LK, Kaye JJ, et al: Occipital condyle fractures: clinical presentation and imaging findings in 76 patients, *Emerg Radiol* 11:342–347, 2005.

Cross-Reference

Emergency Radiology: THE REQUISITES, p 217.

Comment

Occipital condyle fractures were rarely diagnosed prior to the common use of computed tomography (CT) for potential cervical spine injury. The injury is difficult to detect radiologically due to overlapping structures at the craniocervical junction. Prevertebral soft tissue swelling may be the only radiologic clue. It is now appreciated that these may be relatively common, perhaps occurring in 16% to 19% of patients sustaining injuries to the craniocervical junction, and should always be considered in patients with unexplained upper cervical pain. The diagnosis is usually straightforward by CT.

The most common form of the injury (type 1) is a stable fracture of the medial condyle, usually unilateral, from axial loading which produces a vertical split through the condyle and is minimally or nondisplaced. Other axial loading injuries should be sought. The second type (type 2) is a skull base fracture that extends into the condyle, also stable. Type 3 injuries involve high-energy distraction forces that avulse a fragment of the condyle(s). These are considered unstable and are far more likely to have associated neurologic deficits, especially involving the lower cranial nerves or lower medullary and upper cervical cord. With this pattern, other distraction injuries, such as atlanto-occipital and atlantoaxial distractions, should be sought. This Anderson–Montesano classification is being replaced by the Tuli system which includes type 1 (stable, nondisplaced), type 2a (stable with displacement), and type 2b (displaced fragment and unstable) injuries.

Notes

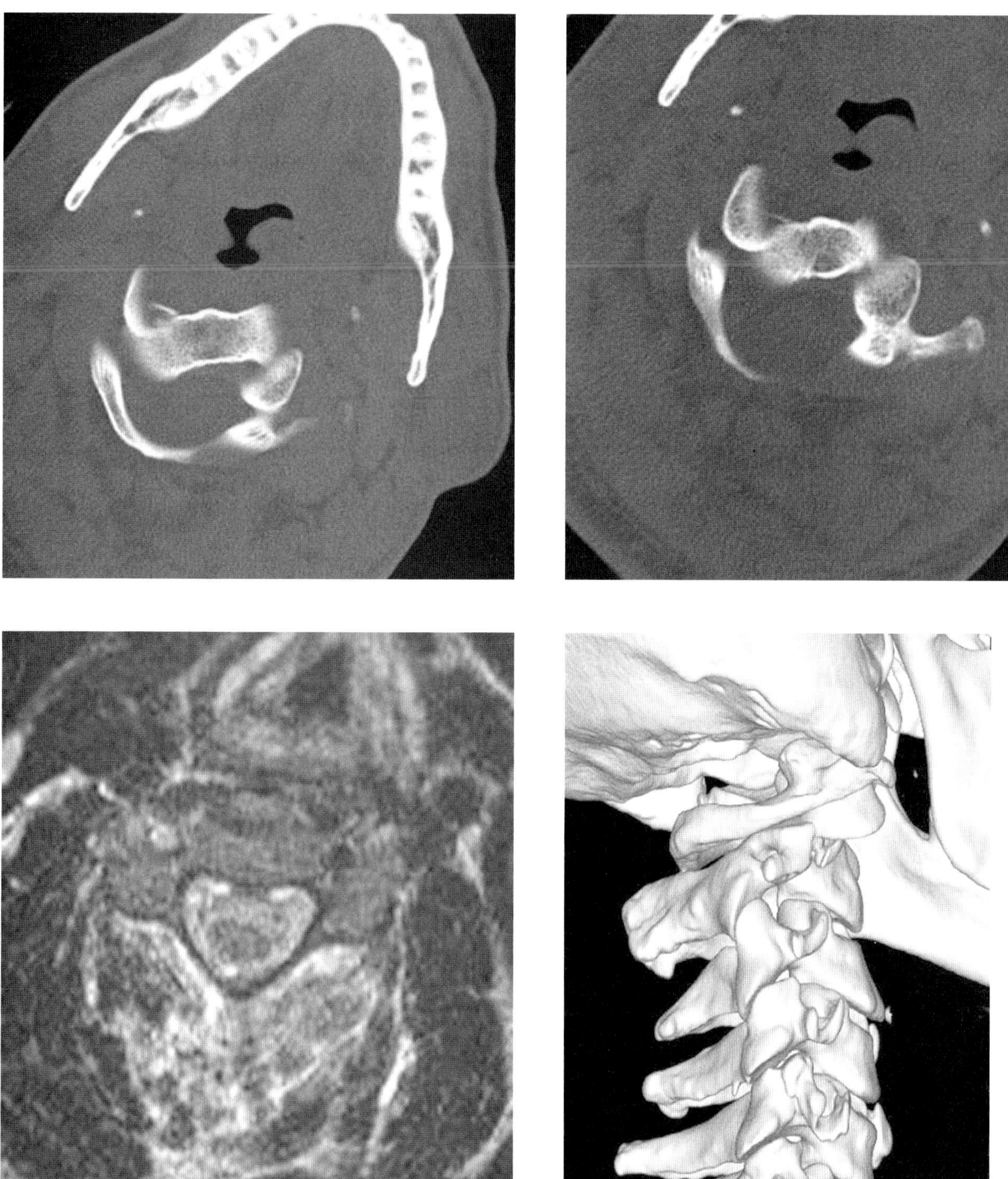

You are shown images of a blunt trauma patient with neck pain.

1. What osseous injury has occurred?
2. What nonosseous injury has occurred?
3. Is this patient able to turn his head in the other direction?
4. In this injury, stability is based mainly on the integrity of which ligament?

CASE 81

Atlantoaxial Rotatory Dislocation

1. Bilateral atlantoaxial rotatory dislocation.
2. Right vertebral artery occlusion.
3. No, this injury is locked in position and requires traction and rotation for reduction.
4. The transverse ligament.

Reference

Hecht AC, Silcox DH, Whitesides TE: Injuries of the cervicocranium. In Browner BD, Jupiter JB, Levine AM, Trafton PG eds: *Skeletal Trauma*, 3rd ed, Philadelphia, WB Saunders, 2003, pp 777–813.

Cross-Reference

Emergency Radiology: THE REQUISITES, p 219.

Comment

Rotational subluxation and dislocation of the atlantoaxial joint is rare. Most cases are nontraumatic, occur in childhood and early adolescence, and are referred to as torticollis or wryneck. The alignment abnormality is usually associated with acute infection of the upper respiratory tract or occasionally relatively minor trauma. This abnormality usually resolves spontaneously. The second form occurs in older adolescents or adults mainly during vehicular impacts and sporting injuries. The head appears tilted in one direction and rotated in the opposite direction. The injury produces disruption of the alar ligaments, which check hyper-rotation, the atlantoaxial joint capsule(s), and potentially the transverse ligament, the main support ligament of the C1-C2 articulation.

On the anteroposterior radiograph, there is likely to be marked asymmetry of the lateral atlantodental spaces. The anterior rotation of a lateral mass of C1 produces narrowing of the C1-C2 lateral articular space, elongation of the C1 lateral mass, and narrowing of the ipsilateral atlantodental space. With posterior displacement, the contralateral lateral mass becomes foreshortened, produces widening of the C1-C2 ipsilateral lateral joint space, and widens the ipsilateral lateral atlantodental space. On the lateral radiograph, the C1 ring shows an elliptical configuration due to tilting, and the anterior arch displays a peculiar contour. On computed tomography, the diagnosis is more easily established, although it is possible for a subluxation to appear reduced depending on head position. If suspected, stress views with maximal head rotation to each side, performed by the patient, may bring out the abnormal alignment. In the case of a "locked" rotation, the C1 lateral mass falls either in front of or completely behind the lateral axis body and cannot be voluntarily reduced. Use of three-dimensional images to show the amount of facet surfaces exposed helps distinguish normal from subluxed to dislocated lateral masses. The injury can be associated with vertebral artery damage as these vessels are stretched by rotation while fixed between the C1 and C2 transverse foramina.

Notes

CASE 82

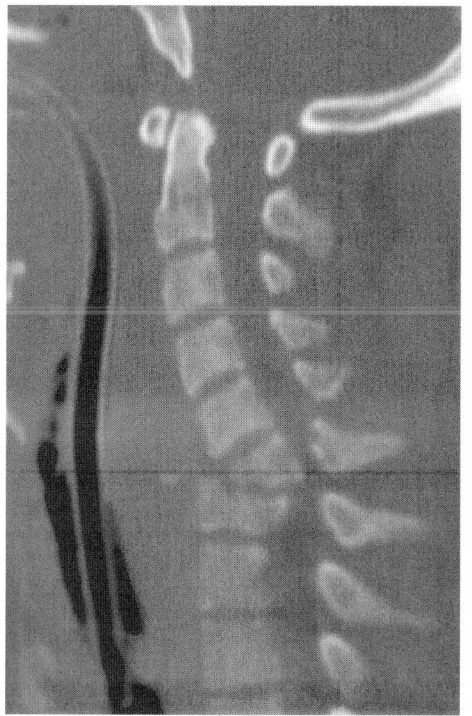

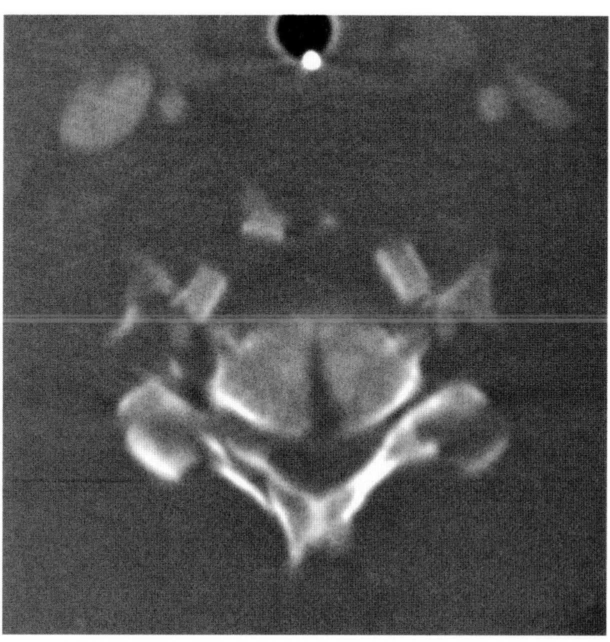

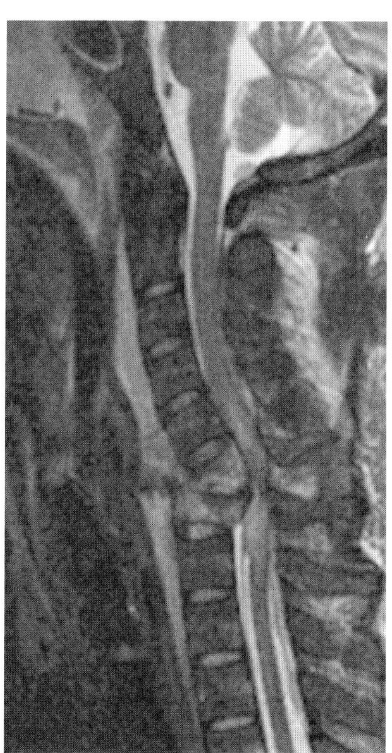

You are shown images of a blunt trauma patient.

1. What is the diagnosis?
2. Is the injury mechanically stable or unstable?
3. What is the mechanism of injury?
4. What is the usual clinical result?

CASE 82

Flexion-Teardrop Fracture-Dislocation

1. Hyperflexion teardrop fracture.
2. Unstable.
3. Axial loading on a flexed spine.
4. Quadriplegia with loss of pain, touch, and temperature sensation.

Reference

Kim KS, Chen HH, Russell EJ, Rogers LF: Flexion teardrop fracture of the cervical spine: radiographic characteristics, *AJR Am J Roentgenol* 152:319–326, 1989.

Cross-Reference

Emergency Radiology: THE REQUISITES, p 220.

Comment

The hyperflexion teardrop fracture is a high-energy injury produced by axial loading on a flexed cervical spine. Typically, the injury involves a lower cervical vertebral body from C4 to C6. The injury produces loss of height of the anterior body with avulsion and anterior displacement of a triangle-shaped bone fragment from the anteroinferior body. This fragment in the lateral radiographic projection has the teardrop shape for which the injury is named. The fragment stays aligned with the anterior spine, while the remaining posterior body is retropulsed into the spinal canal producing cord injury. The focal kyphotic deformity created by the injury contributes to narrowing of the spinal canal, exacerbating the impact of the retropulsed body. Because of posterior distraction forces, there is usually associated widening of the interlaminar spaces and interfacetal joints between the fractured body and the level above. Hyperflexion injuries may also be present at adjacent levels. Also, a sagittal mid-body fracture through the involved vertebral body is common on axial computed tomography (CT), as well as multiple fractures of the anterior superior endplate of the same vertebral body. Laminar and spinous process fractures are common as well but are more likely to be diagnosed on CT than on radiographs.

Most patients, 85% to 90%, will sustain a major neurologic deficit with quadriplegia, in addition to loss of pain, touch, and temperature sensation. Magnetic resonance (MR) imaging is valuable to document the extent of the injury, but mainly it is useful to detect ligament injuries at other levels and to assess both the nature and extent of spinal cord injury. Either CT-angiography or MR angiography with MR imaging can be used to exclude a vertebral artery injury that can occur with significantly displaced cervical spine fractures.

Notes

CASE 83

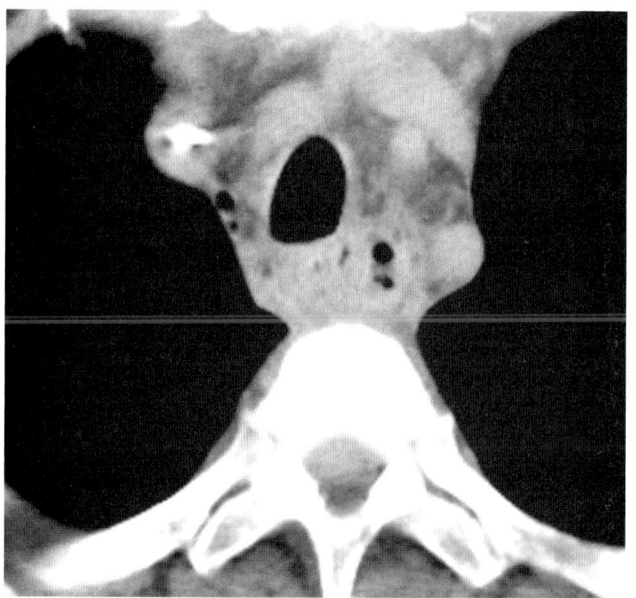

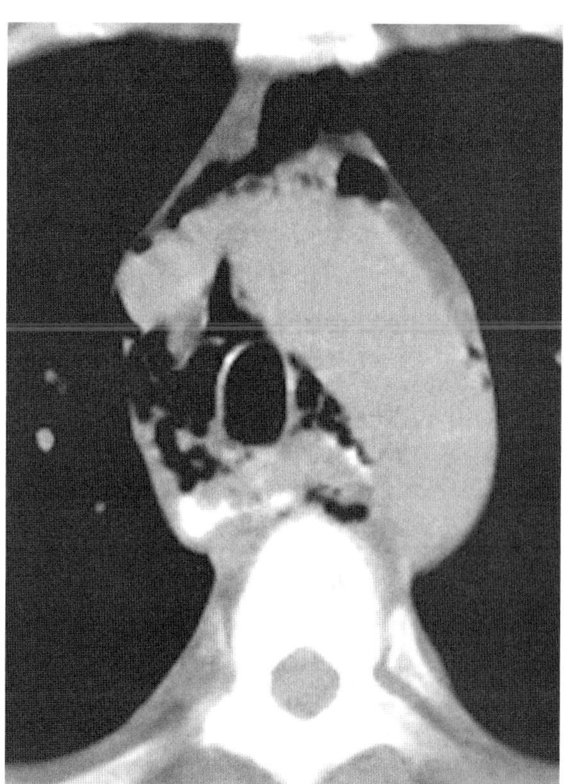

You are shown images of a blunt trauma patient.

1. What is the diagnosis?
2. What studies would be used to confirm the diagnosis?
3. Is the injury more often related to blunt or penetrating injury?
4. Injuries to what other major structures need to be excluded?

CASE 83

Blunt Trauma Esophageal Rupture

1. Esophageal rupture (blunt trauma).
2. Endoscopy or esophagram.
3. Penetrating is far more common.
4. Trachea and major mediastinal vascular structures.

Reference

Mirvis SE: Imaging of acute thoracic injury: the advent of MDCT screening, *Semin Ultrasound CT MR* 26: 305–331, 2005.

Cross-Reference

Emergency Radiology: THE REQUISITES, p 242.

Comment

Esophageal injury from blunt trauma is quite rare with all forms of noniatrogenic trauma accounting for less than 10% of cases. Injuries are most common in the cervical and upper esophagus and above the gastroesophageal junction. Mechanisms of injury may involve crushing between the trachea and spine, hyperextension with longitudinal traction, and direct penetration by a cervical spine fracture fragment. It is important to exclude injuries to the trachea and major mediastinal vessels as these structures are not infrequently also injured concurrently.

With complete esophageal wall disruption, chest radiographic signs can include persistent pneumomediastinum and cervical soft tissue air, left pleural effusion, and an abnormal mediastinal contour related to accumulation of fluid around the injury site or associated mediastinal hemorrhage. Unlike tracheal injury, air leaks from the esophagus tend to remain relatively localized near the tear since there is little positive pressure in the esophagus to force air more distally. Computed tomography (CT) is more sensitive to small amounts of periesophageal air and can show extravasation of small quantities of contrast material. Diagnosis can be verified by contrast esophagram or endoscopy. Performance of chest CT after an apparently negative esophagram may be useful to detect a small quantity of extravasated contrast.

Lack of specific clinical symptoms, the rarity of the injury, and distraction by more apparent injuries often leads to a delayed diagnosis, increasing the occurrence of mediastinitis, empyema, sepsis, and death.

Notes

CASE 84

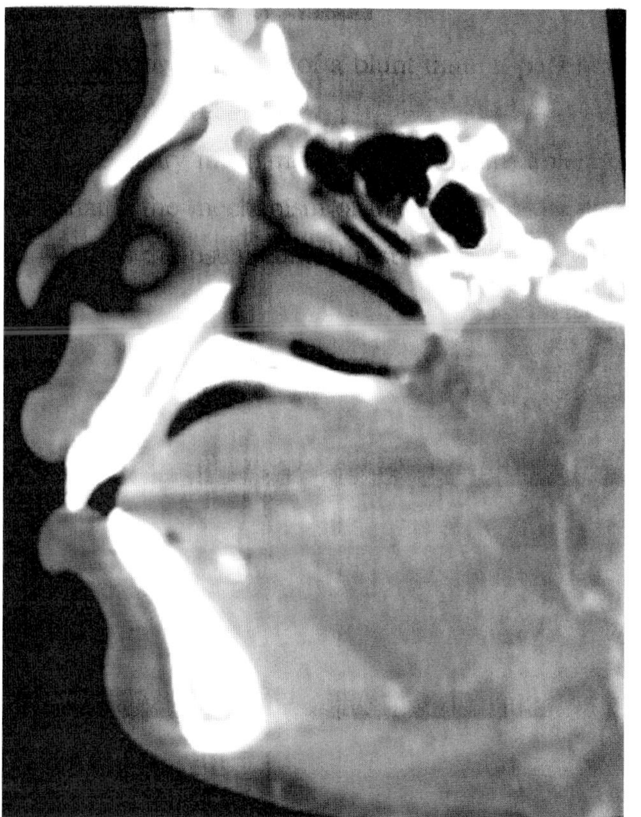

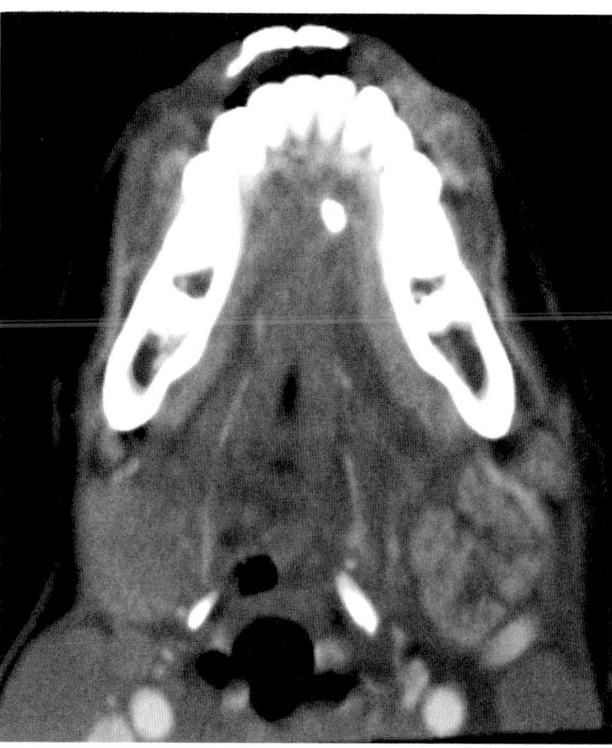

You are shown images of a patient with nontraumatic facial pain.

1. What are the pathologic findings?
2. What symptoms is the patient likely to complain of?
3. What is the most common site for this pathologic process?
4. What other studies can be used to infer or establish the diagnosis?

CASE 84

Obstructive Sialadenitis

1. Dilated Wharton's duct with occluding sialolith, enlarged submandibular gland with increased enhancement.
2. Pain and swelling of salivary gland; warmth and redness over the gland.
3. Submandibular gland.
4. Radiography, MRI, and sonography.

Reference

Yousem DM, Kraut MA, Chalian AA: Major salivary gland imaging, *Radiology* 216:19–29, 2000.

Cross-Reference

Emergency Radiology: THE REQUISITES, p 47.

Comment

Sialolithiasis is the second most common disease of the salivary glands after mumps. Most patients with sialolithiasis will have the cardinal signs of pain and swelling of the gland. The gland may be diffusely or focally enlarged with a sialolith in the proximal duct. Sialolithiasis is predominantly a disease of the submandibular gland where 80% to 82% of sialoliths occur. Sialoliths form more frequently in the submandibular gland because of the more alkaline, thicker, and viscous saliva the submandibular gland produces. Other factors that predispose to stasis in the Wharton duct including an uphill course, a dependent gland, a wider lumen, and a tighter orifice may also play a role. Calculi may be multiple (25%) and may occur within intraglandular ductal tributaries or the main ducts. When in the gland itself, symptoms may be relatively minor, whereas ductal sialoliths usually have a more precipitous presentation.

Imaging helps to define the location of isolated nonpalpable or multiple sialoliths. Most imaging modalities sensitive to calculi, including conventional radiography, computed tomography (CT), and ultrasound, can demonstrate sialoliths with high accuracy. Sonography has been reported to accurately localize up to 94% of major salivary gland calculi as ductal or glandular. However, sonography is less accurate than CT in distinguishing multiple clusters of stones from single large stones. Generally, CT in this setting is best performed without administration of contrast material, since small opacified blood vessels may simulate small sialoliths. If an abscess or inflammatory process is suspected, performing an additional contrast-enhanced scan may be valuable.

Recent investigations have shown that fast T2-weighted thin-section MRI can noninvasively evaluate ductal architecture and identify stones, and it affords the opportunity to visualize the effect the sialolith has on the ductal system. Tiny calculi can be overlooked on MR images because of the signal void associated with the calcified stone. Sialography is contraindicated in the acute setting of sialadenitis because of the possibility of exacerbating symptoms associated with infection.

Notes

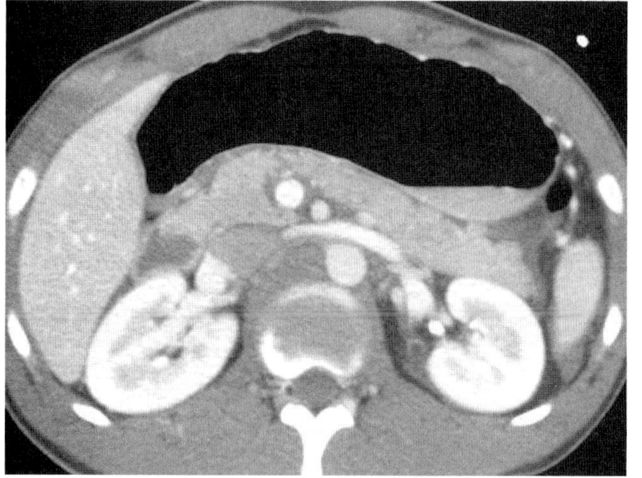

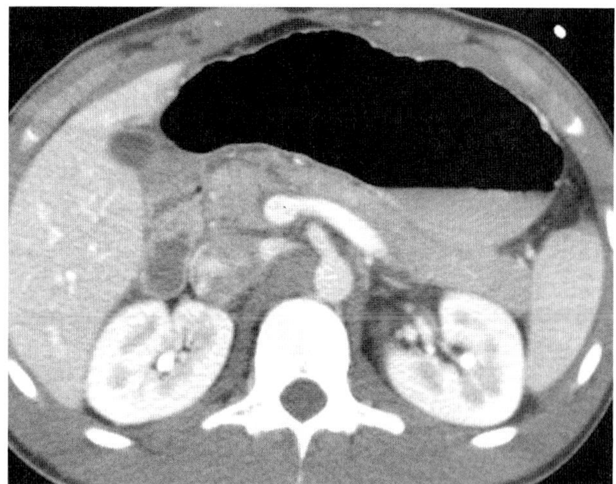

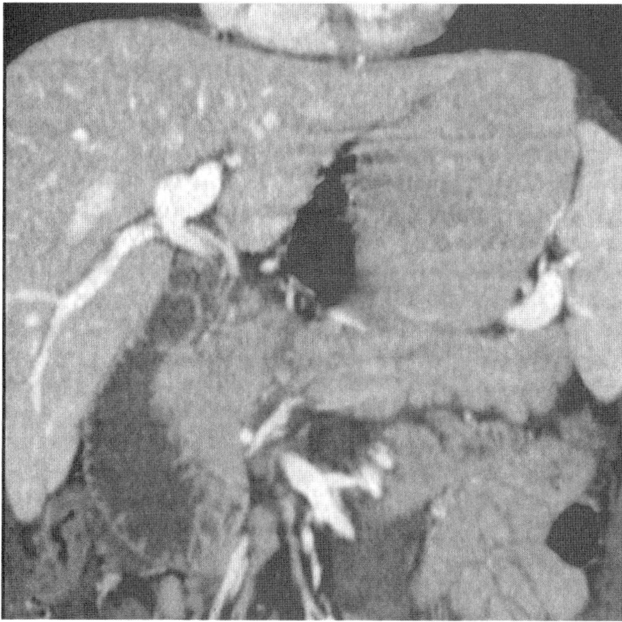

You are shown images of a blunt trauma patient.

1. What is the major injury demonstrated?
2. What are some possible ancillary computed tomography (CT) findings that would support this diagnosis?
3. What is the grading system for these injuries?
4. What other diagnostic test(s) will be needed to complete the workup?

CASE 85

Pancreatic Transection

1. Pancreatic body transection.
2. Peripancreatic fat infiltration, peripancreatic hematoma, fluid between pancreas and splenic vein, and fluid tracking along anterior pararenal fascia.
3. Grade 1: Contusion or laceration of pancreas with intact duct.

   Grade 2: Deep laceration or transection with duct injury.

   Grade 3: Severe laceration or crush injury to head of pancreas.

   Grade 4: Pancreaticoduodenal injuries.
4. Magnetic resonance cholangiopancreatography (MRCP) or endoscopic retrograde cholangiopancreatography (ERCP).

Reference

Gupta A, Stuhfaut JW, Fleming KW, et al: Blunt trauma of the pancreas and biliary tract: a multimodality imaging approach to diagnosis, *Radiographics* 24: 1381–1395, 2004.

Cross-Reference

Emergency Radiology: THE REQUISITES, pp 91–93.

Comment

In the United States, pancreatic injury commonly results twice as often from penetrating as from blunt force trauma. Impact of the abdomen into the steering wheel in motor vehicle crashes is the most common blunt traumatic cause. Due to its retroperitoneal location, pancreatic injury may be clinically silent or may cause minimal symptoms for several days after injury. Given the central location of the pancreas, associated visceral injuries are common and typically involve the liver, spleen, or bowel. These other injuries may dominate the clinical presentation, thereby delaying the recognition of the pancreatic injury. Persistent elevation of pancreatic enzymes can be an indicator of the injury, but does not always occur, particularly soon after admission, and can be seen with injury to other structures, such as the duodenum, stomach, small bowel, and salivary glands.

Computed tomography (CT) has become the mainline diagnostic study for diagnosing pancreatic injuries, and it usually reveals pancreatic edema, peripancreatic or adjacent mesenteric fluid, and, potentially, duct transection. Injuries to the head of the pancreas are twice as lethal as those of the tail or body. A laceration appears as an irregular low attenuation line across the parenchyma. If a laceration crosses less than 50% of the anteroposterior diameter of the pancreas, then the duct is usually intact, but if greater than 50%, duct transection is likely. The diagnosis is more evident if there is separation of the fragments across the laceration. Endoscopic retrograde cholangiopancreatography (ERCP) and magnetic resonance cholangiopancreatography (MRCP) may be needed to assess duct integrity. Complications of pancreatic injury include fistula formation, pseudocyst, and infection and are more common with main duct injury, pancreatic head-duodenal injury, inadequate drainage, and distal pancreatectomy. Injuries can be graded as follows: Grade 1—contusion or laceration of pancreas with intact duct; Grade 2—deep laceration or transection with duct injury; Grade 3—severe laceration or crush injury to head of pancreas; and Grade 4—pancreaticoduodenal injuries.

Notes

CASE 86

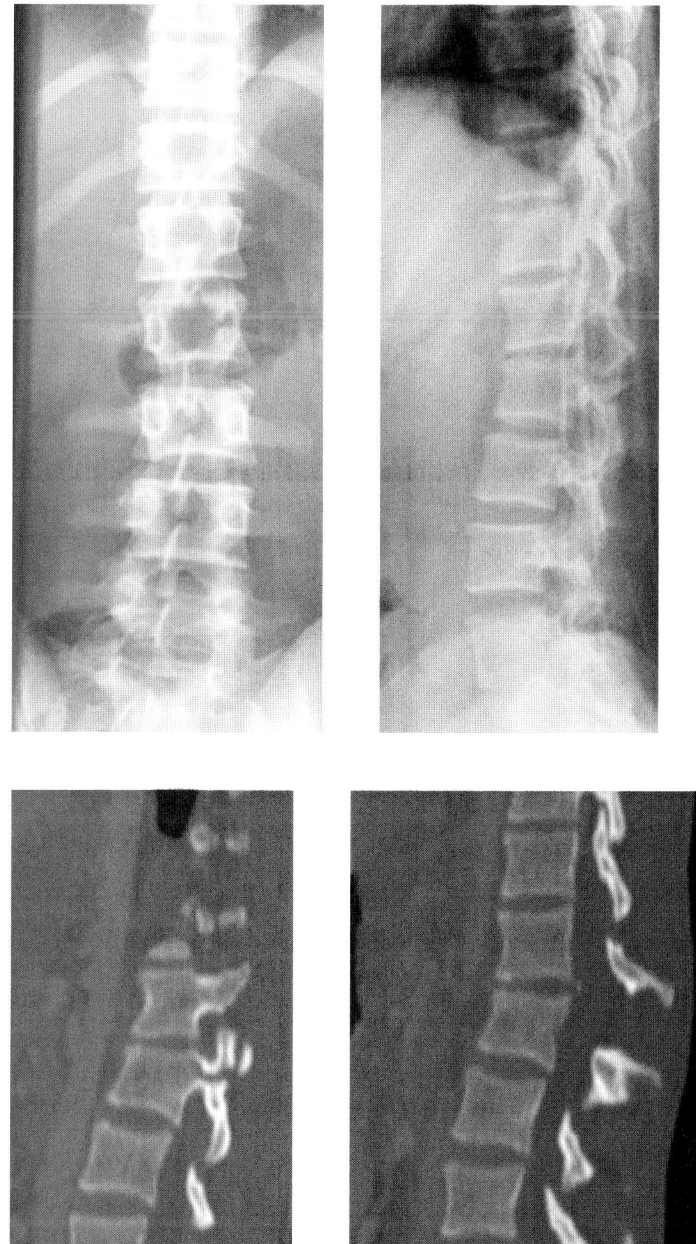

You are shown images of a blunt trauma patient.

1. What is the pathology shown?
2. What is the mechanism of the injury?
3. What other pathology is commonly associated with this finding?
4. Does a neurologic deficit commonly or uncommonly result from this injury?

CASE 86

Chance Fracture

1. Chance fracture of thoracic spine.
2. Hyperflexion-distraction.
3. Intra-abdominal injuries.
4. Uncommonly.

Reference

Bernstein MP, Mirvis SE, Shanmuganathan K: Chance-type fractures of the thoracolumbar spine: imaging analysis in 53 patients, *AJR Am J Roentgenol* 187: 859–868, 2006.

Cross-Reference

Emergency Radiology: THE REQUISITES, p 223.

Comment

The flexion-distraction fracture of the spine, described in 1948 by G.Q. Chance, is a horizontally oriented injury coursing through the posterior elements, pedicles, and vertebral bodies or through the intervertebral ligaments. Injuries can also course obliquely through the osseous and ligamentous structures of the spine. This injury became more common after placement and use of seat belts. By 1970, the connection between spine hyperflexion injuries and intra-abdominal visceral injuries was made, both deemed to result from forces caused by rapid deceleration against a restraining lap belt. The "seat belt syndrome" was designated to include both the characteristic thoracolumbar spine transverse fracture and abdominal injury.

Intra-abdominal injuries most commonly involve perforation or transection of small bowel and mesenteric lacerations, but colonic perforation, splenic rupture, pancreatic rupture, kidney rupture, liver rupture, and gravid uterine rupture have been reported. Intra-abdominal injuries occur in from 40% to 45% of patients with Chance fractures. The association of abdominal injuries with Chance-type fracture patterns is key to avoiding diagnostic delay of either injury.

Flexion-distraction injuries account for 5% to 15% of all thoracolumbar spine injuries occurring predominantly at or near the thoracolumbar junction. Injuries are often subtle radiographically and by computed tomography (CT), are unstable, and usually do not initially cause a neurologic deficit. Imaging findings include a "split pedicle" sign on the anteroposterior radiograph or coronal/sagittal CT MPR, the "dissolving pedicle" sign on axial images resulting from the intrapedicular fracture, the "naked" (uncovered) facet, flaring of or fracture through the spinous processes, increased vertical distance across the posterior intervertebral disc, and, typically, a compression fracture of the superior vertebral body. A common variant fracture demonstrating elements of both a classic Chance and the burst fracture has been reported. CT is more sensitive for the diagnosis since radiographic findings are often obscured by minimal fracture displacement and overlapping osseous structures. Magnetic resonance imaging can verify the extent of ligament injury, typically involving the posterior and middle columns, and assess for cord injury or hematoma.

Notes

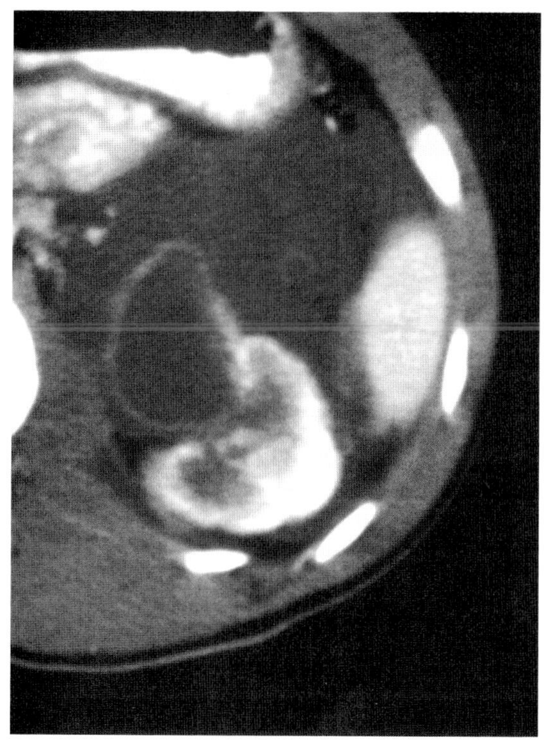

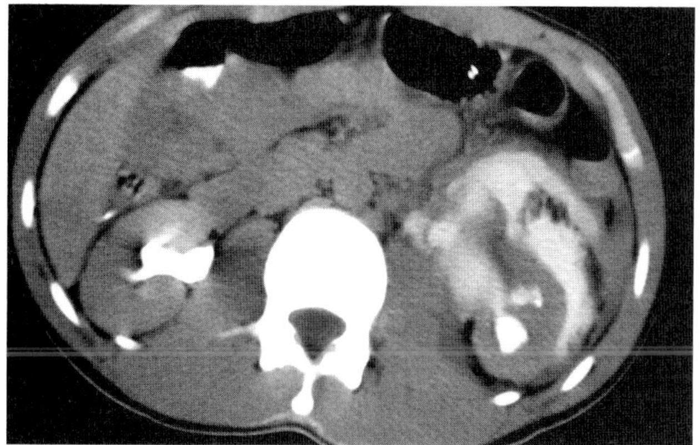

You are shown images of a blunt trauma patient.

1. What is the traumatic injury?
2. What is the most likely underlying pathology?
3. What other preexisting conditions predispose to renal or renal pelvis injury?
4. What is the most appropriate management for this condition?

CASE 87

Renal Pelvic Rupture with Congenital Ureteropelvic Junction Obstruction

1. Rupture of the renal pelvis.
2. Ureteropelvic junction (UPJ) obstruction predisposes to pelvic rupture from sudden increase in pressure at impact.
3. Renal tumor (benign or malignant), renal cysts, ectopic renal position (pelvic kidney, horseshoe), acquired collecting system obstruction (calculus, retroperitoneal fibrosis).
4. Surgical repair of renal pelvis and pyeloplasty. Nephrostomy can provide short-term management.

Reference

Sebastia MC, Rodriguez-Dobao M, Quiroga S, et al: Renal trauma in occult uretero-pelvic junction obstruction: CT findings, *Eur J Radiol* 9:611–615, 1999.

Cross-Reference

Emergency Radiology: THE REQUISITES, p 196.

Comment

Injury to the renal collecting system from blunt trauma typically involves the UPJ. Urine tends to extravasate anterior and medial to the proximal ureter. Absence of gross contrast extravasation on the nephrogram phase of a computed tomography (CT) study does not exclude a major collecting system injury. It is important to perform delayed CT imaging in the excretory phase (5 to 8 minutes after injection of contrast) whenever there is evidence of renal injury or perirenal fluid on the initial arterial CT phase. If the ureter below the injury level is opacified, the injury may often be managed successfully by stenting the injured area, but if there is no contrast seen in the distal ureter, meaning complete ureteral disruption, then surgical repair will be required. In most cases that we have seen in our practice, the renal parenchyma itself is intact in the presence of UPJ injury. Medial perinephric contrast material extravasation is highly suggestive of UPJ injury, and urine may also extend into the anterior pararenal space when Gerota's fascia is breached, as in the current case.

Preexisting renal pathology such as tumors, cysts, congenital or acquired obstruction to antegrade urine flow, and ectopic positioning of the kidney predispose to injury from a given impacting force compared with a normal kidney. In such cases, very careful inspection of the kidney is mandatory.

Notes

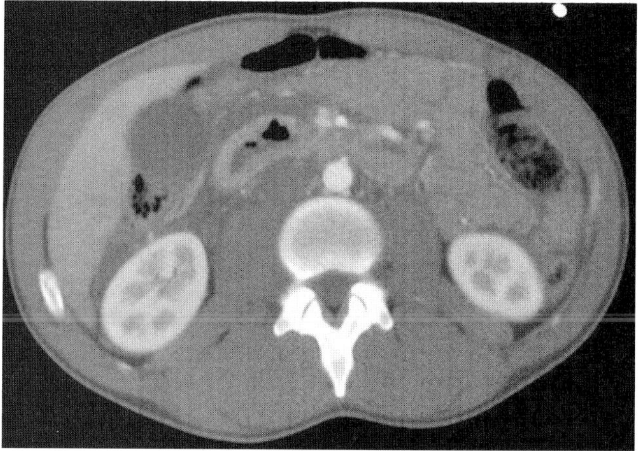

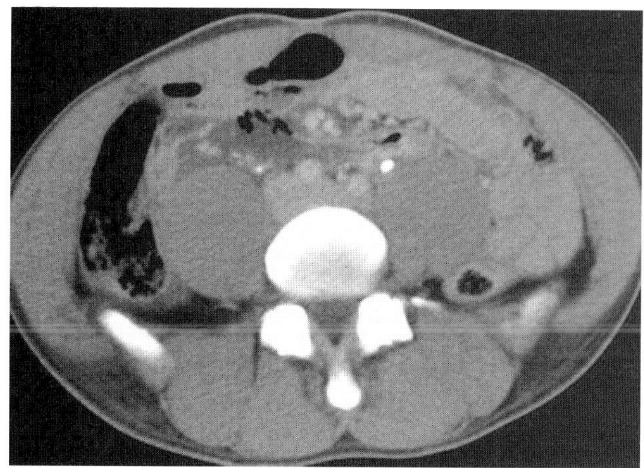

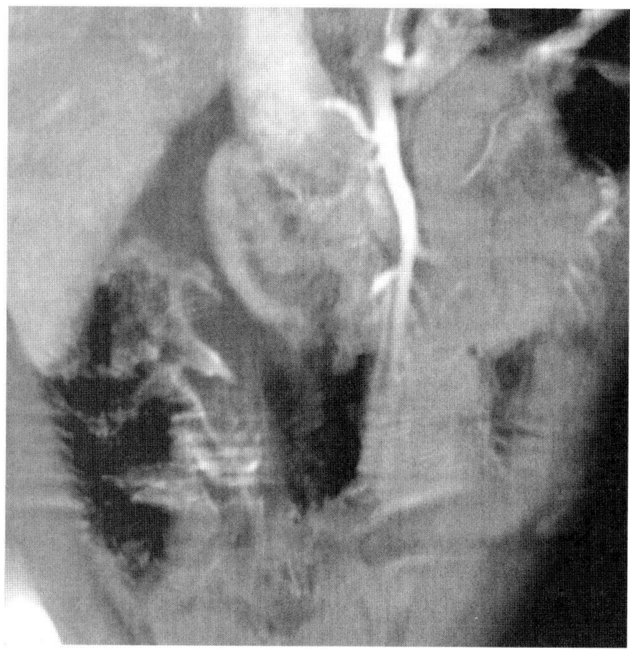

1. What is the diagnosis?
2. What is the mechanism of the injury?
3. What findings are evident on the images that establish the diagnosis?
4. Can computed tomography accurately predict need for surgical versus nonoperative management?

CASE 88

Full-thickness Duodenal Rupture (Blunt Trauma)

1. Duodenal rupture.
2. Crush injury between object impacting upper abdomen (seat belt, bike handlebar) and the spine.
3. Pneumoretroperitoneum and direct visualization of wall disruption.
4. Yes, computed tomography can distinguish duodenal contusion or hematoma from full-thickness injury in most cases.

References

Ballard RB, Badellino MM, Eynon CA, et al: Blunt duodenal rupture: a 6-year statewide experience, *J Trauma* 43:229–233, 1997.

Brofman N, Atri M, Epid D, et al: Evaluation of bowel and mesenteric blunt trauma with multidetector CT, *Radiographics* 26:1119–1131, 2006.

Cross-Reference

Emergency Radiology: THE REQUISITES, pp 93–97.

Comment

Rupture of the bowel from blunt trauma occurs in about 5% of trauma patients undergoing laparotomy. Bowel injury is the third most common abdominal organ injury after those of the liver and spleen. Injuries can result from crushing and shearing forces or are due to sudden increased intraluminal pressure. Injuries are most common in the proximal jejunum, near the ligament of Treitz and in the distal ileum, near the ileocecal valve. In general, areas of transition between relatively fixed and mobile segments of bowel predispose to shearing injury. Duodenal rupture occurs from impacts to the upper abdomen or abdominal compression from high-riding seat belts. It usually occurs from crushing of the duodenum between the spine and steering wheel, handlebar, or some other force applied to the anterior aspect of the abdomen. Patients with duodenal injury have concomitant surgically significant injuries in about 40% of cases including the liver (28%) and pancreas (38%).

Blunt duodenal injury was identified in 206 (0.2%) patients of more than 103,000 patients entered into a statewide trauma registry over a 6-year period. The second portion of the duodenum is the most commonly injured segment, and most blunt duodenal injuries do not result in full-thickness injury, but contusion or hematoma of the wall, which do not require surgical intervention. Computed tomography (CT) signs indicating full-thickness injury include visualization of a direct tear, extravasated air, or oral contrast in the retroperitoneum adjacent to the duodenum (usually right anterior pararenal space). Other findings such as fluid in the retroperitoneum, edema or hematoma of the duodenal wall, stranding of the peripancreatic fat, and pancreatic transection are nonspecific.

Notes

CASE 89

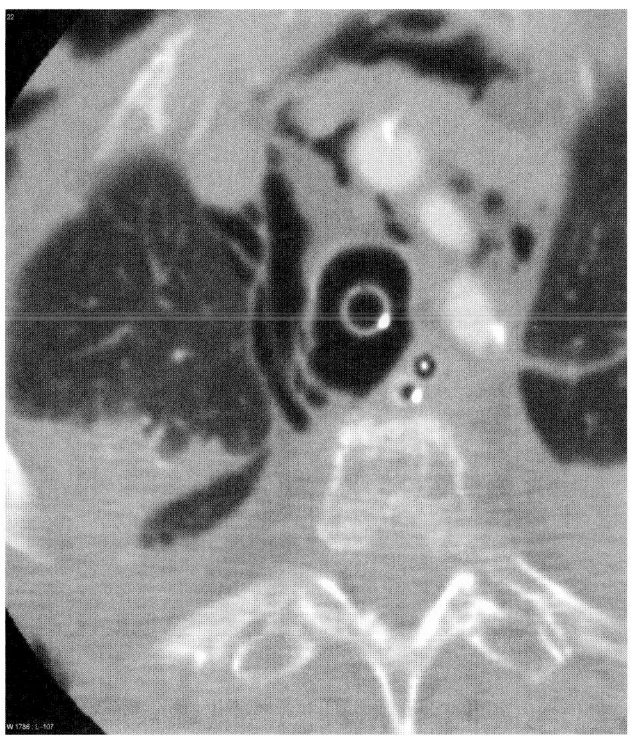

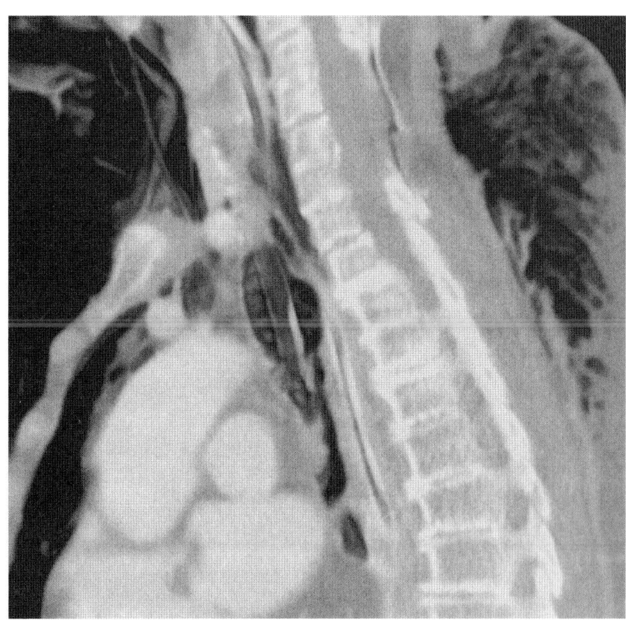

You are shown images of a blunt trauma patient.

1. What is the injury shown?
2. What is a "fallen lung" sign?
3. How can an endotracheal tube assist in the radiologic diagnosis?
4. What are the major proposed mechanisms of injury at this location?

CASE 89

Tracheal Rupture—Blunt Trauma

1. Thoracic tracheal rupture.
2. Complete tear of the mainstem bronchus with a dependent position of the collapsed lung in the pleural cavity.
3. The balloon cuff can be overdistended due to decreased resistance to expansion of injured airway or an ectopic position of the tube in relation to airway.
4. Compression of airway against a closed glottis increasing intraluminal pressure or direct compression of airway between sternum and spine.

Reference

Chen JD, Shanmuganathan K, Mirvis SE, et al: Using CT to diagnose tracheal rupture, *AJR Am J Roentgenol* 176:1273–1280, 2001.

Cross-Reference

Emergency Radiology: THE REQUISITES, pp 66–69.

Comment

Tracheobronchial injury (TBI) is uncommon, occurring in 0.4% to 1.5% of cases of major blunt trauma in clinical series and 2.8% to 5.4% in autopsy series of trauma victims. The majority of patients with this injury (80%) die in the prehospital period, indicating the seriousness of TBI and associated injury. The usual site of TBI is in close proximity to the carina. The thoracic trachea is more commonly involved than the cervical portion. A transverse acting force is far more likely to produce a tracheal disruption than a longitudinal (traction) force with most lacerations occurring in the transverse plane.

Imaging findings include mediastinal and soft tissue air, often severe and rapidly progressive, overdistention of the endotracheal tube (ETT) balloon, ectopic ETT position, direct visualization on computed tomography (CT) of an airway to mediastinal air tract, fractured tracheal ring, abnormal configuration of mainstem bronchus (cut-off or bayonet deformity), atelectasis, and pneumothorax. A rare sign of airway injury, the "fallen lung sign," refers to a dependent position of the collapsed lung in the pleural cavity due to complete tear of the mainstem bronchus.

Overdistention of the ETT balloon cuff results from the lack of resistance to distension by the injured tracheal wall. The diameter of the balloon should not exceed 2.8 cm in men and 2.1 cm in women. Manual rupture of the trachea by overexpansion of the ETT balloon is extremely unlikely, requiring 75 to 80 mL of air and great effort to instill it.

Thin-section CT and virtual "CT tracheography" are helpful in establishing the diagnosis of tracheal disruption. Early diagnosis is critical to improving the chances for a successful primary repair and satisfactory long-term outcome.

Notes

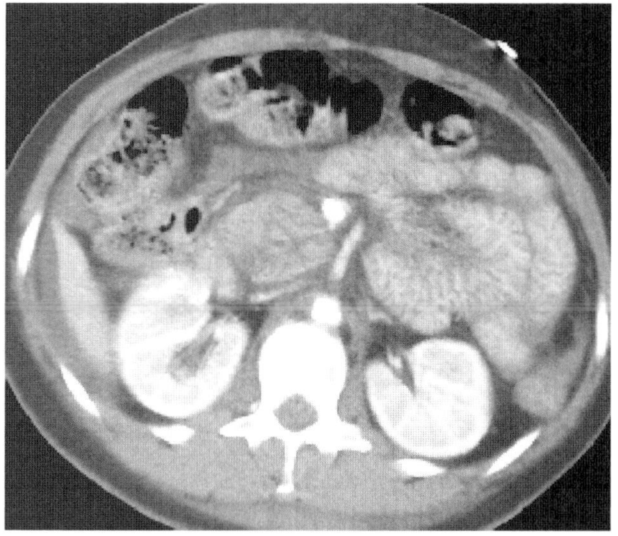

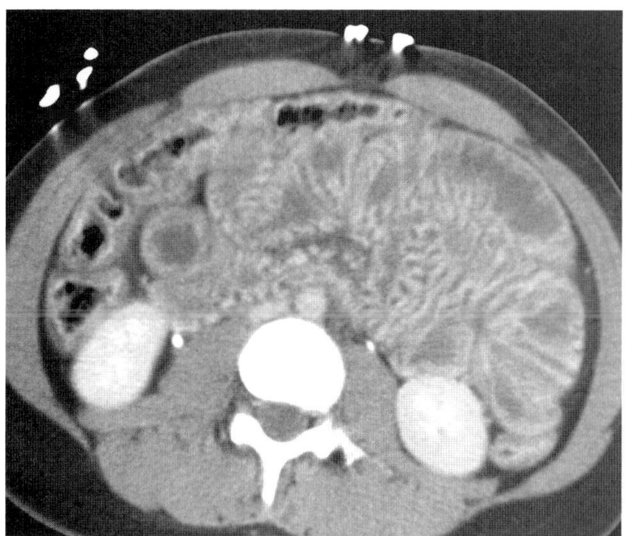

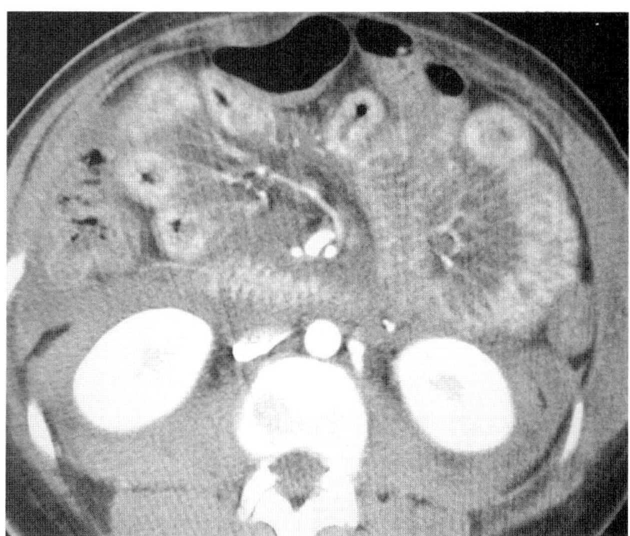

You are shown images of a blunt trauma patient.

1. What are the pathologic findings?
2. What is the etiology of this entity?
3. What other CT findings not shown in these images may be seen in this condition?
4. Does the bowel usually return to normal function with proper treatment of this condition?

CASE 90

Hypovolemic Shock Complex

1. Thickened small bowel wall and increased enhancement of bowel mucosa; dilated and fluid-filled small bowel, a flat inferior vena cava and small abdominal aorta, pancreatic swelling, small amount of retroperitoneal fluid; perihepatic free fluid.
2. Prolonged hypotension (status post cardiac arrest and/or persistent hemodynamic shock).
3. Hyperenhancement of the kidneys, adrenal glands, and major vessels; a halo of low attenuation fluid around the inferior vena cava; under- or nonperfused spleen/pancreas; mesenteric edema; increased enhancement of gallbladder mucosa.
4. Yes.

References

Mirvis SE, Shanmuganathan K, Erb R: Diffuse small-bowel ischemia in hypotensive adults after blunt trauma (shock bowel): CT findings and clinical significance, *AJR Am J Roentgenol* 163:1375–1379, 1994.

Ryan MF, Hamilton PA, Sarrazin J, et al: The halo sign and peripancreatic fluid: useful CT signs of hypovolemic shock complex in adults, *Clin Radiol* 60: 599–607, 2005.

Cross-Reference

Emergency Radiology: THE REQUISITES, p 99.

Comment

The hypoperfusion complex was initially described in severely injured children, typically under 2 years of age, and is usually associated with high morbidity. Findings indicate inadequate volume resuscitation and possible ongoing bleeding. The condition was subsequently recognized in older children and adults. A canine model of bowel hypoperfusion indicates that the bowel mucosa becomes increasingly permeable to albumin after blood flow is reduced to a point at which oxygen consumption is 50% or less than normal. Increased permeability to macromolecules develops after 1 to 4 hours of ischemia. Oxygen consumption is maintained, despite hypoperfusion, by an increase in oxygen extraction through diffusion and recruitment of capillary beds. The reduction in blood flow for periods of 2 hours does not affect oxygen consumption, so usually no permanent mucosal damage occurs.

The increase in capillary permeability coupled with initial resuscitation with crystalloid fluids and low intravascular volume probably explains the generalized increase in density of perfused mucosa (reflecting contrast leak and slow perfusion), the high density of vessels, and the generalized loss of low attenuation fluid into the bowel wall, mesentery, retroperitoneum, and peritoneal cavity. Usually with adequate restoration of intravascular volume and oxygen delivery no permanent injury to hypoperfused abdominal organs occurs.

Notes

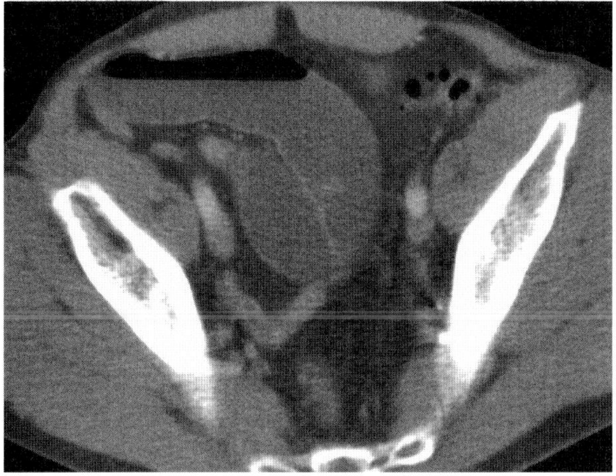

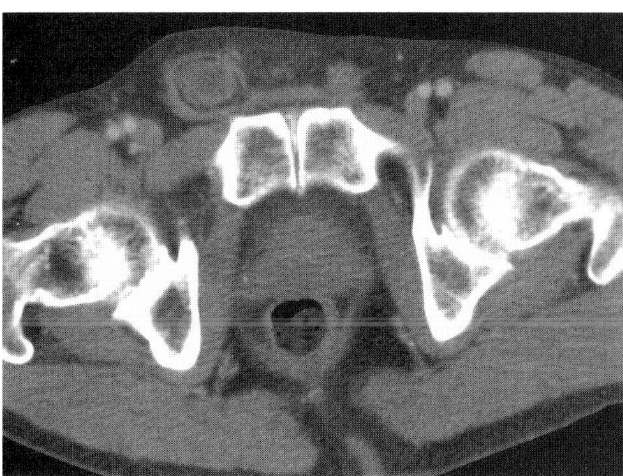

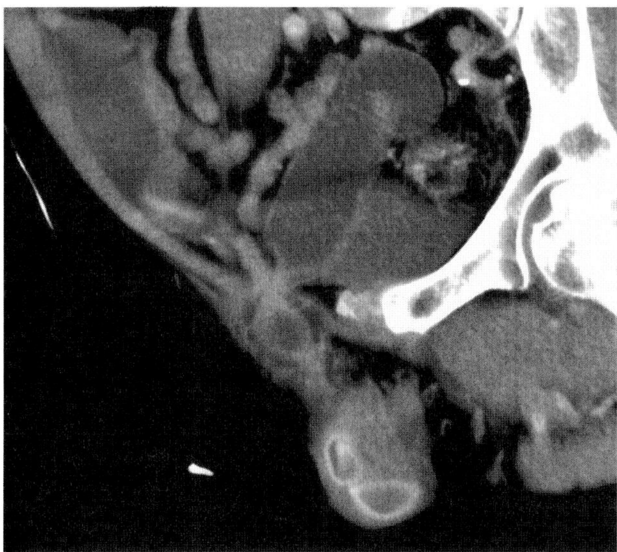

You are shown images of a nontrauma patient with lower abdominal pain and vomiting.

1. What is the diagnosis?
2. Name several CT signs of intestinal ischemia.
3. What is the most common cause of the entity shown in this case?
4. Is bowel contrast usually required for this diagnosis to be established?

CASE 91

Small Bowel Obstruction/Incarcerated Indirect Inguinal Hernia

1. Small bowel obstruction due to incarcerated indirect inguinal hernia.
2. Thickened bowel wall, ascites, "target" sign (trilaminar appearance of bowel wall resulting from IV contrast enhancement of the mucosal and muscularis layers, plus submucosal edema), poor or absent enhancement of bowel wall on IV contrast-enhanced scans, pneumatosis intestinalis and gas in mesenteric or portal veins, the "whirl" sign (twisting of mesenteric vasculature signifying volvulus), tortuous engorged mesenteric vessels, mesenteric hemorrhage, increased attenuation of bowel wall on noncontrast computed tomography.
3. Adhesions responsible for at least 60% to 70% of cases of small bowel obstruction.
4. No, fluid retained in the small bowel serves as intraluminal contrast. With complete obstruction the contrast is diluted by small bowel fluid, has prolonged transit time, and is difficult for the patient to consume.

References

Furukawa A, Yamasak M, Furuich K, et al: Helical CT in the diagnosis of small bowel obstruction, *Radiographics* 21:341–355, 2001.

Nicolaou S, Kai B, Ho S, et al: Imaging of acute small-bowel obstruction, *AJR Am J Roentgenol* 185: 1036–1044, 2005.

Cross-Reference

Emergency Radiology: THE REQUISITES, pp 276–279.

Comment

Typically, radiography is the first imaging procedure used in patients with possible bowel obstruction. Diagnostic accuracy of this modality in determining the presence of obstruction is only 46% to 80%, and accuracy in diagnosing the site and cause of obstruction and strangulation is even lower. Computed tomography (CT) clearly depicts pathologic processes involving the bowel wall, mesentery, mesenteric vessels, and peritoneal cavity. CT confirms the diagnosis (site and level) and cause of small bowel obstruction with 94% to 100% sensitivity and 90% to 95% accuracy. Causes of small bowel obstruction include extrinsic lesions, intrinsic lesions, intussusception, and intraluminal lesions. The most common cause of obstruction is adhesion (up to 75% of cases), followed by hernia and neoplasm. External hernia is produced by prolapse of viscera through a defect in the abdominal or pelvic wall. It usually involves a specific site of congenital weakness or previous surgery. Although visible or palpable hernias account for 95% of obstructive hernias, CT is useful in detecting hernias in unsuspected sites and in obese patients.

Identification of dilated proximal bowel and collapsed distal bowel is diagnostic for bowel obstruction. Small bowel with a caliber greater than 3 cm is considered dilated. The degree of bowel dilatation alone is not a reliable criterion for distinguishing bowel obstruction from an adynamic ileus. If a transition zone between the dilated proximal and collapsed distal bowel is detected, the diagnosis is more certain. The transition point often resembles a beak. The "small bowel feces" sign is another less common but reliable indicator of small bowel obstruction. The sign is a result of stasis and mixing of small bowel contents and is present in 82% of small bowel obstructions. The "string-of-pearls" sign may also be identified, caused by slow resorption of intraluminal air leaving small bubbles trapped between the folds of the valvulae conniventes.

Notes

CASE 92

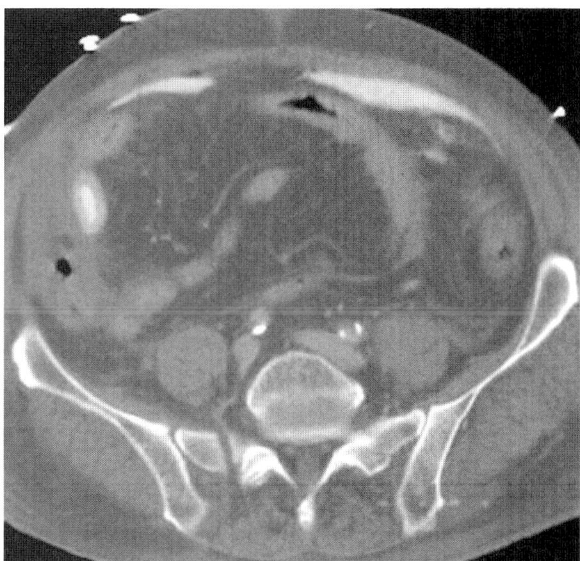

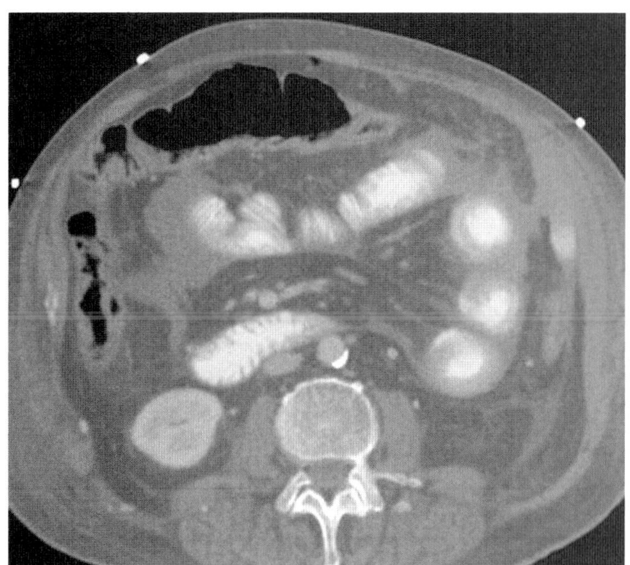

You are shown images of a blunt abdominal trauma patient.

1. What abnormal findings are present in this patient?
2. Does the patient require surgery?
3. What is the most likely site of injury, accounting for the nonskeletal abnormalities?
4. What two other entities commonly seen in blunt trauma cases could mimic or mask computed tomography signs of the pathology shown in this patient?

CASE 92

Full-thickness Bowel Perforation

1. Pneumoperitoneum, bowel wall thickening, extravasated oral contrast, intraperitoneal free fluid, mesenteric fluid around bowel loops, and right sacral fracture.
2. Yes.
3. Proximal jejunum.
4. Overexpansion of intravascular volume from resuscitation and prolonged shock can both produce some computed tomography findings that mask or mimic full-thickness bowel injury.

Reference

Brofman N, Atri M, Epid D, et al: Evaluation of bowel and mesenteric blunt trauma with multidetector CT, *Radiographics* 26:1119–1131, 2006.

Cross-Reference

Emergency Radiology: THE REQUISITES, pp 93–97.

Comment

Bowel and mesenteric injuries occur in approximately 5% of blunt trauma patients who sustain blunt abdominal trauma. Delay in diagnosis and treatment worsens prognosis with delays beyond 24 hours often leading to peritonitis, sepsis, uncontrolled hemorrhage, and potentially death. Physical findings of major bowel injury are often delayed in development, and classic symptoms such as rigidity, local tenderness, and decreased or absent bowel sounds are present as a triad in less than one third of patients. Computed tomography (CT) has become the major diagnostic study to diagnose bowel injury with a sensitivity ranging from 84% to 94% and accuracy from 84% to 99% for full-thickness tears. It is imperative that bowel injuries that require surgical repair be reliably excluded before attempting nonsurgical management of selected solid visceral injuries, as is increasingly becoming common practice.

CT findings of full-thickness injury in blunt trauma include pneumoperitoneum (without an extra-abdominal source), extravasastion of oral contrast material, if utilized, and direct identification of a bowel wall defect. Findings that are suspicious for bowel injury include intraperitoneal free fluid, bowel wall thickening, mesenteric contusion, and hematoma. The use of oral contrast prior to CT of the abdomen in trauma is controversial as regards improvement in diagnostic accuracy. However, it can help distinguish hematoma from unopacified bowel loops, outlines the stomach, duodenum, and pancreas clearly, and is very specific, but it is insensitive for full-thickness bowel injury. It is vital that abdominal CT images be reviewed in "CT windows" for the lung, to improve detection of small amounts of pneumoperitoneum. The location of the pneumoperitoneum is usually near the site of the bowel perforation, such as duodenal perforation leading to air in the porta hepatis. Air in the bowel wall, mesentery, and portal venous system also typically indicates wall disruption.

Notes

CASE 93

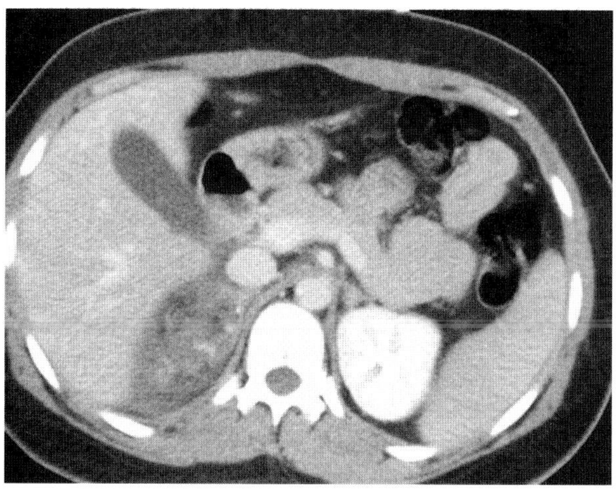

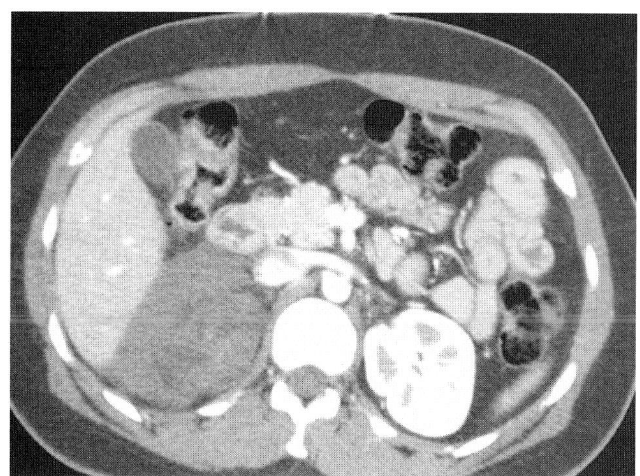

You are shown images of a patient with nontraumatic flank pain.

1. What is the diagnosis?
2. What therapeutic options are available?
3. Is the underlying lesion typically symptomatic?
4. What other typical pathologic feature is often present, but is not shown in this case?

CASE 93

Hemorrhage of Adrenal Myelolipoma

1. Spontaneous hemorrhage of right adrenal myelolipoma.
2. Observation, angiographic embolization, surgical excision.
3. No, it is usually incidentally diagnosed.
4. Calcifications.

References

Catalano O: Retroperitoneal hemorrhage due to a ruptured adrenal myelolipoma. A case report, *Acta Radiol* 37:688–690, 1996.

Rao P, Kenney PJ, Wagner BJ, Davidson AJ: Imaging and pathologic features of myelolipoma, *Radiographics* 17:1373–1385, 1997.

Cross-Reference

Emergency Radiology: THE REQUISITES, p 345.

Comment

Adrenal myelolipoma is a benign tumor composed of fat and bone marrow tissues and is usually found incidentally. Spontaneous rupture and bleeding of the myelolipoma is an infrequent complication, and can result in hematoma or, less commonly, a massive retroperitoneal hemorrhage compressing adjacent structures such as the inferior vena cava. Rarely, hemorrhagic tumors may produce life-threatening shock. Typically, patients present with sudden onset of flank pain. Microscopically, the tumor consists mainly of mature adipose tissue with scattered islands of hemopoietic cells. They are usually unilateral but may be bilateral (10%) and may also develop in extra-adrenal sites like the retroperitoneum, thorax, and pelvis. Hemorrhage is more common in larger lesions (diameter > 10 cm). Vascular embolization may be useful in treating or stabilizing the patient prior to definitive surgery.

These lesions are usually diagnosed incidentally on computed tomography (CT). A characteristic mass is lucent on plain radiographs, echogenic on ultrasound (US), shows fat attenuation on CT, is avascular at angiography, and has signal intensity similar to that of fat on T1-weighted magnetic resonance images. On T2-weighted images, myelolipomas were slightly hypointense to fat and either hypo- or isointense to the liver. Myelolipomas large enough to be detected by CT or US often contain macroscopic fat. In some cases a myelolipoma containing macroscopic quantities of nonfatty material (blood, calcium, and myeloid tissue) may have a nonspecific CT/US appearance, due to the fat inside being obscured by these elements. An absence of fat can render imaging findings nonspecific, requiring percutaneous needle biopsy. Other adrenal lesions in a differential diagnosis include renal angiomylolipoma, cystic teratoma, and liposarcoma.

Notes

CASE 94

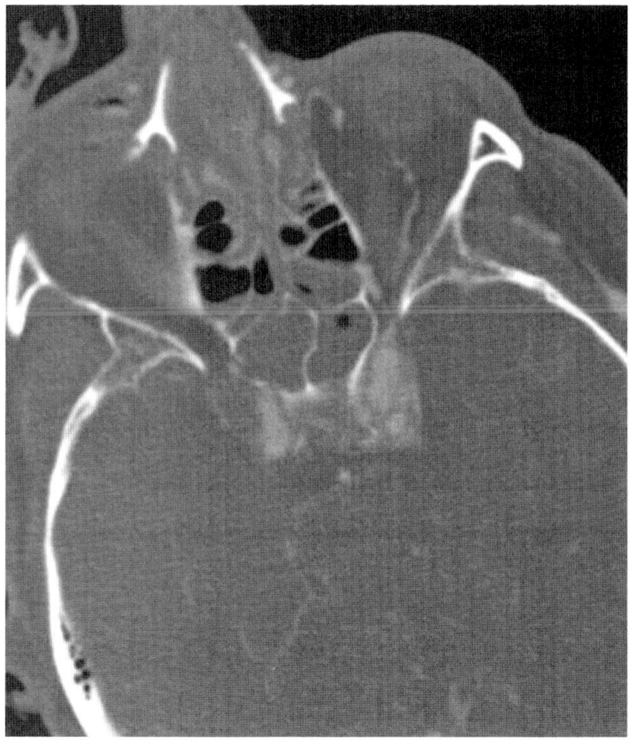

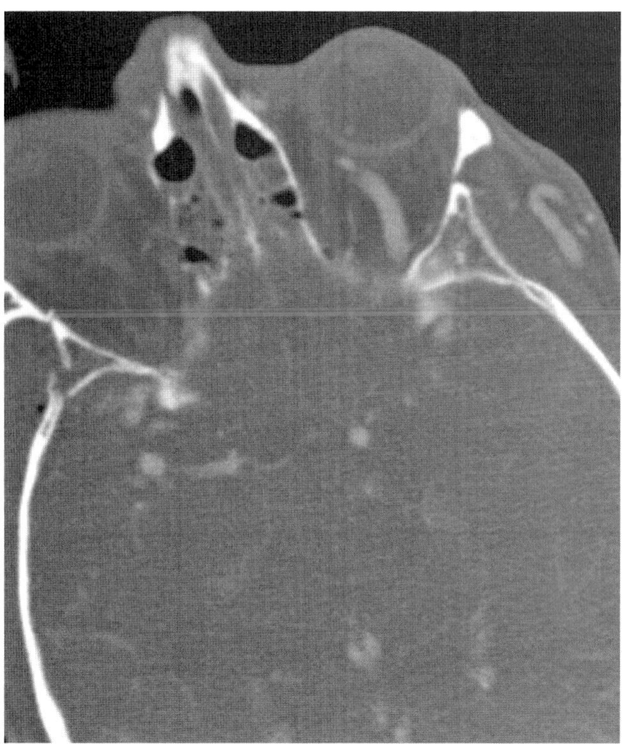

You are shown images of a blunt trauma patient.

1. What is the diagnosis?
2. What clinical signs and symptoms might be manifest?
3. Indications for urgent treatment of this injury include what?
4. What is the most common treatment for this injury?

CASE 94

Traumatic Carotid Cavernous Fistula

1. Traumatic carotid cavernous sinus fistula.
2. Chemosis, exopthalmous, headache, vision disturbance, diplopia, increased ocular pressure, and transcavernous cranial nerve palsies.
3. Increased intracranial pressure, cortical venous hypertension, deterioration in vision, increasing ocular pressure, and worsening proptosis.
4. Balloon or coil cavernous sinus occlusion of the fistula via arterial or venous route.

References

Halbach VV, Hieshima GB, Higashida RT, Reicher M: Carotid cavernous fistulae, *AJR Am J Roentgenol* 149:587–593, 1987.

Stallmeyer MJB: Vascular injury of the head and neck. In Mirvis SE, Shanmuganathan K, eds: *Imaging in Trauma and Critical Care*, Philadelphia, WB Saunders, 2003, pp 119–126.

Cross-Reference

Emergency Radiology: THE REQUISITES, p 20.

Comment

Traumatic carotid cavernous fistula (TCCF) is a rare vascular complication of brain and facial injury. Direct connections between the internal carotid artery and cavernous sinus may also develop as a consequence of ruptured intracavernous carotid aneurysms, collagen deficiency syndromes, arterial dissection, fibromuscular dysplasia, and direct surgical trauma. The mechanism of injury is thought to be a laceration of the cavernous carotid artery or one of its intracranial branches either by spicules of bone associated with fracture or penetrating injury or by rupture of the dural attachments located between the foramen lacerum and the anterior clinoid process. A relatively high incidence of TCCF occurs in trauma patients with middle fossa fractures, especially with a transverse or oblique orientation. Clinical signs and symptoms include headache, chemosis, exophthalmos, cranial nerve palsy, increased intraocular pressure, diplopia, and impaired vision. Cortical venous drainage from a TCCF is secondary to occlusion or absence of the normal venous outflow pathways and is associated with signs and symptoms of increased intracranial pressure and an increased risk of intraparenchymal hemorrhage.

Computed tomography and catheter angiographic findings include near simultaneous opacification of the cavernous carotid artery and cavernous sinus. Venous drainage occurs to the ipsilateral superior opthalmic vein and inferior petrosal sinus and to the contralateral venous sinus via the intercavernous sinus. Rarely, the arterialized venous drainage can lead to bilateral superior ophthalmic venous enlargement. Also, though infrequently, venous drainage to the cerebral cortical veins, mainly the sphenoparietal sinus or uncal vein, can produce cerebral venous hypertension and result in cortical venous ischemia or infarct. Surgical and angiographic techniques that have been described for the closure of CCFs include carotid occlusion; trapping procedures; direct surgical exposure and closure; and embolization with muscle, glue, thrombus, wires, and, more recently, detachable balloons. The transvenous coil occlusion of the superior and inferior ophthalmic veins and the cavernous sinus is also a highly efficient and safe treatment.

Notes

CASE 95

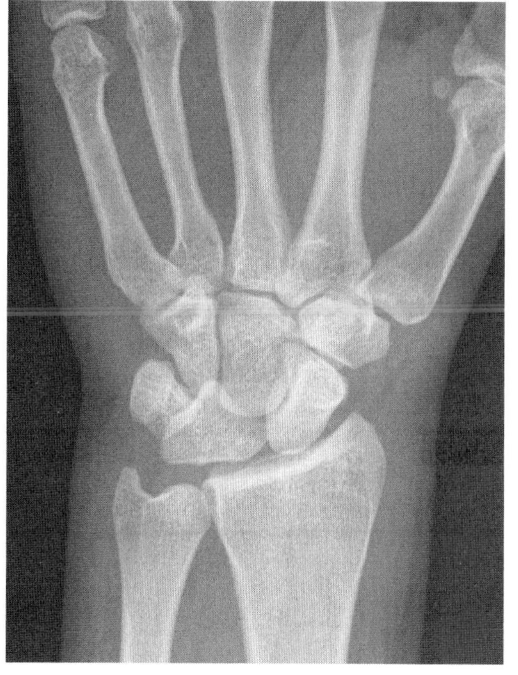

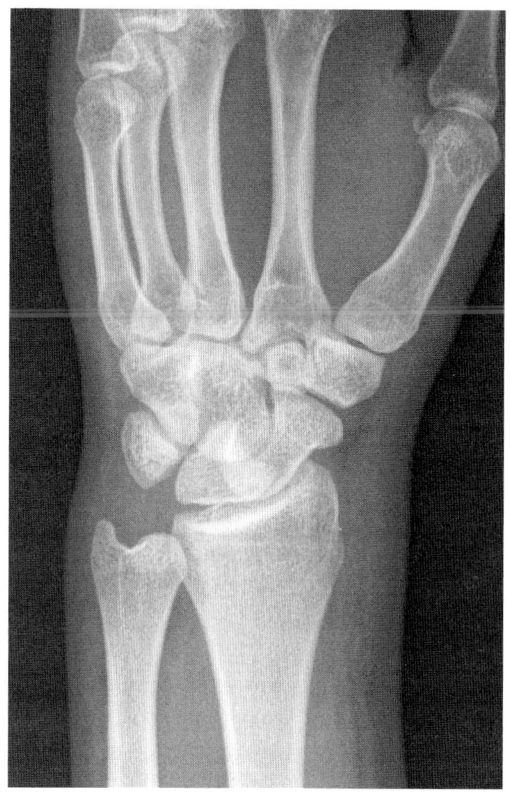

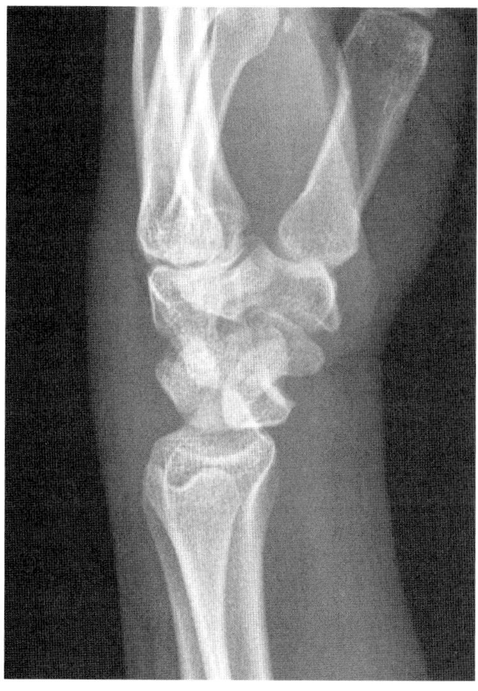

1. What is the diagnosis?
2. What is the mechanism of the injury?
3. Name three potential complications.
4. What is the most commonly associated fracture?

CASE 95

Lunate Dislocation

1. Lunate dislocation.
2. Hyperextension (fall on outstretched hand).
3. Residual ligamentous instability, lunate avascular necrosis, osteoarthrosis.
4. Trans-scaphoid fracture.

Reference

Barron D, Branfoot T: Imaging trauma of the appendicular skeleton, *Imaging* 15:324–340, 2003.

Cross-Reference

Emergency Radiology: THE REQUISITES, pp 131–133.

Comment

A lunate dislocation is a very rare injury, but is the most severe of carpal instabilities. It involves all the intercarpal joints with disruption of most of the carpal ligaments. When the injury is misdiagnosed, the prognosis is poor. The injury is most commonly associated with a trans-scaphoid fracture. The dislocation is caused by an acute hyperextension injury typically resulting from falls from heights.

Radiographs of the wrist are diagnostic. The key to identifying these injuries is careful inspection of the lateral radiograph. On a true lateral radiograph the middle metacarpal, the capitate, the lunate, and the radius should all line up. Any disruption in this pattern raises the possibility of a dislocation. In a true lunate dislocation the lunate rotates 90 degrees in a volar plane (facing anteriorly), thus losing both its radiolunate and capitolunate articulations. As a result of this the lunate comes to lie anterior to the line of the radius and capitate. All lunate dislocations show up on the anteroposterior radiograph, but this is much more difficult to interpret; usually the lunate loses its normal shape and adopts a "pie," or triangular, shape. The injury requires surgical reduction, ligament repair, and wire fixation. Complications include residual instability, osteoarthrosis, and lunate avascular necrosis.

In perilunate dislocation there is dislocation of the capitate, usually dorsally relative to the lunate, which maintains a normal relationship with the radius. Midcarpal dislocation is midway between lunate and perilunate with volar tilt of the lunate and slight dorsal dislocation of capitates; the lunate is not dislocated with respect to the distal radius.

Notes

CASE 96

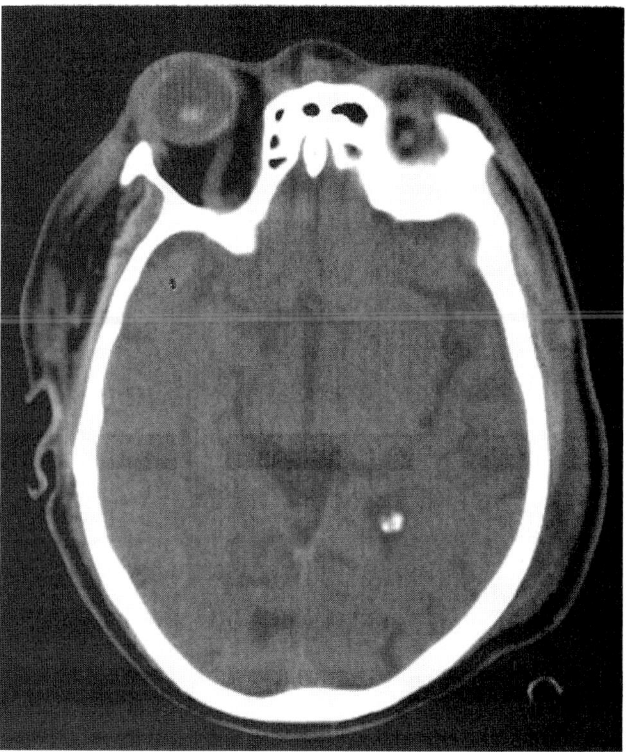

1. What is the diagnosis?
2. What symptoms may this patient have?
3. What is the mechanism of injury?
4. What are three potential complications of this injury?

CASE 96

Lens Dislocation

1. Lens dislocation.
2. The patient may be asymptomatic, have distorted or blurry vision, or have unilateral blindness.
3. Acceleration of the lens relative to the suspensory ligament with resultant tearing of the ligament and dislocation of the lens.
4. Retinal detachment, secondary glaucoma, and uveitis.

Reference

Asbury CC, Castillo M, Mukherji SK: Review of computed tomographic imaging in acute orbital trauma, *Emerg Radiol* 2:367–375, 1995.

Cross-Reference

Emergency Radiology: THE REQUISITES, p 39.

Comment

Trauma accounts for approximately 50% of all lens dislocations. Dislocation occurs due to acceleration of the lens relative to the suspensory ligament. The lens is most commonly displaced posterior into the vitreous humor. Less commonly, the lens dislocates into the anterior chamber.

Clinically, the patient may be asymptomatic, have blurry vision, or unilateral blindness. On noncontrast head or face computed tomography, the hyperdense biconvex lens is easily seen within the hypodense vitreous. The lens commonly settles into the dependent portion of the globe, but may be floating in the vitreous if still partially attached to the suspensory ligament. If there has been direct orbital trauma, periorbital soft tissue swelling, orbital fractures, or hemorrhage within the orbit or globe may be seen. Apparent mild retropulsion of the lens or "deepening" of the anterior chamber usually indicates rupture of the posterior sclera rather than true lens dislocation. Complications may develop, including retinal detachment, secondary glaucoma, or uveitis. These complications are due to rupture of the lens capsule and leakage of irritating material from the lens into the vitreous. Treatment of a lens dislocation may require surgical relocation or removal of the lens in order to salvage vision.

Notes

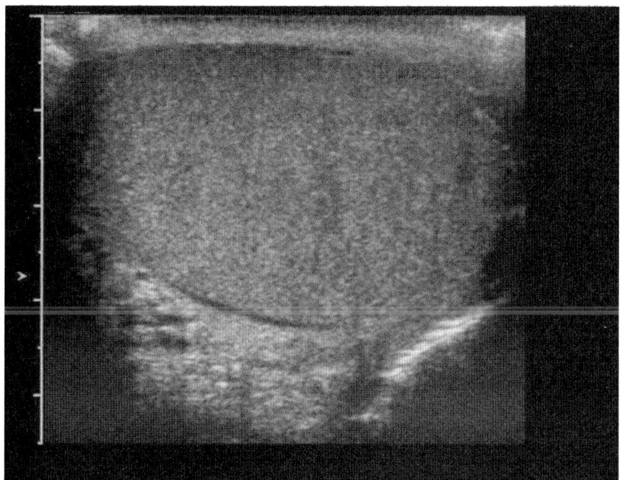

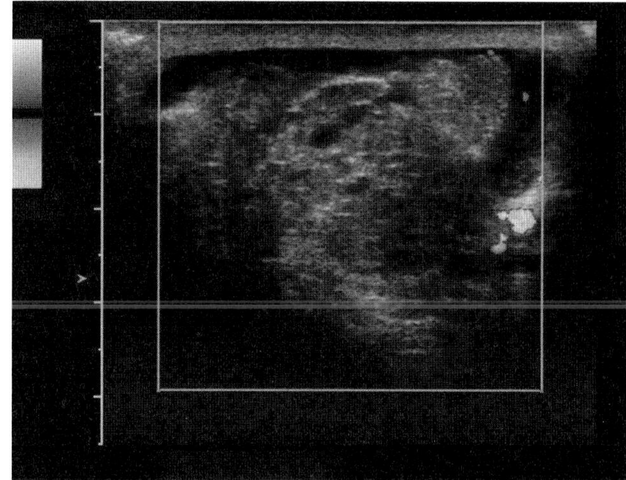

See also Color Plate

1. What are the findings on this testicular ultrasound of a 28-year-old male with acute onset of left-sided testicular pain?
2. What other radiologic test could be used to make this diagnosis?
3. What is the surgical salvage rate if the correct diagnosis is made within 6 hours of onset of symptoms?
4. What are two testicular ultrasound findings that may be seen if the correct diagnosis is not made promptly?

CASE 97

Testicular Torsion

1. Absence of vascular flow in the left testicle, indicating testicular torsion.
2. ^{99m}Tc pertechnetate radionuclide imaging.
3. 100%.
4. Complete absence of Doppler flow and heterogeneity within the testicle.

Reference

Dogra VS, Gottlieb RH, Oka M, et al: Sonography of the scrotum, *Radiology* 227:18–36, 2003.

Cross-Reference

Emergency Radiology: THE REQUISITES, pp 310–311.

Comment

Testicular torsion is most commonly seen in adolescent boys but can occur at any age. In teens and adults, torsion occurs within the tunica vaginalis. A predisposing factor for torsion is bell-clapper deformity, an anatomical variant in which the tunica vaginalis completely envelopes the testicle, distal spermatic cord, and epididymis rather than attaching to the posterior testicle. The testicle is then free to rotate and twist within the tunica vaginalis. Once the testicle torses, first venous and then arterial obstruction occurs, leading to testicular ischemia.

Symptoms of testicular ischemia include acute pain and swelling of the affected hemiscrotum, nausea, vomiting, and low-grade fever. Findings on clinical exam include a swollen, tender, and inflamed hemiscrotum. These signs and symptoms are similar to those seen in acute epididymo-orchitis, a major differential diagnosis. Testicular ultrasound is used to differentiate between these two entities and avoid unnecessary surgical exploration.

Both color ultrasound and power Doppler ultrasound should be used for maximum sensitivity in detection of vascular flow signal. Grey scale images may be completely normal in early cases or show only mild edema with increased echogenicity, both nonspecific findings. The finding of absence of intratesticular blood flow is considered diagnostic of testicular ischemia. However, due to intermittent or transient torsion, testicular torsion cannot be totally excluded in the presence of color or power Doppler signal in a patient with signs or symptoms highly suggestive of torsion. Ultrasound findings of a missed torsion include absence of Doppler flow and heterogeneity within the testicle, indicating hemorrhage and infarction.

Prompt and accurate diagnosis of testicular torsion is essential. The surgical salvage rate is 100% if the correct diagnosis if made within 6 hours of onset of symptoms, but drops to 20% if symptoms have been present for 12 to 24 hours.

Notes

CASE 98

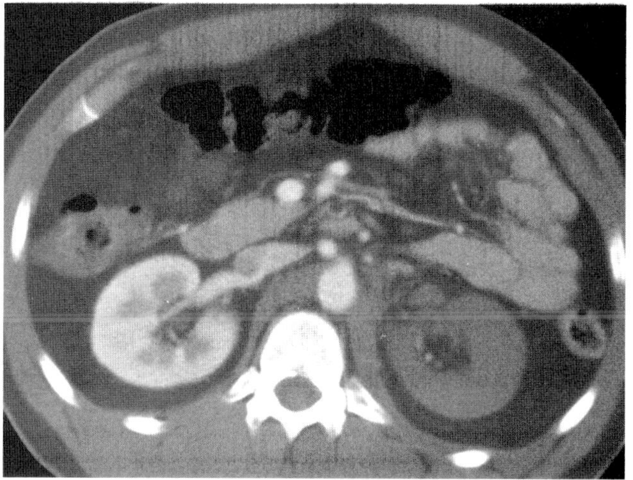

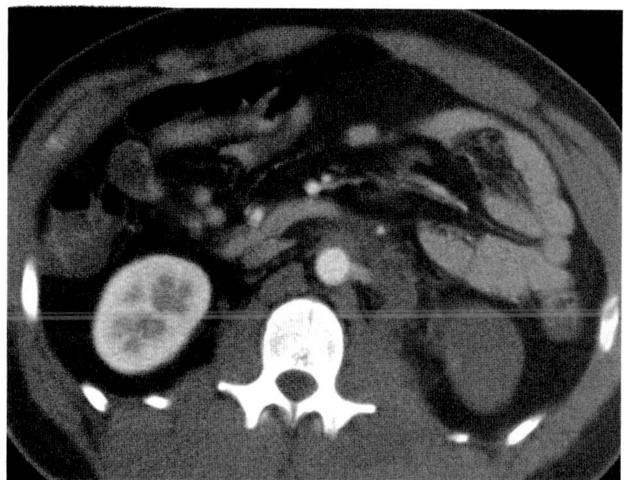

1. What is the diagnosis in this patient involved in a high-speed motor vehicle collision?
2. What is the computed tomography "rim" sign?
3. Irreversible ischemic changes within the kidney can be seen how soon after injury?
4. Name three treatment options for this injury.

CASE 98

Left Renal Infarction

1. Total left renal infarction due to renovascular injury.
2. Peripheral cortical enhancement of an otherwise infarcted kidney.
3. One hour.
4. Surgical revascularization, angiographic stenting, and expectant management.

References

Dowing JM, Lube MW, Smith CP, et al: Traumatic renal artery occlusion in a patient with a solitary kidney: case report of treatment with endovascular stent and review of the literature, *J Am Surg* 73:351–353, 2007.

Nunez D Jr, Becerra JL, Fuentes D, et al: Traumatic occlusion of the renal artery: helical CT diagnosis, *AJR Am J Roentgenol* 167:777–780, 1996.

Cross-Reference

Emergency Radiology: THE REQUISITES, pp 100–102, 344.

Comment

Renovascular injury is considered a major renal injury. This injury is rare, occurring in less than 1% of all patients sustaining blunt abdominal trauma. The mechanism of injury is usually sudden deceleration with stretching of the relatively inelastic intima leading to intra-arterial thrombosis or dissection. A direct blow to the abdomen can also cause renovascular injury due to compression of the renal artery against the vertebral column.

On clinical exam, there may be a flank contusion or abdominal/flank tenderness. Hematuria is absent in up to 25% of patients with a major renal injury and is thus a poor predictor of renal trauma.

Computed tomography (CT) with intravenous contrast is the modality of choice in evaluation of blunt renal injury. On CT, the infarcted kidney may be intact but smaller in size due to the lack of perfusion. There will be decreased or absent enhancement, depending on the presence of accessory renal arteries. Subtotal renal infarctions are wedge-shaped, with straight margins, and involve both the cortex and the medulla. A "rim" sign may be seen and refers to a thin rim of peripheral cortical enhancement in an otherwise nonenhancing kidney. The rim sign is a result of patent cortical arteries that originate from the renal artery proximal to the site of injury. The arterial injury or dissection typically occurs within the proximal third of the renal artery, and the exact site of injury can often be seen on axial or multiplanar reformatted images.

Prompt radiographic diagnosis of renovascular injury can decrease the warm ischemic time, an important factor in renal salvage. Irreversible ischemic changes can be seen in as little as 1 hour after injury. Treatment should generally occur within 4 hours of injury. The optimal treatment is unclear due to the rarity of this injury. Surgical revascularization, angiographic stenting, and expectant management have all been tried, with mixed results. Return of complete renal function is the exception in the vast majority of cases. Surgery or angiographic stenting is always attempted in those patients with a solitary kidney or those patients with bilateral renal artery injuries.

Notes

CASE 99

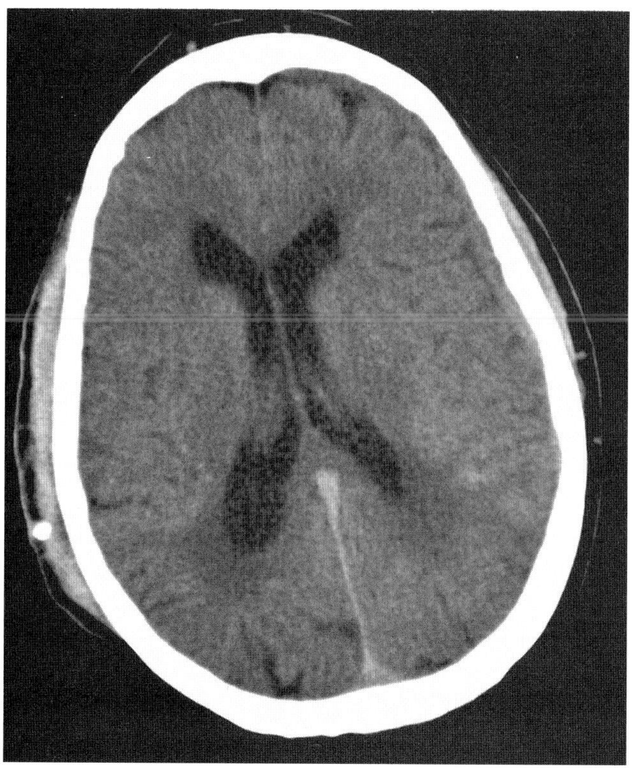

1. What kind of extra-axial collection is shown?
2. Based on the computed tomography density, approximately how long ago did the head trauma occur?
3. Name three other instances in which such a collection may be isodense to the brain.
4. What are the three most common intracranial locations where this type of collection is seen?

CASE 99

Subacute Left Subdural Hematoma

1. Left subdural hematoma.
2. One to three weeks prior.
3. Anemia, admixture of blood with cerebrospinal fluid, and hyperacute subdural hematomas only a few hours old. In the latter case, there may be isodense regions within the subdural hematoma due to the presence of uncoagulated blood.
4. Cerebral convexities, falx cerebri, and the tentorium cerebelli.

Reference

Provenzale J: CT and MR imaging of acute cranial trauma, *Emerg Radiol* 14:1–12, 2007.

Cross-Reference

Emergency Radiology: THE REQUISITES, pp 2–5.

Comment

Subdural hematomas (SDH) are accumulations of blood between the dura and arachnoid meningeal layers. They are often the result of tearing of bridging cortical veins at the time of trauma but may also result from rupture of an adjacent intraparenchymal hematoma into the subdural space. Subdural blood extends along the cerebral convexities and may also spread along the tentorium or falx. Acute subdural blood (less than 1 week from time of trauma) will be hyperdense on computed tomography (CT) in comparison to the underlying brain and measure 50 to 100 Hounsfield units (HU) in density. At 1 to 3 weeks after injury the SDH is categorized as subacute and will appear isodense to brain parenchyma and measure 25 to 45 HUs in density. A chronic SDH is more than 3 weeks old and will appear hypodense (HU = 0–25) due to lysis of red blood cells.

CT is the test of choice to evaluate for the presence of a SDH. The three most common sites for a SDH are the cerebral convexities, the falx cerebri, and the tentorium cerebelli. A SDH along the convexity is typically crescent shaped and will not cross the midline. In contrast to epidural hematomas, subdural hematomas will cross suture lines. On CT, the junction between the inner table of the skull and the cortex of the brain should be carefully examined to detect a small isodense SDH. The peripheral sulci may be effaced or abnormally separated from the inner table of the skull. Additional signs to look for include the presence of midline shift without apparent cause and inward displacement of cortical veins if contrast-enhanced head CT images have been performed. In questionable cases, the use of magnetic resonance imaging (MRI) can be advantageous in detection of very small or isodense subdural hematomas due to its superior multiplanar imaging capabilities. On MRI, subacute SDHs are often hyperintense to brain on T1-weighted images and of variable signal intensity compared with brain on T2-weighted images.

Notes

CASE 100

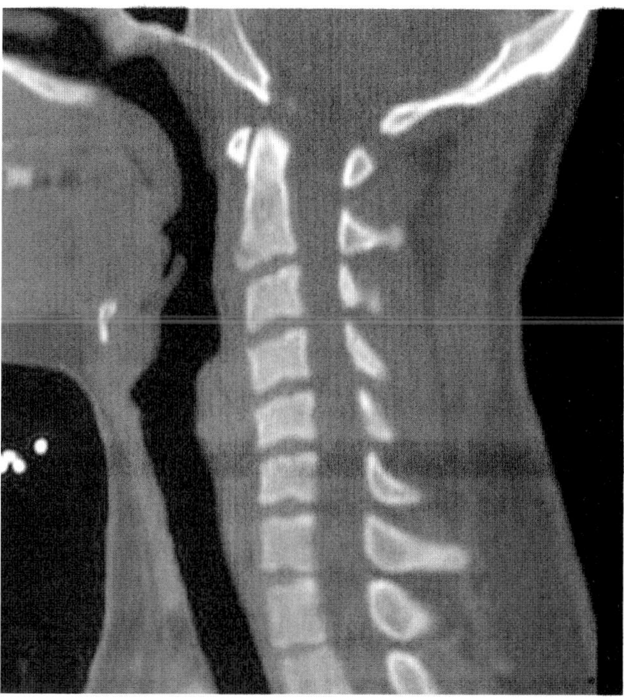

1. What is the mechanism responsible for this cervical spine injury?
2. How does this injury differ between young and elderly patients with regard to cervical level typically affected and likelihood of neurological deficit?
3. Name three types of preexisting cervical spine conditions that predispose a patient to a cervical spine hyperextension injury.
4. What is acute central cord syndrome?

CASE 100

C2 Hyperextension Teardrop Fracture

1. Hyperextension.
2. If this injury occurs in an elderly patient, it will most commonly involve the C2 vertebra. In this case, there is often little prevertebral soft tissue swelling or neurological deficit. In younger patients, it will more commonly occur in the lower cervical spine, with extensive prevertebral soft tissue swelling and a high rate of spinal cord injury.
3. Ankylosing spondylitis, diffuse idiopathic skeletal hyperostosis (DISH), and severe degenerative disc disease.
4. Acute central cord syndrome is characterized by loss of motor function affecting the upper extremities much more than the lower extremities and loss of distal upper extremity pain and temperature sensation.

Reference

Rao SK, Wasyliw C, Nunez DB Jr: Spectrum of findings in hyperextension injuries of the neck, *Radiographics* 25:1239–1254, 2005.

Cross-Reference

Emergency Radiology: THE REQUISITES, pp 220–221.

Comment

Hyperextension injuries account for up to 26% of all cervical spine injuries. They result from a direct anteroposterior force striking the head or face. A hyperextension teardrop fracture is an avulsion of an anteroinferior vertebral endplate. The anterior longitudinal ligament remains intact and the bone to which it is attached fractures, resulting in a characteristic teardrop-shaped bone fragment.

This fracture most commonly occurs at the C2 level in elderly patients and is stable in the vast majority of cases. If this injury occurs in a younger patient it frequently involves the lower cervical spine and there is a higher rate of cord injury. Up to 80% of those patients with a neurological deficit from cord injury will present with acute central cord syndrome.

A lateral cervical spine radiograph will show the triangular fracture fragment adjacent to the involved vertebral endplate. The height of this fracture fragment is characteristically greater than its width. Anterior disc space widening and prevertebral soft tissue swelling may also be present. Concurrent hyperextension injuries such as hangman fracture or posterior C1 arch fractures are common. Cervical spine computed tomography may be especially useful in younger patients to better characterize the fracture and evaluate for additional fractures. Magnetic resonance imaging is used to evaluate the integrity of the cervical spine ligaments and determine the presence or extent of spinal cord injury.

Notes

CASE 101

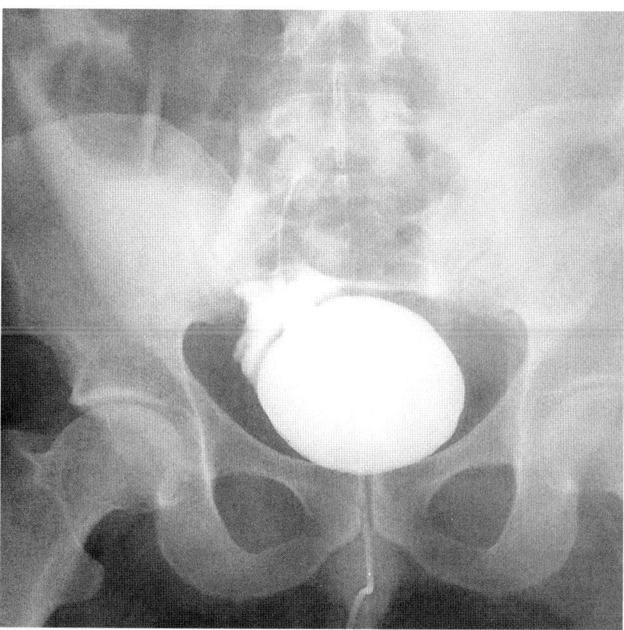

1. What are the findings?
2. Name two radiologic methods used to make the diagnosis of bladder rupture.
3. What is the treatment for intraperitoneal bladder rupture? Extraperitoneal rupture?
4. What volume of contrast material must be instilled into the bladder to reliably exclude a bladder rupture?

CASE 101

Intraperitoneal Bladder Rupture

1. There is extravasation of contrast from the right superior urinary bladder, with contrast material surrounding bowel loops in the lower abdomen.
2. Standard cystography and CT-cystography.
3. Intraperitoneal bladder rupture is treated surgically while extraperitoneal rupture is treated with Foley catheter placement.
4. 250 to 300 mL.

References

Chan DP, Abujudeh HH, Cushing GL Jr, et al: CT cystography with mulitplanar reformation for suspected bladder rupture: experience in 234 cases, *AJR Am J Roentgenol* 187:1296–1302, 2006.

Mirvis SE: Trauma. In Advances in Uroradiology II, *Radiol Clin North Am* 34:1225–1257, 1996.

Cross-Reference

Emergency Radiology: THE REQUISITES, pp 103–105.

Comment

Urinary bladder rupture occurs in up to 10% of patients sustaining pelvic fractures. Rupture may be categorized as intraperitoneal, extraperitoneal, or mixed intraperitoneal-extraperitoneal. Intraperitoneal rupture accounts for 15% to 45% of all bladder ruptures. Typically, the dome ruptures after a full bladder has sustained blunt force, with subsequent urine extravasation into the peritoneal cavity. Gross hematuria may or may not be present.

The diagnosis of bladder rupture can be made with cystography or computed tomography (CT)–cystography. In standard cystography, at least 250 mL of 30% iodinated contrast material is instilled into the bladder via a Foley catheter. In male patients, urethral injury must first be excluded. Scout, full bladder, and postvoid anteroposterior views of the pelvis are obtained. If a pelvic angiogram is anticipated for treatment of active pelvic bleeding, the cystogram should be performed after the angiogram. This avoids retained soft tissue or intraperitoneal contrast-obscuring visualization during the angiographic procedure.

CT-cystography has been found to be more sensitive compared with standard cystography in detection of bladder rupture. While techniques vary, at our institution, CT-cystography is done immediately following a standard CT of the abdomen and pelvis that has been performed for evaluation of intra-abdominal trauma. 40 mL of nonionic IV contrast material is instilled into a 500-mL IV bag of normal saline. At least 250 mL of this mixture is then infused into the bladder via a Foley catheter. The Foley is clamped and a CT of the pelvis is then performed. The bladder is drained and a postvoid scan through the pelvis is completed.

Intraperitoneal bladder rupture is diagnosed on both standard cystography and CT-cystography by the presence of contrast material within the peritoneal cavity. Contrast material will be seen outlining loops of bowel and layering in the peritoneal recesses. Treatment of intraperitoneal bladder rupture is surgical. Delay in diagnosis and treatment may lead to acidosis, uremia, or peritonitis.

Notes

CASE 102

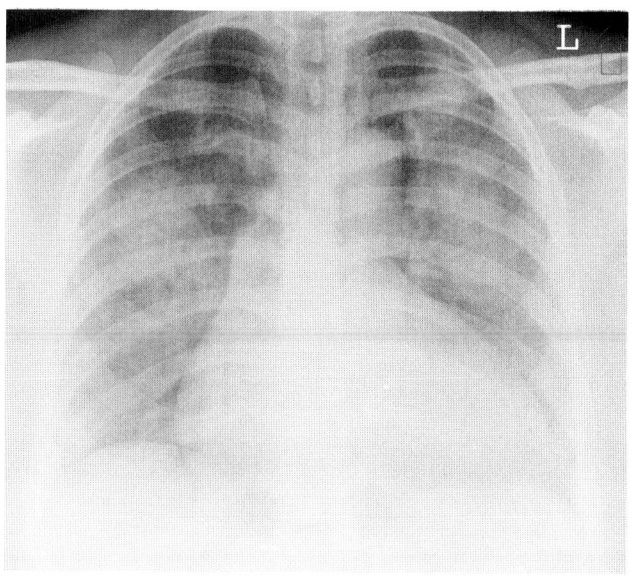

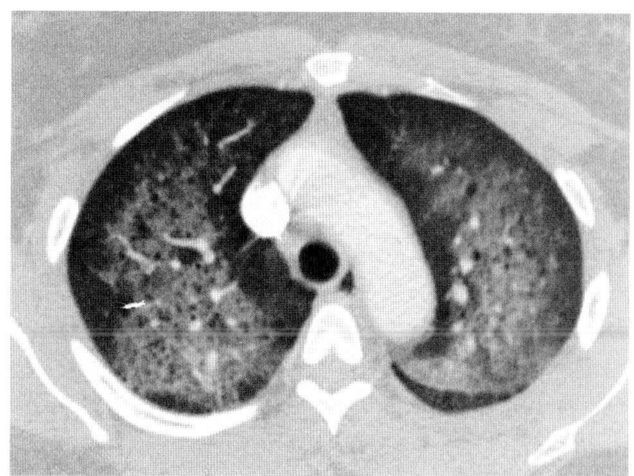

1. What are the findings on the chest radiograph and chest CT of this 49-year-old HIV-positive patient with a cough and hypoxia?
2. What is the most likely diagnosis?
3. What is the differential diagnosis?
4. True or false: The incidence of this condition has steadily increased in the AIDS population in the past 10 years.

CASE 102

Pneumocystis Pneumonia

1. Bilateral perihilar ground glass densities.
2. Pneumocystis pneumonia (PCP).
3. Community-acquired or bacterial pneumonia, cryptococcal pneumonia, or aspergillus infection.
4. False. The incidence of PCP has declined due to widespread use of antibiotic prophylaxis.

References

Boiselle PM, Crans CA Jr, Kaplan MA: The changing face of *Pneumocystis carinii* pneumonia in AIDS patients, *AJR Am J Roentgenol* 172:1301–1309, 1999.

Waite S, Jeudy J, White CS: Acute lung infections in normal and immunocompromised hosts, *Radiol Clin North Am* 44:295–315, 2006.

Cross-Reference

Emergency Radiology: THE REQUISITES, p 236.

Comment

Pneumocystis pneumonia (PCP) is caused by *Pneumocystis jiroveci*, previously known as *Pneumocystis carinii. P. jiroveci* is thought to be a fungus rather than a protozoan as initially classified. PCP is rare in the general population and mainly affects immunocompromised patients such as those with AIDS, organ transplant recipients, or patients on long-term steroid therapy. PCP is considered an AIDS-defining illness. It is estimated that up to 60% of all AIDS patients will present with PCP. Overall, the incidence of PCP has declined due to widespread use of antibiotic prophylaxis.

The typical clinical presentation is an immunocompromised patient, with a CD4 cell count less than 200/μL, who presents with hypoxia. Gradual onset of malaise, weight loss, fever, dry cough, and dyspnea may also be present. Classic chest radiographic findings are bilateral perihilar air space disease or increased reticular markings. Chest computed tomography is more sensitive than radiography in demonstrating parenchymal changes. In addition to perihilar ground glass density, a "crazy paving" pattern may be seen and is due to thickened interlobular septae. Upper lobe pneumatoceles are common and predispose the patient to spontaneous pneumothorax. There is a characteristic absence of pleural effusion. Definitive diagnosis of PCP is made by sputum or bronchoscopic sampling for microscopy and culture.

Notes

CASE 103

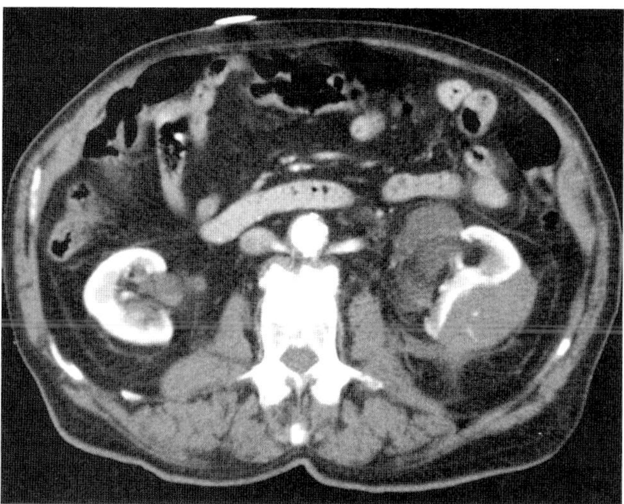

1. What is the diagnosis?
2. Name two other solid organs in which this condition can be seen.
3. True or false: A kidney with a preexisting abnormality, such as a horseshoe kidney, renal cell carcinoma, or angiomyolipoma, is at increased risk for renal trauma compared with a completely normal kidney.
4. What is a Page kidney?

CASE 103

Left Renal Subcapsular Hematoma with Active Bleeding

1. Renal subcapsular hematoma with focus of active bleeding.
2. Liver and spleen.
3. True.
4. A Page kidney is a rare complication of a renal subcapsular hematoma in which the hematoma results in hypertension.

References

Al-Qudah HS, Santucci RA: Complications of renal trauma, *Radiol Clin North Am* 41:1019–1035, 2003.
Miller LA, Shanmuganathan K: Multidetector CT evaluation of abdominal trauma, *Radiol Clin North Am* 43:1079–1095, 2005.

Cross-Reference

Emergency Radiology: THE REQUISITES, pp 99–100.

Comment

Renal subcapsular hematomas are infrequently seen due to the strong attachment between the renal capsule and the underlying parenchyma. Etiologies include blunt or penetrating trauma or iatrogenic injury from renal biopsy or lithotripsy. Patients may have flank pain or tenderness, hematuria, or be completely asymptomatic. On contrast-enhanced computed tomography, a subcapsular hematoma is crescent shaped and indents the underlying kidney. There may be an associated renal laceration or perirenal hematoma. Delayed renal perfusion may be seen due to increased resistance to arterial perfusion. Active bleeding within the subcapsular hematoma may be seen rarely and may require angiographic embolization or surgery for control of bleeding.

A Page kidney is an unusual complication of a renal subcapsular hematoma that results from compression of the kidney by the hematoma. Local ischemia causes activation of the renin angiotensin aldosterone axis resulting in hypertension from salt and water retention. The vast majority of subcapsular hematomas resolve without treatment. Treatment of a patient with hypertension due to a Page kidney will depend on the age of the hematoma. If the hematoma is acute, the patient may be started on angiotensin-converting enzyme inhibitors to control blood pressure while waiting for the hematoma to resolve. For those cases in which the hematoma does not resolve and the patient remains hypertensive, a subcapsular hematoma may be drained percutaneously if the blood within the hematoma is still in a liquid state. If the chronic subcapsular hematoma becomes calcified a partial or total nephrectomy may be required for control of blood pressure.

Notes

CASE 104

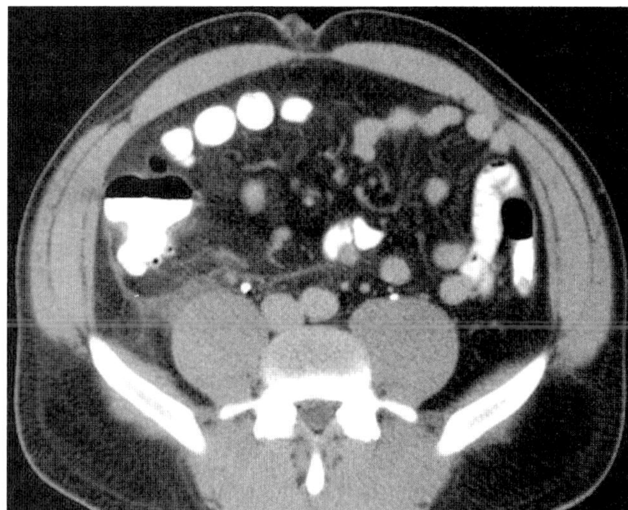

1. What are the computed tomography findings?
2. What is the pathogenesis of this condition?
3. What is the "halo" sign?
4. True or false: This condition is self limited in the vast majority of cases.

CASE 104

Cecal Diverticulitis

1. Pericecal fat stranding and fluid seen adjacent to a few cecal diverticuli consistent with the diagnosis of cecal diverticulitis.
2. A colonic diverticulum is a herniation of the mucosa through the muscularis propria. If the neck of the diverticulum becomes obstructed (usually from a fecalith) diverticulitis may result.
3. This is a computed tomography (CT) sign that suggests cecal diverticulitis rather than malignancy. The "halo" sign refers to preservation of the normal colonic wall layers on CT despite the inflammatory changes. In malignancy, the normal colonic wall layers may be disrupted or indistinct.
4. True. Treatment is generally conservative.

References

Jhaveri KS, Harisinghani MG, Wittenberg J, et al: Right-sided colonic diverticulitis: CT findings, *J Comput Assist Tomogr* 26:84–89, 2002.

Junge K, Marx A, Peiper C, et al: Caecal diverticulitis: a rare differential diagnosis for right-sided lower abdominal pain, *Colorectal Dis* 5:241–245, 2003.

Cross-Reference

Emergency Radiology: THE REQUISITES, p 285.

Comment

Although uncommon compared with conditions such as appendicitis or enteritis, cecal diverticulitis should not be forgotten as a possible etiology of acute onset of right lower quadrant pain. Up to 14% of all colonic diverticuli are localized to the right colon, usually near the ileocecal valve. In contrast to sigmoid diverticulitis, cecal diverticulitis usually results from a solitary diverticuli and is more common in younger patients, with up to 50% occurring in patients less than 30 years old. Right-sided diverticulitis is also more common in the Asian population.

Although not always possible, it is important to differentiate cecal diverticulitis, cecal malignancy, and acute appendicitis on computed tomography (CT) since the treatment of each of these conditions is different. The best way to exclude acute appendicitis is to see a normal appendix. The characteristic appearance of cecal diverticulitis on contrast-enhanced CT is an inflamed diverticulum that enhances more than the remainder of the adjacent normal colonic wall. Pericolonic fat stranding and focal colonic wall thickening are frequently present. Abscess or extraluminal air from a microperforation of the diverticulum may also be seen. These findings can also be seen in cecal malignancy. The CT "halo" sign can help to differentiate cecal diverticulitis and malignancy. This sign refers to preservation of the normal colonic wall layers on CT despite the inflammatory changes. In malignancy, the normal colonic wall layers may be disrupted or indistinct.

Notes

CASE 105

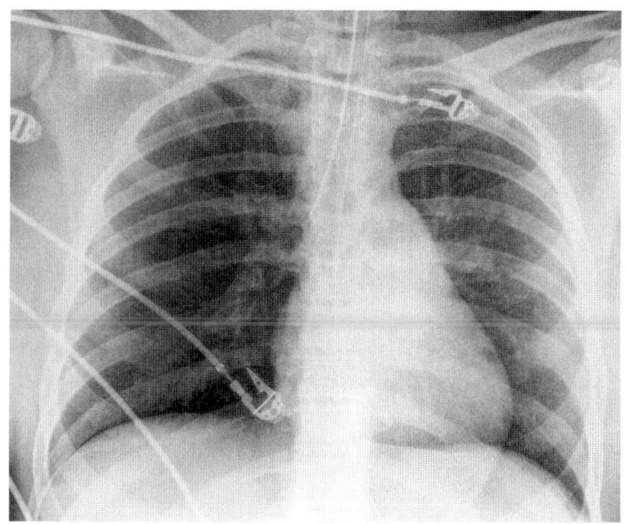

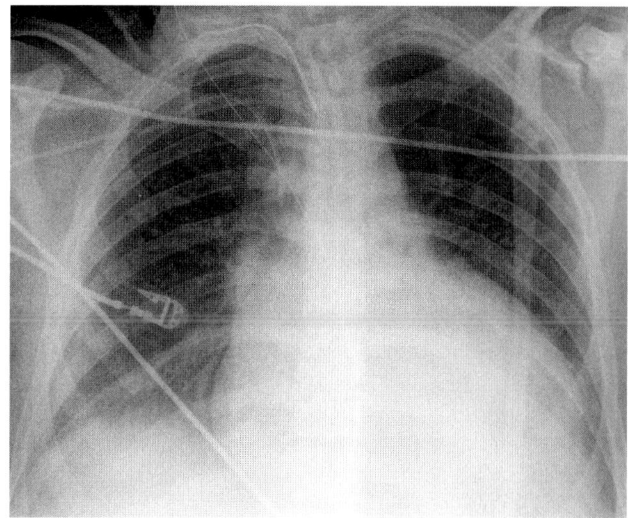

1. What is the finding on the second chest radiograph of a 19-year-old trauma patient who demonstrated new signs of low cardiac output on hospital day 16? The first radiograph was taken on the day of admission.
2. What are three causes of this condition?
3. With computed tomography, how could the use of Hounsfield unit (HU) measurements of this condition help narrow the differential diagnosis?
4. If this patient exhibits tachycardia, muffled heart tones, and distended neck veins, what clinical diagnosis should be suspected?

CASE 105

Pericardial Effusion

1. "Water bottle" enlargement of the cardiac silhouette due to pericardial effusion. This finding can also be seen with dilated cardiomyopathy.
2. Causes of simple pericardial effusions include heart failure, renal insufficiency, pericarditis, and collagen vascular disease. Hemopericardium may be the result of penetrating trauma, aortic dissection, or myocardial infarction.
3. A simple or serous effusion will have Hounsfield units (HU) of 0 to 15. HUs higher than this indicate hemorrhage, pus, or complex fluid due to malignancy.
4. Cardiac tamponade.

References

Goldstein L, Mirvis SE, Kostrubiak IS, et al: CT diagnosis of acute pericardial tamponade after blunt chest trauma, *AJR Am J Roentgenol* 152:739–741, 1989.

Wang ZJ, Reddy GP, Gotway MB, et al: CT and MRI imaging of pericardial disease, *Radiographics* 23: S167–S180, 2003.

Cross-Reference

Emergency Radiology: THE REQUISITES, p 244.

Comment

A pericardial effusion refers to accumulation of fluid between the parietal and visceral layers of the pericardium. This space normally contains less than 50 mL of serous fluid. Abnormal collection of fluid is due to obstruction of the venous or lymphatic drainage from the heart muscle. Common causes of serous pericardial effusions include heart failure, renal insufficiency, pericarditis, and collagen vascular disease. Causes of hemopericardium include penetrating and blunt chest trauma, aortic dissection, and myocardial infarction. The classic chest radiograph finding associated with pericardial effusion is a "water bottle" shaped cardiomediastinal silhouette. This term refers to symmetric enlargement of the heart shadow. Chest computed tomography (CT) is often used in the emergency/trauma setting for evaluation of a suspected pericardial effusion on chest radiograph. A simple or serous effusion will have Hounsfield units (HU) of 0 to 15. HUs higher than this indicate hemorrhage, pus, or complex fluid due to malignancy.

If enough fluid collects in the pericardial space, generally greater than 150 to 200 mL, cardiac tamponade may result, with a critically diminished cardiac output. Clinical signs of cardiac tamponade include tachycardia, muffled heart tones, and distended neck veins. CT signs of cardiac tamponade include a large pericardial effusion with flattening of the underlying heart muscle, distention of the vena cava or renal veins, and periportal edema.

Notes

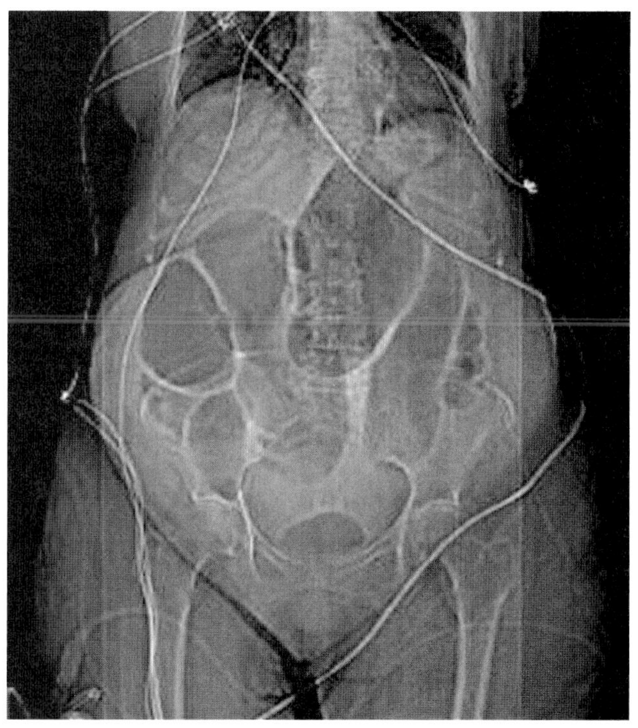

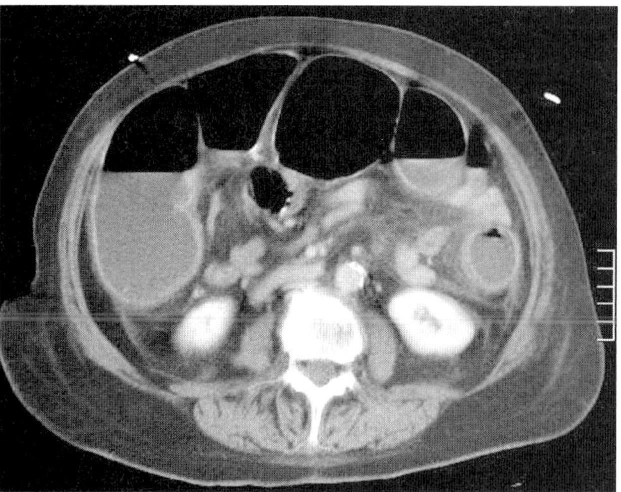

1. What is the likely cause of the findings in this 50-year-old female patient who developed abdominal pain, diarrhea, and abdominal distention 48 hours after being placed on antibiotics for treatment of pneumonia?
2. What is the "accordion" sign?
3. What is the "target" sign?
4. Name three additional findings that can be seen on abdominopelvic computed tomography with this disease process.

CASE 106

Toxic Megacolon

1. Toxic megacolon in association with pseudomembraneous colitis.
2. The "accordion" sign describes the computed tomography appearance seen when oral contrast is trapped between folds of thickened colon.
3. The "target" sign refers to two layers of different density within the thickened colonic wall. The mucosa enhances due to hyperemia and is high density while the submucosa is low density due to edema.
4. Colonic distension greater than 6 cm, pericolonic stranding, ascites, pneumoperitoneum, and segmental or pancolonic wall thickening.

References

Imbriaco M, Balthazar EJ: Toxic megacolon: role of CT in evaluation and detection of complications, *Clin Imaging* 25:349–354, 2001.

Kawamoto S, Horton KM, Fishman EK: Pseudomembraneous colitis: spectrum of imaging findings with clinical and pathologic correlation, *Radiographics* 19: 887–897, 1999.

Cross-Reference

Emergency Radiology: THE REQUISITES, p 279.

Comment

Toxic megacolon is a serious, potentially life-threatening complication of colitis. The condition is characterized by diffuse nonobstructive colonic dilatation in association with colitis and systemic sepsis. Although toxic megacolon has traditionally been seen as a complication of ulcerative colitis, it can be a complication of any inflammatory or infectious condition of the colon. More recently, the widespread use of broad-spectrum antibiotics has led to a steady increase in toxic megacolon associated with pseudomembraneous colitis. The mortality rate can be as high as 64%.

The most common finding on an abdominal radiograph is distension of the colon greater than 6 cm, usually involving the ascending and transverse portions of the colon. "Thumb printing" of the colon may also be seen, a term reflecting thickening of the colonic haustral folds. Additional radiographic findings include colonic air–fluid levels and gastric or small bowel distention. Pneumoperitoneum may be seen if colonic perforation has occurred.

Computed tomography (CT) is more sensitive compared with radiographs in detecting small amounts of free air in cases of colonic perforation, and also better displays the length and severity of the colitis. Additional CT findings seen in toxic megacolon include ascites, pericolonic stranding, and colonic wall thickening. The "accordion" sign refers to the appearance of oral contrast trapped in folds of thickened colon. The "target" sign may also be seen and describes the appearance of two layers of different density within the thickened colonic wall: the high-density enhancing mucosa due to hyperemia and the edematous low-density submucosa.

In cases of toxic megacolon due to pseudomembraneous colitis, definitive diagnosis is made once *Clostridium difficile* toxins are detected in a stool sample. Treatment includes oral metronidazole or vancomycin.

Notes

CASE 107

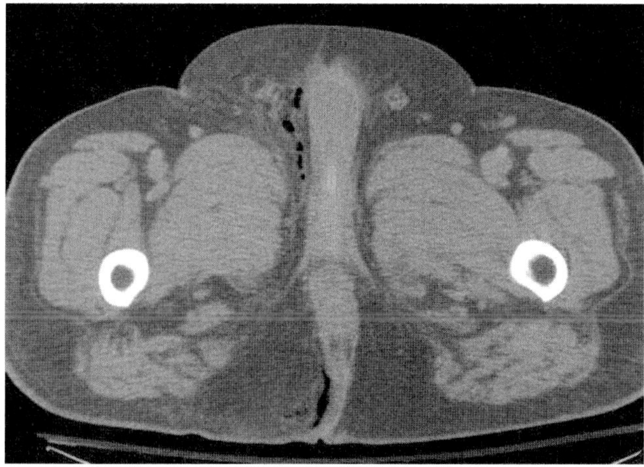

1. What are the findings?
2. In the absence of penetrating trauma, what is the likely diagnosis?
3. True or false: Computed tompgraphy will accurately define the anatomical extent of tissue involvement of this condition.
4. What are risk factors for this disease?

CASE 107

Fournier Gangrene

1. Fat stranding, skin thickening, and soft tissue gas within the medial right buttock. Soft tissue gas is also seen in the right side of the penis.
2. Fournier gangrene.
3. False. Macroscopic findings, including mushy or obviously necrotic tissue, lack of bleeding, and noncontracting muscle are typically used at time of surgery to guide the extent of débridement.
4. Injection drug use, diabetes mellitus, obesity, and immunosuppression are risk factors, but up to 50% of cases occur in previously healthy patients.

References

Anaya DA, Dellinger EP: Necrotizing soft tissue infection: diagnosis and management, *Clin Infect Dis* 44:705–710, 2007.

Cainzos M, Gonzalez-Rodriguez FJ: Necrotizing soft tissue infection, *Curr Opin Crit Care* 13:433–439, 2007.

Cross-Reference

Emergency Radiology: THE REQUISITES, pp 174–175.

Comment

Necrotizing soft tissue infection (NSTI) is the term given to an infection of any layer of the soft tissues including the dermis, subcutaneous fat, fascia, or muscle. The infection is characterized by widespread necrosis and is typically rapidly progressive. Fournier gangrene is a form of NSTI, which affects the penis, scrotum, or perineum.

Although uncommon, NSTI is highly lethal, carrying a mortality rate of 24%, and is a radiologic and surgical emergency. Patients often have a recent history of a trivial wound and present with swelling, erythema, and pain out of proportion to the appearance of the affected site. The infection can progress rapidly to blister formation, ecchymosis, crepitus due to subcutaneous gas, and signs of sepsis.

Establishing the diagnosis can be challenging since the early findings are similar to more common soft tissue infections like cellulitis or abscess. On radiographs, the presence of subcutaneous gas is a specific but late sign of NSTI and may not be present in all cases. Contrast-enhanced computed tomography can better determine the extent of subcutaneous gas and may demonstrate thickened, enhancing fascia and fat stranding. Ultrasound of the scrotum can be used in the diagnosis of Fournier gangrene and will show scrotal thickening, soft tissue edema, and hyperechoic foci of gas in the subcutaneous tissue. NSTI is treated with aggressive surgical débridement.

Notes

CASE 108

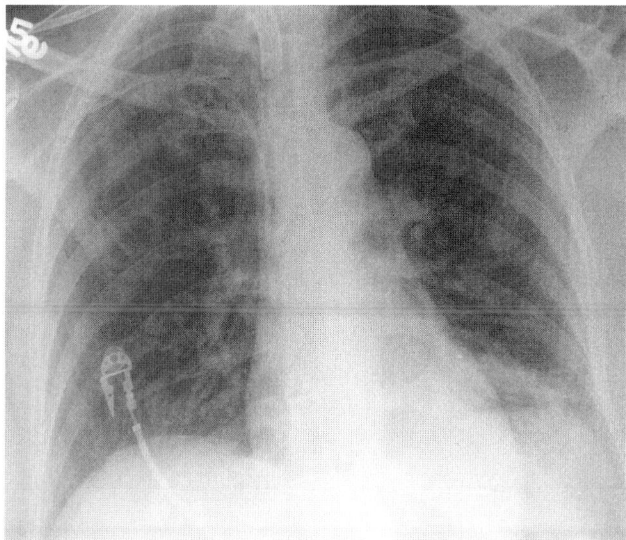

1. What are the findings on this chest radiograph of a 69-year-old patient with a chronic cough?
2. What is the most common material associated with this condition?
3. Foreign bodies usually lodge in what airway locations in the adult population?
4. True or false: No further workup is needed in cases of suspected foreign body aspiration if the radiologic evaluation is normal.

CASE 108

Aspirated Foreign Body

1. Patchy opacity in the left lower lung zone with a punctate radiopaque foreign body overlying the left cardiac border. These findings represent an aspirated foreign body with left lower lobar atelectasis.
2. Food. In children, peanuts are the most common foreign body aspirated. In adults, additional considerations often include pills, teeth, or dental work.
3. The right lower lobe bronchus or bronchus intermedius due to the vertical course of the right-sided airway.
4. False. In all cases of suspected aspiration with inconclusive radiologic findings, bronchoscopy must be performed to exclude the diagnosis.

References

Kavanaugh PV, Mason AC, Muller NL: Thoracic foreign bodies in adults, *Clin Radiol* 54:353–360, 1999.

Patel S, Kazerooni EA: Case 31: foreign body aspiration—chicken bone, *Radiology* 218:523–525, 2001.

Cross-Reference

Emergency Radiology: THE REQUISITES, pp 202–203.

Comment

In the United States, 500 to 2000 deaths per year are caused by foreign body aspiration. Seventy-five percent of all cases of foreign body aspiration occur in children younger than 3 years old. In this population, the foreign body usually lodges in the central airway and is often a non-radiopaque organic material, most commonly a peanut. In adults, the peak incidence of foreign body aspiration is in the sixth decade. Risk factors in adults include neurologic dysfunction, facial trauma, intubation, and alcohol consumption. The foreign body usually lodges in the peripheral airway in adults and is most commonly food, dental work, teeth, or pills. The diagnosis may be remote to the aspiration event and may be undetected for weeks or years, or misdiagnosed as bronchitis or asthma.

All cases of suspected foreign body aspiration should initially be evaluated with lateral neck and posteroanterior and lateral chest radiographs. Radiographic findings in the acute setting include hyperinflation, atelectasis, and visualization of the foreign body. The films may also be completely normal. Chronic chest radiograph findings include atelectasis, post-obstructive pneumonia, bronchiectasis, lung abscess, or empyema. Computed tomography (CT) is far more sensitive than radiographs in demonstrating a radiolucent foreign body. In children, CT is of limited usefulness since sedation is often required, putting the child at risk of airway compromise. In all cases of suspected aspiration with inconclusive radiologic findings, bronchoscopy is used as the next step in the diagnosis, and ultimately the treatment, of this condition.

Notes

CASE 109

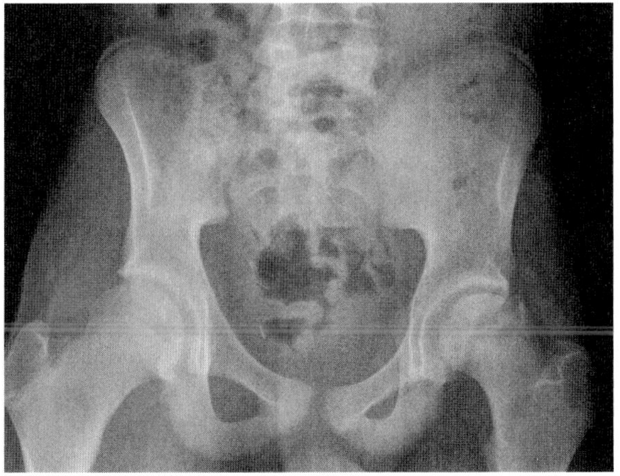

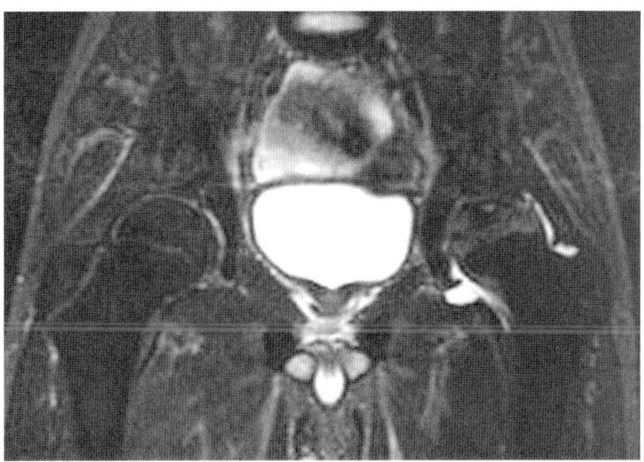

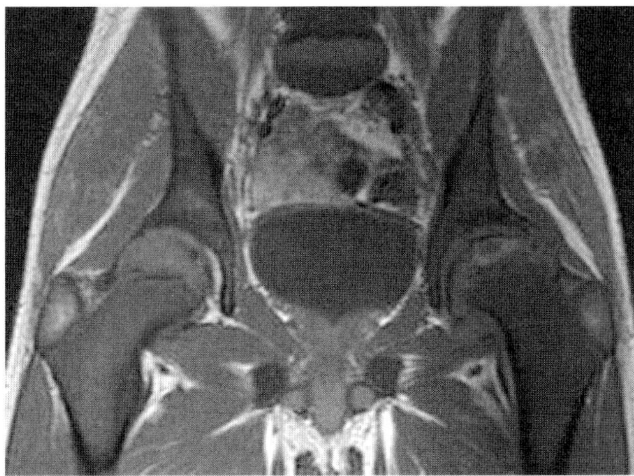

1. What are the findings in this patient with sickle cell disease and a gradual onset of left hip pain?
2. What are some etiologies of this condition?
3. What is the "crescent" sign?
4. What is the FICAT staging system?

CASE 109

Avascular Necrosis of Bilateral Femoral Heads

1. Frontal view of the pelvis shows sclerosis and subchondral cyst formation in the right femoral head. The left hip shows similar findings as well as flattening and cortical disruption of the femoral head. T1- and T2-weighted images of the pelvis demonstrate a small left hip effusion with flattening of the left femoral head. A geographic subchondral lesion with a rim of low T1 signal is seen in the left femoral head, consistent with avascular necrosis (AVN). Chronic flattening of the right femoral head due to AVN is also noted.
2. Trauma is the most common cause. Other etiologies include hemoglobinopathies, corticosteroid use, pregnancy, collagen vascular disorders, and alcoholism.
3. The "crescent" sign is a thin subchondral linear lucency in the superior portion of the femoral head seen on radiographs. This sign indicates a subchondral microfracture of the femoral head and is a late finding of AVN.
4. FICAT stages are used to classify the radiographic appearance of AVN. Briefly, stage I is characterized by the presence of symptoms without radiographic findings. In stage II, osteopenia, subchondral sclerosis, and cyst formation are seen. Stage III findings include the "crescent" sign with or without flattening of the femoral head. In stage IV, the femoral head is flattened and deformed with a decrease in the hip joint space.

References

Imhof H, Breitenseher M, Trattnig S, et al: Imaging of avascular necrosis of bone, *Eur J Radiol* 7:180–186, 1997.

Watson RM, Roach NA, Dalinka MK: Avascular necrosis and bone marrow edema syndrome, *Radiol Clin North Am* 42:207–219, 2004.

Cross-Reference

Emergency Radiology: THE REQUISITES, pp 170–172.

Comment

Avascular necrosis (AVN) is most commonly seen in the femoral head in patients with a displaced femoral neck fracture or hip dislocation. AVN is also seen in the scaphoid, capitate, humeral head, vertebral body, talus, and knee. The epiphyseal region of bone is affected by AVN due to limited arterial and venous flow at this site. Multiple microinfarctions from decreased blood flow or occlusion lead to edema, necrosis, subchondral microfractures, and eventual flattening of the femoral head. Insufficient healing causes rapid wear of the uneven joint space and further bony destruction.

In cases of nontraumatic AVN of the hip, the symptoms are usually intermittent groin pain of gradual onset. Imaging evaluation typically starts with radiographs of the hip. Visualization of the superior portion of the femoral head is often limited due to the superimposed acetabulum; a "frog-leg" lateral view should be performed to further evaluate this region. Radiographic findings of AVN include osteopenia, subchondral sclerosis and cyst formation, the "crescent" sign, flattening of the femoral head, and decrease in joint space. The radiographs may also be normal. Magnetic resonance imaging is more sensitive in detection of early AVN; findings include a geographic subchondral lesion in the anterosuperior femoral head with a low T1 linear rim. A "double line" sign may also be seen, and consists of parallel stripes of outer hypointensity and inner hyperintensity along the margin of the femoral head lesion.

Treatment of AVN may include anticoagulation, bisphosphonates, surgical drilling and core compression, rotational osteotomy, or total hip replacement.

Notes

CASE 110

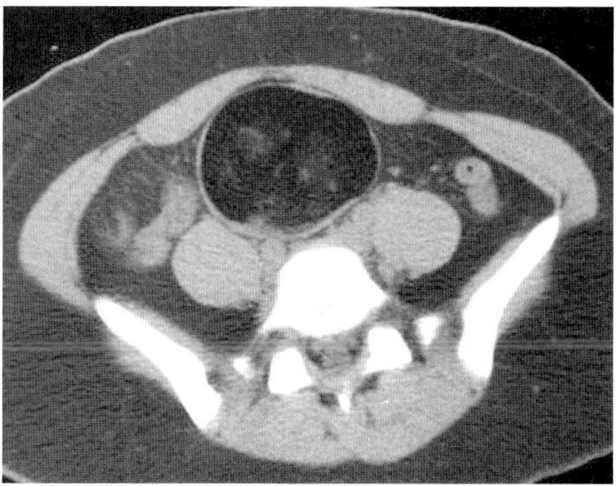

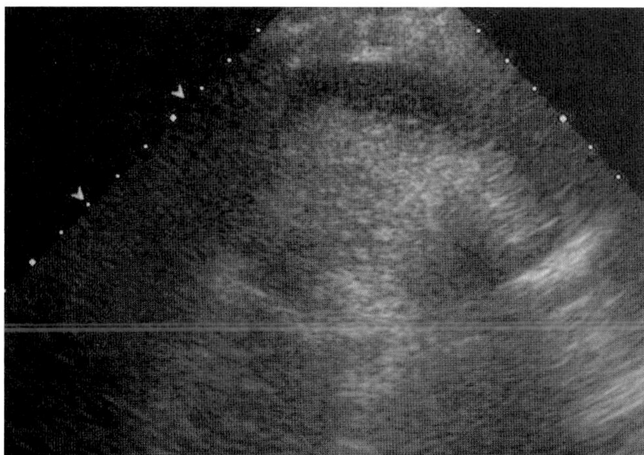

1. What are the findings in this 29-year-old female patient with vague mid-abdominal pain?
2. What percentage of these tumors contain teeth?
3. What percentage of these tumors are bilateral?
4. What is the most common complication seen with this condition?

CASE 110

Mature Cystic Teratoma

1. Computed tomography shows a well-circumscribed round lesion in the midline of the mid abdomen containing a few foci of soft tissue density and a large amount of fat density. Ultrasound demonstrates echogenic material within the lumen of the mass. These findings are consistent with a mature cystic teratoma.
2. 31%.
3. 10%.
4. Torsion of the teratoma. This usually occurs in teratomas greater than 11 cm in diameter.

References

Foshager MC, Hood LL, Walsh JW: Masses simulating gynecological diseases at CT and MR imaging, *Radiographics* 16:1085–1099, 1996.

Outwater EK, Siegelman ES, Hunt JH: Ovarian teratomas; tumor types and imaging characteristics, *Radiographics* 21:475–490, 2001.

Comment

Teratomas make up 20% of all ovarian tumors in adults and 50% of all ovarian tumors in children. Ovarian teratomas include mature cystic teratomas, also known as dermoid cysts, immature teratomas, and monodermal teratomas such as struma ovarii. Mature cystic teratomas are made up of mature derivations of at least two of the three germ cell layers. Most mature cystic teratomas are filled with liquid sebaceous material. Squamous epithelium lines the walls of the tumor. Hair follicles, skin glands, and muscle are located in the wall. A Rokitansky nodule may be seen projecting into the lumen and may contain bone or teeth.

At sonography, a mature cystic teretoma may have a variety of appearances, including a cystic mass containing an echogenic nodule (i.e., Rokitansky nodule), an echogenic mass with posterior acoustic attenuation caused by internal fat or hair, or a mass with diffuse internal echogenic bands caused by hair. With computed tomography and fat-saturated magnetic resonance imaging, the diagnosis of a mature cystic teratoma is frequently straightforward due to the presence of fat in the mass. However, only 65% to 75% of mature cystic teratomas contain fat, which can complicate the diagnosis.

Mature cystic teratomas are slow growing, enlarging less than 2 mm per year, and most are asymptomatic. Both abdominal pain and pelvic pain are exhibited by a minority of patients with uncomplicated tumors. Complications are rare, and they include torsion, malignant degeneration, or rupture with leakage of sebaceous material into the peritoneal cavity.

Notes

CASE 111

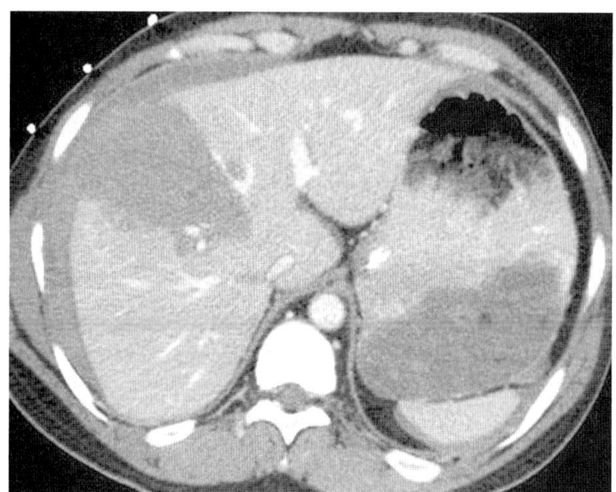

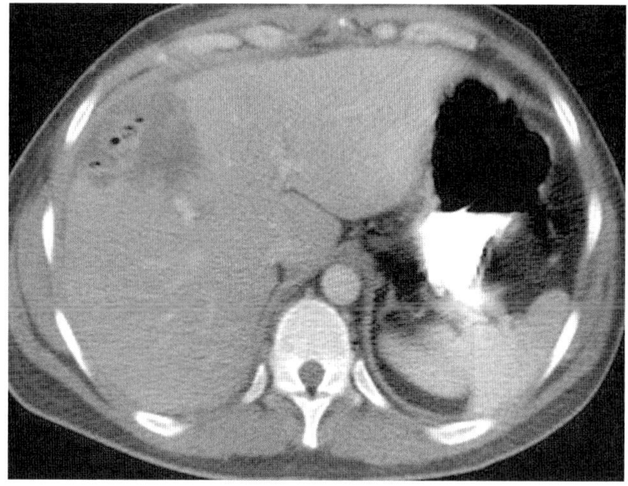

1. What are the findings on the admission (left) and hospital day 13 (right) abdominal computed tomography views of this patient initially involved in a motor vehicle collision and now complaining of worsening right upper quadrant pain?
2. What is the "double rim" sign?
3. What findings on magnetic resonance imaging are thought to be characteristic of this condition?
4. What is the first line of treatment of this condition?

CASE 111

Liver Injury with Post-traumatic Liver Abscess

1. The admission abdominal computed tomography (CT) shows a focal area of liver contusion and laceration and a small amount of perihepatic and perisplenic blood. The follow-up CT demonstrates interval decrease in the size of the liver injury and new foci of gas within the injured parenchyma consistent with liver abscess.
2. The "double rim" sign is seen on contrast-enhanced CT and consists of wall enhancement of a pyogenic liver abscess with a surrounding rim of low density due to edema around the abscess.
3. Early intense and persistent wall enhancement and perilesional enhancement.
4. Antibiotics and image-guided percutaneous aspiration and/or drainage.

References

Doyle DJ, Hanbidge AE, O'Malley ME: Imaging of hepatic infections, *Clin Radiol* 61:737–748, 2006.

Mortele KJ, Segatto E, Ros PR: The infected liver: radiologic-pathologic correlation, *Radiographics* 24: 937–955, 2004.

Cross-Reference

Emergency Radiology: THE REQUISITES, pp 297–298.

Comment

Pyogenic liver abscesses are most commonly caused by ascending cholangitis. Additional causes include hematogenous dissemination, penetrating trauma, transcatheter arterial chemoembolization, percutaneous radiofrequency ablation, or, as in this case, superinfection of necrotic tissue. More than 50% of pyogenic liver abscesses are polymicrobial. *Escherichia coli* is the most common microorganism isolated from abscesses. Symptoms vary from vague abdominal discomfort to high fever, rigors, and severe right upper quadrant pain.

Pyogenic abscesses have a wide range of appearances on computed tomography (CT) and sonography. On ultrasound, an abscess may be hypoechoic to hyperechoic, may have varying degrees of internal debris or gas, and usually has poorly defined walls. When present, posterior acoustic enhancement is thought to be the most reliable sign of a liver abscess. On contrast-enhanced CT, a pyogenic liver abscess is usually a well-defined, low-density lesion that may be unilocular or contain multiple septae. Gas, rim enhancement, or the "double rim" sign may be seen. On magnetic resonance imaging, the pyogenic liver abscess has a variable appearance but is usually low signal intensity on T1-weighted images and high signal on T2-weighted images. Signal voids from air and perilesional edema may be seen. On gadolinium-enhanced images, early, intense, and persistent wall enhancement and perilesional enhancement are thought to be characteristic of a pyogenic liver abscess.

Notes

CASE 112

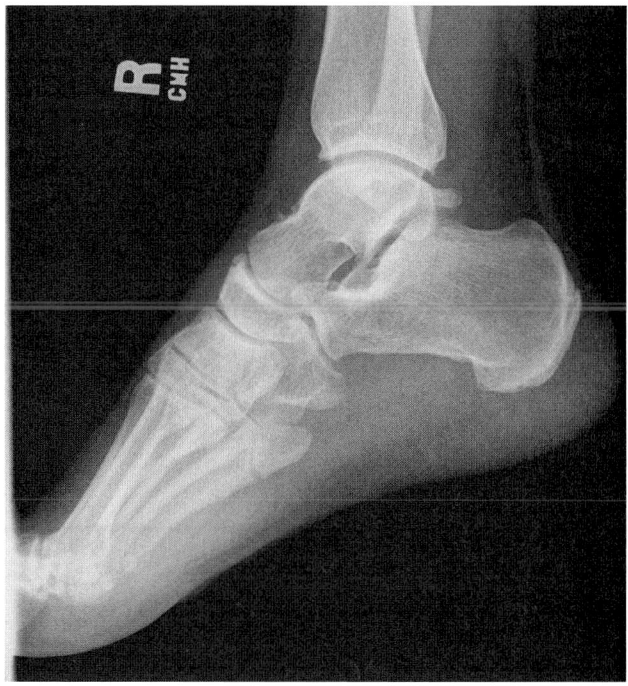

1. What is the finding in this patient with a history of acute onset of lateral foot pain after twisting his ankle?
2. What are the three types of fractures seen at the base of the fifth metatarsal?
3. At what age is the normal apophysis seen at the base of the fifth metatarsal?
4. What are radiographic signs of delayed or nonunion of a fracture?

CASE 112

Minimally Displaced Avulsion Fracture at the Base of the Fifth Metatarsal

1. Minimally displaced avulsion fracture through the base of the fifth metatarsal.
2. Avulsion fracture, Jones fracture, and stress fracture.
3. Ages 9 to 14 years. The normal apophysis is often confused with a fracture of the base of the fifth metatarsal. The apophyseal line runs parallel to the shaft of the metatarsal, while a fracture is transversely oriented and may extend into the cuboid–metatarsal joint space.
4. Widened fracture margins, periosteal reaction or callus formation, intramedullary canal sclerosis.

References

Fetzer GB, Wright RW: Metatarsal shaft fractures and fractures of the proximal fifth metatarsal, *Clin Sports Med* 25:139–150, 2006.

Nunley JA: Fractures of the base of the fifth metatarsal, *Orthop Clin North Am* 32:171–180, 2001.

Cross-Reference

Emergency Radiology: THE REQUISITES, pp 158–159.

Comment

Avulsion fracture, Jones fracture, and stress fracture are the three different types of fractures involving the proximal fifth metatarsal. Although radiographically similar, these three fractures occur at slightly different sites of the proximal fifth metatarsal, have different mechanisms of injury, and have significant differences in treatment and prognosis.

An avulsion fracture occurs at the tubercle at the base of the fifth metatarsal at the site of attachment of the peroneus brevis tendon. There is usually history of acute inversion injury. These fractures typically heal with conservative therapy and do not require surgical fixation.

A Jones fracture refers to a transverse fracture at the junction of the metaphysis and diaphysis within 1.5 cm of the tuberosity. The mechanism is thought to be due to a large adduction force applied to the forefoot with the ankle plantar flexed. The patient may present with acute pain or with a history of chronic pain along the lateral margin of the foot. Because of poor blood supply at the site of the fracture, Jones fractures are typically slow to heal and often require surgery.

Stress fractures occur at the proximal diaphyseal shaft and are due to repeated applications of normal loads over a short period of time. Stress fractures may present acutely or with delayed union or nonunion from a chronic fracture. In the latter case, surgical fixation is often required for management of the injury.

Notes

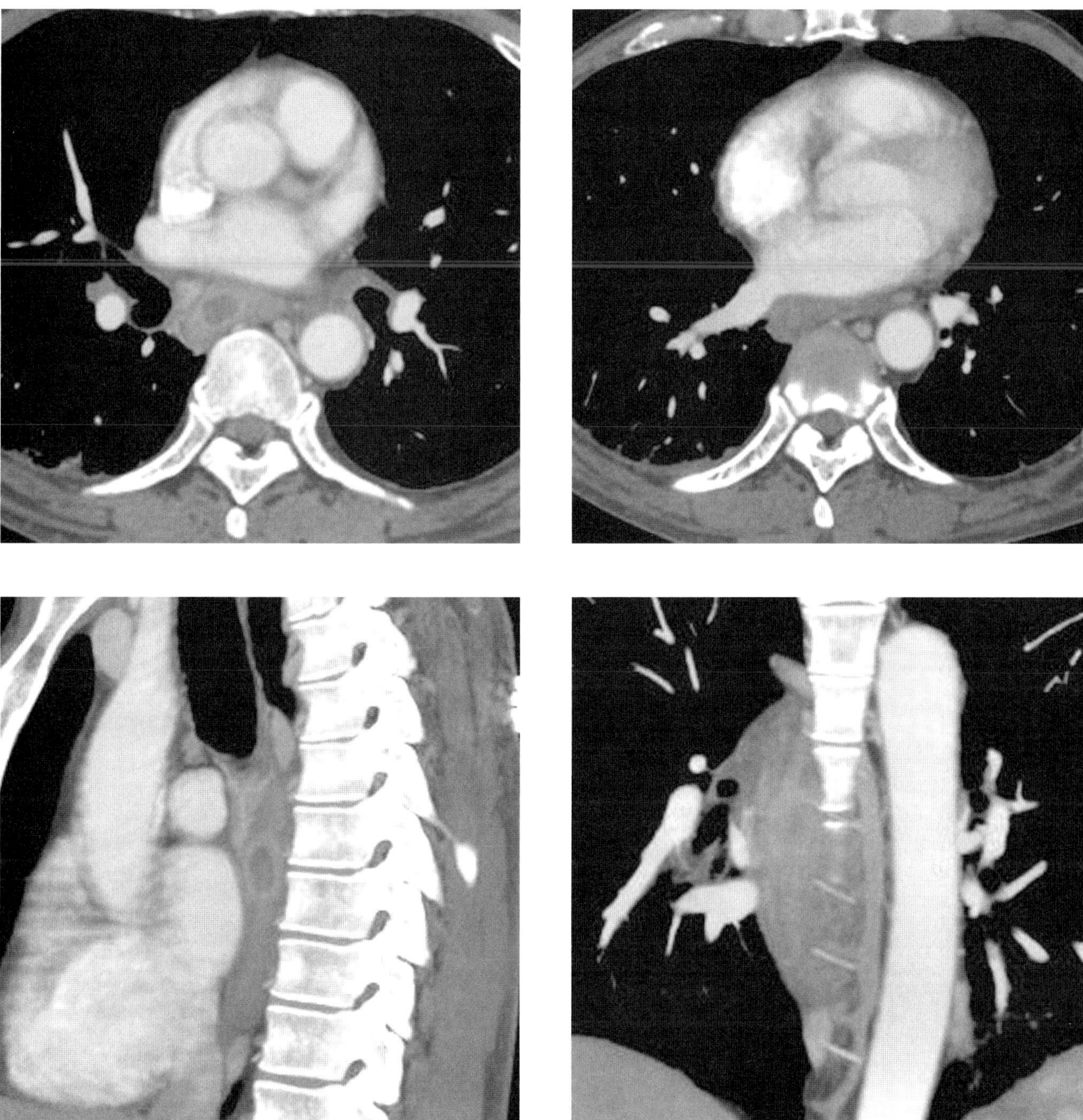

You are shown images of a 55-year-old man infected with HIV who presented to the emergency department (ED) with acute chest pain.

1. What are the abnormalities?
2. What is the diagnosis?
3. Given the patient's medical history, what are the two most likely etiologies?
4. What is the most common cause of noncardiac chest pain in patients who present to the ED with acute chest pain?

CASE 113

Infectious (*Candida*) Esophagitis

1. Circumferential esophageal wall thickening, mucosal enhancement, submucosal edema, and an intraluminal mass or retained food bolus.
2. Esophagitis.
3. Gastroesophageal reflux disease and infection, especially by *Candida.*
4. Gastroesophageal reflux disease.

References

Pace F, Pallotta S, Antinori S: Nongastroesophageal reflux disease-related infectious, inflammatory and injurious disorders of the esophagus, *Curr Opin Gastroenterol* 23:446–451, 2007.

Young CA, Menias CO, Bhalla S, Prasad SR: CT features of esophageal emergencies, *Radiographics* 28: 1541–1553, 2008.

Comment

Among patients who present to the ED, the most frequent and potentially life-threatening causes of acute chest pain are acute myocardial infarction and unstable angina. However, noncardiac causes of chest pain are frequent, occurring in as many as 55% of cases. Causes of noncardiac chest pain that may or may not be immediately life-threatening include acute aortic dissection, pulmonary embolism, pneumothorax, pneumonia, esophagitis, and pericarditis. Typically, the correct diagnosis can be suspected and rapidly diagnosed with detailed history, physical examination, electrocardiography, blood tests, and/or chest radiography. When suspected, the diagnosis of some diseases, such as pulmonary embolism or aortic dissection, requires additional evaluation with imaging studies (e.g. multidetector computed tomography [MDCT], magnetic resonance imaging, etc.).

Esophagitis is a common cause of noncardiac chest pain with gastroesophageal reflux disease accounting for 60% of cases. Other types of esophagitis that include infectious, eosinophilic, chemical-induced (chemotherapy or caustic ingestion) esophagitides are not uncommon. In particular, infectious esophagitis is common in patients who are immunosuppressed due to human immunodeficiency virus infection or organ transplantation, and *Candida* esophagitis is especially common. Although they may present with chest pain, patients with candidal esophagitis may not exhibit dysphagia or oral candidiasis, so the diagnosis may not be suspected clinically.

Standard means for diagnosing esophagitis include esophagography and endoscopy. However, because the diagnosis may not be initially apparent based on clinical means, it may be first suspected due to findings exhibited by MDCT obtained to evaluate for other diseases of more immediate clinical consequence. Consequently, the radiologist must maintain a high index of suspicion when reviewing an MDCT obtained to evaluate a patient with acute chest pain. MDCT signs of esophagitis include diffuse esophageal mural thickening, low attenuation submucosal edema, and mucosal enhancement. At times, there may be retained intraluminal food fragments secondary to food impaction.

Notes

CASE 114

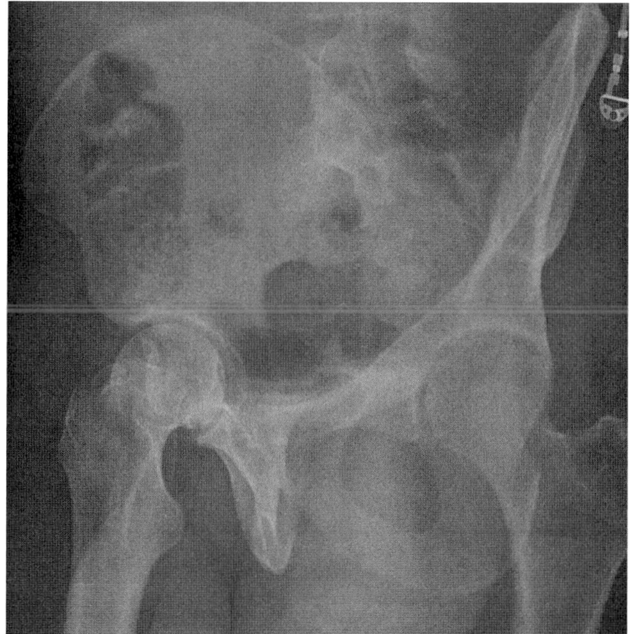

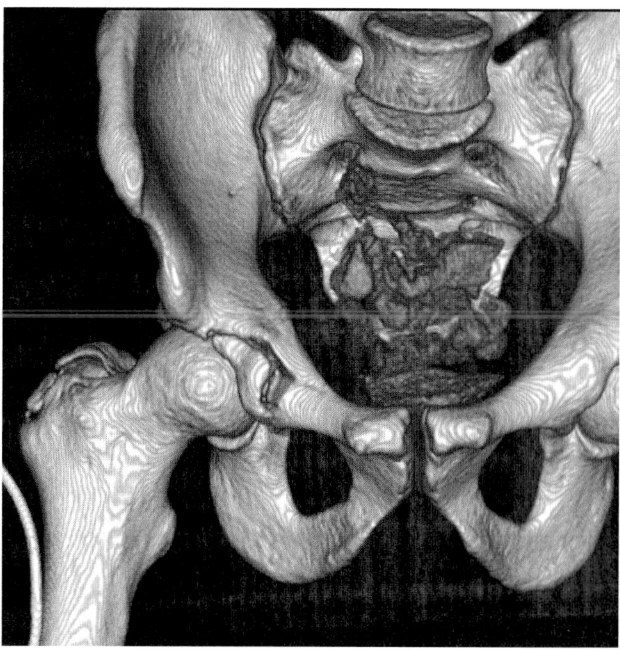

See also Color Plate

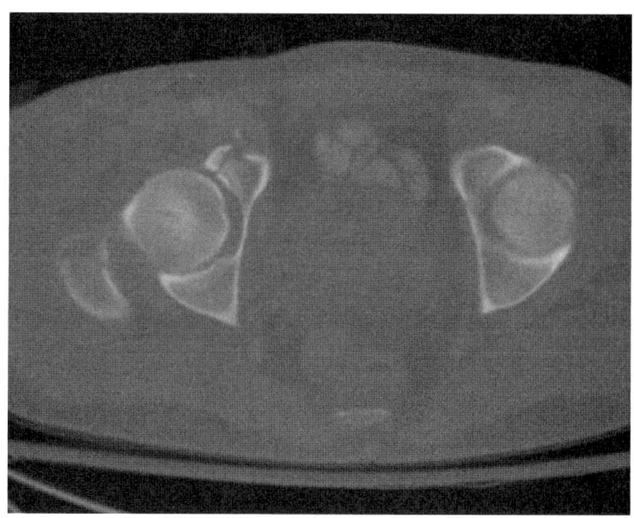

1. What part of the acetabulum is fractured?
2. In the Letournel classification system, is an isolated fracture of this structure common?
3. What important information does classification of acetabulum fractures attempt to convey?
4. What imaging studies are required to classify fractures with the Letournel system?

CASE 114

Acetabulum Anterior Wall Fracture

1. The acetabulum anterior wall.
2. No. It is the least common type of fracture.
3. Integrity of weight-bearing structures.
4. Anteroposterior and bilateral Judet radiographs, although multidetector computed tomography with 3-D reconstructions may supplant Judet radiographic views.

References

Ohashi K, El-Khoury GY, Abu-Zahra KW, Berbaum KS: Interobserver agreement for Letournel acetabular fracture classification with multidetector CT: are standard Judet radiographs necessary? *Radiology* 241: 386–391, 2006.

Potok PS, Hopper KD, Umlauf MJ: Fractures of the acetabulum: imaging, classification, and understanding, *Radiographics* 15:7–23, 1995; discussion 23–24.

Cross-Reference

Emergency Radiology: THE REQUISITES, pp 140–141.

Comment

Acetabulum fractures are important subsets of pelvic fractures given the role of the acetabulum in weight bearing and ambulation. Structurally, the weight-bearing acetabular roof is supported by anterior and posterior columns that join at an inverted angle just superior to the roof. Treatment of acetabular fractures targets primarily preservation of the weight-bearing function. Classification of acetabular fractures communicates information about the integrity of the acetabulum's weight-bearing components, thereby facilitating surgical planning. Among the classification systems, the Letournel classification system is the most widely recognized. In Letournel system "elementary fractures," one component of the acetabulum is detached from the others, whereas in "associated fractures," several elementary fractures combine to form one fracture pattern. Elementary fractures include posterior wall, transverse, anterior column, posterior column, and anterior wall fractures. Associated fractures include transverse and posterior wall, both column, T-shaped, anterior wall and posterior hemi-transverse, and posterior column and posterior wall fractures. The most frequently encountered fracture patterns are the posterior wall, transverse and posterior wall, both column, and transverse fractures. The least commonly encountered fracture is the isolated anterior wall fracture.

The Letournel classification system is based on the use of anteroposterior and bilateral posterior oblique (i.e., Judet view) radiographs. However, high-quality Judet views can be difficult to obtain and painful to the acutely injured patient. Traditionally, computed tomography (CT) was considered an important, but supplemental, imaging technique in the evaluation of acetabulum fractures. However, since classification of acetabulum fractures based on results of multidetector CT with multiplanar and three-dimensional reconstructed images can be performed with greater interobserver agreement than classification with radiographs, CT has emerged as the primary means to characterize acetabulum fractures, and the role of Judet view radiographs in acute fracture diagnosis and classification now appears limited.

Notes

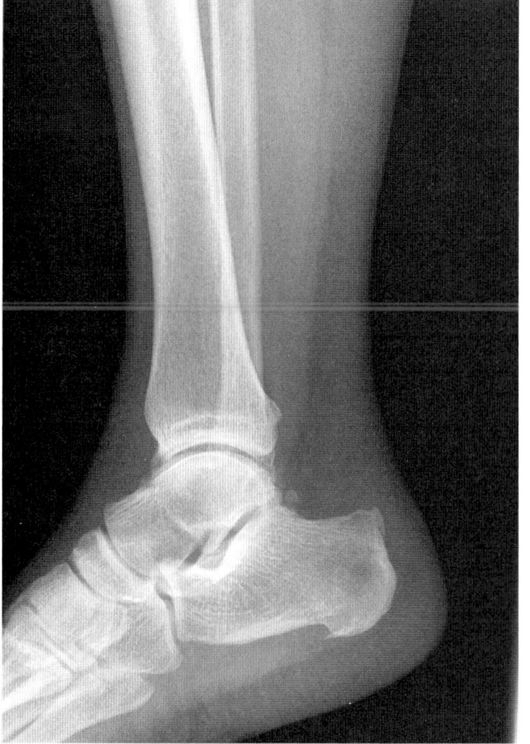

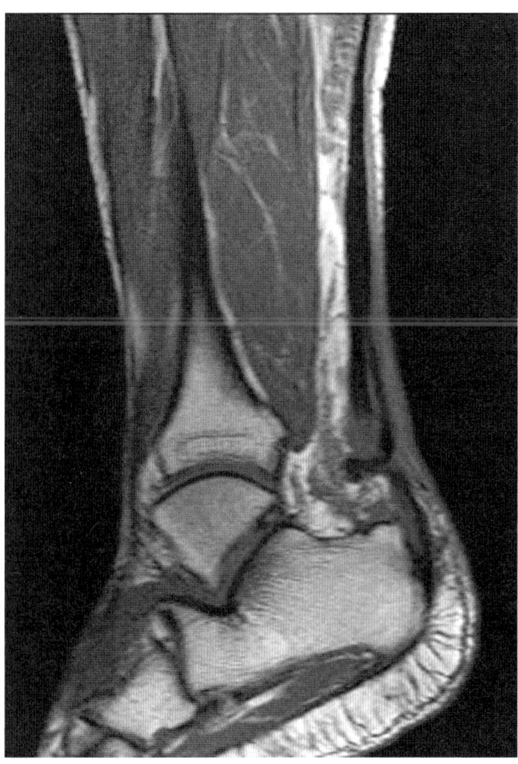

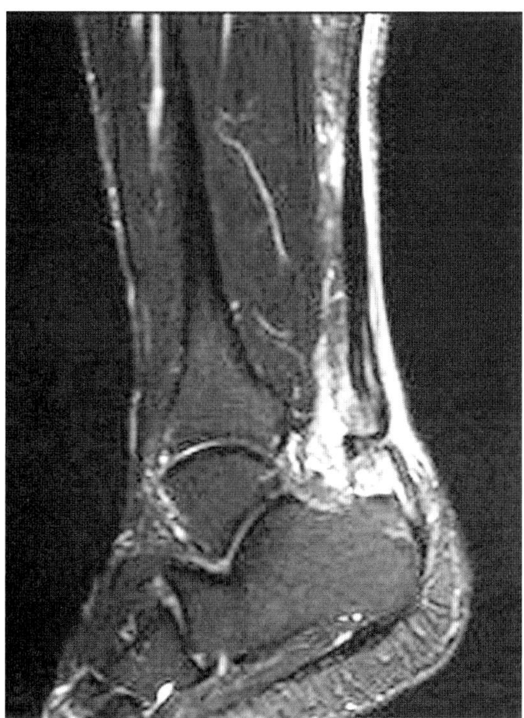

1. What is the usual mechanism of injury?
2. How is this injury treated?
3. What is the role of imaging in the evaluation of these injuries?
4. What are the diagnostic magnetic resonance imaging findings?

CASE 115

Achilles Tendon Rupture

1. Sudden, forceful dorsiflexion of the ankle.
2. Surgery or casting with the ankle in plantar flexion.
3. To exclude other injuries and confirm Achilles tendon rupture in clinically equivocal cases; assess apposition of tendon ends when patient is treated with cast.
4. Loss of normal hypointense tendon signal, hyperintense T2-weighted signal in and around the tear, and abnormal tendon contour.

References

Kaplan PA, Helms CA, Dussault R, et al: Foot and ankle. In *Musculoskeletal MRI*, Philadelphia, WB Saunders, 2001, pp 395–397.

Schweitzer ME, Karasick D: MR imaging of disorders of the Achilles tendon, *AJR Am J Roentgenol* 175: 613–625, 2000.

Comment

Acute Achilles tendon ruptures typically occur in men between the ages of 30 and 50 years as a consequence of forceful, sudden dorsiflexion. Tears usually occur 2 to 3 cm proximal to the tendon's calcaneal insertion, although some may occur at the myotendinous junction. Typically, rupture occurs as a result of sudden, forceful dorsiflexion of the ankle during sporting events, although it can be caused by direct trauma to the tendon itself (as was the case with this patient). Treatment consists of either surgery or casting with the ankle in plantar flexion.

Clinical diagnosis is usually straightforward. However, in clinically equivocal cases, imaging may exclude alternative injuries and/or confirm clinically suspected tendon rupture. In addition, magnetic resonance imaging (MRI) can be used to assess the need for open Achilles tendon repair by demonstrating the overall state of the tendon and, when the patient is casted, the adequacy of tendon reapposition.

Typically, lateral radiographs may demonstrate a thickened, ill-defined Achilles tendon. Edema and hemorrhage may blur Kager's fat pad. With complete tears, the normal curved posterior contour of the tendon is lost, and there may be a small notch.

MRI may demonstrate partial longitudinal (interstitial), partial transverse, or complete tears with replacement of the normally hypointense tendon signal by a hyperintense T2-weighted signal related to edema and hemorrhage. An abnormal signal may also be demonstrated in the peritendinous soft tissues. The normal tendon contour may be lost. Occasionally, a complete tear is associated with wide separation of the tendon ends due to retraction of the proximal tendon segment. Given the possibility of tendon retraction or a high tear at the myotendinous junction, sagittal imaging should be performed with an extended field of view.

Notes

CASE 116

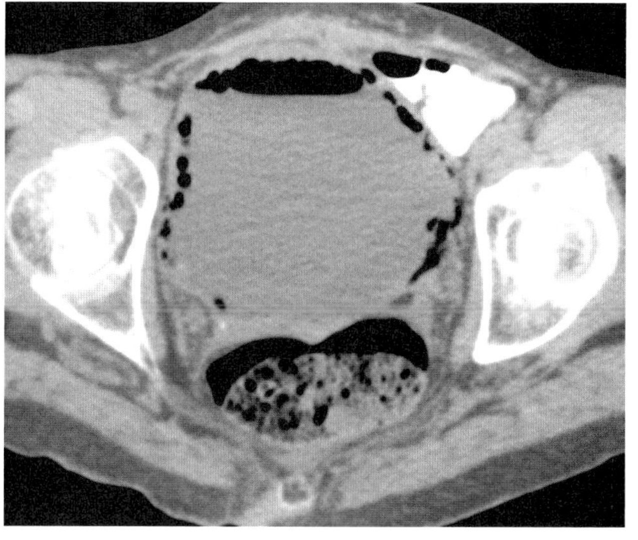

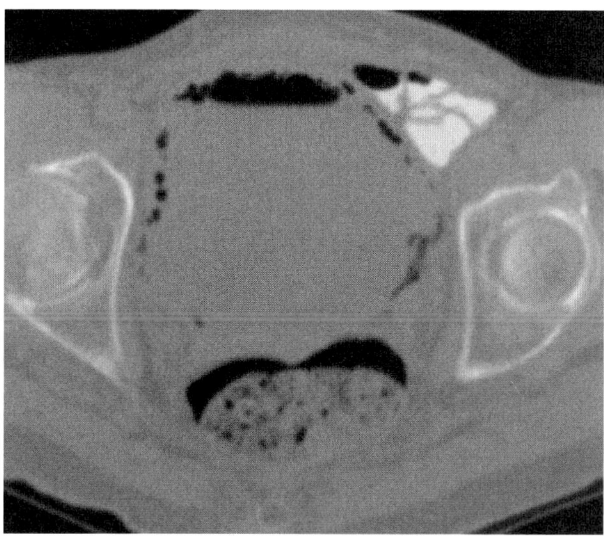

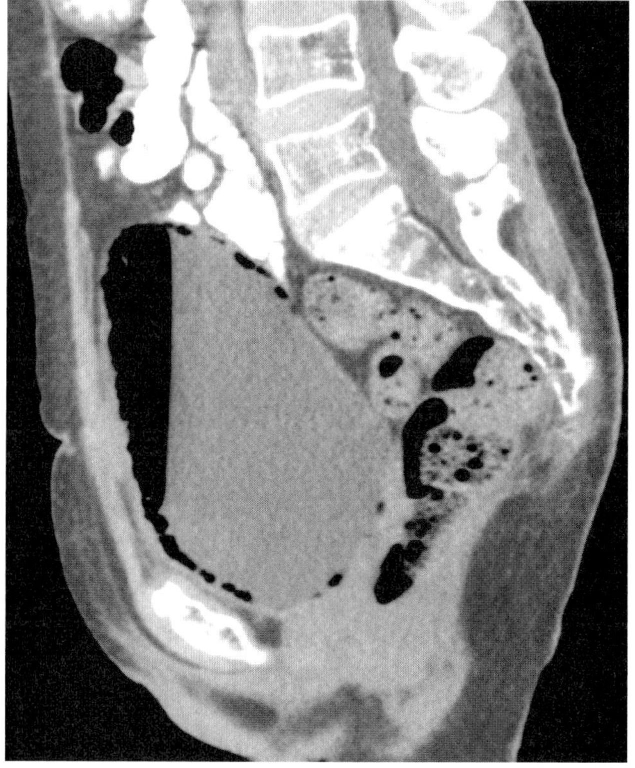

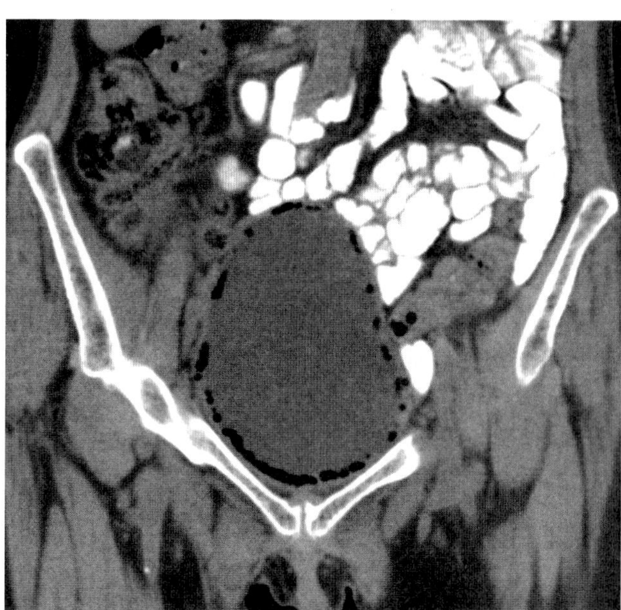

You are shown images of a patient who presented with abdominal pain and fever.

1. What are the computed tomography findings?
2. What is the best diagnosis?
3. What is the differential diagnosis?
4. What factors predispose to developing this entity?

CASE 116

Emphysematous Cystitis

1. There is air within the wall and lumen of the urinary bladder.
2. Emphysematous cystitis.
3. Recent bladder instrumentation, vesicocolic or vesicovaginal fistula.
4. Elderly females with uncontrolled diabetes mellitus, chronic urinary tract infection, bladder outflow obstruction, and neurogenic bladder.

References

Grayson DE, Abbott RM, Levy AD, et al: Emphysematous infections of the abdomen and pelvis: a pictorial review, *Radiographics* 22:543–561, 2002.

Thomas AA, Lane BR, Thomas AZ, et al: Emphysematous cystitis: a review of 135 cases, *BJU Int* 100: 17–20, 2007.

Cross-Reference

Emergency Radiology: THE REQUISITES, pp 302–303.

Comment

Emphysematous cystitis is a rare life-threatening acute inflammation of the bladder mucosa and the underlying musculature. It is characterized by gas within the wall and lumen of the bladder. The gas is produced by bacterial fermentation of glucose. The majority of the patients are middle-aged females (median age 66 years) with underlying poorly controlled diabetes mellitus. Other predisposing conditions include chronic urinary tract infection, bladder outflow obstruction, and neurogenic bladder.

The most commonly isolated organism is *Escherichia coli.* Other gas-producing organisms, including *Enterobacter aerogenes,* Clostridia species, and fungal species are occasionally isolated. Gas within the bladder wall may also be due to noninfectious etiologies, such as recent bladder instrumentation, trauma, vesicocolic or vesicovaginal fistula, and pneumatosis cystoidies intestinalis. Clinical symptoms are nonspecific, and patients commonly present with dysuria, urinary frequency, and hematuria. Pneumaturia is rare.

On abdominal radiographs, emphysematous cystitis can be seen as curvilinear or mottled radiolucent collections in the region of the urinary bladder. The intraluminal gas can be seen as an air fluid level in the pelvis. Gas gangrene of the uterus or gas within the vaginal wall may mimic this entity and require further anatomical localization. Computed tomography is highly sensitive for gas and allows early demonstration of small quantities of gas within the bladder wall and lumen. Use of either lung or bone windows and levels to view the images may help to differentiate small amounts of gas within the bladder wall from intraluminal or free intraperitoneal air.

Most patients with emphysematous cystitis are treated with medical management alone. They require broad spectrum antibiotics, control of hyperglycemia, and adequate drainage of bladder outflow obstruction. The mortality rate is 7% with prompt diagnosis and treatment.

Notes

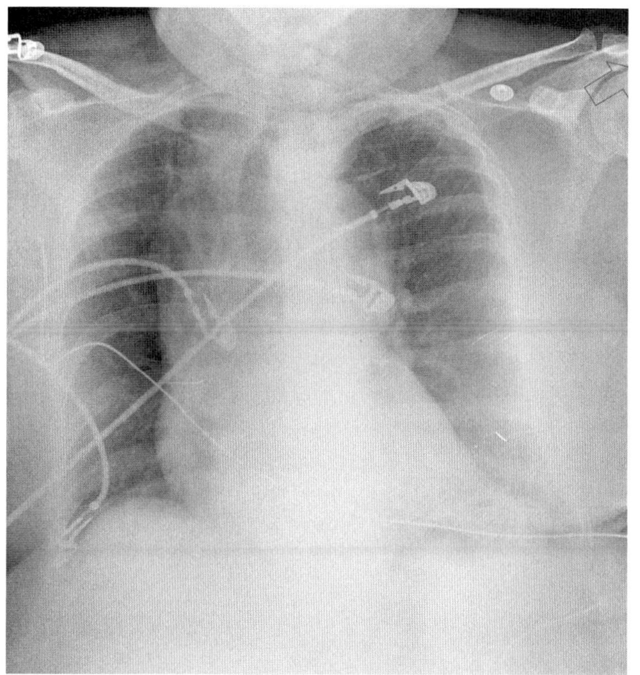

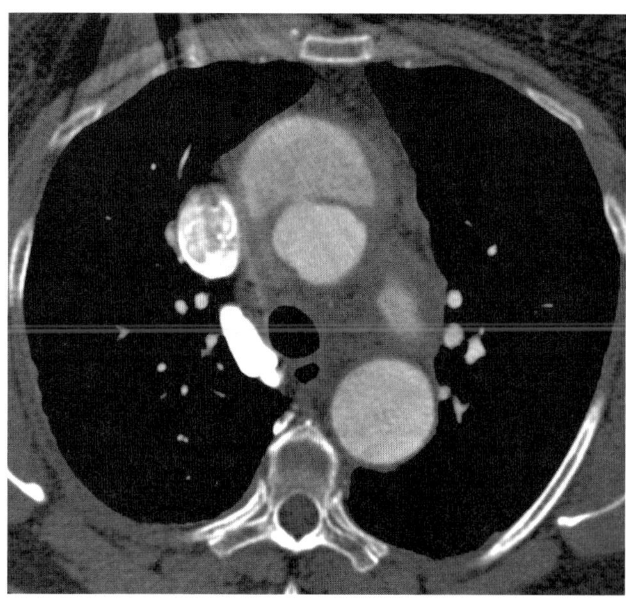

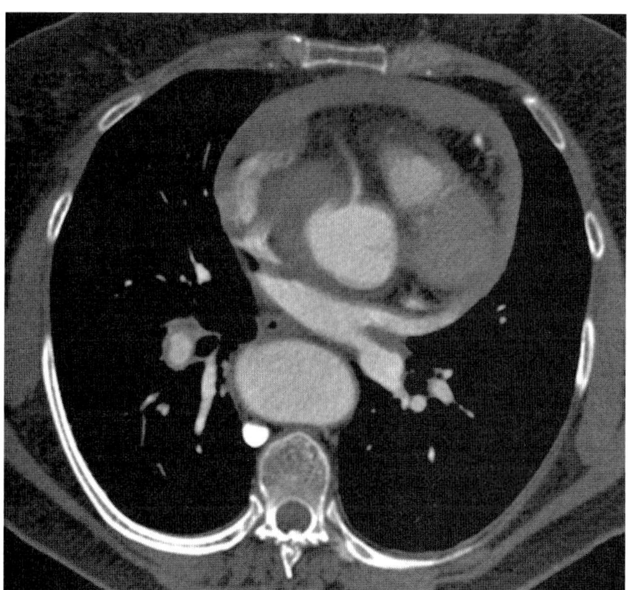

1. What is the diagnosis?
2. What are the potentially fatal complications of this disease?
3. What may the pericardial fluid indicate?
4. If untreated, what is the mortality of this disease?

CASE 117

Aortic Dissection (Stanford Type A) with Hemopericardium

1. Stanford type A aortic dissection.
2. Rupture into the mediastinum or pleural space, rupture into the pericardium with cardiac tamponade, acute aortic regurgitation, and end organ ischemia due to aortic branch vessel involvement.
3. Rupture into the pericardial space.
4. 70% by 7 days.

References

Castaner E, Andreu M, Gallardo X, et al: CT in nontraumatic acute thoracic aortic disease: typical and atypical features and complications, *Radiographics* 23 (Suppl):S93–S110, 2003.

Yoshida S, Akiba H, Tamakawa M, et al: Thoracic involvement of type A aortic dissection and intramural hematoma: diagnostic accuracy—comparison of emergency helical CT and surgical findings, *Radiology* 228:430–435 2003.

Cross-Reference

Emergency Radiology: THE REQUISITES, pp 240–242.

Comment

Aortic dissection occurs when an intimal tear permits blood to enter the medial layer of the aortic wall, thereby resulting in both a true lumen and a false lumen. Aortic dissection typically affects patients with hypertension, but other predisposing factors include Marfan syndrome and other connective tissue diseases, aortic coarctation, aortitis, pregnancy, and cocaine use. Patients usually present with chest and/or back pain. Most deaths from aortic dissection occur within 2 weeks of initial symptoms.

Aortic dissections are classified based on the aortic segment involved. Utilizing the Stanford classification system, a type A dissection involves the ascending aorta or aortic arch. With a Stanford type B dissection, the aortic involvement is distal to the subclavian artery. Accurate classification is necessary to direct management as uncomplicated type B dissections are generally managed with medical control of blood pressure, whereas type A dissections generally warrant immediate surgical repair due to high rates of fatal complications. The mortality of untreated type A dissections may be as high as 70% by 7 days.

Lethal complications of type A dissection include rupture into the mediastinum, pleural space, or pericardium, branch vessel occlusion with ischemia (e.g., coronary arteries and great vessels), or acute aortic regurgitation. Up to 90% of type A dissections are complicated by rupture. With rupture into the pericardium, the resulting hemopericardium frequently results in fatal cardiac tamponade (as was the case in this patient). Although pericardial fluid is a nonspecific finding, a pericardial effusion, especially when high attenuation suggests hemorrhage, is a poor sign in patients with type A dissection.

Acute aortic dissection can be diagnosed with computed tomography (CT), magnetic resonance imaging, and transesophageal echocardiography. CT is the favored imaging technique given its widespread availability and speed. CT without the use of intravenous contrast may demonstrate signs of aortic dissection or related intramural hematoma, but a definitive diagnosis and characterization of acute aortic dissection requires intravenous contrast. Contrast-enhanced CT diagnoses acute aortic dissection with sensitivity and specificity that both approach 100%. The accuracies of CT for detecting extension into the aortic arch branch vessels and pericardial fluid are 98% and 91%, respectively.

Notes

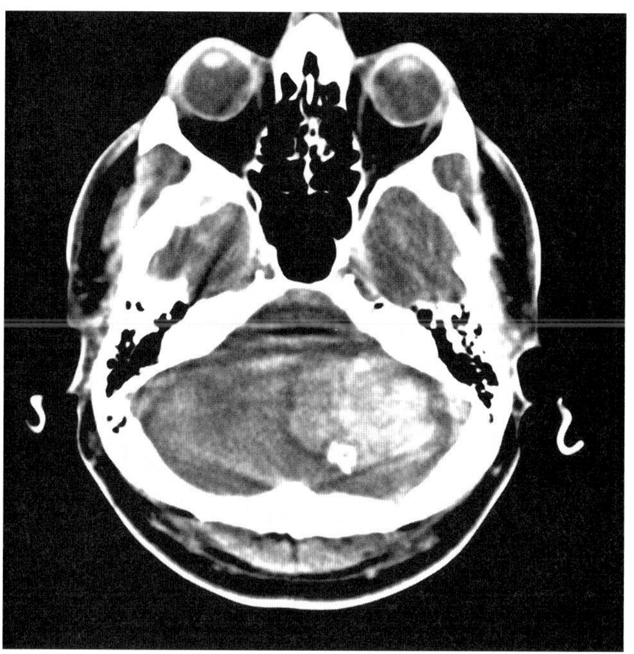

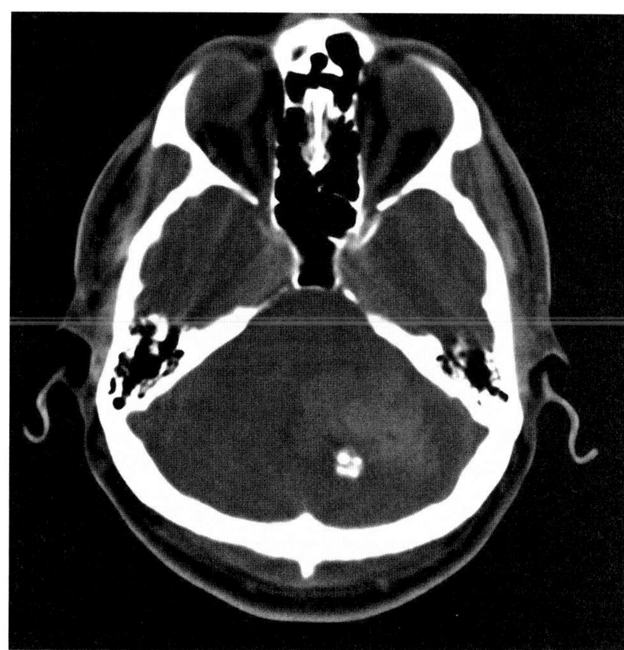

1. Are most of the lesions demonstrated infratentorial or supratentorial?
2. What percentage of these lesions exhibits calcifications?
3. What is the usual initial presentation of this pathology?
4. Are aneurysms commonly associated with this pathology?

CASE 118

Acute Cerebellar Hemorrhage Secondary to Arteriovenous Malformation

1. Supratentorial.
2. 25% to 30%.
3. Spontaneous intracranial hemorrhage.
4. Yes.

References

Byrne JV: Cerebrovascular malformations, *Eur Radiol* 15:448–452, 2005.

Osborn AG: Arteriovenous malformation. In Osborn AG, ed: *Diagnostic Imaging,* vol 4. Brain. Salt Lake City, UT, Amirsys, 2004, pp 4–6.

Cross-Reference

Emergency Radiology: THE REQUISITES, pp 1–2, 6–7, 20.

Comment

Arteriovenous malformations (AVM) are developmental abnormalities that consist of collections of abnormal feeding arteries and draining veins without an intervening capillary bed. Arteriovenous shunting is present. Nearly all are isolated. Most (85%) are supratentorial. Although many may remain asymptomatic, the majority are thought to become symptomatic during the patient's lifetime. Most present between the ages of 20 and 40 years. The most common clinical presentation at first diagnosis is a spontaneous intracranial hemorrhage. Other common signs and symptoms include headache, seizure, and focal neurologic deficit. Digital subtraction angiography, the diagnostic reference standard, demonstrates associated feeding artery aneurysms in 10% to 20% of patients with an AVM.

In addition to intracranial hemorrhage, computed tomography may demonstrate tortuous hyperdense dilated vessels that enhance following intravenous contrast administration. Focal calcifications are demonstrated in 25% to 30% of cases. Absent an acute hematoma, mass effect is characteristically absent.

Notes

CASE 119

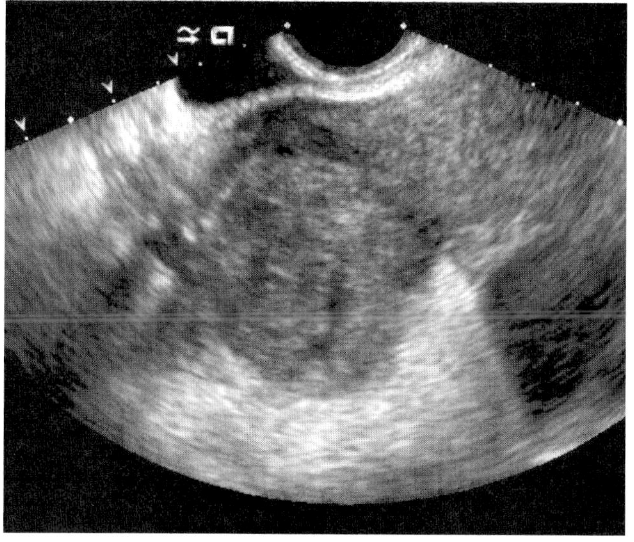

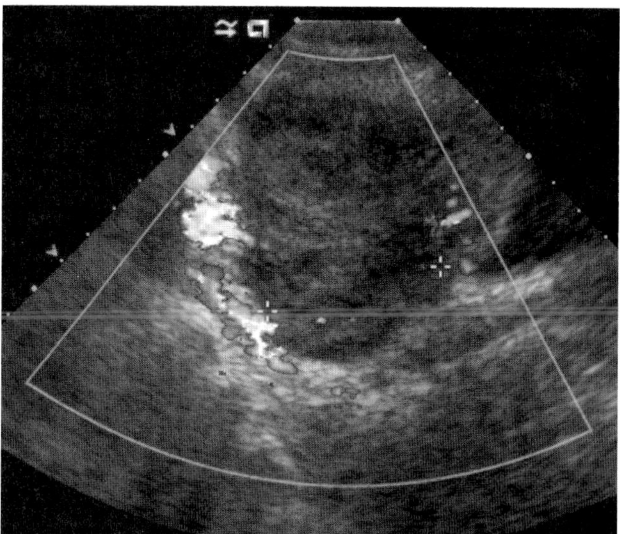

See also Color Plate

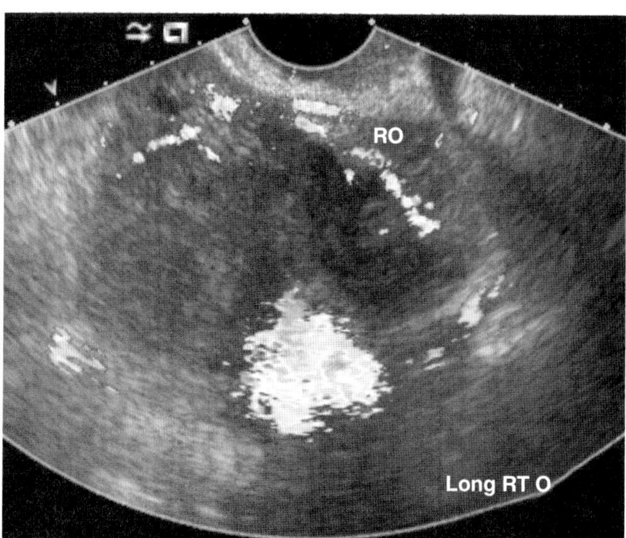

See also Color Plate

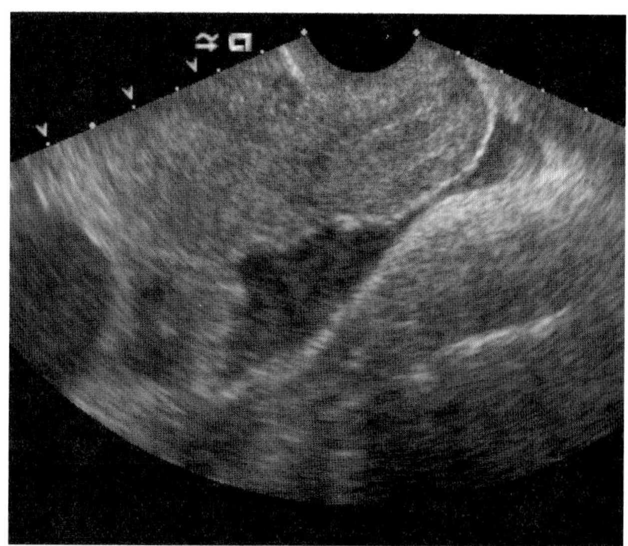

1. This 25-year-old woman with a history of tubal ligation presents with low abdominal pain. With these ultrasound findings, what should be the primary diagnostic consideration?
2. What clinical information would support the imaging diagnosis?
3. What sonographic finding would render the diagnosis definite rather than probable?
4. What does the echogenic fluid in the cul-de-sac represent?

CASE 119

Ruptured Ectopic Pregnancy

1. Ectopic pregnancy.
2. A maternal serum β-HCG level over 1500 mIU/mL (this patient's level was 1940 mIU/mL).
3. A defined embryo within an ectopic gestational sac.
4. Hemoperitoneum.

References

Dilbaz S, Caliskan E, Dilbaz B, et al: Predictors of methotrexate treatment failure in ectopic pregnancy, *J Reprod Med* 51:87–93, 2006.

Morin L, Van den Hof MC: SOGC clinical practice guidelines: ultrasound evaluation of first trimester pregnancy complications, *Int J Gynaecol Obstet* 93: 77–81, 2006.

Cross-Reference

Emergency Radiology: THE REQUISITES, p 317.

Comment

Ectopic pregnancy is a common cause of maternal death that may account for up to 80% of early pregnancy deaths. In women of reproductive age who present with lower abdominal pain, it should be a diagnostic consideration until pregnancy is excluded. Women with suspected ectopic pregnancy and clinical signs of hemodynamic instability are managed surgically. However, many clinically stable patients with early ectopic pregnancy can be successfully treated medically with intramuscular methotrexate therapy.

Transvaginal ultrasound (TV-US) facilitates accurate early diagnosis and treatment of ectopic pregnancy. The TV-US signs of an ectopic pregnancy include a simple adnexal cyst, complex adnexal mass, an echogenic tubal ring, an extrauterine embryo or fetus, or an empty uterus without other findings. Isolated free fluid in the cul-de-sac is an uncommon finding. Correlation of the TV-US findings with the timing of the last menstrual period and the maternal serum β-HCG levels promotes accurate diagnosis. Generally, by 5 weeks gestational age, TV-US should demonstrate a normal intrauterine gestational sac with an echogenic decidua, and a diameter of 2 to 3 mm should be visible. Similarly, a gestational sac should be seen when maternal serum β-HCG levels reach 1500 mIU/mL. If a normal intrauterine gestational sac is not seen by a serum β-HCG level of 2000 mIU/mL, an ectopic pregnancy should be suspected. If maternal serum β-HCG levels are greater than 1000 mIU/mL and a complex adnexal mass, with or without an echogenic tubal ring, is demonstrated, an ectopic pregnancy is probable. If TV-US demonstrates an adnexal or extraendometrial gestational sac, the diagnosis of ectopic pregnancy is assured. When diagnostic criteria are appropriately coupled with serum markers of pregnancy, the sensitivity of TV-US for ectopic pregnancy is 87% to 93% compared with laparoscopy.

In addition to confirming the diagnosis of ectopic pregnancy, TV-US can provide prognostic information. A subchorionic hematoma and/or a formed embryo in the ectopic gestational sac have been reported as predictors of methotrexate treatment failure. Although echogenic fluid in the cul-de-sac or Morrison's pouch may indicate hemoperitoneum from tubal rupture, the latter may also be due to leakage from the fimbrial end of the fallopian tube, and it does not necessarily contraindicate medical therapy in the hemodynamically stable patient.

Notes

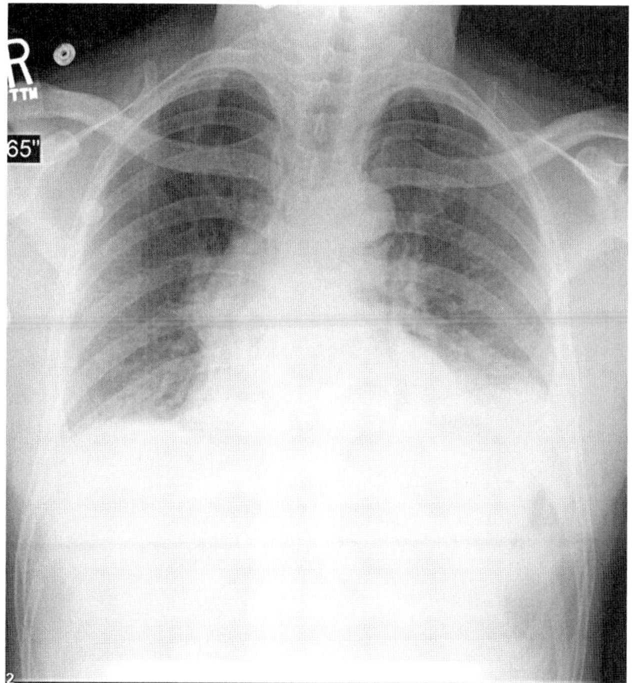

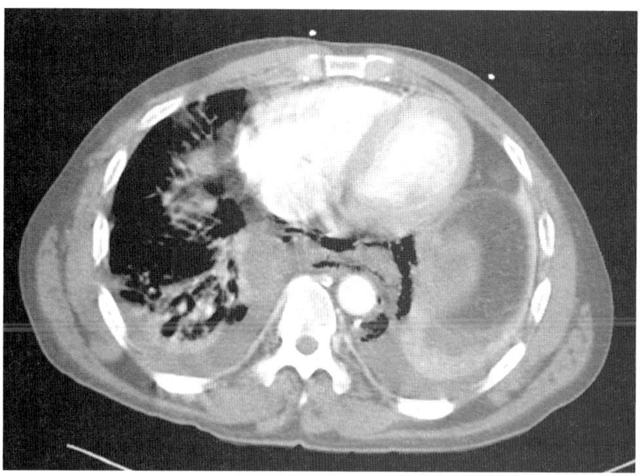

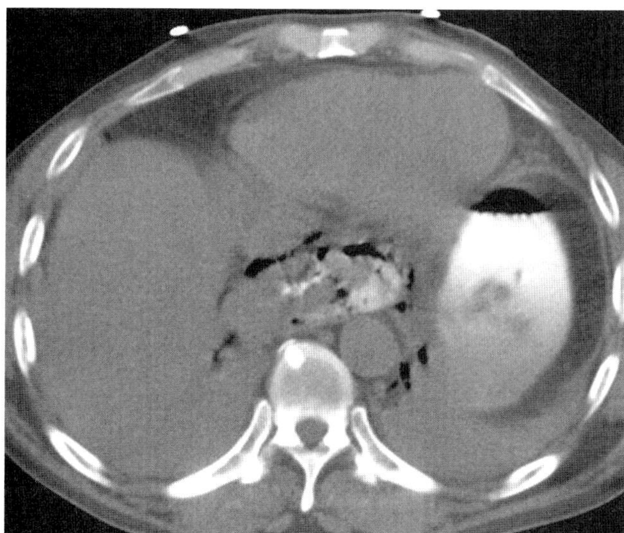

1. What is the source of the mediastinal gas and pleural fluid?
2. When this injury occurs as a consequence of violent emesis, by what eponym is it known?
3. If untreated, what is the mortality rate of the postemetic form of this entity?
4. What computed tomographic abnormalities are typical of this entity?

ANSWERS

CASE 120

Postemetic Esophageal Rupture (Boerhaave's Syndrome)

1. An esophageal tear.
2. Boerhaave's syndrome.
3. Nearly 100%.
4. Esophageal wall thickening, mediastinal fluid, pleural effusion, pneumomediastinum.

Reference

White CS, Templeton PA, Attar S: Esophageal perforation: CT findings, *AJR Am J Roentgenol* 160:767–770, 1993.

Cross-Reference

Emergency Radiology: THE REQUISITES, pp 60, 62.

Comment

Esophageal perforation may result from many causes, and esophageal rupture caused by violent emesis is known as Boerhaave's syndrome. Regardless of the etiology, oral and gastric secretions leaking through the esophageal rent cause fulminant mediastinitis, although the inflammatory response in Boerhaave's syndrome is particularly severe. Patients characteristically progress to sepsis and multiorgan system failure. The mortality rate of untreated Boerhaave's syndrome approaches 100%, but a survival rate of 80% is possible if surgical repair is rendered within 24 hours of the onset of symptoms.

Patients with Boerhaave's syndrome classically present with postemetic chest pain and fever, and clinical examination may suggest pleural effusion or pneumomediastinum. However, the clinical picture is frequently nonspecific, and esophageal rupture can mimic entities such as pneumonia, myocardial infarction, aortic dissection, or an acute upper abdominal disorder.

Chest radiography may demonstrate pneumomediastinum and a pleural effusion (usually left-sided), although a normal radiograph does not preclude the diagnosis. Esophagography is the imaging reference standard that both confirms and localizes the leak, which is usually left-sided and just proximal to the esophageal hiatus. In cases when the diagnosis is not initially suspected, or when an esophagram cannot be performed, chest computed tomography (CT) may be diagnostic. CT signs of esophageal perforation are usually localized to the region of the esophageal tear and include: focal esophageal wall thickening, mediastinal fluid and/or edema, pneumomediastinum, and pleural effusion. When the location of the esophageal tear is in doubt, CT scanning following administration of water-soluble contrast may facilitate localization.

Notes

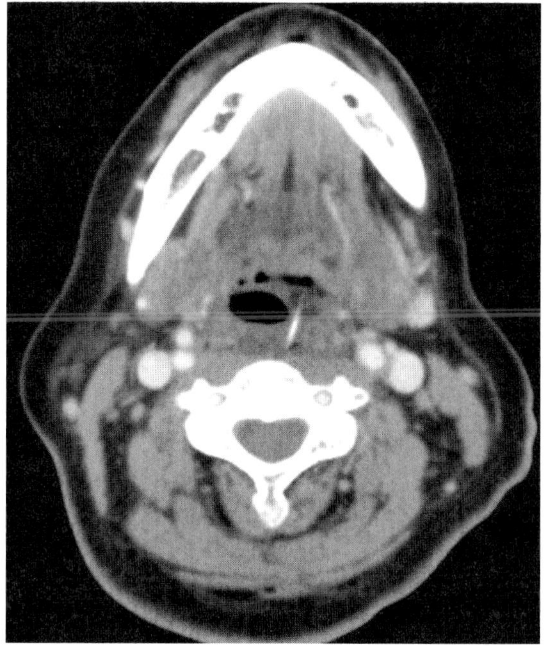

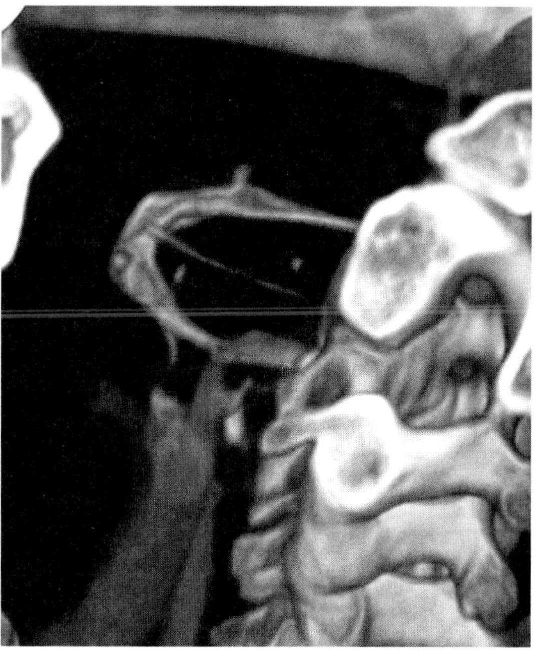

See also Color Plate

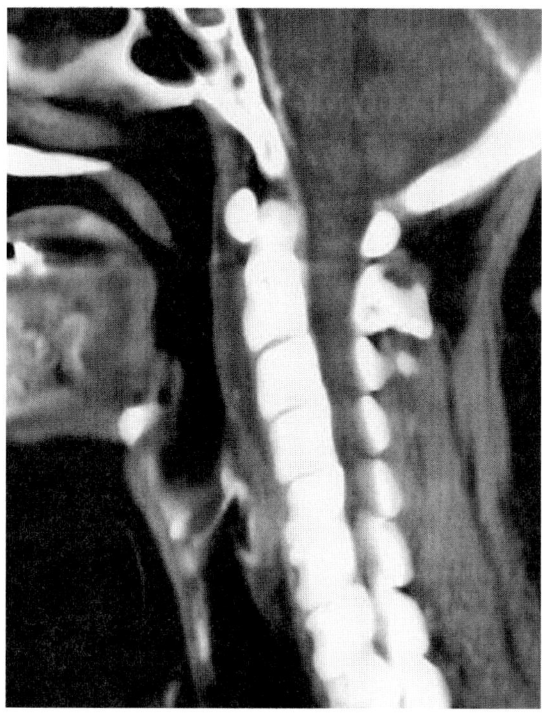

You are shown images of a patient who presents with a 2-day history of dysphagia following a meal of homemade sushi.

1. What is the primary abnormality?
2. What is the most likely reason that endoscopy failed to identify the primary abnormality?
3. What complication of the primary abnormality is demonstrated?
4. What is the sensitivity of radiographs for detecting the primary abnormality?

CASE 121

Retained Foreign Body (Fish Bone) with Pharyngeal Perforation

1. Retained fish bone.
2. The bone is submucosal.
3. Posterior submucosal abscess secondary to perforation.
4. The sensitivity of radiographs for detecting retained fish bones in the neck is 25% to 39%.

References

Lue AJ, Fang WD, Manolidis S: Use of plain radiography and computed tomography to identify fish bone foreign bodies, *Otolaryngol Head Neck Surg* 123: 435–438, 2000.

Marco De Lucas E, Sádaba P, Lastra García-Barón P, et al: Value of helical computed tomography in the management of upper esophageal foreign bodies, *Acta Radiol* 45:369–374, 2004.

Cross-Reference

Emergency Radiology: THE REQUISITES, pp 202–203.

Comment

Foreign body ingestion is a frequently encountered problem in the emergency department. It is usually seen in young children and the elderly. Among adults, fish bones are the most common foreign bodies to lodge in the upper gastrointestinal tract, with dentures and rapid eating predisposing to fish bone ingestion. The event is frequently unnoticed, and the bone passes spontaneously. Although complications are uncommon, ingested fish bones can cause gastrointestinal perforation with resulting abscess or perforation of adjacent vital structures. Common sites of impaction include the vallecula, hypopharynx, and cervical esophagus. Thorough physical examination and indirect laryngoscopy identify many pharyngeal foreign bodies, yet they are insensitive to cervical esophageal foreign bodies.

Neck radiographs are frequently used to search for impacted upper aerodigestive foreign bodies. However, the sensitivity of radiographs for detecting fish bones impacted in the neck is only 25% to 39%. Although fish bones are relatively radiolucent, with some interspecies variability, the characteristically very small diameter of retained fish bones is most likely the primary reason for the relative insensitivity of radiographs. Contributing to the low sensitivity, the bones are frequently oriented parallel to the film cassette or detector, thereby further reducing their conspicuity. Moreover, at the common sites of impaction, radiographic conspicuity can be further compromised by overlap with prominent soft tissues, thyroid cartilage and cricoid calcification, or the hyoid bone.

Computed tomography (CT) has a 90% to 100% sensitivity for detecting retained fish bones, with a specificity and a negative predictive value (NPV) of 91% and 100%, respectively. Since no impacted foreign body is found in over half of those patients suspected of harboring one, the high NPV of CT makes it a useful means to limit the diagnostic workup of this patient population. One advantage of CT over other diagnostic options, including barium swallow and endoscopy, is its ability to more readily diagnose foreign bodies that have perforated and migrated beyond the mucosa, as well as the complications of perforation, including abscesses. In addition, in most emergency departments, CT can be rapidly obtained. A disadvantage of CT is the associated radiation dose. Therefore, in patients with suspected impaction of an ingested foreign body, its use should be limited to those patients in whom clinical examination fails to reveal a suspected impacted fish bone or other potentially radiolucent foreign body.

Notes

CASE 122

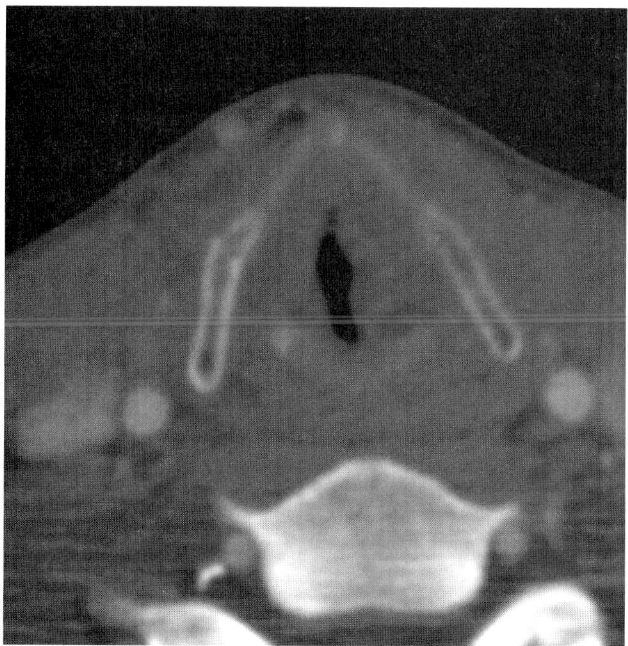

1. What structure is injured?
2. What is the probable mechanism of injury in this case?
3. What acute complication may result from this injury?
4. What is the imaging modality of choice for diagnosing this injury?

CASE 122

Laryngeal Fracture

1. The right thyroid cartilage is fractured.
2. Motor vehicle collision. Sports injuries, assault, and gunshot wounds are other common causes.
3. Fatal acute airway compromise.
4. Computed tomography.

Reference

Lee WT, Eliashar R, Eliachar I: Acute external laryngotracheal trauma: diagnosis and management, *Ear Nose Throat J* 85:179–184, 2006.

Cross-Reference

Emergency Radiology: THE REQUISITES, p 44.

Comment

Laryngeal fractures are rare and are encountered in anywhere from 1 in 5000 to 1 in 42,000 emergency room visits. Blunt injuries occur as a consequence of a direct blow to the larynx, such as in this patient, who was punched in the neck. Blunt injury most commonly occurs due to a motor vehicle collision. Other common causes include sports injuries and assault. Penetrating injuries are usually caused by gunshot wounds. Laryngeal injuries can result in acute airway compromise and death. Late complications include chronic breathing difficulties, chronic dysphonia or dysphagia, and aspiration.

Symptoms include dyspnea, dysphonia, hoarseness, dysphagia, odynophagia, neck pain, and hemoptysis. Clinical examination may reveal subcutaneous emphysema, tenderness, edema, hematoma, ecchymosis, and laryngeal distortion. However, clinical clues to laryngeal injury are frequently overlooked because they are subtle or are masked by other craniofacial injuries with which they are frequently associated.

Diagnosis of laryngeal injury is made with a combination of endoscopy and imaging. Computed tomography (CT) is the imaging modality of choice. Thin-section CT can demonstrate disruption of the laryngeal structures, although the diagnosis may be difficult in younger patients without calcification of the laryngeal components. In some instances, soft tissues gas and submucosal edema are demonstrated. A high index of suspicion facilitates the diagnosis, and the larynx warrants close scrutiny in all patients with anterior neck and/or craniofacial trauma who undergo evaluation with cervical spine CT or neck CT angiography.

Notes

CASE 123

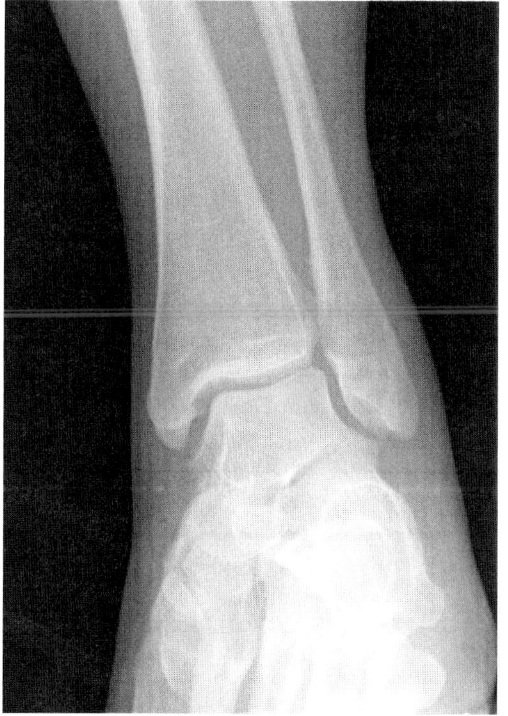

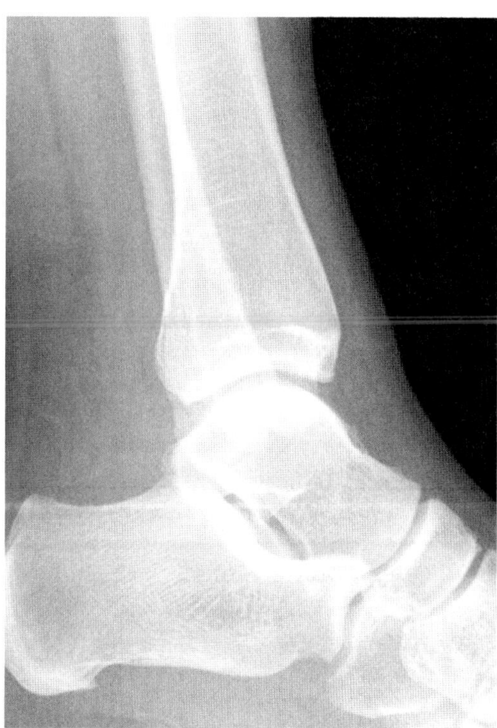

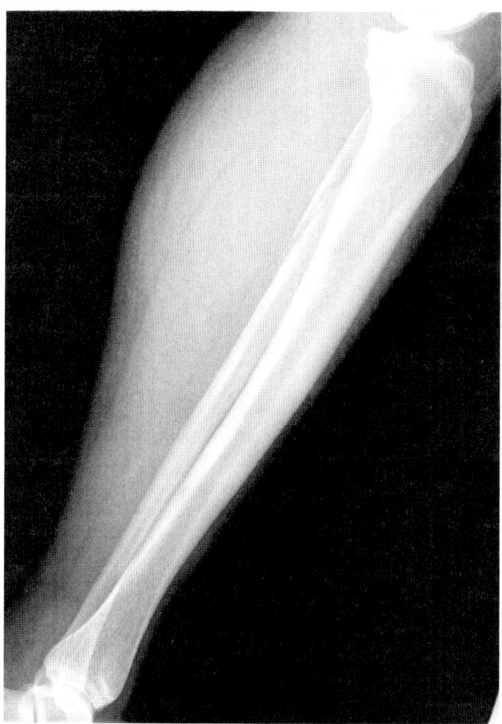

1. By what name is the proximal fibula fracture known?
2. What is the clinical significance of the proximal fibula fracture?
3. What is the treatment of this injury?
4. What radiographic signs of injury should prompt radiographic evaluation of the lower leg in addition to the ankle?

CASE 123

Maisonneuve Fracture

1. Maisonneuve fracture.
2. It is associated with extensive ankle ligamentous injuries.
3. Screw stabilization of the syndesmosis and ligamentous repair.
4. An isolated fracture of the posterior tibial margin, an isolated displaced medial malleolus fracture, widening of either the medial or lateral clear spaces of the ankle without an associated fibula fracture, or either anteromedial or syndesmotic tenderness without radiographic evidence of injury.

References

Babis GC, Papagelopoulos PJ, Tsarouchas J, et al: Operative treatment for Maisonneuve fracture of the proximal fibula, *Orthopedics* 23:687–690, 2000.

Wilson AJ: The ankle. In Rogers LF, ed: *Radiology of Skeletal Trauma*, 3rd ed, Philadelphia, Churchill Livingstone, 2002, p 1270.

Cross-Reference

Emergency Radiology: THE REQUISITES, pp 154, 155.

Comment

A Maisonneuve fracture is a proximal fibula fracture that occurs in stages as a consequence of forced external rotation of the foot. First, the anterior talofibular, anterior inferior tibiofibular, and interosseous ligaments rupture with varying degrees of injury to the interosseous membrane. Second, there is rupture of the posterior talofibular ligament or fracture of the posterior tibial tubercle (usually involving less than 25% of the articular surface). Third, the anteromedial joint capsule ruptures. Fourth, the proximal fibula fractures. Fifth, either the medial malleolus fractures or the medial collateral ligament ruptures. Since it is associated with ligamentous injuries at the ankle, a Maisonneuve fracture is best appreciated as part of a constellation of injuries rather than as an isolated fracture. The extensive ankle ligament disruption associated with Maisonneuve fracture renders this an unstable injury. Typically, it is internally fixated with screw stabilization of the syndesmosis and repair of the anterior inferior tibiofibular ligament.

Given the need for surgical repair, it is important to recognize this injury, although it can be easily overlooked clinically, since the injuries at the ankle are usually more painful and obvious than the fibula fracture. Radiographic clues to a Maisonneuve fracture on routine ankle radiographs (anteroposterior, lateral, and "mortise" views) include an isolated fracture of the posterior tibial margin, an isolated displaced medial malleolus fracture, widening (greater than 3 to 4 mm) of either the medial or lateral clear spaces of the ankle without an associated fibula fracture, or anteromedial or syndesmotic tenderness without radiographic evidence of an injury. If any of these radiographic criteria are met, routine ankle radiographs should be supplemented with full-length anteroposterior and lateral radiographs of the lower leg in order to assess for a proximal fibula fracture that would indicate Maisonneuve fracture.

Notes

CASE 124

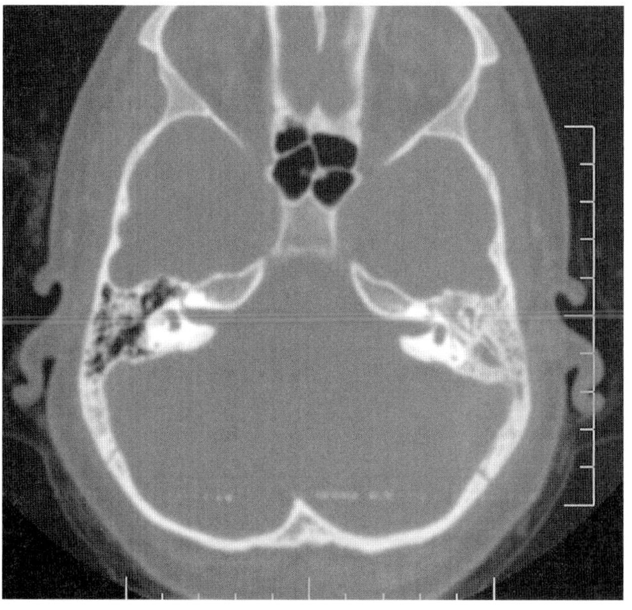

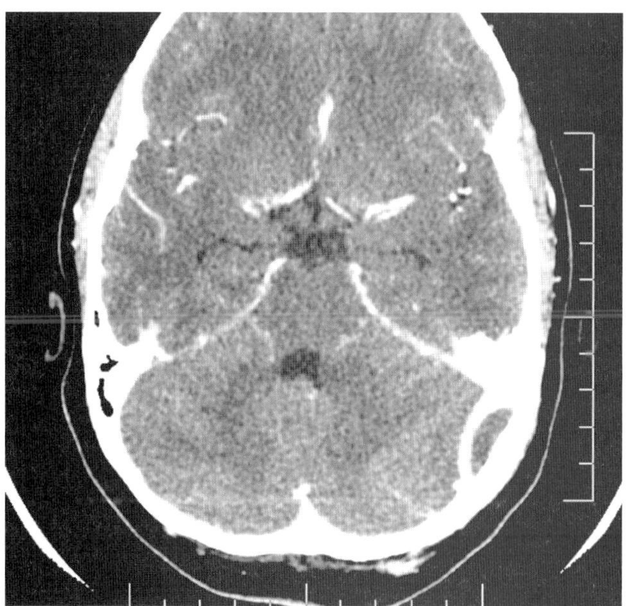

1. Acute mastoiditis is a complication of what common childhood infectious process?
2. What intracranial complication of acute mastoiditis is demonstrated in this patient?
3. What are computed tomographic findings of incipient mastoiditis?
4. Subperiosteal abscesses complicating mastoiditis are usually seen in what age group?

CASE 124

Acute Mastoiditis Complicated by Epidural Abscess

1. Otitis media.
2. Epidural abscess.
3. Middle ear fluid and high attenuation within the mastoid air cells without bone resorption.
4. Children under 11 years old.

Reference

Migirov L: Computed tomographic versus surgical findings in complicated acute otomastoiditis, *Ann Otol Rhinol Laryngol* 112:675–677, 2003.

Cross-Reference

Emergency Radiology: THE REQUISITES, pp 27, 54, 56, 208.

Comment

While acute otitis media typically responds in short order to adequate antibiotic therapy, untreated or inadequately treated cases can be complicated by acute mastoiditis. Even with adequate antibiotic therapy, the mortality rate for acute mastoiditis remains high at 8% to 19%. Surgery may be required to adequately address local or intracranial infection in 25% to 34% of cases. Mastoiditis is suspected when pain, fever, and/or otorrhea persist despite adequate antibiotic therapy for otitis media. Other signs include retroauricular swelling, erythema, and auricular protrusion. Signs of complicated mastoiditis include deep facial pain, cranial nerve palsies, altered mental status, and nuchal rigidity.

The sensitivity of computed tomography (CT) for detecting acute mastoiditis ranges from 87% to 100%. CT detects the complications of mastoiditis with a sensitivity of 97% and a positive predictive value of 94%. CT signs of uncomplicated, or incipient, mastoiditis include middle ear fluid and high attenuation within the mastoid air cells without bone resorption.

Complications of mastoiditis localized to the temporal bone include coalescent mastoiditis (with bone erosion/resorption), petrous apicitis, labyrinthitis, facial nerve paralysis, and hearing loss. Spread of infection through the superficial mastoid cortex causes subperiosteal abscess formation, most common in children under 11 years old, which may extend into the face, the external auditory canal, or the deep neck soft tissues. Intracranial complications include epidural empyema (i.e., abscess), dural venous thrombophlebitis, and subdural empyema.

Notes

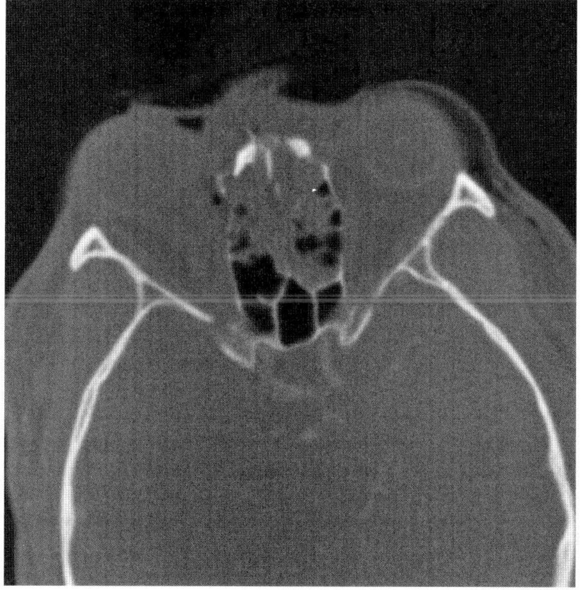

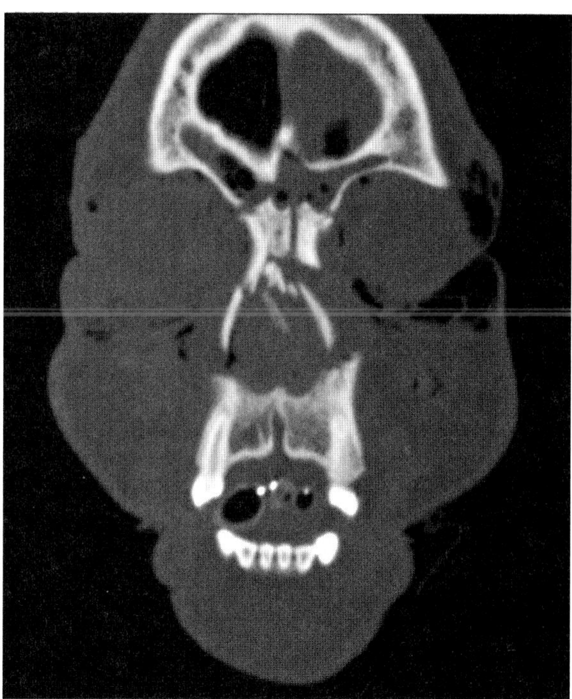

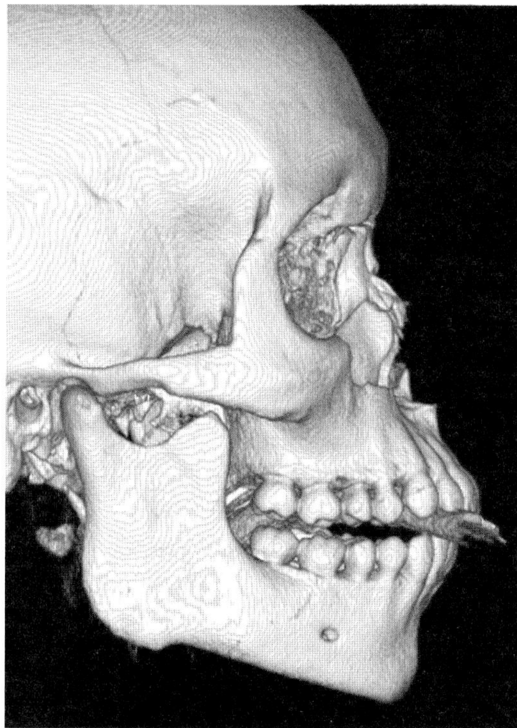

See also Color Plate

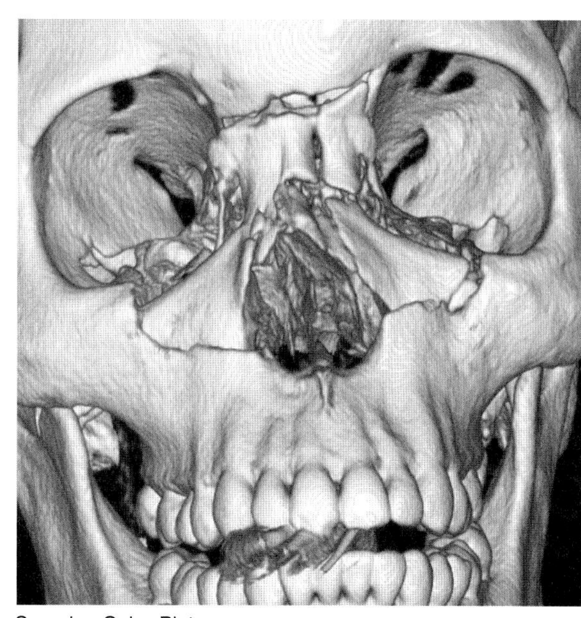

See also Color Plate

1. What region of the midface is fractured?
2. Fracture of what structure, commonly associated with this injury, is the source of the pneumocephalus?
3. What are common complications of this injury?
4. How may three-dimensional computed tomographic (3D-CT) reconstructions benefit this patient?

CASE 125

Naso-orbital Ethmoidal Fracture

1. Naso-orbital ethmoidal complex.
2. Cribiform plate.
3. Vision loss, cerebrospinal fluid rhinorrhea, and telecanthism.
4. 3D-CT reconstructions can assist with surgical planning.

Reference

Sargent LA, Rogers GF: Nasoethmoid orbital fractures: diagnosis and management, *J Craniomaxillofac Trauma* 5:19–27, 1999.

Cross-Reference

Emergency Radiology: THE REQUISITES, p 39.

Comment

The naso-orbital ethmoidal complex comprises the interorbital facial skeleton bounded by the medial orbital walls, lacrimal bones, and maxillary frontal processes on either side, the floor of the anterior cranial fossa superiorly, and the ethmoidal labyrinths posteriorly. Direct trauma to this region may result in complex disruption of these structures. Naso-orbital ethmoid fractures characteristically involve the nasal bones, the junction of the frontal bone with the maxillary frontal process, the maxillary frontal process, the medial orbital wall, the inferior orbital rim, and the piriform aperture (i.e., the superomedial anterior maxillary wall). Fragments may be displaced posteriorly, laterally, or in both directions; rarely, there may be superior displacement. Disruption of the cribiform plate, pneumocephalus, and intracranial hemorrhage are common conse-quences of posterior displacement. Lateral displacement may be associated with ocular injury, or fracture extension into either the nasolacrimal or nasofrontal ducts.

Essentially nondisplaced fractures can be addressed nonoperatively; however, the complicated anatomy, the confluence of major facial structural struts in this region, and the high frequency of complex, comminuted fractures typically require open reduction and internal fixation of the injury in order to limit cosmetic deformity and preserve function of the affected structures. Still, visual impairment and cerebrospinal fluid rhinorrhea are common complications. Disruption of the medial canthal ligaments or their insertions may lead to telecanthism.

Computed tomography with axial and coronal reconstructed images is vital to accurate diagnosis and surgical planning. Thin image reconstruction (1.5 mm to 2.0 mm) is important. While not essential to diagnosis, three-dimensional reconstructions may provide valuable information for treatment planning.

Notes

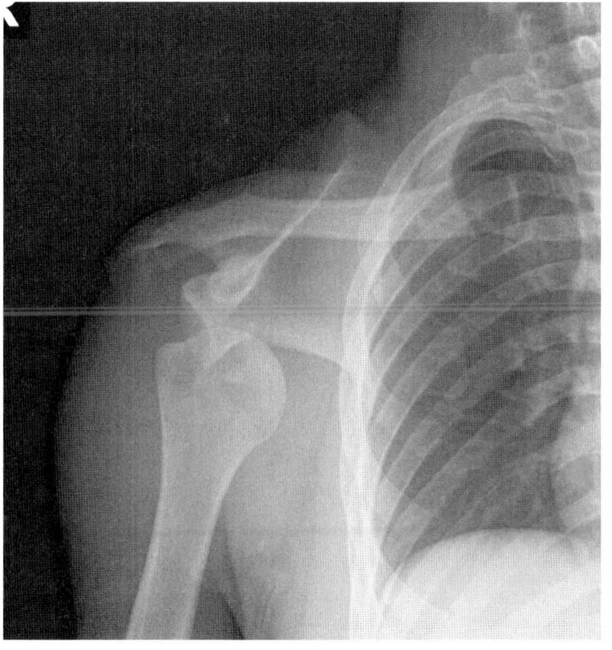

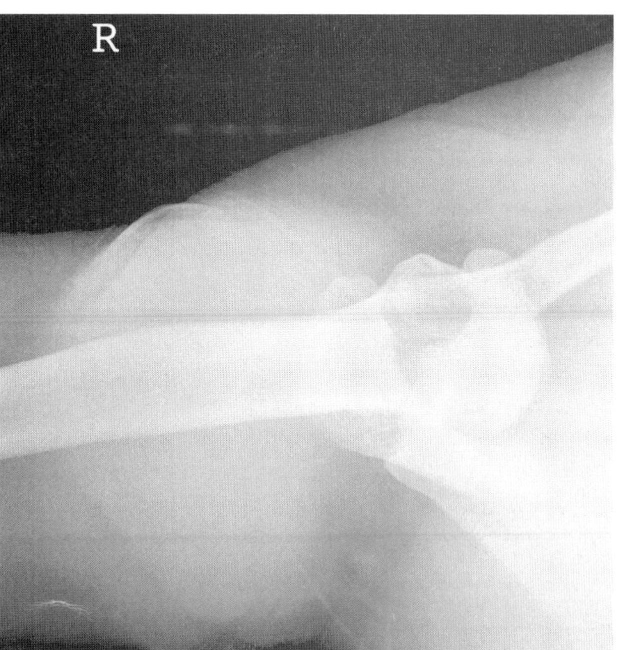

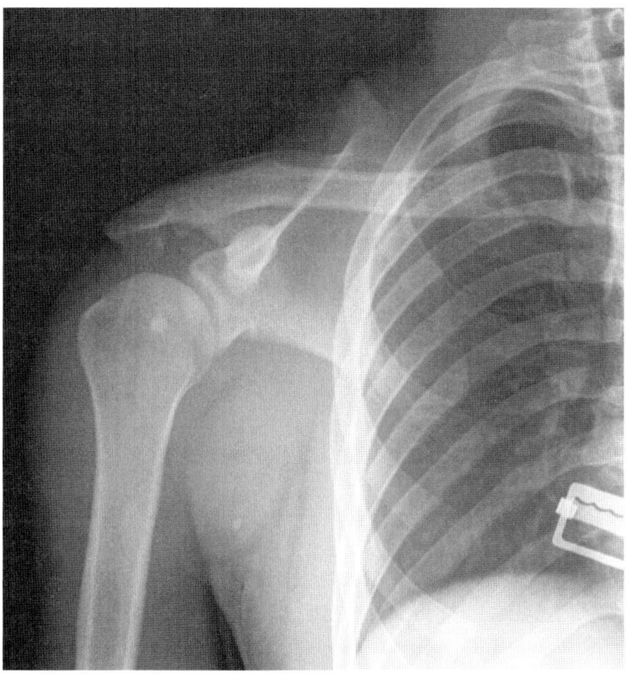

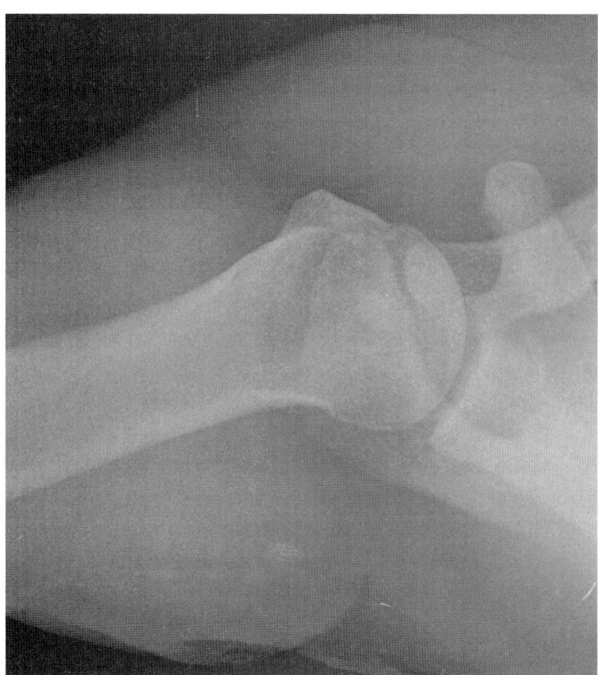

1. What type of shoulder dislocation is this?
2. Is this a common injury?
3. What associated injury is there?
4. What is the risk of obtaining an axillary projection during radiographic evaluation of an acute glenohumeral dislocation?

CASE 126

Anterior Shoulder (Glenohumeral Joint) Dislocation with Bankart Lesion

1. Anterior.
2. Yes.
3. Bony Bankart lesion.
4. The shoulder dislocation may recur.

References

Postacchini F, Gumina S, Cinotti G: Anterior shoulder dislocation in adolescents, *J Shoulder Elbow Surg* 9:470–474, 2000.

Rogers LF, Lenchik L: The shoulder and humeral shaft. In Rogers LF, ed: *Radiology of Skeletal Trauma*, 3rd ed, Philadelphia, Churchill Livingstone, 2002, pp 650–658.

Cross-Reference

Emergency Radiology: THE REQUISITES, pp 116–117.

Comment

The glenohumeral joint is the most commonly dislocated joint in the body. Humeral head displacement may be anterior, posterior, inferior, or superior. Anterior dislocations account for 95% of dislocations, and the humeral head is typically displaced anteromedially into a subcoracoid location. Since the clinical diagnosis is usually obvious, radiographs are generally obtained to confirm the clinical diagnosis and evaluate for associated injuries including greater tuberosity fractures, anterior glenoid rim fractures (bony Bankart lesions), and posterolateral humeral head impaction fractures (Hill-Sachs defects).

Anterior shoulder dislocations tend to recur. The incidence of recurrence is inversely proportional to patient age with recurrence rates ranging from 80% to 92% of adolescents to 10% to 15% of patients older than 40 years. Hill-Sachs defects and Bankart lesions, particularly large ones, predispose to recurrent dislocation.

Anteroposterior radiographs with the arm held in internal and external rotation not only identify dislocations but may also identify Hill-Sachs defects and greater tuberosity fractures. Axillary views help characterize the dislocation as either anterior or posterior while evaluating the anterior glenoid rim for a bony Bankart lesion. Axillary views should be obtained with caution following acute dislocation since zealous positioning of the arm for the exam may induce a recurrent dislocation or further displace associated fractures. Other views that may be obtained to assess the direction of the dislocation include scapular-Y and Grashey views, with the latter providing additional information regarding the integrity of the inferior and superior glenoid rim.

Notes

CASE 127

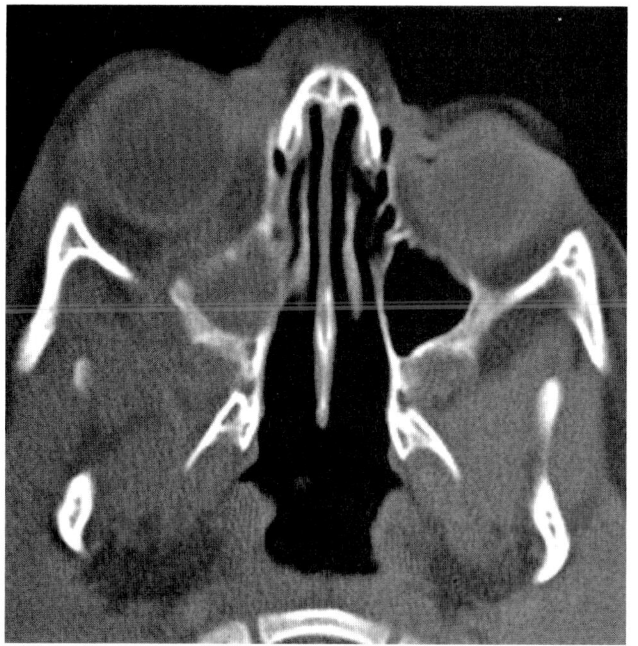

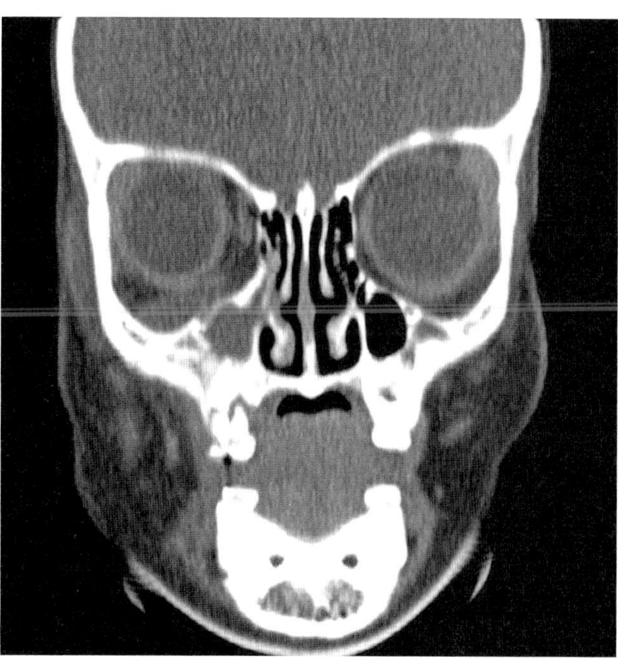

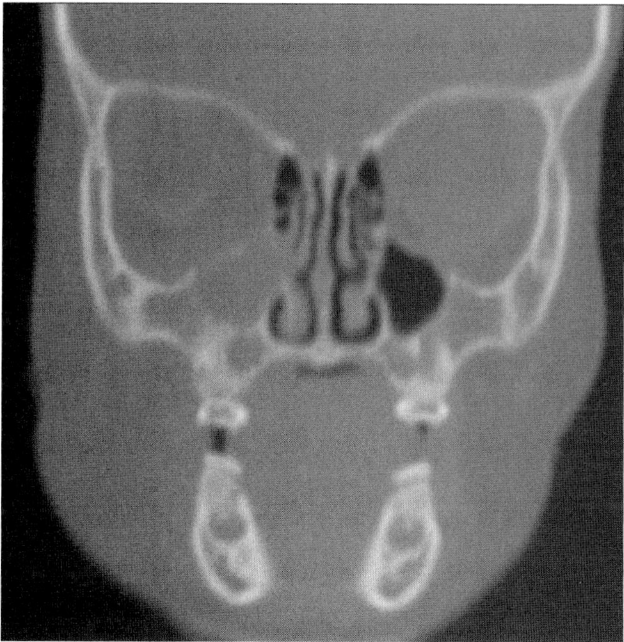

1. What is the diagnosis?
2. What is the usual treatment?
3. What are the consequences of inadequate treatment?
4. This is usually a complication of sinusitis at which site?

CASE 127

Subperiosteal Orbital Abscess

1. Subperiosteal orbital abscess.
2. Intravenous antibiotics and surgical drainage.
3. Impaired vision, spread to deep compartments of the face, intracranial extension.
4. The ipsilateral ethmoid air cells.

Reference

Pereira FJ, Velasco e Cruz AA, Anselmo-Lima WT, Elias J Jr: Computed tomographic patterns of orbital cellulitis due to sinusitis, *Arq Bras Oftalmol* 69: 513–518, 2006.

Cross-Reference

Emergency Radiology: THE REQUISITES, p 50.

Comment

Most orbital infections occur as a complication of acute sinusitis. Infection can extend from any of the paranasal sinuses, but most frequently occurs at the ethmoid air cells. When intraorbital involvement is limited to cellulitis, medical treatment with intravenous antibiotics is usually sufficient. However, subperiosteal and orbital abscesses generally require the addition of surgical drainage to promote adequate response to antibiotics. In addition, an abscess can result in a rapid increase in the orbital contents that may threaten vision. Intraorbital infection may demonstrate intracranial extension or spread into the deep compartments of the face.

Orbital infections can be diagnosed clinically with an accuracy of 81%, whereas computed tomography (CT) demonstrates an accuracy of 91%. On contrast-enhanced CT, orbital cellulitis manifests as diffuse, ill-defined, orbital fat infiltration. Subperiosteal abscesses are well defined by the elevated periosteum, although there may be associated orbital fat infiltration. An orbital abscess is recognized as a well-defined fluid collection within the confines of the orbit itself. When intracranial infection complicating sinusitis or orbital cellulitis is suspected, the sensitivity of CT is 92%, while the accuracy of magnetic resonance imaging approaches 100%.

Notes

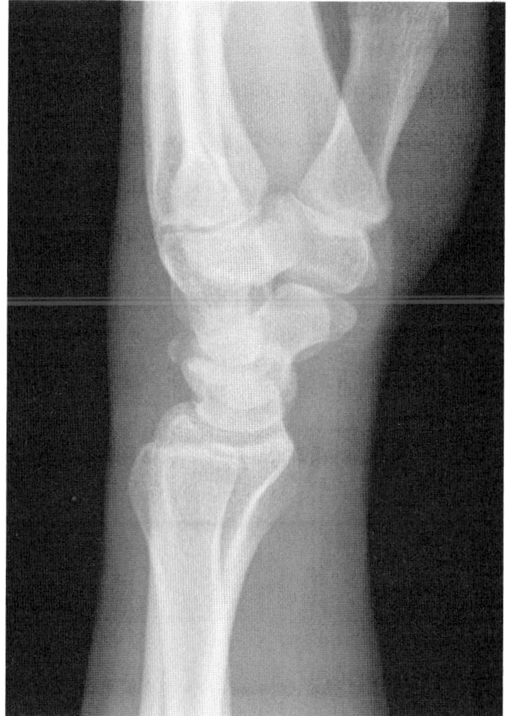

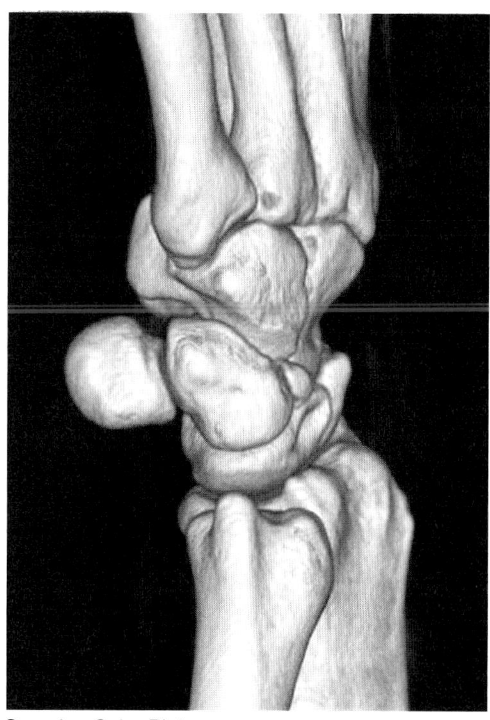

See also Color Plate

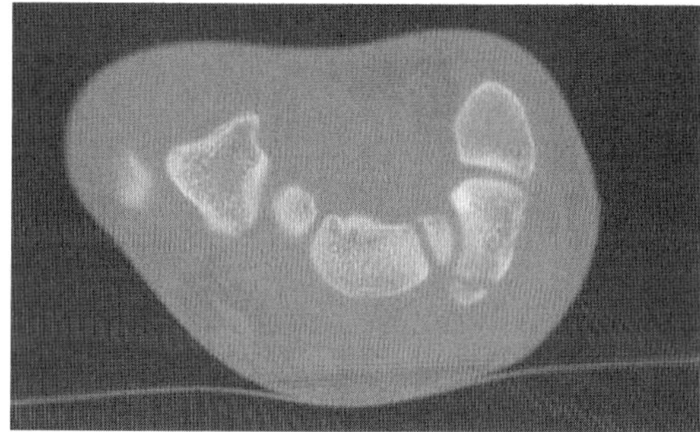

1. What is fractured?
2. What is the usual mechanism of injury for fractures of this bone?
3. What two types of fracture can be encountered in this bone?
4. Among carpal bones, in what order of frequency is this bone fractured?

CASE 128

Triquetral Fracture

1. Triquetrum.
2. Backwards fall onto the dorsiflexed hand with ulnar deviation of the wrist.
3. Avulsion of the radiocarpal ligament at its attachment on the dorsum of the triquetrum and either transverse or vertical transtriquetral fractures.
4. It is the second most frequently fractured carpal bone.

References

Beer JD, Hudson DA: Fractures of the triquetrum, *J Hand Surg Br* 12:52–53, 1987.

Eustace S, Keogh C, Bergin D: The wrist. In Rogers LF, ed: *Radiology of Skeletal Trauma*, 3rd ed, Philadelphia, Churchill Livingstone, 2002, pp 839, 841.

Cross-Reference

Emergency Radiology: THE REQUISITES, pp 129–131.

Comment

The triquetrum is the second most commonly fractured carpal bone, following the scaphoid, with an incidence between 3.5% and 20%. Fractures may occur in isolation or in association with other carpal injuries. Most patients with triquetral fractures present with dorsal soft tissue swelling and pain with ulnar-sided carpal tenderness following a backwards fall onto the dorsiflexed hand with ulnar deviation of the wrist. Fractures usually represent avulsion of the radiocarpal ligament at its attachment on the dorsum of the triquetrum. Transverse or vertical transtriquetral fractures may result from compression of the bone between the ulna and hamate. Treatment with prompt external immobilization with a cast typically results in adequate healing. However, delayed diagnosis can result in nonunion and chronic wrist pain.

Radiographs of the wrist typically demonstrate dorsal soft tissue swelling. Compressive-type fractures are generally apparent on the posteroanterior projection. Avulsion-type fractures are characteristically visible only on the lateral projection as small bone fragments at the dorsal triquetral margin. Computed tomography facilitates differentiation of a triquetral avulsion fracture from a lunate avulsion fracture in radiographically equivocal cases, although it is usually unnecessary since treatment of both types of injury is identical.

Notes

CASE 129

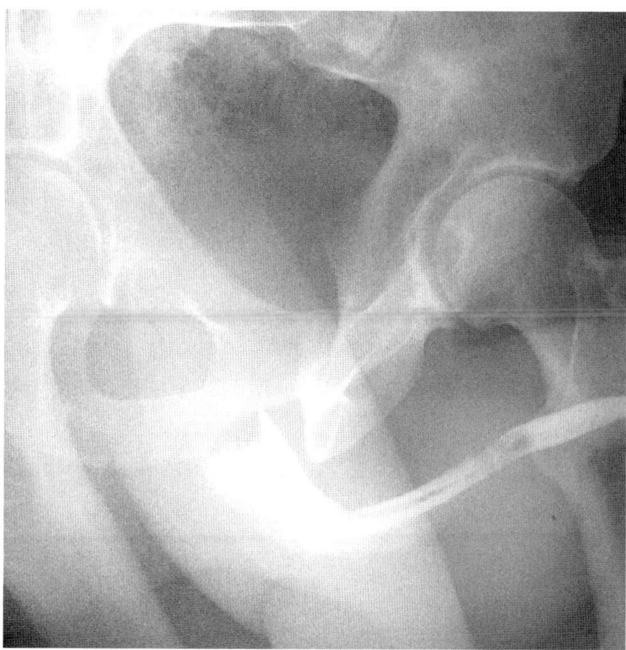

1. What urethral segment is injured?
2. What is the mechanism of injury?
3. What typical clinical signs mandate a retrograde urethrogram prior to urethral catheterization?
4. What is a long-term complication of this injury?

ANSWERS

CASE 129

Anterior Urethral Disruption

1. Bulbar urethra.
2. Straddle injury with urethra crushed against the pubic symphysis.
3. Blood at the meatus and gross hematuria.
4. Urethral stricture.

Reference

Park S, McAninch JW: Straddle injuries to the bulbar urethra: management and outcomes in 78 patients, *J Urol* 171:722–725, 2004.

Cross-Reference

Emergency Radiology: THE REQUISITES, pp 105–107.

Comment

Anterior urethral injuries typically occur as a consequence of a straddle injury when the bulbar urethra is crushed against the pubic symphysis. They are uncommon injuries which should be suspected with signs of significant perineal or penile trauma. Given their shorter urethras, anterior urethral injuries are distinctly uncommon in women. In contrast to posterior urethral injuries, associated pelvic fractures are uncommon.

Blood at the meatus and gross hematuria are typical clinical signs that should prompt a retrograde urethrogram to evaluate for injury before urethral catheterization is performed. Injuries can be characterized as contusions, incomplete disruptions, and complete transections. Disruptions may require urinary diversion with suprapubic bladder catheterization to limit inflammation prior to surgical repair. Even with prompt urinary diversion and surgery, anterior urethral injury can lead to urethral strictures requiring delayed surgical intervention.

Notes

CASE 130

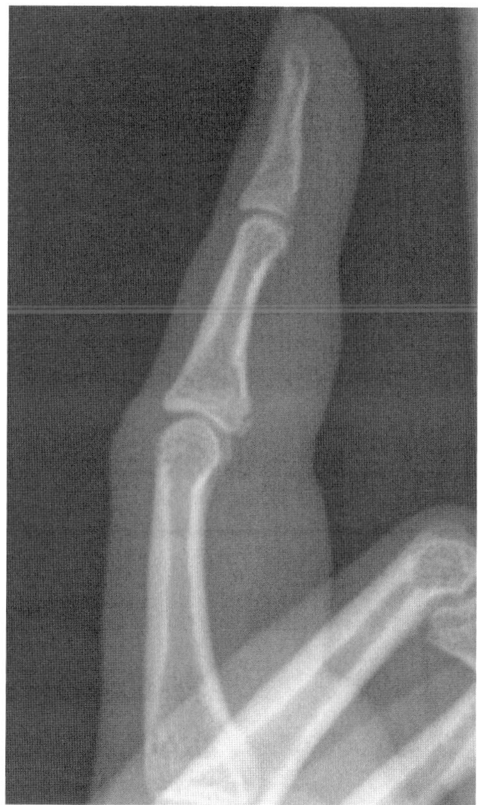

1. What structure is avulsed from the base of the middle phalanx?
2. What is the typical mechanism of injury?
3. Is the small size of the avulsed fragment typical for this injury?
4. What are potential long-term consequences if this injury is not treated?

CASE 130

Volar Plate Avulsion Fracture

1. The volar plate.
2. Hyperextension.
3. Yes.
4. Accelerated arthritis, chronic joint instability, deformity.

Reference

Nance EP Jr, Kaye JJ, Milek MA: Volar plate fractures, *Radiology* 133:61–64, 1979.

Cross-Reference

Emergency Radiology: THE REQUISITES, p 137.

Comment

The volar plate is a dense fibrous ligament that forms the palmar aspect of the proximal interphalangeal joint capsule. Distally, it firmly attaches to the volar aspect of the middle phalanx base. Disruption of the volar plate is a common type of hyperextension injury most commonly seen as a consequence of athletic injuries, particularly in football and basketball. Usually, the diagnosis can be suspected clinically, although up to 20% may go unappreciated on clinical exam. Closed reduction usually promotes satisfactory healing, although large fragments may require open reduction and internal fixation. Untreated injuries may lead to accelerated arthritis, chronic joint instability with recurrent subluxation, flexion contracture, or swan neck deformity.

Volar plate disruption may occur anywhere along its length, or it may avulse a fragment from its insertion on the middle phalanx. The avulsed fracture fragment is usually minimally displaced and best seen on either a lateral or an oblique radiograph. Fragments are typically very small and subtle with appearances ranging from a small dot to a sliver of bone with a diameter commonly less than 1 mm.

Notes

CASE 131

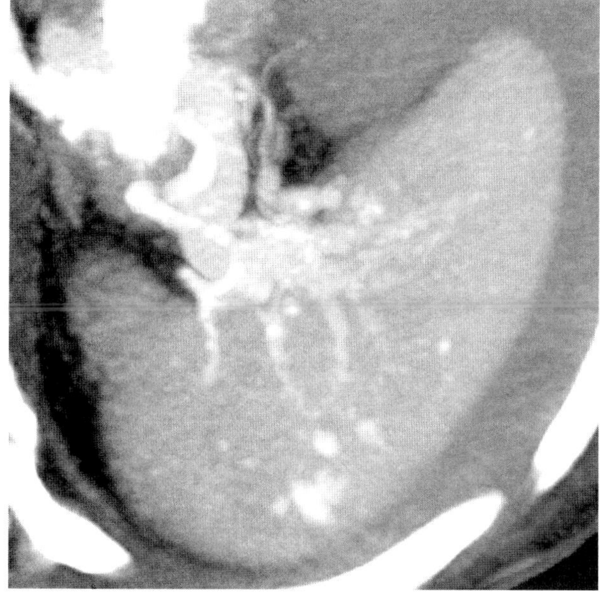

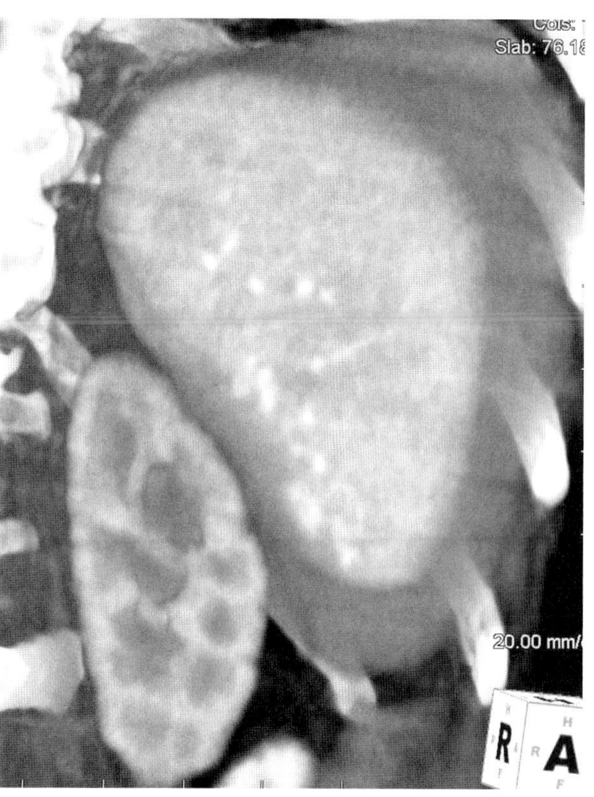

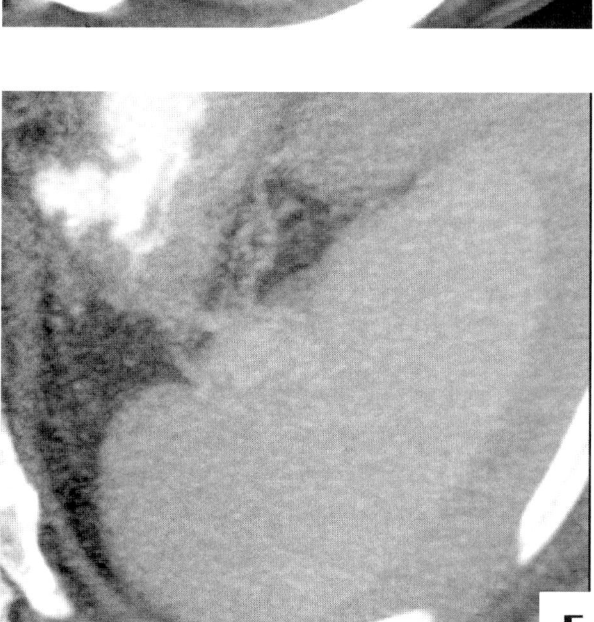

You are shown portal venous and excretory phase multidetector computed tomographic (MDCT) images of a patient admitted following blunt abdominal trauma.

1. What is the diagnosis?
2. What are the two types of splenic vascular injuries?
3. Can MDCT differentiate this injury from splenic active bleeding?
4. What is the significance of this injury?

CASE 131

Splenic Vascular Injury

1. Splenic vascular injury.
2. Pseudoaneurysms and post-traumatic arteriovenous fistula (AVF).
3. Yes.
4. Delayed hemorrhage may occur in up to 82% of untreated splenic vascular injuries.

References

Gavant ML, Schurr M, Flick PA, et al: Predicting clinical outcome of nonsurgical management of blunt splenic injury: using CT to reveal abnormalities of splenic vasculature, *AJR Am J Roentgenol* 173:855–856, 1999.

Hann JM, Biffle W, Knudson M, et al: Splenic embolization revisited: a multicenter review, *J Trauma* 56: 542–547, 2004.

Cross-Reference

Emergency Radiology: THE REQUISITES, pp 89, 90.

Comment

Splenic vascular injuries or active bleeding are seen in about 22% of patients with splenic injury. A pseudoaneurysm or AVF appears as a well-circumscribed lesion of contrast material of attenuation similar to an adjacent contrast-enhanced artery. These vascular lesions may be surrounded by a low-attenuation area. On delayed imaging during the excretory phase, vascular lesions typically lose density from washout of intravenous contrast material and become similar to or slightly higher in attenuation than adjacent normal parenchyma. This helps to differentiate vascular injuries from active bleeding, which is typically a linear or irregular area of contrast material enhancement, with an attenuation value similar to or greater than an adjacent major artery. The area of active bleeding identified during the initial images may appear to expand on renal excretory phase imaging because of continuing bleeding.

On contrast-enhanced multidetector computed tomography (MDCT), pseudoaneurysm and AVF have the same appearance and can be differentiated only on splenic arteriography. Studies report that up to 80% of these lesions may fail nonoperative management due to delayed splenic hemorrhage. Identifying and treating these lesions with transcatheter splenic artery embolization in a prospective fashion helps to increase the number of patients who can be managed nonoperatively. Transcatheter main or distal splenic artery embolization decreases the splenic perfusion pressure and provides hemostasis. Splenic salvage rates are similar for main splenic artery and subselective embolization groups. Splenic surgery is the treatment of choice if the patient is hemodynamically unstable or if splenic arteriography is not available.

Notes

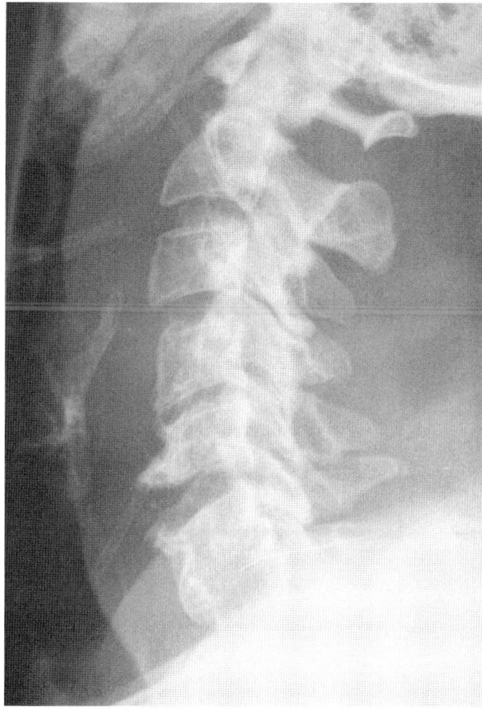

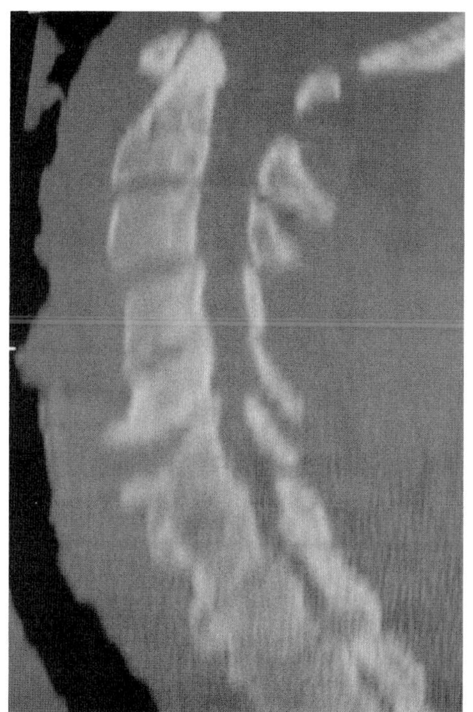

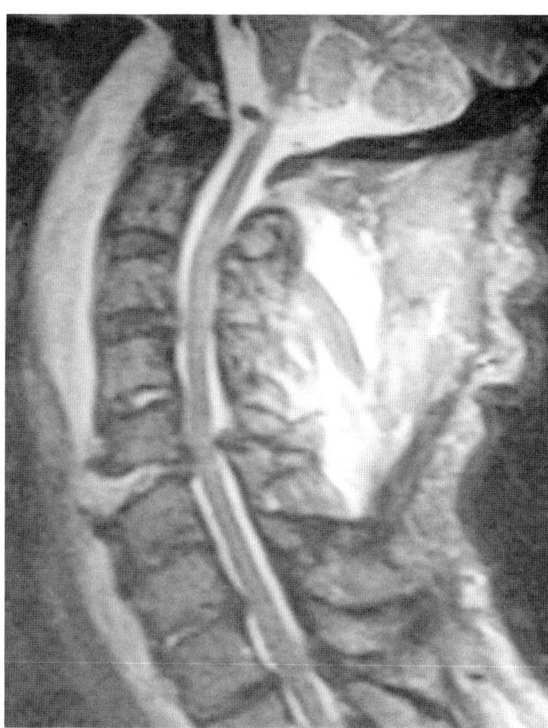

You are shown images of a patient who complained of neck pain after trauma.

1. Describe the radiographic findings.
2. What is the diagnosis?
3. What is the role of magnetic resonance (MR) imaging in this injury?
4. Which MR sequence optimally demonstrates cord contusions?

CASE 132

Hyperextension Dislocation Injury at the C5-C6 Level

1. Diffuse prevertebral and posterior soft tissue of the neck edema, widening of the anterior disc space at the C5-C6 level, retrolisthesis of C5 vertebra in relation to the C6 vertebra, and a step-off in the spinolaminar line at the C5-C6 level are seen.
2. Hyperextension dislocation injury at the C5-C6 level.
3. Magnetic resonance imaging demonstrates extramedullary bleeds, ligament, disc, and cord injuries.
4. Fat suppressed inversion recovery images (STIR).

References

Davis SJ, Teresi LM, Bradley WG, et al: Cervical spine hyperextension injuries: MR findings, *Radiology* 180: 245–251, 1991.

Edeiken-Monroe B, Wagner LK, Harris JH Jr: Hyperextension dislocation of the cervical spine, *AJR Am J Roentgenol* 146:803–806, 1986.

Cross-Reference

Emergency Radiology: THE REQUISITES, pp 220, 221.

Comment

Hyperextension dislocation is caused by an impact force to the forehead or mid-face that drives the cervical spine into hyperextension. This force injures the anterior longitudinal and intervertebral disc horizontally. The injury may even extend more posteriorly to involve the posterior longitudinal ligament with impingement of the cord between the posterior cortex of the vertebral body anteriorly and the ligamentum flavum and lamina posteriorly. In the literature this injury has been described as spinal cord injury without radiographic abnormalities (SCIWORA). Clinically, an acute central cervical cord syndrome may result. The asymmetric neurological deficit involves the upper extremity to a greater extent than the lower extremity.

Radiographic and computed tomographic (CT) signs of this injury may be extremely subtle and occur without any apparent skeletal fractures or dislocation. The posterior dislocation may reduce itself by antagonistic muscle action or by the application of a cervical collar. Lateral radiographs and sagittal reformatted CT images may demonstrate diffuse prevertebral soft tissue swelling usually extending over multiple vertebral segments, an avulsion fracture arising from the anteroinferior aspect of the vertebral body, widening of the anterior intervertebral disc space, and a vacuum disc in young patients. The avulsion fracture fragment is usually wider in width than its vertical height.

Magnetic resonance imaging (MRI) is the imaging modality of choice to demonstrate this injury. The various MR sequences used to image the cervical spine help to optimally demonstrate injuries to the spinal ligaments, intervertebral disc, and spinal cord. Ligaments are visualized as linear low-signal intensity regions on all sequences, but are optimally visualized on proton density images. An acute injury is seen as an interruption to the normal flow of the low-signal structure with an associated adjacent high signal representing edema. An injury to the intervertebral disc is seen as an abnormal high signal within the disc space or acute disc herniation. An abnormal signal may also be seen within the spinal cord due to edema and hemorrhage resulting from the impingement between the posterior vertebral body and the lamina and ligamentum flavum. MRI signal characteristics of the acute cord injury may vary depending on the presence of edema or hemorrhage. Several investigators have reported a worse prognosis in those patients with hemorrhagic cord contusion.

Notes

CASE 133

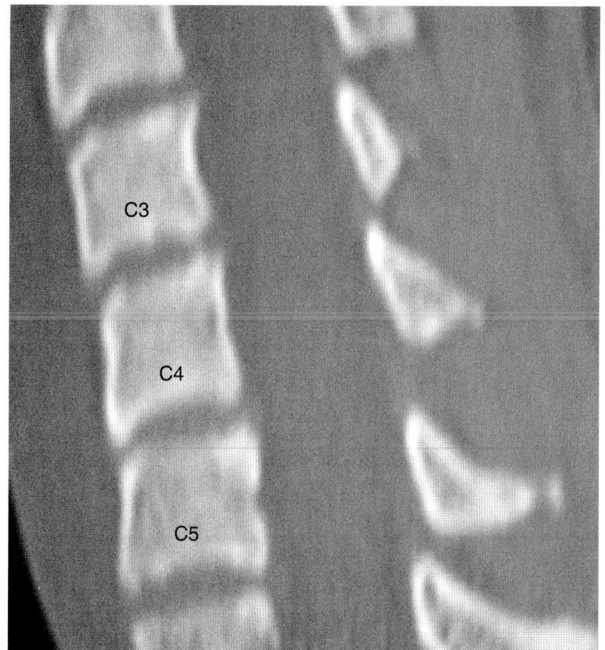

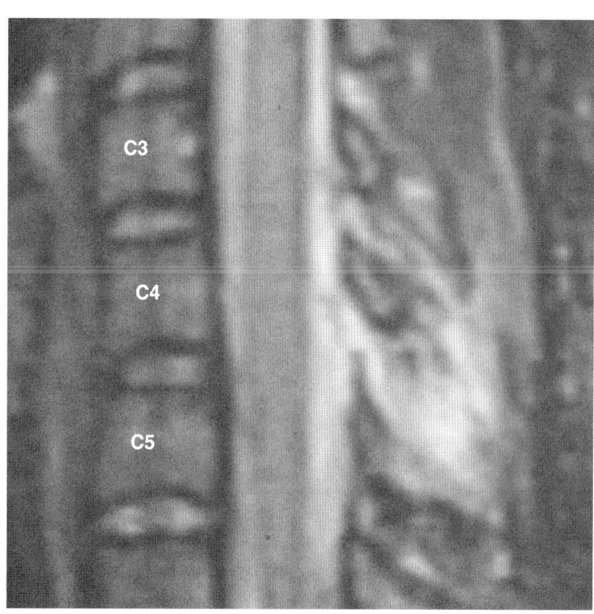

You are shown images of a patient with persistent lower neck pain and tenderness caused by a motor vehicle collision.

1. What are the radiographic and computed tomographic findings?
2. What are the magnetic resonance imaging findings?
3. What is the best diagnosis?
4. How do lateral flexion and extension assist in the diagnosis of this injury?

CASE 133

Hyperflexion Sprain Injury at the C3-C4 and C4-C5 Levels

1. Widening of the interspinous and interlaminar distances and a kyphous deformity at the C4-C5 level.
2. Discontinuity of the ligamentum flavum at the C3-C4 and C4-C5 levels; edema in the posterior soft tissues of the neck and interspinous ligament at the C3-C4 and C4-C5 levels.
3. Hyperflexion sprain injury at the C3-C4 and C4-C5 levels.
4. Application of stress (performed under the direct supervision of a physician) during flexion helps to demonstrate the injury.

References

Braakman M, Braakman R: Hyperflexion sprain of the cervical spine. Follow-up of 45 cases, *Acta Orthop Scand* 58:388–393, 1987.

Ronnen HR, de Korte PJ, Brink PR, et al: Acute whiplash injury: is there a role for MR imaging? A prospective study of 100 patients, *Radiology* 201:93–96, 1996.

Cross-Reference

Emergency Radiology: THE REQUISITES, p 220.

Comment

Hyperflexion sprain injuries are commonly caused by rear-end motor vehicle collisions. The abrupt deceleration force causes the head and neck to go into hyperextension followed by hyperflexion. The soft tissue injury to the cervical spine often results from the flexion component.

The disruption of the posterior ligament complex may include the supraspinous and interspinous ligaments, the ligamentum flavum, and the capsules of the facet joint. Usually, with an increase in the magnitude of the flexion force, the soft tissue injury may extend anteriorly to disrupt the posterior longitudinal ligament, annulus of the disc, and posterior aspect of the intervertebral disc. Clinically patients with hyperflexion sprain injury have neck and interscapular pain, limited range of cervical spine flexion and extension, and point tenderness over the involved interspinous space.

Radiographic findings may be subtle on the neutral lateral view. At the level of injury the interspinous and interlaminar distance is increased compared with the subadjacent levels above and below the injury. A kyphous deformity in the alignment of the spine is noted at the level of injury. Anterior subluxation and widening of the posterior disc space is seen in patients with disruption of the posterior longitudinal ligament and the disc.

Patients who have persistent symptoms and normal or equivocal radiographs require further imaging with magnetic resonance imaging (MRI) or lateral flexion and extension views performed under physician supervision. MRI protocol should include sagittal fat-suppressed inversion recovery (STIR), proton density, and T2-weighted fast spin echo sequences to demonstrate this injury. Ligament disruption optimally visualized on the proton-weighted sequence is seen as an interruption in the normal linear low signal of the ligament. A high-intensity signal representing edema may be seen on STIR, proton density, and T2-weighted images within the posterior neck muscles, facet joints, disc space, and interspinous and interlaminar ligaments. Flexion and extension views help to "stress" the posterior ligament complex and demonstrate the radiographic signs of the injury on flexion view. On the extension view the signs usually return to normal.

Notes

CASE 134

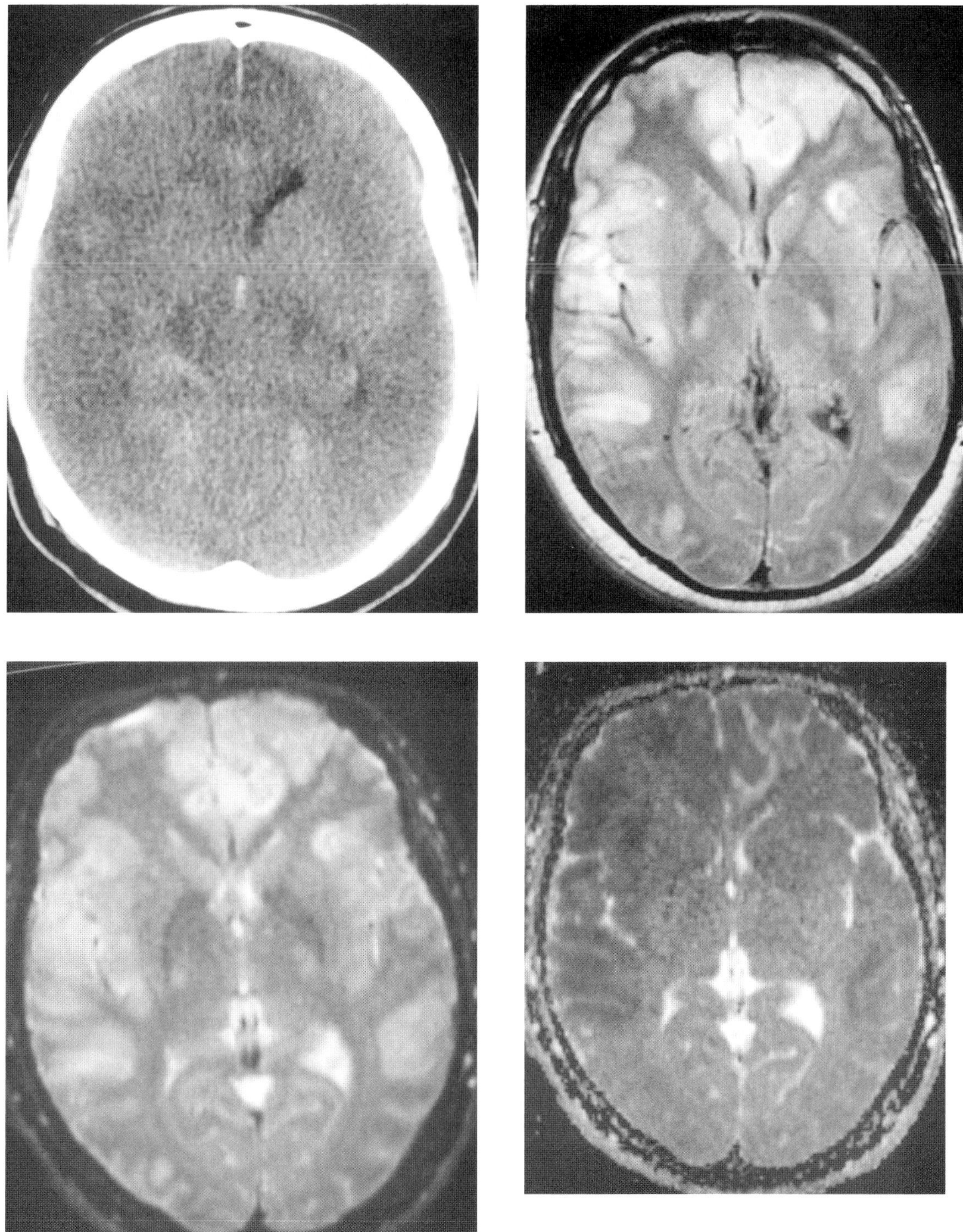

You are shown images of a brain-injured patient unresponsive after a motorcycle collision: CT, FLAIR, diffusion-weighted, and ADC images obtained 5 days post admission.

1. What are the computed tomographic findings?
2. What are the magnetic resonance imaging findings?
3. What is the diagnosis?
4. What are the different causes for this injury?

CASE 134

Anoxic Brain Injury

1. CT image shows loss of gray matter–white matter differentiation, with low attenuation areas in the right temporal lobe external capsules and frontal lobes bilaterally.
2. FLAIR image shows predominantly high signal intensity in the cortical gray matter, some white matter and bilateral external capsules. Diffusion-weighted and ADC images show restricted diffusion in the areas of high signal intensity noted on FLAIR.
3. Anoxic brain injury.
4. Anoxic anoxia (lack of oxygen), anemic anoxia (not enough blood or hemoglobin), stagnant anoxia (circulatory collapse).

References

Chao CP, Zaleski CG, Patton AC: Neonatal hypoxic-ischemic encephalopathy: multimodality imaging findings, *Radiographics* 26(Suppl):S159–S172, 2006.

Takahashi S, Higano S, Ishii K, et al: Hypoxic brain damage: cortical laminar necrosis and delayed changes in white matter at sequential MR imaging, *Radiology* 189:449–456, 1993.

Comment

Anoxic brain injury results from the inadequate supply of oxygen, which is unable to meet the metabolic requirements of the brain. Sustained anoxia usually leads to both neuronal cell and glial cell injury or death. In the trauma setting systemic hypotension, low cardiac output, and respiratory arrest are common causes for cerebral anoxia. The extent of injury depends on the duration and severity of these systemic factors and coexisting vascular disease.

Imaging findings of global hypoxic brain damage are time dependent and vary with the severity of the initial insult. Changes may not be seen on computed tomography within the first few hours. Early changes may include subtle loss of gray matter–white matter differentiation, decreased attenuation of the gray matter, and effacement of the cerebral sulci from mass effect. The amount of cerebral edema may reflect the severity of the time of anoxic insult. The areas of infarction are usually seen in the arterial boundary zones (watershed) in the cerebral cortex and cerebellum. Metabolically active areas including the lateral thalamus, posterior putamina, hippocampi, and sensorimotor cortex are vulnerable to infarction. Experimental studies report the gray matter is much more vulnerable to ischemia compared with the white matter.

Magnetic resonance imaging (MRI) is the most sensitive and specific technique to demonstrate changes due to anoxic brain injury. Newer MR techniques including diffusion-weighted images (DWI) and spectroscopy are more sensitive than conventional MRI in depiction and detection of the ischemic event within the first few hours to days. Early subtle changes may only be seen in the boundary zone in the cortex at the occipitoparietotemporal region as hyperintense signal areas on FLAIR and T2-weighted images and areas of restricted diffusion on DWI. Characteristic cortical laminar enhancement on post-contrast and hyperintense areas on unenhanced T1-weighted sequences are seen in the subacute phase.

Notes

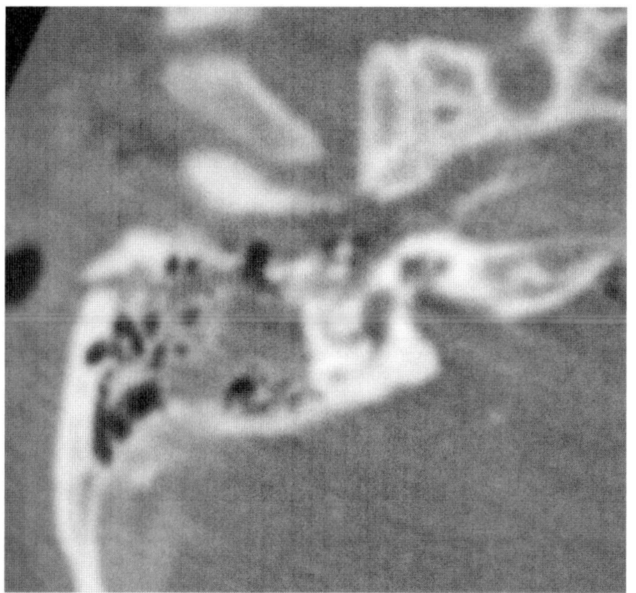

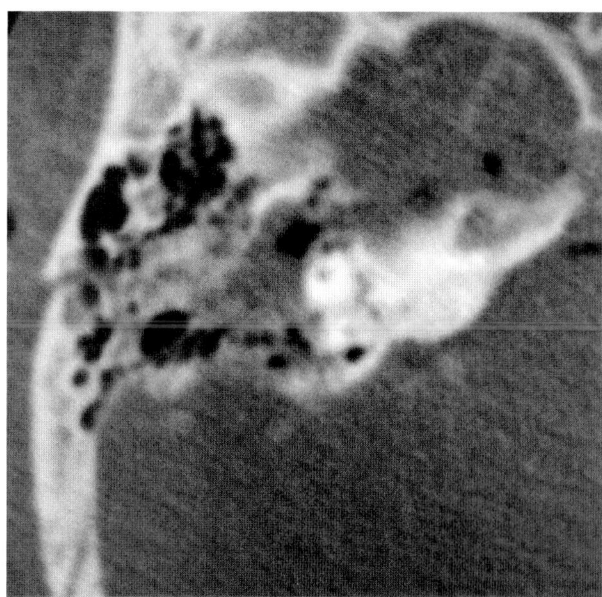

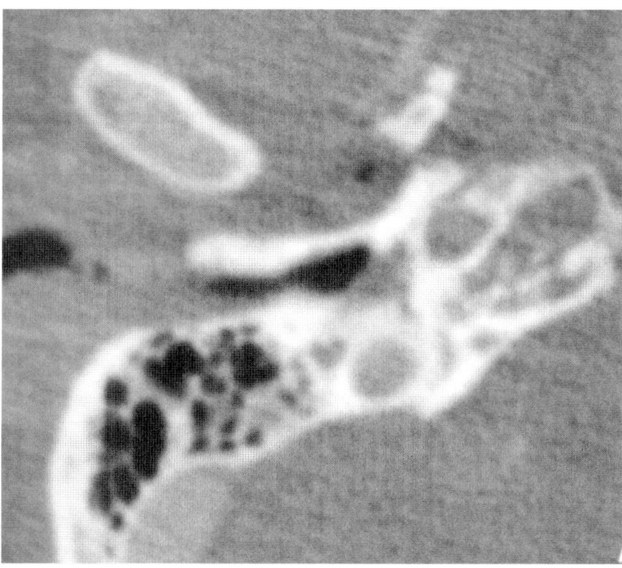

You are shown images of a patient bleeding from the right ear after trauma.

1. What are the computed tomographic findings?
2. What is the diagnosis?
3. What are the different types of fractures seen in this entity?
4. Name three complications related to this injury.

CASE 135

Longitudinal Fracture of the Petrous Temporal Bone

1. Blood is seen within the middle ear and mastoid air cells. Pneumocephalus and air is also seen within the temporomandibular joint, and a fracture of the petrous temporal bone is also seen.
2. Longitudinal fracture of the petrous temporal bone.
3. Longitudinal fracture, transverse fracture, and complex or mixed fracture.
4. Conductive hearing loss, cerebrospinal fluid otorrhagia, and facial nerve palsy.

References

Betz BW, Wiener DM: Air in the temporomandibular joint fossa: CT sign of temporal bone fracture, *Radiology* 180:463–466, 1991.

Fatterpekar GM, Doshi AH, Dugar DM: Role of 3D CT in the evaluation of the temporal bone, *Radiographics* 26(Suppl):S117–S132, 2006.

Cross-Reference

Emergency Radiology: THE REQUISITES, pp 41–43.

Comment

Temporal bone fractures may be difficult to visualize on multidetector computed tomography (MDCT). They account for 20% of all skull fractures. Temporal bone fractures are categorized into three types depending on their orientation relative to the longitudinal axis of the petrous temporal bone. Longitudinal fractures usually extend from the squamous temporal bone medially toward the tympanic cavity, parallel to the long axis of the petrous pyramid. The typical impact site is at the temporoparietal region of the skull. Transverse fractures are oriented perpendicular to the long axis of the petrous temporal bone and result from a blow to the occipital bone. Transverse fractures are seen medially extending through the fundus of the internal carotid artery or the bony labyrinth. Complex or mixed fractures have both longitudinal and transverse components. The majority of the patients (75% to 80%) have a longitudinal fracture.

High-resolution temporal bone MDCT images are required to demonstrate the fracture. Indirect CT findings of temporal bone fracture include opacification of the mastoid air cells, blood within the auditory canal and middle ear, air within the temporomandibular joint (TMJ), pneumocephalus seen adjacent to the petrous pyramid, air in the soft tissue superficial to the temporal bone, and air within the labrynthine system. The air enters the TMJ because the longitudinal fracture extends through the adjacent air-containing bony external auditory canal or tympanic cavity.

Clinical findings associated with temporal bone fractures include blood within the external auditory canal, hearing loss, cerebrospinal fluid ottorrhagia, facial nerve palsy, postaricullar ecchymosis, and hematotympanum. With longitudinal fractures the facial nerve palsy is usually partial and temporary and is seen in about 15% of patients. Transverse fractures are associated with permanent facial nerve palsy and are seen in about 80% of patients. A conductive hearing loss occurs with longitudinal fractures due to blood within the middle ear or from ossicular disruption. In contrast, transverse fractures may involve the labyrinth and cause sensorineural hearing loss. Vestibular dysfunction is more likely to be seen following transverse fractures. Three-dimensional (3D) volume rendered images are useful to demonstrate ossicular dislocation and extension of fractures into the region of the round and oval windows. A degree of permanent hearing loss may result from scarring due to healing of fractures that involve the oval window. Hence, 3D images may be useful to predict the outcome of surgery performed to correct the hearing loss following ossicular disruption.

Notes

CASE 136

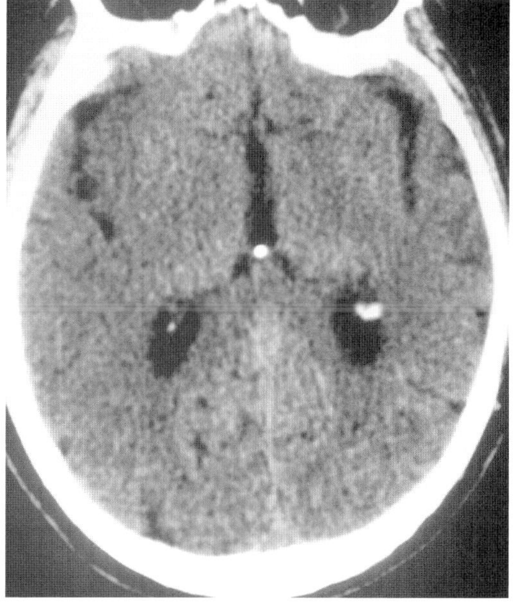

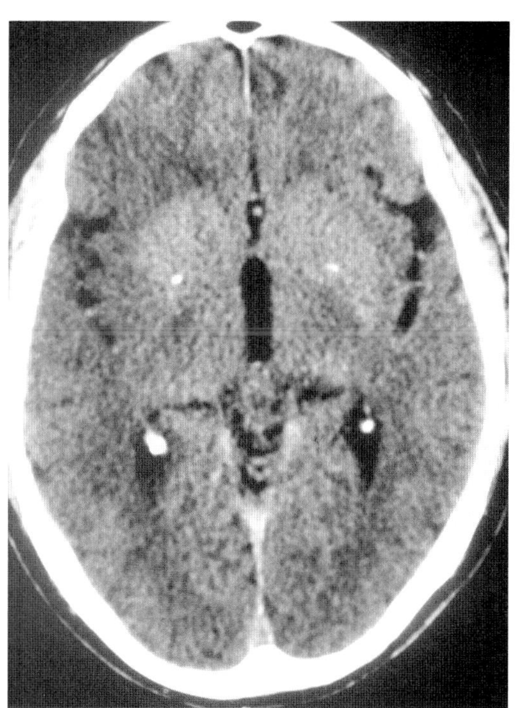

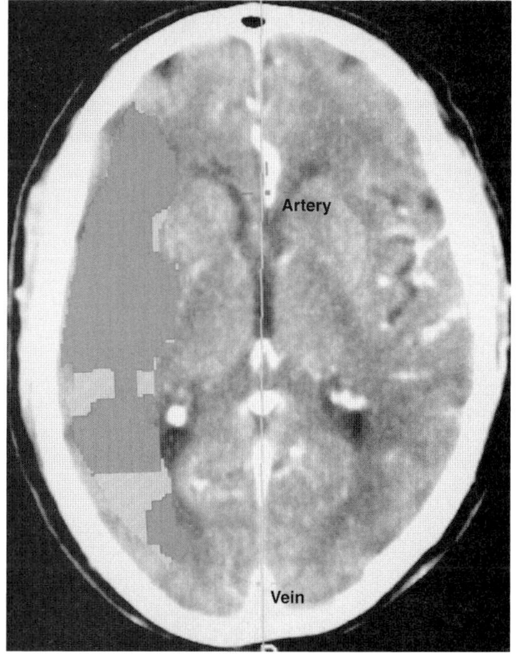

See also Color Plate

You are shown images of a patient who complains of an inability to move the left upper and lower extremities.

1. What is the diagnosis?
2. What study has been demonstrated in the bottom left image? What are the findings?
3. Describe three early findings seen in this entity on unenhanced computed tomography (CT).
4. What are the key three CT techniques used to image this entity?

CASE 136

Nonhemorrhagic Right Middle Cerebral Artery Infarct

1. Nonhemorrhagic right middle cerebral artery infarct.
2. Computed tomography (CT) perfusion study shows a large right middle cerebral artery infarct (red) with a small penumbra (green).
3. Hyperdense vessel sign, "insular ribbon" sign or effacement of salci at the insular cortex, and obscuration of the lentiform nucleus.
4. Unenhanced CT, perfusion CT, and CT angiogram of the head.

References

Srinivasan A, Goyal M, Al Azri F: State-of-the-art imaging of acute stroke, *Radiographics* 26(Suppl): S75–S95, 2006.

Wintermark M, Fischbein NJ, Smith WS, et al: Accuracy of dynamic perfusion CT with deconvolution in detecting acute hemispheric stroke, *AJNR Am J Neuroradiol* 26:104–112, 2005.

Cross-Reference

Emergency Radiology: THE REQUISITES, p 17.

Comment

The primary role of stroke imaging is to establish the diagnosis as early as possible, and to demonstrate the intracranial vasculature and brain perfusion in order to plan optimal treatment. The most common imaging modality performed is an unenhanced computed tomography (CT) scan of the head because it is quick and available in most emergency rooms in the United States. Using standard windows the sensitivity and specificity of unenhanced CT in demonstrating an ischemic stroke is 52% to 57% and 94%, respectively. The early CT findings of obscuration of the lentiform nucleus and the "insular ribbon" sign are due to loss of contrast between the gray and white matter from cytotoxic edema. By using a variable window width and level (10 HU [Hounsfield units] and 30 HU, respectively) to view the unenhanced CT images, the sensitivity of early acute ischemic stroke detection may be improved to about 72%. Unenhanced CT is also used to demonstrate any intracranial hemorrhage.

CT angiography is routinely performed in most centers as part of the stroke workup to demonstrate the intracranial and neck vessels. Axial, maximum intensity reformatted, and three-dimensional volume rendered images are used in the evaluation. An acute ischemic stroke with a large thrombus burden may favor intra-arterial or mechanical thrombolysis. The location of the thrombus may also help to predict outcome. Early improvement is usually seen in patients with peripheral arterial occlusions.

CT perfusion is used to quantitatively and qualitatively measure the mean transit time (MTT), cerebral blood flow (CBF), and cerebral volumes (CBV). This technique can be performed quickly on any helical CT scanner. The perfusion maps are generated on an independent workstation within a short period of time. The maps help to identify the area of cerebral infarction from the more peripheral parenchyma, called the penumbra, an area that could be potentially salvaged by early thrombolytic therapy. Infarcted tissue shows a severely decreased CBF (<10 mL/g/min) and CBV (<3 mL/100 g), and an increased MTT. The penumbra shows an increased MTT, normal or increased CBV, and moderately decreased CBF due to preservation of autoregulation. The MTT maps are the most sensitive and the CBV maps are the most specific indicators of a stroke.

The preference to use CT or magnetic resonance imaging to work up patients with acute stroke may depend on the clinical circumstances, and on the availability and expertise of the staff at the institution.

Notes

CASE 137

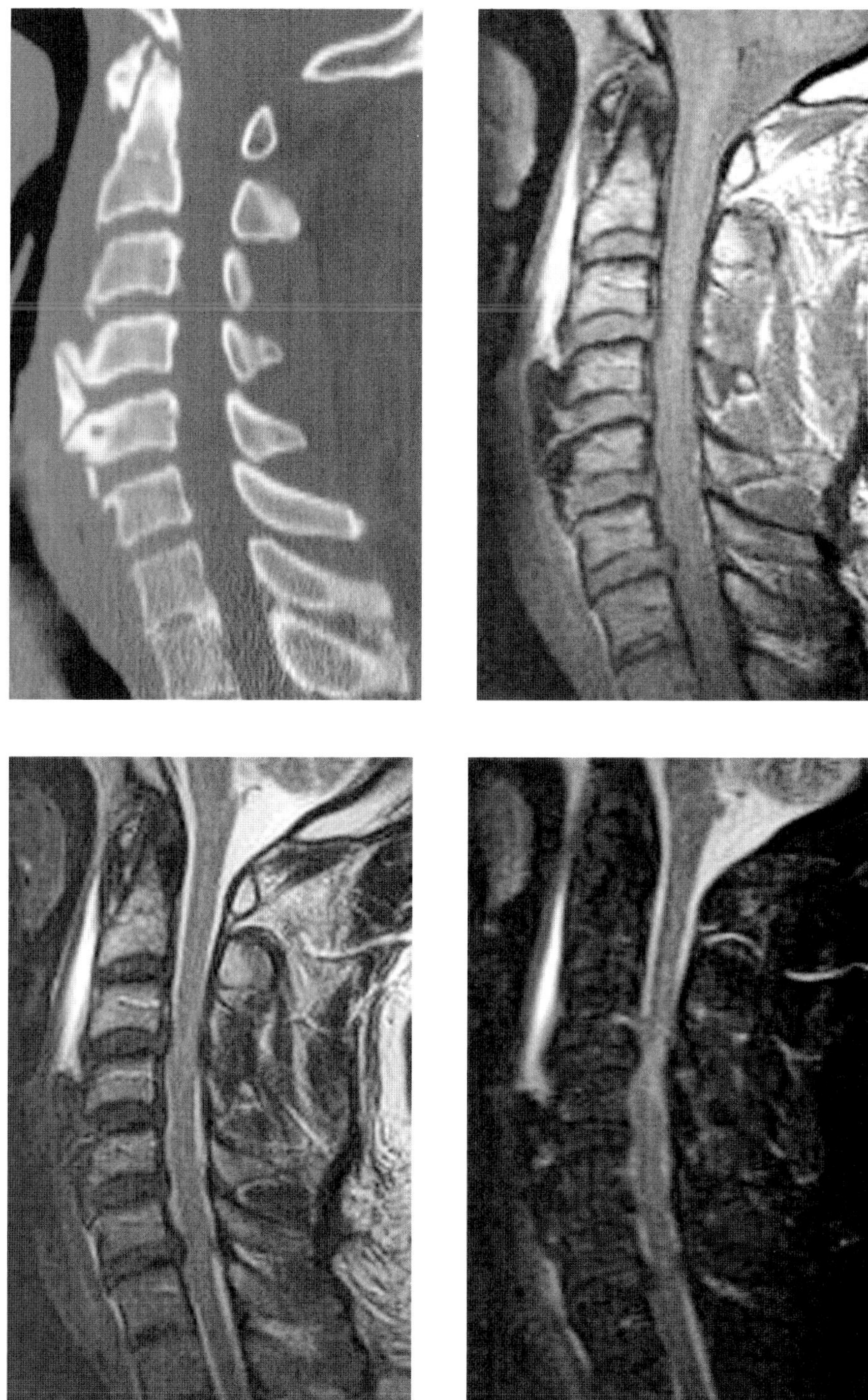

You are shown images of a patient with neck pain and bilateral upper and lower extremity weakness following trauma.

1. What are the three parts of a normal intervertebral disc?
2. What are the normal signals of intensity of a normal disc on T1- and T2-weighted spin echo images?
3. What is the diagnosis?
4. How can this entity be classified?

CASE 137

Acute Disc Herniation

1. The annulus fibrosus, nucleus pulposus, and cartilaginous end plates.
2. On T1-weighted images the disc is slightly hypointense and on T2-weighted images it is hyperintense compared with the vertebral body marrow.
3. Acute disc herniation at C3-C4 and C6-C7 levels. Disc bulges are seen at all other levels of the cervical spine. A cord contusion is seen at the C3-C4 level.
4. Bulging disc, prolapsed disc, extruded disc, and free disc fragment.

Reference

Czervionke LF, Daniels DL: Degenerative disease of the spine. In Atlas SW, ed: *Magnetic Imaging of the Brain and Spine*, New York, Raven Press, 1991, pp 795–864.

Cross-Reference

Emergency Radiology: THE REQUISITES, p 222.

Comment

In the normal disc the annulus fibrosis is formed of complex collagen fibers called lamellae. The anterior annulus is thicker than the posterior annulus. The peripheral annuli that attach to the end plates are called the *Sharpey's fibers*. The remnant cells of the notochord form the nucleus pulposus and help the disc to resist compressive forces.

Disc herniation may be classified as follows: A disc bulge represents extension of the disc diffusely beyond the margins of the vertebral body resulting from laxity of the annulus fibrosis. The nucleus pulposus extends into a tear of the inner fibers of the annulus and results in a prolapsed disc. A focal deformity in the disc may not be seen. The outer fibers of the annulus are intact. Disc extrusion occurs when the nucleus extends through a focal tear involving all the layers of the annulus. A "free disc fragment" consists of a fragment of nucleus that is discontinuous with the nucleus pulposus.

The various types of disc herniation described above are not always possible to differentiate with magnetic resonance imaging (MRI) or multidetector computed tomography (MDCT). Often it is difficult to differentiate between a disc prolapse and an extruded disc. A diffuse extension of the disc beyond the vertebral body margin is called a "bulging disc" on MRI. A focal extension of the disc is called a "herniated disc." The disc herniation may occur at the anterior or posterior aspect of the disc. The vast majority of the disc herniations occur posteriorly in a central or paracentral location. The disc may be seen subligamentously or extend through the posterior longitudinal ligament.

On MRI the herniated disc is usually contiguous with the residual disc material in the intervertebral disc space. The disc material may displace the epidural fat, epidural veins, dural sac, nerve root, or the spinal cord. The herniated disc is typically isointense on T1-weighted and slightly hyperintense on T2-weighted images compared with the intervertebral disc. Low signal intensity within the herniated disc may represent calcification or gas. Most disc material in the absence of surgery will not enhance following administration of intravenous Gd-DTPA. Free disc fragments are typically demonstrated on sagittal images to migrate inferiorly, anteriorly, or posteriorly to the posterior longitudinal ligament. Rarely, the fragment may migrate superiorly or penetrate the dura and will be seen in the subarachnoid space.

Far lateral disc herniation usually compresses the exiting nerve root within the neural foramen at the same level, obscuring the epidural fat. Posterolateral and midline disc herniation usually causes mass effect on the dural sac at the same level and will compress the nerve root exiting at the level below.

Notes

CASE 138

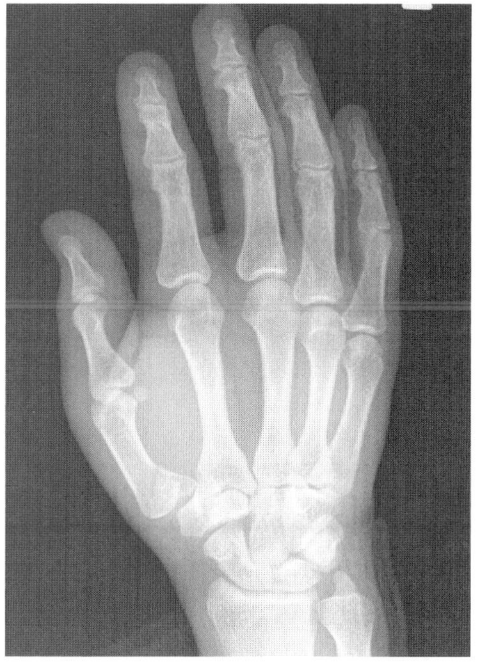

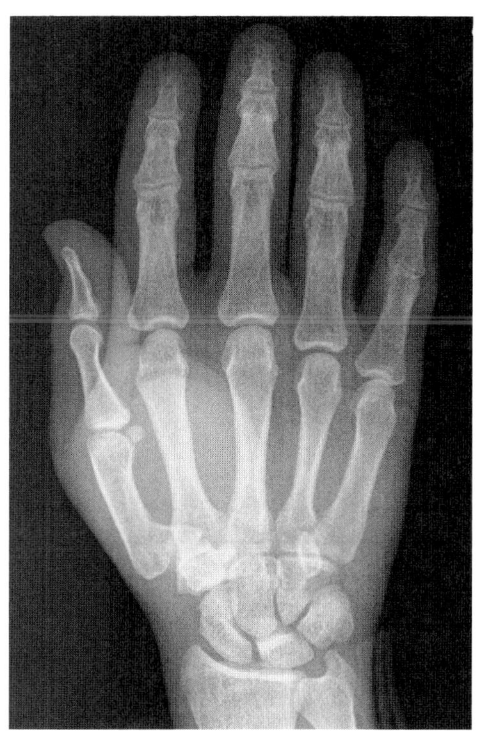

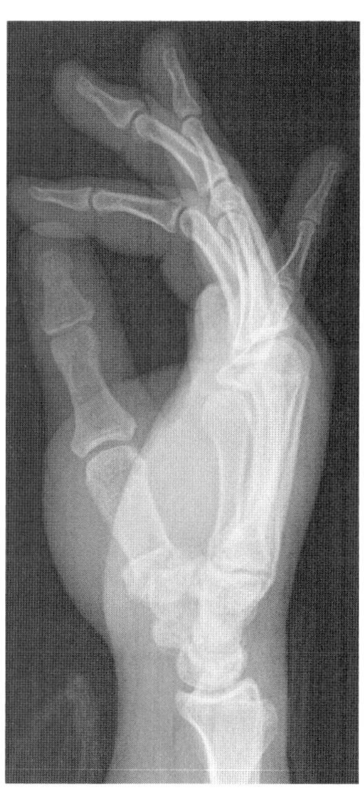

You are shown images of a patient in pain due to trauma to the hand.

1. What is the diagnosis?
2. What are the four types of basal fractures of the metacarpal bone of the thumb?
3. How does this fracture differ from a Rolando fracture?
4. Name the muscle that causes displacement of the metacarpal basal bone fragment.

CASE 138

Bennett's Fracture

1. Bennett's fracture.
2. Epibasal extra articular, Bennett's, Rolando, and a comminuted basal fracture are the four fractures of the base of thumb.
3. The base of the metacarpal bone is fractured into two parts in a Bennett's and three parts in a Rolando fracture.
4. The abductor pollicis longus pulls the metacarpal base dorsally with rotation into supination.

Reference

Jupiter JB, Axelrod TS, Belsky MR: Fractures and dislocation of the hand. In Browner BD, Jupiter JB, Levine A, Trafton PG, eds: *Skeletal Trauma*, Philadelphia, WB Saunders, 1998, pp 1270–1277.

Cross-Reference

Emergency Radiology: THE REQUISITES, p 133.

Comment

More than 80% of the fractures of the metacarpal bone of the thumb involve the base. Four types of fracture are seen. Extra-articular epibasal fractures are usually transverse in orientation. The vast majority of these fractures are stable and only require protective cast immobilization. Intra-articular fractures are more common than extra-articular fractures of the base of the thumb. These fractures are often seen in the dominant hand in males.

Routine radiographs of the hand may not demonstrate the true anatomy and displacement of the bone fragments of the metacarpal bone of the thumb well. This is because of the oblique orientation of the metacarpal bone in reference to the palm. A true lateral and an anteroposterior view of the thumb on computed tomography are required to determine the previous displacement of the fracture fragments.

Bennett's fracture is an intra-articular injury involving the carpo-metacarpal joint of the thumb. The two-part fracture splits off the medial volar beak of the base of the metacarpal bone. The intracapsular volar oblique ligament is essential for stability of this joint. This ligament is attached to the volar beak of the metacarpal base on the ulnar aspect. The metacarpal base is displaced dorsally and rotated into supination by the pull of the abductor pollicis longus muscle. The metacarpal head is pulled into the palmar aspect by the adductor pollicis muscle.

Rolando's fracture is a three-part intra-articular injury of the carpo-metacarpal joint of the thumb. This injury could result in a Y or T fracture pattern. These fractures are less common compared with the Bennett's fracture and have a poor prognosis. When more than three bony fragments are seen the fracture is called a comminuted fracture. They are difficult to treat and more than 50% of patients will develop post-traumatic arthritis on follow-up.

Surgical treatment is required for Bennett's fracture depending on location, amount of displacement of fracture fragments following closed reduction, and impaction at the metacarpal base. No general consensus is reported in the orthopedic literature regarding the optimal method to treat this fracture.

Notes

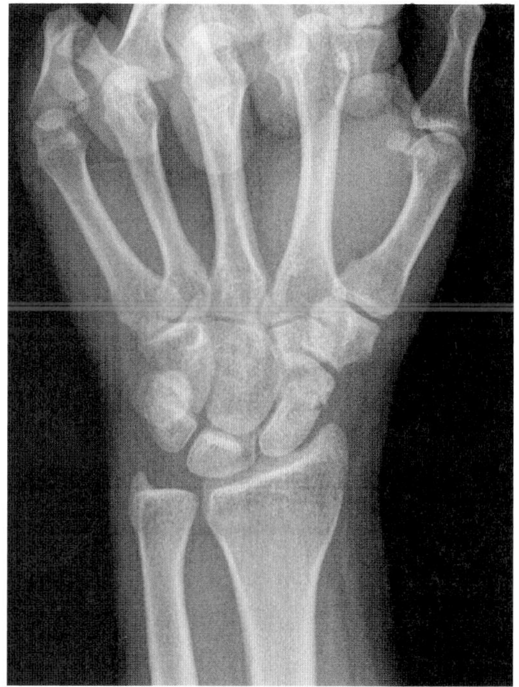

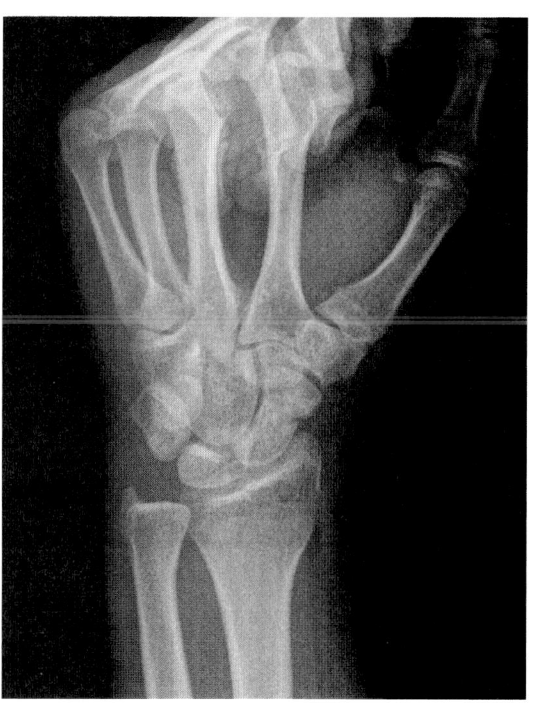

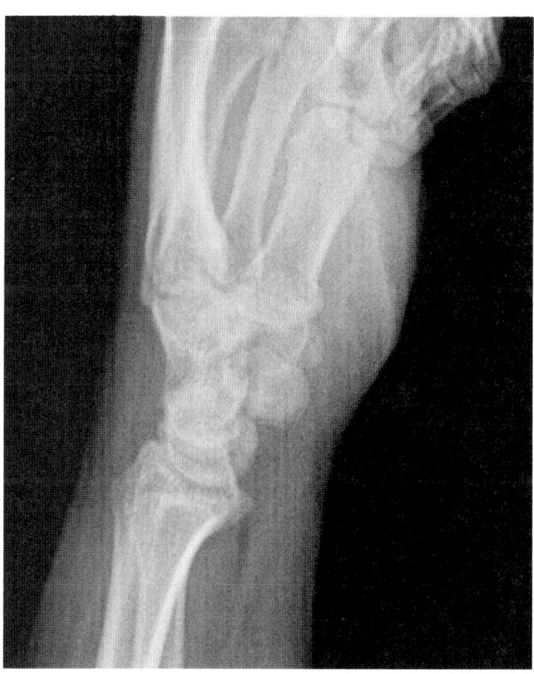

You are shown images of a patient with wrist pain caused by a fall on the outstretched hand.

1. What is the diagnosis?
2. Name two complications of this fracture.
3. What are the factors that affect the healing of this fracture?
4. Why do proximal pole fractures of the scaphoid heal poorly?

CASE 139

Scaphoid Fracture

1. Comminuted displaced fracture of the distal and mid scaphoid.
2. Nonunion and avascular necrosis.
3. Late diagnosis, fracture of proximal pole of scaphoid, displacement or angulation at fracture site, and obliquity of fracture line.
4. The majority of the blood supply enters the bone distal to the waist of the scaphoid. Proximal pole fractures interrupt the blood supply required for healing. This leads to avascular necrosis and nonunion.

References

Memarsadeghi M, Breitenseher MJ, Schaefer-Prokop C, et al: Occult scaphoid fractures: comparison of multidetector CT and MR imaging—initial experience, *Radiology* 240:169–176, 2006.

Welling RD, Jacobson JA, Jamadar DA, et al: MDCT and radiography of wrist fractures: radiographic sensitivity and fracture patterns, *AJR Am J Roentgenol* 190: 10–16, 2008.

Cross-Reference

Emergency Radiology: THE REQUISITES, p 129.

Comment

Fractures of the scaphoid bone account for 60% to 70% of all carpel bone fractures. They are second only to fractures to the distal radius in frequency of wrist fractures. Though many different radiographic views are recommended, the routine initial radiographic views may include a posteroanterior (PA), true lateral, ulnar deviation PA, and 45 degrees pronation PA. The ulnar deviation view orients the scaphoid parallel with the radiographic cassette and helps to demonstrate fracture lines well.

Up to 65% of the scaphoid fractures may be occult immediately following injury on initial radiography. It is common practice to place patients with a high index of suspicion in a scaphoid cast for 6 weeks. Follow-up radiographs are obtained at regular intervals at 2, 4, and 6 weeks to demonstrate the scaphoid fracture prior to discontinuing the cast immobilization.

To avoid this long period of immobilization, other imaging modalities including scintigraphy, multidetector computed tomography (MDCT), and magnetic resonance imaging (MRI) have been used to image the wrist to demonstrate the fracture immediately following injury. Both MRI and MDCT are superior to radiographs in demonstrating scaphoid fractures. MRI is very sensitive in localizing and demonstrating trabecular injury, which is seen as a linear area of bone marrow edema. However, only 38% of cortical fractures are seen on MRI. When compared with MRI, the excellent spatial resolution of MDCT is superior in demonstrating cortical fractures. Purely trabecular fractures are usually missed by MDCT. The benefits in the outcome of early diagnosis of purely trabecular scaphoid fractures have not been clinically evaluated.

Negative prognostic factors associated with healing of the scaphoid fractures include delay in diagnosis, fractures involving the proximal pole, and displacement of more than 2 mm or greater than 45 degrees of scapholunate angulation on the lateral radiograph. The interruption of the blood supply from the branches of the radial artery that enter the bone distal to the waist of the scaphoid by the fracture has been attributed to the poor healing and avascular necrosis fractures of the proximal pole.

Notes

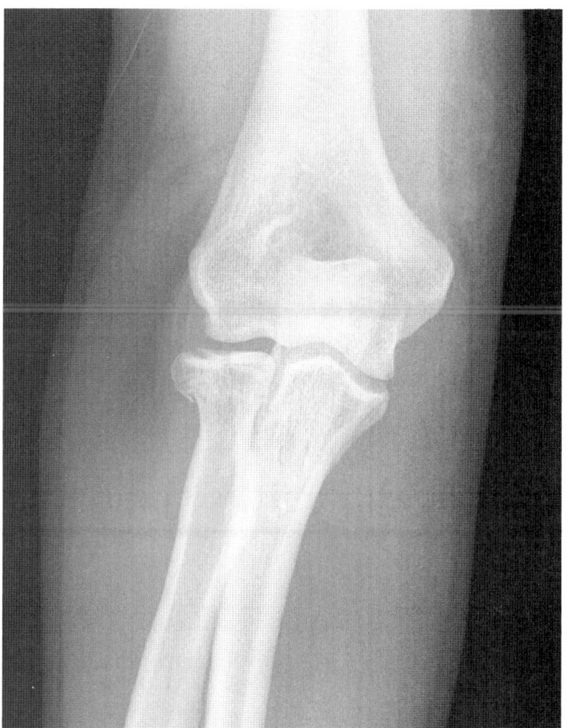

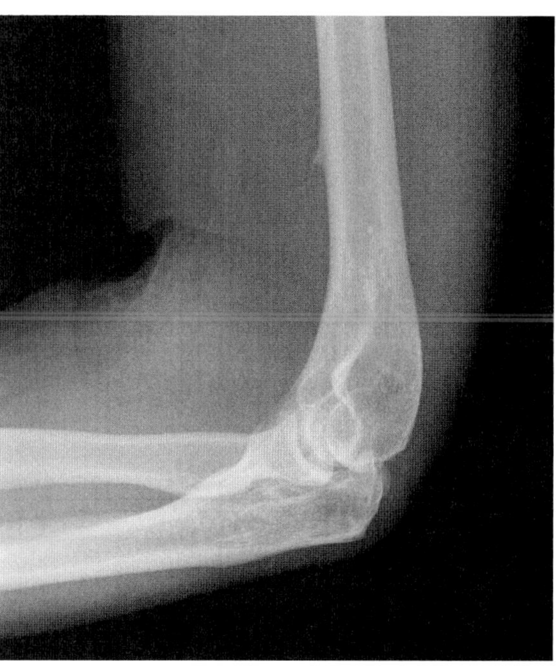

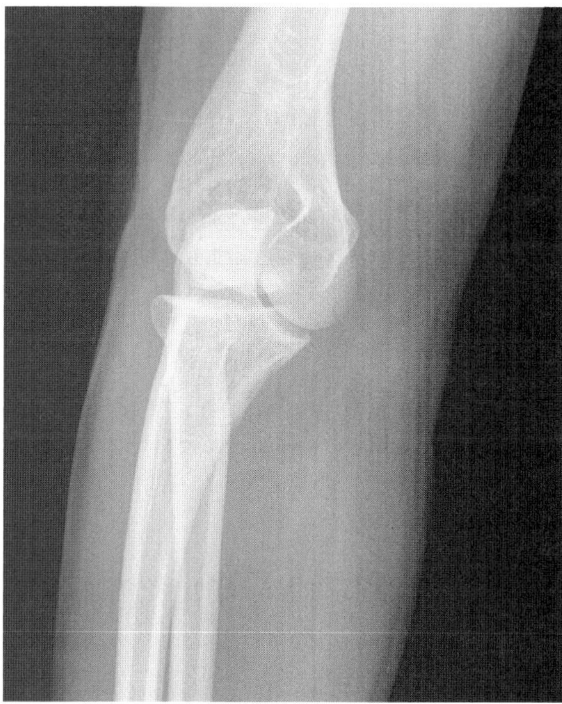

You are shown images of a patient with elbow pain caused by a fall on an outstretched hand.

1. What is the diagnosis?
2. Name two soft tissue abnormalities seen on radiographs with this fracture.
3. Name three associated fractures that may be seen with this injury.
4. What are the injuries seen in an Essex-Lopresti fracture?

CASE 140

Radial Head Fracture

1. Fracture of the radial head.
2. An effusion of the elbow joint and displacement or obliteration of the supinator facial plane.
3. Colles' fracture, scaphoid fracture, and distal radius fracture.
4. A comminuted radial head fracture, proximal migration of the radius, and subluxation of the distal radioulnar joint.

Reference

Cox D, Sonin A: The elbow and forearm. In Rogers LF, ed: *Radiology of Skeletal Trauma*, New York, Churchill Livingstone, 2002, pp 696–705.

Cross-Reference

Emergency Radiology: THE REQUISITES, pp 122–124.

Comment

Fractures of the radial head account for 20% of all injuries that occur at the elbow joint. The classification of these fractures has undergone considerable evolution and is based on the amount of displacement, comminution, and associated injuries. Up to 50% of all radial head and neck fractures are nondisplaced, and the fracture may be difficult to visualize on radiographs.

Tenderness on palpation over the radial head is the clue to the presence of a fracture. On routine anteroposterior and lateral radiographs the fracture may not be visualized. Patients with secondary soft tissue abnormalities on these two views, including the posterior "fat pad" sign on the true lateral radiograph and displacement or obliteration of the supinator fascial plane, require additional oblique or the radial head–capitellum view to demonstrate the fracture. Follow-up radiographs may demonstrate a fracture in 17% to 76% of patients with a "fat pad" sign.

The fracture line is usually located on the lateral aspect of the radial head and is vertically oriented. A step-off, abrupt angulation of the articular surface, and a double line of cortical bone due to depression of the articular surface, are other findings seen on radiographs. Impaction fractures are best seen on the lateral radiograph and are visualized as obliteration of the gentle curve between the anterior radial head and neck. Multidetector computed tomography, magnetic resonance imaging, and scintigraphy are adjunct imaging techniques that may be utilized to evaluate patients with post-traumatic elbow effusion. These techniques have a higher sensitivity, specificity, and accuracy in demonstrating radiographically occult fractures in the immediate postinjury period.

Displaced fractures account for 20% of all radial head fractures. They are usually displaced at least 2 mm and are easily recognized. Comminuted fractures account for another 20% of the fractures. Severely comminuted radial head fractures may be associated with proximal migration of the radius and distal radioulnar joint injuries. Injury to the distal radioulnar joint allows the proximal migration. The combination of these two injuries is called the Essex-Lopresti fracture. Comparison radiographs of the normal wrist should be obtained in all patients with severely comminuted fracture of the radial head to evaluate for this injury.

A small number of patients with radial head fracture may have an elbow joint dislocation. Other associated fractures seen in patients with radial head fracture include Colles' fracture, scaphoid fracture, and distal radius and ulnar fractures. Avulsion fracture of the capitellum may be seen typically occurring superiorly and ventrally to the radial head.

The vast majority of the radial head fractures are treated conservatively. Resection of the radial head for comminuted fractures is controversial.

Notes

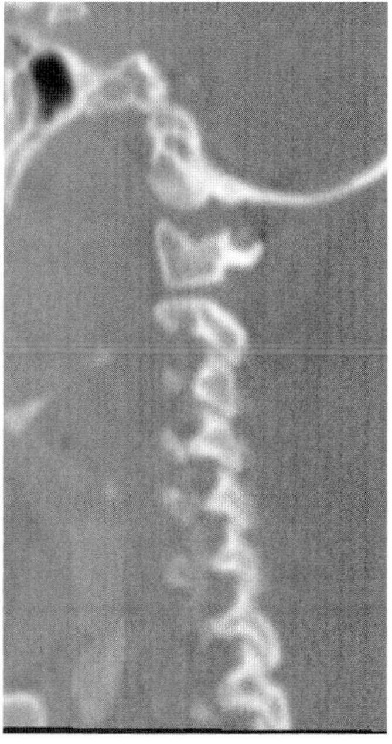

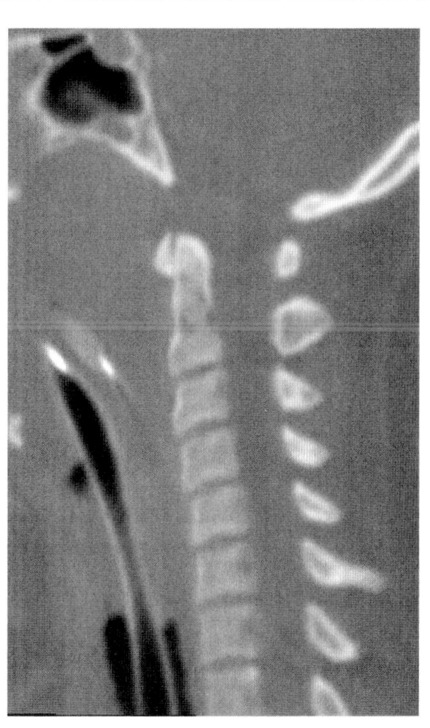

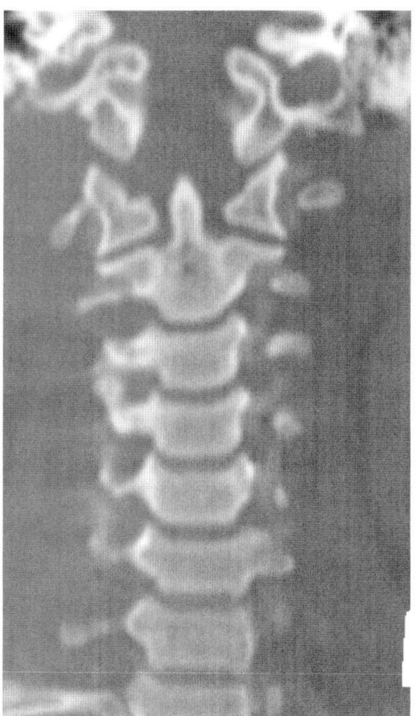

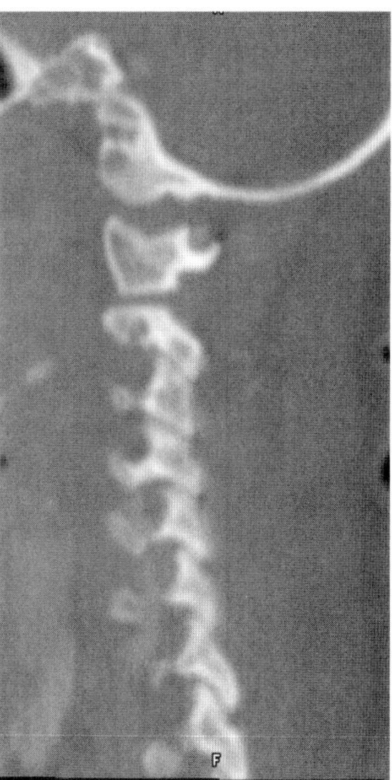

You are shown multidetector computed tomographic images in an obtunded patient admitted after a high-speed motor vehicle collision.

1. What is the diagnosis?
2. What are the four patterns of this injury?
3. Name two methods used to evaluate the cranio–cervical relationship.
4. What is the measurement of the basion-axial (BAI) and basion-dental (BDI) intervals in a normal adult?

CASE 141

Occipitoatlantal Dislocation

1. Anterior and distracted occipitoatlantal dislocation.
2. They include purely anterior, purely distractive, concomitant anterior and distractive, and purely posterior occipitoatlantal dislocation.
3. BAI and BDI distances and Power's ratio.
4. Both of these measurements are less than 12 mm in normal adults.

References

Harris JH Jr, Carson GC, Wagner LK: Radiologic diagnosis of traumatic occipitovertebral dissociation: normal occipitovertebral relationships on lateral radiographs of supine subjects, *AJR Am J Roentgenol* 62:881–886, 1994.

Harris JH Jr, Carson GC, Wagner LK, et al: Radiologic diagnosis of traumatic occipitovertebral dissociation: comparison of three methods of detecting occipitovertebral relationships on lateral radiographs of supine subjects, *AJR Am J Roentgenol* 62:887–892, 1994.

Cross-Reference

Emergency Radiology: THE REQUISITES, p 217.

Comment

Injuries to the occipitovertebral or occipitoatlantal junction occur following high-energy trauma. They are commonly seen in patients suffering fatal craniofacial trauma, but the survival of an increasing number of patients with this injury has been reported. Partial or complete disruption of occipitoatlantal articulation may occur. Four distinct patterns of injury are seen based on the relationship between the skull base and the dens. The most common pattern seen is the concomitant anterior and distractive occipitoatlantal dislocation.

Evaluation of the alignment of the craniocervical junction may be made in multitrauma patients using the lateral radiographs or multidetector computed tomographic images of the cervical spine. The various methods used to determine the normal relationship include the Power's ratio, the X-line method, and measuring the basion-axial and basion-dental intervals (BAI and BDI). All these methods require accurate identification of the various anatomical landmarks at the craniocervical junction. This can be extremely difficult on the lateral radiograph, and often requires high-resolution sagittal and coronal reformatted computed tomography (CT) images to help confidently diagnose this injury.

The BAI and BDI provide the easiest and most accurate methods to radiologically diagnose this injury. The distance between the basion and cranial extension of the posterior cortical margin of the dens and body of the axis is the BAI. The distance between the basion and the inferior point of the clivus to the tip of the superior cortex of the dens is the BDI. In adults, measurements less than 12 mm are considered normal.

Indirect findings seen on radiographs or CT in patients with this injury include prevertebral soft tissue swelling, seen in the region of the upper cervical spine, abnormally separated condyles from the superior facets of the atlas, and subtle fracture fragments near the craniocervical junction. These fracture fragments result from impaction fractures arising from the occipital condyles or superior facets of the C1 vertebra or avulsion fractures by intact ligaments. Concurrent bony and ligament injuries at the level of the atlas and axis are not uncommon in these patients. Injuries to the vertebral and carotid arteries at the skull base may potentially be seen if intravenous contrast material is administered routinely to evaluate the cervical spine. Magnetic resonance imaging is helpful in demonstrating the various injuries to ligaments, the spinal cord, and the lower brain stem.

Notes

CASE 142

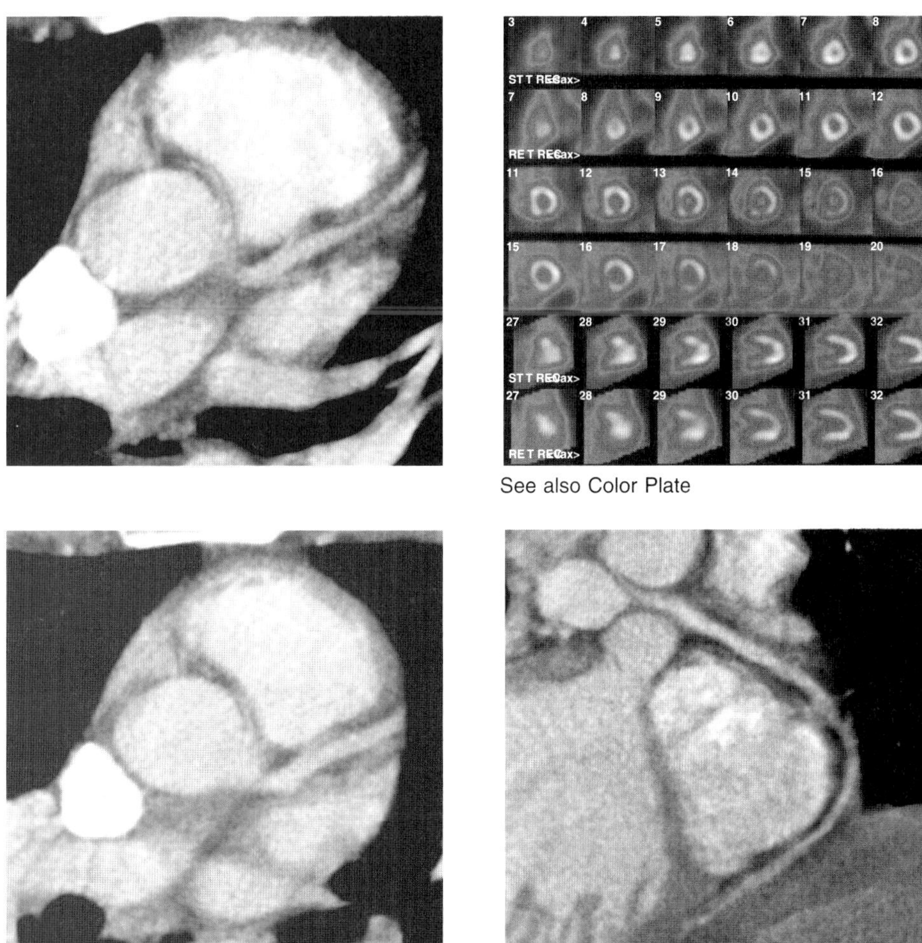

See also Color Plate

You are shown images of a 37-year-old man who presented to the emergency department with increasingly frequent substernal chest pain after he began a weightlifting program.

1. What is the cause of the scintigraphic perfusion abnormality?
2. Is this a common abnormality?
3. What are the typical presentations of patients with this abnormality?
4. In what patient populations is this abnormality a common cause of sudden cardiac death?

CASE 142

Interarterial Anomalous Right Coronary Artery

1. Anomalous right coronary artery.
2. No.
3. Exercise-induced anginal chest pain, syncope, and sudden cardiac death.
4. Young athletes and military recruits.

References

Budoff MJ, Ahmed V, Gul KM, et al: Coronary anomalies by cardiac computed tomographic angiography, *Clin Cardiol* 29:489–493, 2006.

Kim SY, Seo JB, Do KH, et al: Coronary artery anomalies: classification and ECG-gated multi-detector row CT findings with angiographic correlation, *Radiographics* 26:317–333, 2006.

Cross-Reference

Emergency Radiology: THE REQUISITES, pp 266, 350–353.

Comment

Coronary artery anomalies have been reported in 0.6% to 1.3% of patients undergoing cardiac catheterization and as incidental findings in 0.3% to 1% of healthy individuals. Anomalous arteries include those with aberrant origin, course, or termination. While many are clinically insignificant, up to 20% of coronary artery abnormalities may induce life-threatening consequences, such as arrhythmias and myocardial infarction. Patients with significant coronary artery anomalies may present with anginal chest pain, syncope, or sudden cardiac death that is frequently exercised induced. Sudden cardiac death may be the initial presentation of a coronary artery anomaly. After hypertrophic cardiomyopathy, they are the most common cause of sudden death due to structural heart disease in young athletes. Coronary artery abnormalities should be suspected in young athletes who present with exertional syncope, chest pain, or near-fatal arrhythmias.

Of particular clinical significance are coronary artery anomalies associated with an anomalous origin and interarterial course, that is, a course passing between the main pulmonary artery and aorta above the plane of the pulmonic valve. Anomalous right coronary arteries (RCA) and left coronary arteries (LCA) arising from the left and right sinuses of Valsalva, respectively, are rare. Anomalous RCAs are seen in 0.03% to 0.17% and anomalous LCAs are seen in 0.09% to 0.11% of patients who undergo cardiac catheterization. However, they frequently are associated with sudden cardiac death, which can occur in up to 13% to 30% of patients with an anomalous RCA or LCA origin. Ischemia and infarction in these patients most likely result from a combination of the acutely angulated and slit-like origins typical of these arteries couple with compression of the anomalous artery between the aorta and main pulmonary artery. The deleterious consequences of this anatomic arrangement are exacerbated by exercise with the subsequent aortic dilation that causes stretching, and consequent greater narrowing, of the coronary artery ostium, while also increasing compression of the proximal coronary artery against the main pulmonary artery.

Although cardiac catheterization is considered the reference standard for most acquired coronary artery diseases, using it accurately to diagnose and characterize coronary artery anomalies can be difficult. Because of the complex configuration of the coronary arteries, cardiac catheterization may incorrectly classify 50% of anomalous vessels. In contrast, electrocardiogram (ECG)-gated coronary artery multidetector computed tomographic (MDCT) angiography has a reported accuracy of 97% for classifying anomalous coronary arteries. When an anomalous coronary artery is suspected, an ECG-gated coronary artery MDCT angiogram should be obtained. Moreover, with the increased utilization of MDCT angiography to evaluate for other causes of acute chest pain, the course of the coronary arteries should be carefully scrutinized, especially in young patients.

Notes

CASE 143

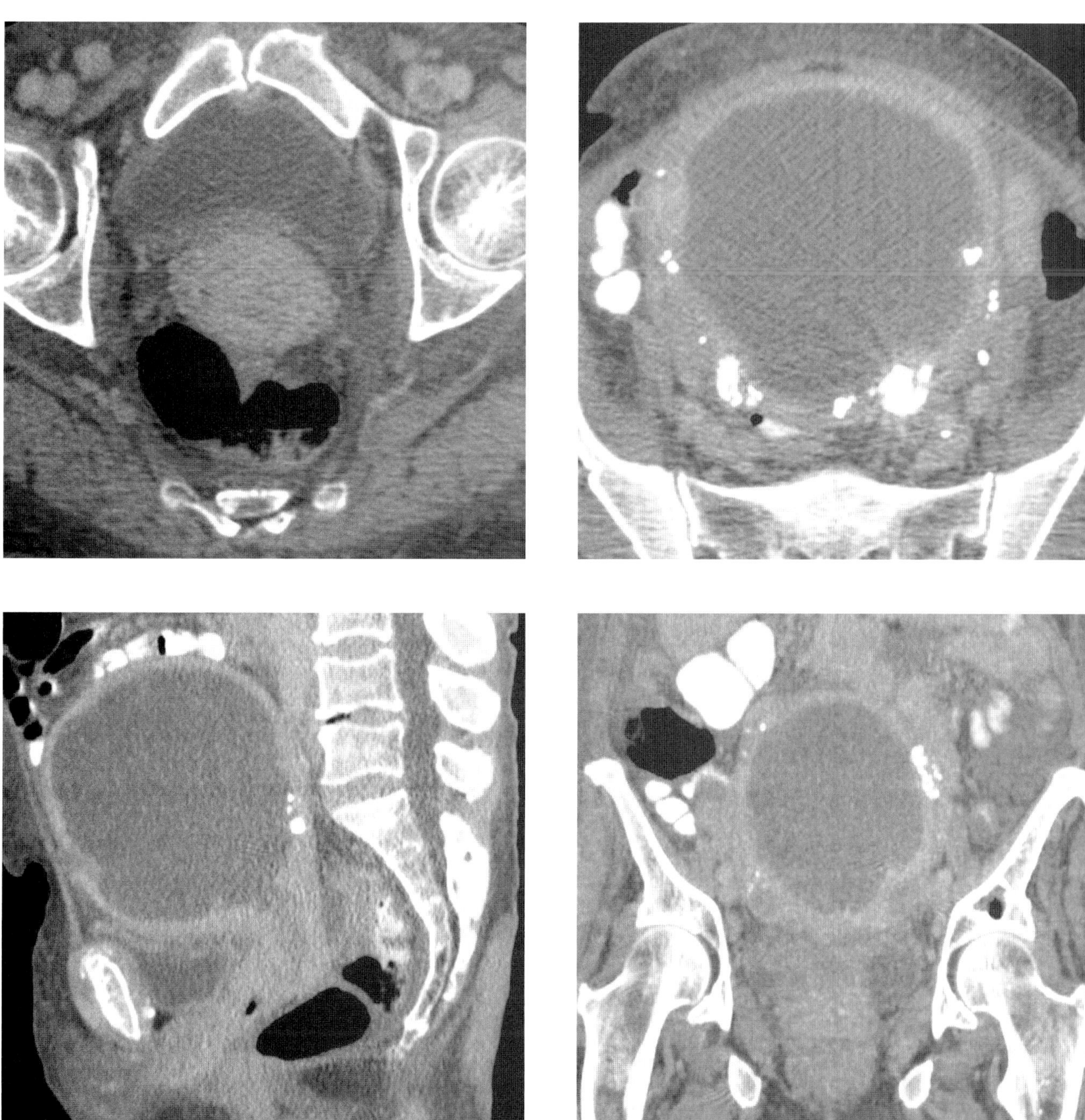

You are shown images of a 67-year-old woman who presented with lower abdominal pain.

1. What are the CT findings?
2. Name two malignant entities that may cause these uterine abnormalities in postmenopausal women.
3. Name five nonmalignant entities that may cause the same uterine abnormalities in postmenopausal women.
4. What types of uterine fluid collections are seen in postmenopausal women?

CASE 143

Pyometra Due to Cervical Carcinoma

1. A large intrauterine fluid collection causing uterine enlargement, an enlarged cervix, left femoral venous thrombus, and multiple calcified degenerated fibroids.
2. Cervical carcinoma and carcinoma of the low uterine segment.
3. Low uterine or cervical stenosis due to radiation therapy, postsurgical stenosis, infection, and either an endometrial polyp or cystic endometrial hyperplasia.
4. Pyometria, hematometria, or serosanguinous fluid collections.

References

Breckenridge JW, Kurtz AB, Ritchie WGM, et al: Postmenopausal uterine fluid collection: indicator of carcinoma, *AJR Am J Roentgenol* 139:529–534, 1982.

Nalaboff KM, Pellerito JS, Ben-Levi E: Imaging the endometrium: disease and normal variants, *Radiographics* 21:1409–1424, 2001.

Comment

The etiology of intrauterine fluid may vary with the age of the patient. Hematometrium or hematocolpos may be seen in infancy or at menarche. Intrauterine fluid collections developing between menarche and menopause are typically related to pregnancy or its complications, pelvic inflammatory disease, or menstruation. Hematometrium, pyometrium, and serosanguinous fluid in the postmenopausal patient are commonly due to carcinoma of the cervix or uterus. Cervical stenosis due to radiation therapy, surgery, or chronic infection could also cause fluid to accumulate within the uterine cavity. Less common benign causes include cystic endometrial hyperplasia and endometrial polyps.

Patients with intrauterine fluid collections usually have intermittent postmenopausal bleeding or serous discharge. They may also present with lower abdominal pain and a new palpable mass. Transabdominal and endovaginal ultrasound examination is the imaging modality of choice for confirming diagnosis, and, potentially, determining the cause for fluid accumulation.

In addition to being signs of malignancy and sources of pain and discomfort, intrauterine fluid collections may become superinfected. The infections are usually due to anaerobic bacteria. Air bubbles may be seen from bacterial gas formation. While clinical diagnosis is not always clear, accurate diagnosis is vital since surgical drainage of the pyometrium is mandatory. Therefore, it is imperative that the radiologist clearly communicate both the malignant potential of endometrial fluid collections and, when clinical factors suggest infection, the possibility of a pyometrium.

Notes

CASE 144

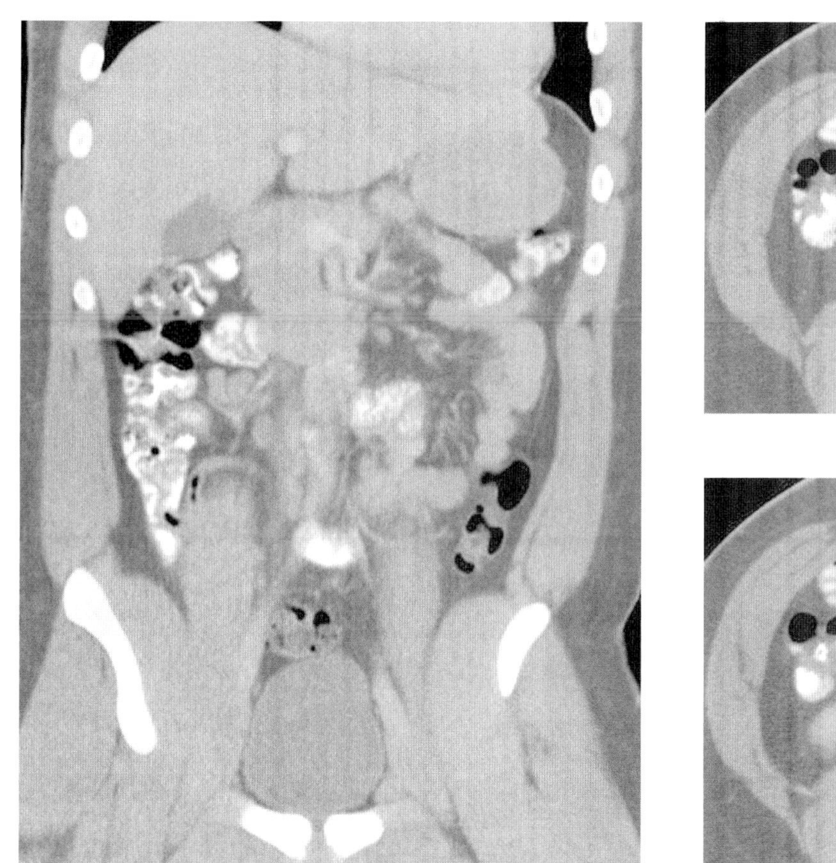

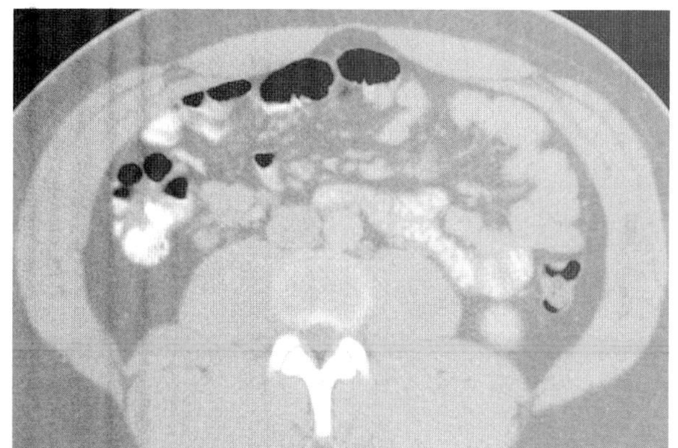

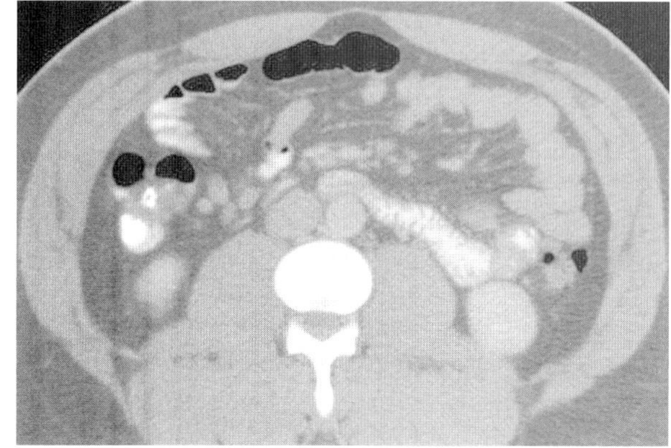

You are shown images of a patient who presented with right lower quadrant pain, vomiting, and fever.

1. What are the computed tomography (CT) findings?
2. What is the best diagnosis?
3. Give three causes for secondary mesenteric adenitis.
4. What is the role of CT in patients with mesenteric adenitis?

CASE 144

Primary Mesenteric Adenitis

1. A cluster of lymph nodes are seen in the right iliac fossa anterior to the psoas muscle. The normal appendix is visualized on the reformatted image.
2. Primary mesenteric adenitis.
3. Appendicitis, Crohn's disease, and right-sided diverticulitis.
4. Evaluate for a specific cause for the mesenteric adenitis.

References

Macari M, Hines J, Balthazar E, et al: Mesenteric adenitis: CT diagnosis of primary versus secondary causes, incidence, and clinical significance in pediatric and adult patients, *AJR Am J Roentgenol* 178:853–858, 2002.

Rao RM, Rhea JT, Novelline RA: CT diagnosis of mesenteric adenitis, *Radiology* 202:145–149, 1997.

Cross-Reference

Emergency Radiology: THE REQUISITES, p 195.

Comment

Mesenteric adenitis can be classified into two distinct groups: primary (without an identifiable associated inflammatory process) and secondary (detectable associated inflammatory process). Primary mesenteric adenitis is seen more commonly in children than in adults. It is a relatively uncommon cause for right lower quadrant abdominal pain in adults. The reported frequency of primary mesenteric adenitis varies between 2% and 7%. An underlying infectious terminal ileitis is thought to be the cause in most cases. The clinical presentation of mesenteric adenitis, which includes right lower quadrant abdominal pain, fever, nausea, vomiting, and leukocytosis, can make it difficult or impossible to differentiate from appendicitis.

The computed tomography (CT) findings of primary mesenteric adenitis include a cluster (three or more) of lymph nodes anterior to the right psoas muscle or in the right lower quadrant small bowel mesentery. The largest lymph nodes usually measure between 5 and 15 mm (short axis) in diameter. Some patients may have mild thickening of the terminal ileum (<5 mm) due to the underlying terminal ileitis. It is important to demonstrate a normal appendix and no other inflammatory conditions.

Secondary mesenteric adenitis occurs in patients with appendicitis, right-sided diverticulitis, and Crohn's disease, but it has also been reported in patients with infective colitis, pseudomembranous colitis, ulcerative colitis, and systemic lupus erythematosis. CT can identify several of the underlying causes of secondary mesenteric adenitis. Secondary mesenteric adenitis is associated with a cluster of right lower quadrant lymph nodes measuring 5 to 20 mm short axis diameter. The terminal ileum wall thickening is more obvious in patients with Crohn's disease than infectious ileitis. At times, identifying the cause of secondary mesenteric adenitis requires endoscopic biopsy, stool cultures, or small bowel barium studies.

Primary mesenteric adenitis is a nonsurgical entity and is treated conservatively. Most patients with primary mesenteric adenitis do not require hospitalization. In patients with mild thickening of the terminal ileum and who do not respond to conservative treatment, endoscopy may be required to exclude Crohn's disease.

Notes

CASE 145

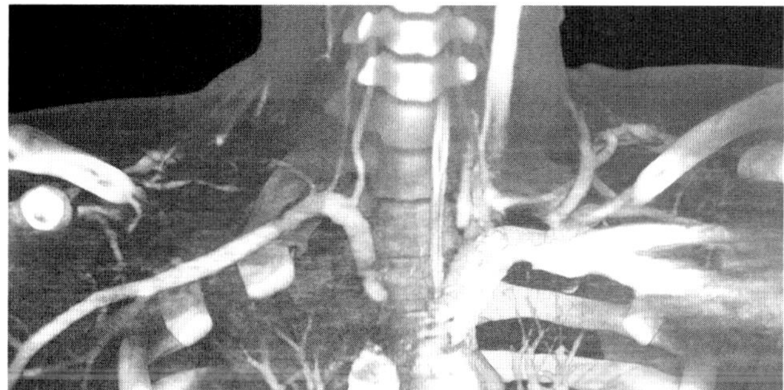

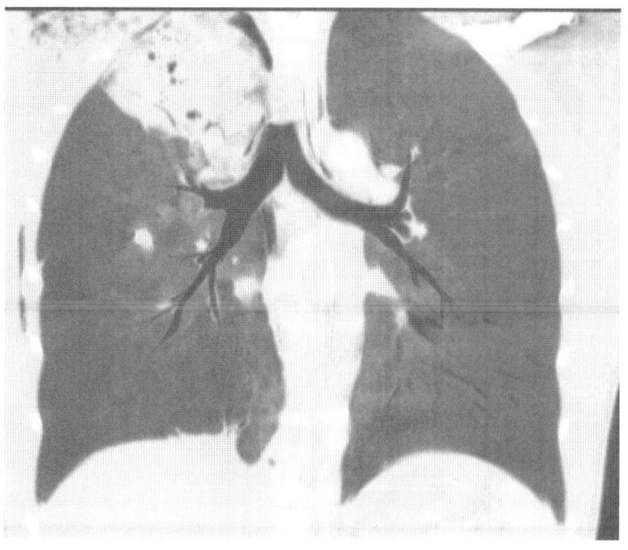

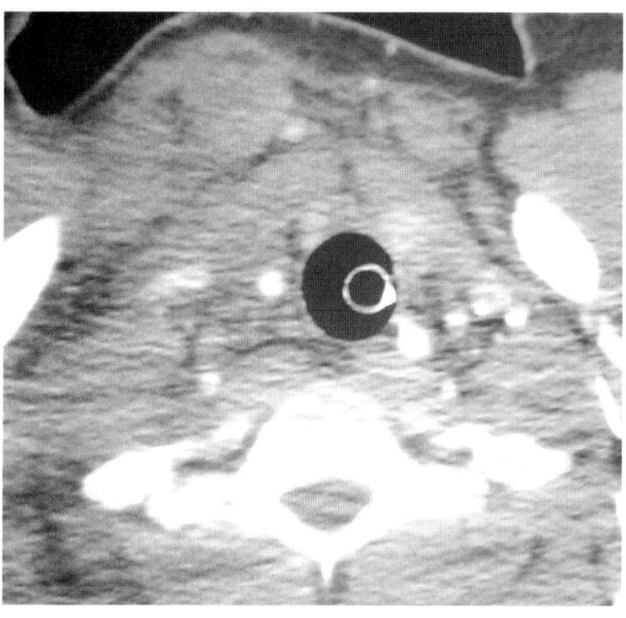

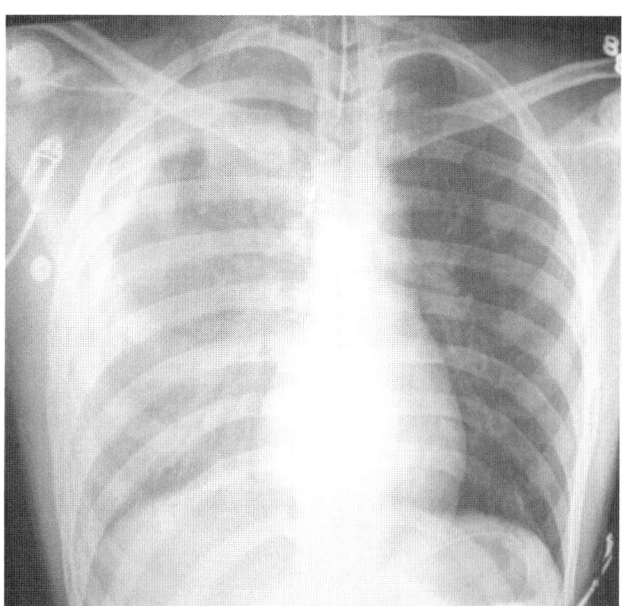

You are shown images of a patient with a history of a gunshot wound with entry site at right thoracic inlet.

1. What are the chest radiographic abnormalities?
2. Name three injuries seen on multidetector computed tomography.
3. Name four life-threatening mediastinal injuries caused by transmediastinal gunshot wounds.
4. What is the established diagnostic tool used to evaluate for suspected airway injury?

CASE 145

Transmediastinal Gunshot Wound

1. Right hemopneumothorax, right upper lobe pulmonary contusion, soft tissue and mediastinal emphysema, and bullet fragments projected over the mediastinum.
2. Right subclavian artery (medial to the first rib), right lung contusion with laceration, and soft tissue hematoma at the thoracic inlet.
3. Injuries to the esophagus, heart, and thoracic aorta or great vessels.
4. Fiber-optic bronchoscopy.

References

Cornwell EE, Kennedy F, Ayad IA, et al: Transmediastinal gunshot wounds: a reconsideration of the role of aortography, *Arch Surg* 131:929–933, 1996.

Hanpeter DE, Demetriades D, Asensio JA, et al: Helical computed tomographic scan in the evaluation of mediastinal gunshot wounds, *J Trauma* 49:689–695, 2000.

Comment

Due to the close proximity of many vital mediastinal structures, especially in the superior and middle mediastinum, transmediastinal penetrating injuries (TMPI) require a rapid and intensive approach to diagnose injuries. Those vital mediastinal structures that require rapid assessment include the heart, thoracic aorta, great vessels, esophagus, and tracheobronchial tree. The thoracic spine and spinal cord are also at risk for injury.

Most patients sustaining TMPI to the heart and great vessels will die at the scene of trauma or arrive at the hospital in a hemodynamically unstable condition requiring immediate surgery. A substantial number of patients with TMPI will arrive hemodynamically stable and require expeditious diagnostic workup to avoid unnecessary surgery or to plan the most optimal surgical approach.

The most common imaging study obtained in patients with TMPI is a portable anteroposterior chest radiograph. The admission chest radiograph is helpful to demonstrate extra-alveolar air in the mediastinum or pleura, hemothorax, injury to lung (contusion and lacerations), and fractures. The thoracic aortic and mediastinal contours should be carefully evaluated for abnormalities that may indicate hemorrhage.

Multidetector computed tomography (MDCT) is optimally suited to demonstrate the trajectory of the bullet and its proximity to individual mediastinal structures. The wound tract is typically outlined by air, hemorrhage, and bone or bullet fragments. High-resolution axial and multiplanar reformatted images should be used in evaluation of the trajectory of the wound tract in all patients. When the wound tract is clearly shown by MDCT not to be in close proximity to vital mediastinal structures, more intensive evaluation of the mediastinum can be deferred. Similarly, if MDCT clearly demonstrates an injury, definitive treatment can be expedited. Otherwise, extensive evaluation with angiography, endoscopy, echocardiography, and contrast swallow are required. Proximity of the wound tract to a given structure directs the need for diagnostic evaluation and the type of test to be performed. For example, a wound tract adjacent to an otherwise normal aorta is an indication for angiography.

Evaluation of the esophagus can be challenging, and it may require both contrast swallow and endoscopy. The length of time to repair an esophageal injury has been shown to be directly correlated to morbidity and mortality related to prolonged leakage of fluid through the esophageal tear with resulting mediastinitis and sepsis. Consequently, evaluation of a potential esophageal injury should be expedited. Hemodynamically stable patients should undergo evaluation of the esophagus prior to angiography.

Notes

CASE 146

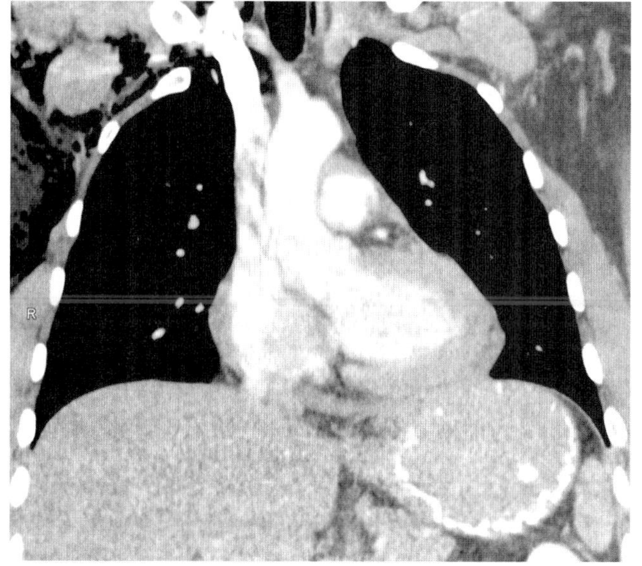

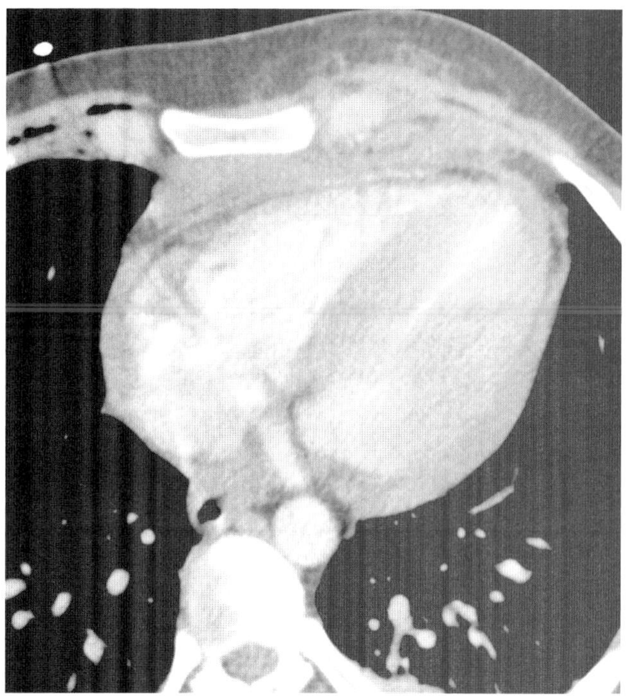

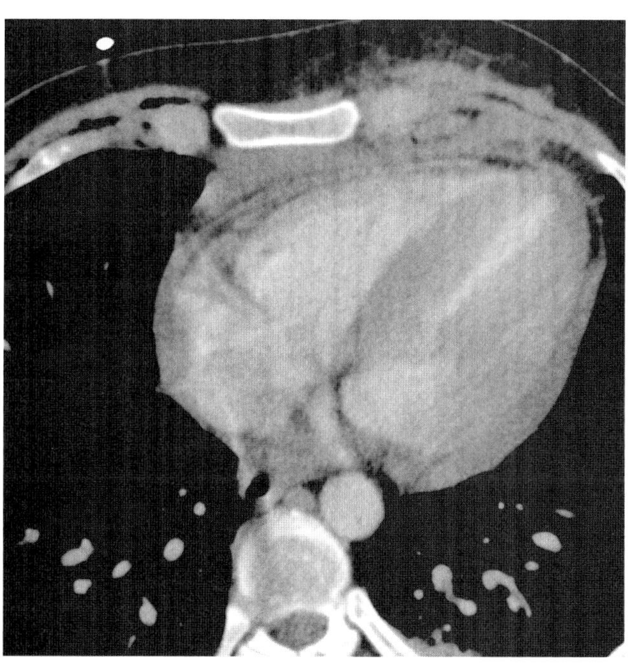

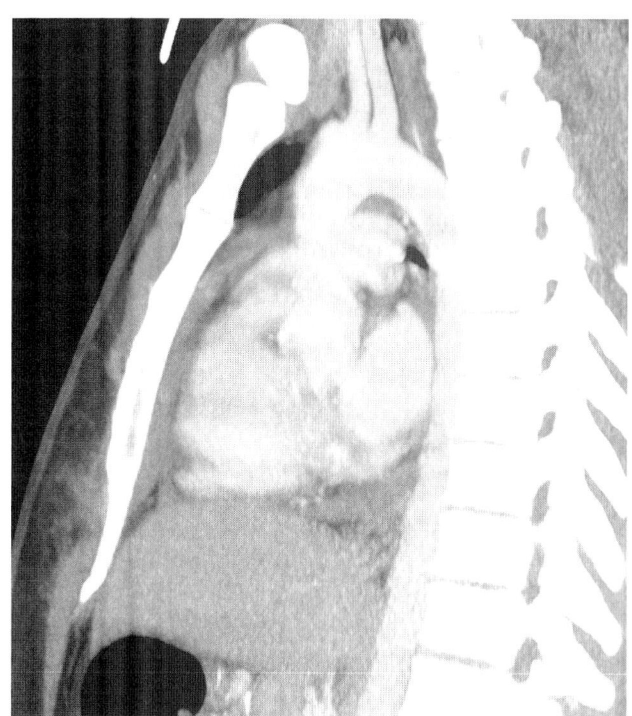

You are shown images of a stab wound to the anterior chest wall.

1. What are the multidetector computed tomography findings?
2. What are the anatomical landmarks of the "cardiac box"?
3. What are the clinical signs that constitute Beck's triad?
4. What other techniques are used to diagnose cardiac injury?

CASE 146

Stab Wound to the Pericardium

1. Subcutaneous wound tract on the anterior chest wall outlined by hematoma, anterior mediastinal hematoma, and pericardial blood.
2. The anterior chest wall bounded superiorly by the clavicles, bilaterally by the mid-axillary lines, and inferiorly by the costal cartilage.
3. Muffled heart sounds, low blood pressure, and elevation of central venous pressure.
4. Subxiphoid pericardial window and evaluation of the pericardium and heart with either ultrasound or echocardiography.

References

Killeen KL, Poletti PA, Shanmuganathan K, Mirvis SE: CT diagnosis of cardiac and pericardial injuries, *Emerg Radiol* 6:339–344, 1999.

Kimberly NK, Corinna L, Dong OK, et al: Role of echocardiography in the diagnosis of occult penetrating cardiac injury, *J Trauma* 38:859–862, 1995.

Comment

The majority of the patients with penetrating injuries to the heart will die at the scene or present to the hospital in shock. Mortality from cardiac injuries ranges from 71% to 83%. While most patients with penetrating cardiac injuries present to the hospital with unstable or absent vital signs, about 20% have no obvious clinical evidence of hemorrhage or tamponade. The most frequently injured chambers are the ventricles (right = 35% and left = 25%) with the atria (right = 33% and left = 14%) less frequently injured. Early diagnosis and optimal treatment of injuries in this group has been reported to result in a survival rate up to 89%.

Up to 80% of mediastinal stab wounds that involve the heart have a precordial entry wound. There is a high likelihood of cardiac injury in patients with stab wounds with entry site within the "cardiac box," which is the region of the anterior chest wall bounded superiorly by the clavicles, bilaterally by the mid-axillary lines, and inferiorly by the costal cartilage. Unlike stab wounds, only 46% of gunshot wounds that injure the heart have an entry wound at the "cardiac box." Any patients with a transmediastinal gunshot wound or a stab wound within the "cardiac box" should be aggressively evaluated for a cardiac injury.

The typical workup of hemodynamically stable patients with suspected penetrating cardiac injuries frequently includes a subxiphoid pericardial window. This invasive technique, ideally performed under general anaesthesia, has been shown to be reliable and safe in diagnosing cardiac injuries. Noninvasive diagnostic techniques, including cardiac ultrasound and formal echocardiography, can detect pericardial effusions or hemopericardium as markers of cardiac injury in hemodynamically stable patients.

Multidetector computed tomography (MDCT) is frequently used to evaluate patients with penetrating thoracic trauma, and, when cardiac injury is highly likely, cardiac gating facilitates evaluation of the heart by limiting cardiac motion. MDCT findings of cardiac and pericardial injury include a wound tract extending to the pericardium, a defect in the pericardium or myocardium, hemopericardium, pneumopericardium, herniation of the heart through a pericardial rent, and, following a gunshot wound, an intrapericardial or intracardiac bullet. Demonstration of a low-attenuation area within the myocardium, a defect in the atrioventricular septum, and extravasation of intravenous contrast material from the atrium, ventricle, or coronary arteries into the pericardium are rare, specific CT signs of cardiac injury.

Notes

CASE 147

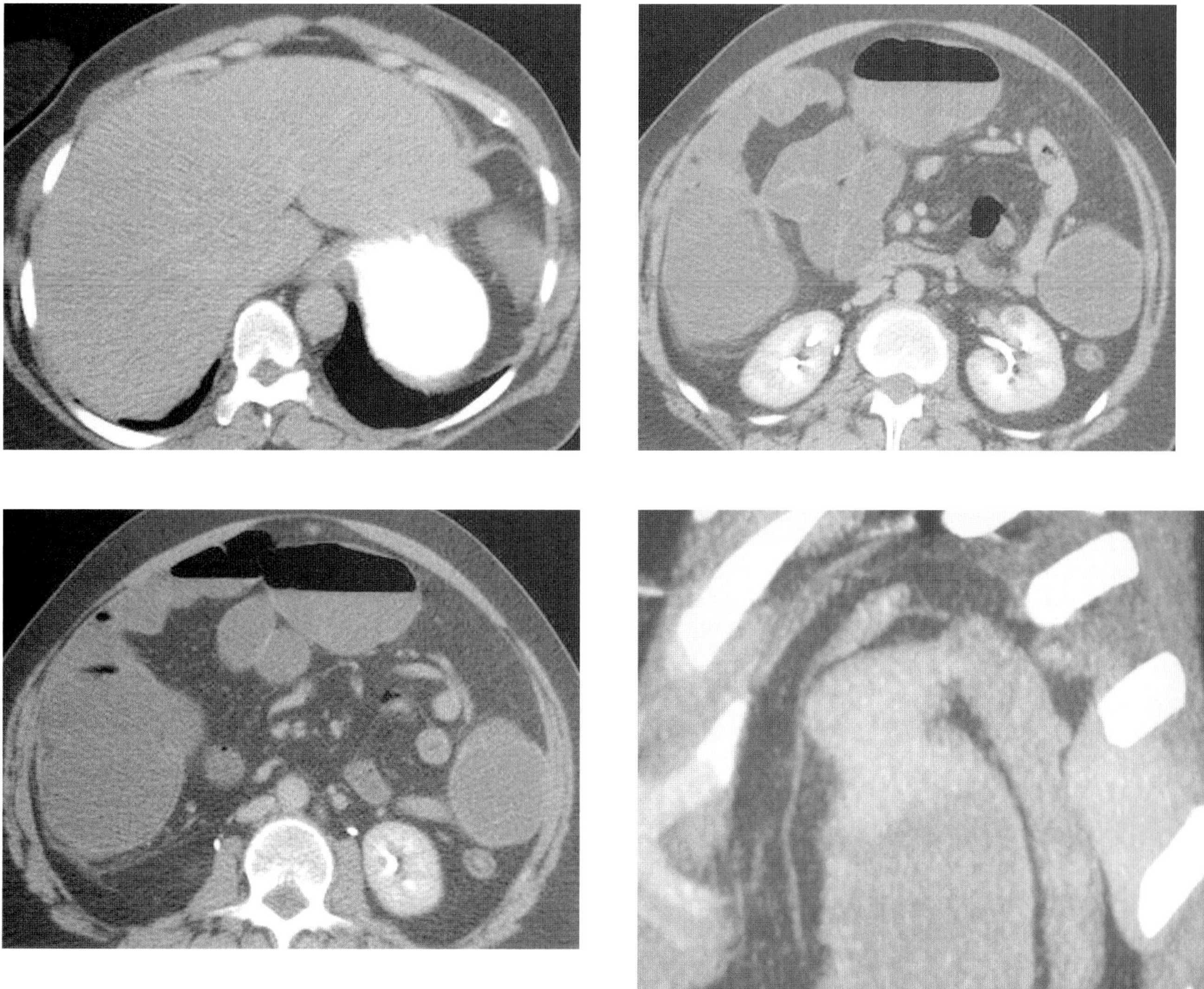

You are shown images of a patient who presented with abdominal pain and distention.

1. What are the multidetector computed tomography abnormalities?
2. What is the best diagnosis?
3. Name three causes for colonic stricture.
4. What is the role of self-expanding colonic stents in colonic obstruction?

CASE 147

Annular Carcinoma with Colonic Obstruction

1. Dilated small bowel and colon with a splenic flexure annular soft tissue mass at the transition point to decompressed descending colon.
2. Annular carcinoma of colon with high-grade colonic obstruction.
3. Crohn's disease, diverticulitis, and ischemic colitis.
4. Relief of obstruction prior to elective surgery or, rarely, palliation in patients who are poor candidates for surgery.

References

Binkert CA, Ledermann H, Jost R, et al: Acute colonic obstruction: clinical aspects and cost-effectiveness of preoperative and palliative treatment with self-expanding metallic stents—a preliminary report, *Radiology* 206:199–203, 1998.

Khurana B, Ledbetter S, McTavish J, et al: Bowel obstruction revealed by multidetector CT, *AJR Am J Roentgenol* 178:1139–1144, 2002.

Cross-Reference

Emergency Radiology: THE REQUISITES, pp 279, 280.

Comment

Acute large bowel obstruction is an emergency that usually requires surgical treatment. Together, small and large bowel obstruction account for 20% of all surgical admissions in patients who present with an acute abdomen. Common causes for large bowel obstruction include neoplasm, sigmoid diverticulitis, and volvulus. Less common causes include radiation colitis, Crohn's disease, intussusception, and strictures related to inflammatory bowel disease, ischemic colitis, or diverticulitis.

Conventional abdominal radiographs accurately demonstrate intestinal obstruction in 46% to 80% of patients. Multidetector computed tomography (MDCT) accurately determines the presence of obstruction. MDCT also demonstrates other information important for therapeutic planning, including the anatomical site of the transition point, the cause of obstruction, the severity of obstruction, and signs of threatened bowel viability. Oral contrast material may not be required because fluid and air within distended loops of bowel can be used as contrast. Intravenous contrast material helps to assess bowel viability.

On MDCT, large bowel obstruction is generally associated with a cecal caliber greater than 9.0 cm, measured from outer wall to outer wall, and a colonic caliber greater than 6.0 cm. In patients with a competent ileocecal valve and large bowel obstruction, the cecum is often the most distended bowel segment. Dilated loops of small bowel, with calibers greater than 2.5 cm, may be seen if the ileocecal valve is incompetent. A systematic approach should be used to determine the transition point, which is identified by abrupt change in caliber between distended proximal and collapsed distal bowel. Multiplanar reformatted images may be helpful to demonstrate the transition point in more difficult cases. Complete versus partial obstruction may be determined by the degree of collapse of the distal bowel. Delayed imaging may be required to demonstrate the passage of oral contrast material past the transition point to determine the severity of obstruction.

It is also important to evaluate for complications such as perforation, incarceration, or strangulation (i.e., ischemia). Increased intraluminal pressure as a function of distention causing venous outflow obstruction is the most common cause of bowel ischemia. The ischemic bowel wall may be thickened by edema or hemorrhage, while a severely ischemic or infarcted bowel may demonstrate a poorly enhancing, thin wall. Fat stranding seen within the affected mesentery may indicate hemorrhage or mesenteric congestive changes related to vascular compromise.

Most patients with acute large bowel obstruction, because of their poor general condition, are poor candidates for general anaesthetic. Self-expanding metallic stents may be used preoperatively to relieve the obstruction and prepare the patient for elective surgery. Studies report that this minimally invasive, cost-effective technique is ideally suited for patients with less than 3-cm-long malignant obstructions. At times, if the patient's clinical status does not improve enough to render surgery a safe option, stents can be used strictly for palliative therapy.

Notes

CASE 148

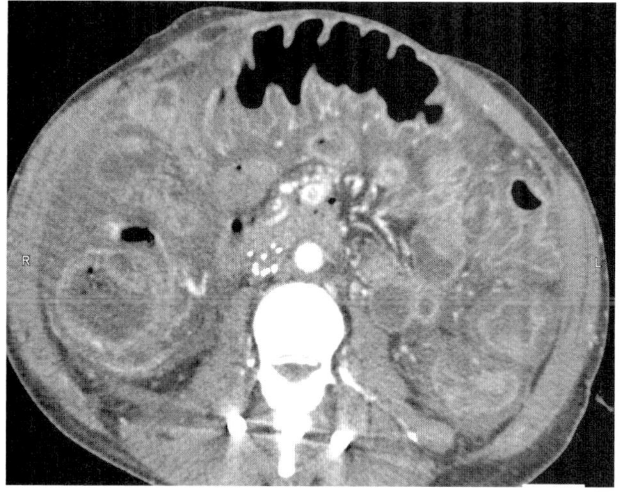

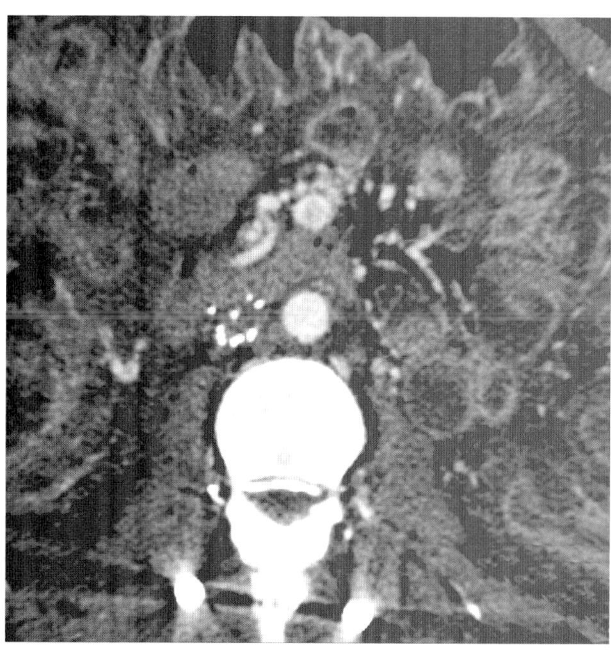

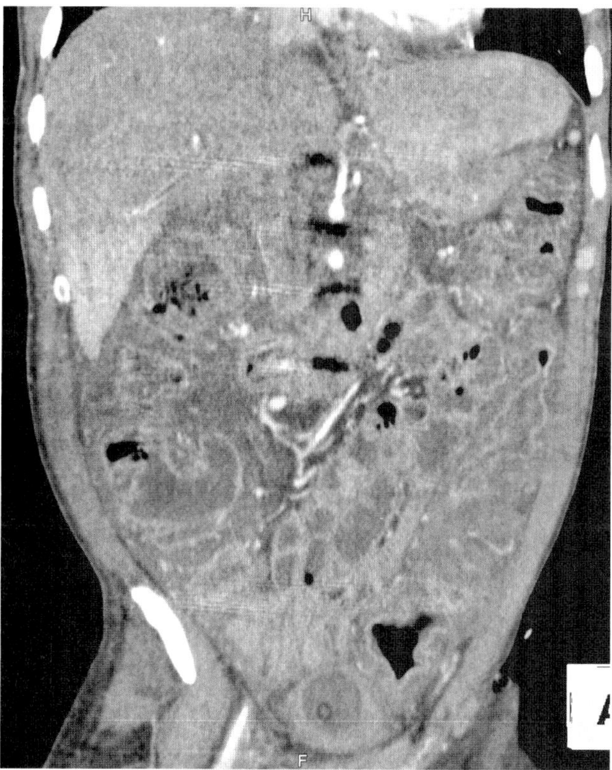

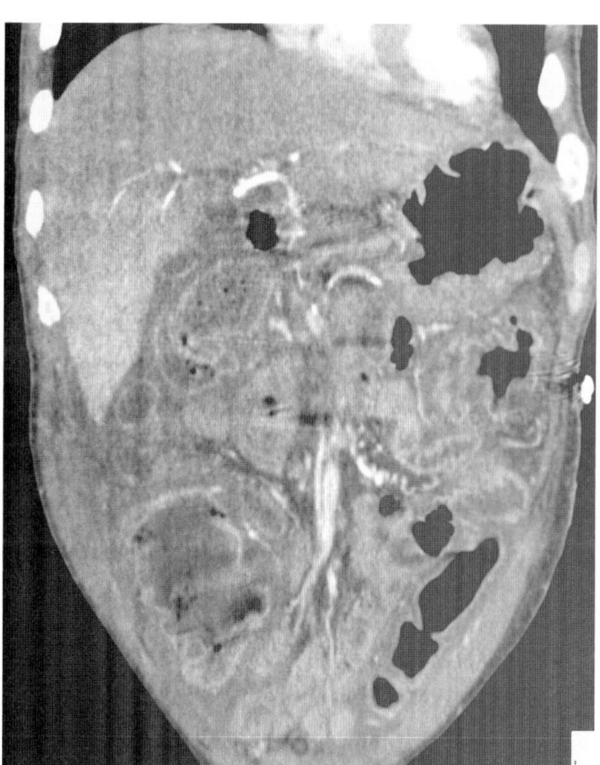

You are shown images of a patient who presented with abdominal pain.

1. What are the multidetector computed tomography findings?
2. What is the best diagnosis?
3. What is the optimal timing for data acquisition during CT angiography to visualize the splanchnic veins?
4. What are the treatment options for this entity?

CASE 148

Superior Mesenteric Vein Thrombosis

1. Ascites, diffuse small and large bowel wall edema, and central low attenuation filling defect within the superior mesenteric vein.
2. Superior mesenteric vein thrombosis.
3. Data acquisition should be performed with an imaging delay of 55 to 70 seconds from the start of intravenous contrast administration.
4. Anticoagulation, surgical thrombectomy, and transcatheter delivery of thrombolytics.

References

Bradbury MS, Kavanagh PV, Bechtold RE, et al: Mesenteric venous thrombosis: diagnosis and noninvasive imaging, *Radiographics* 22:527–541, 2002.

Warshauer DM, Lee JKT, Mauro MA, et al: Superior mesenteric vein thrombosis with radiologically occult cause: a retrospective study of 43 cases, *AJR Am J Roentgenol* 177:837–841, 2001.

Comment

Superior mesenteric vein thrombosis may have an acute or subacute presentation. It often mimics acute mesenteric arterial ischemia since a small percentage (10% to 15%) of patients with mesenteric ischemia will have splanchnic venous occlusive disease. Most patients with superior mesenteric vein thrombosis are symptomatic at the time of presentation. The symptoms are nonspecific and nonlocalizing, hence often the diagnosis is delayed. Factors predisposing to mesenteric venous thrombosis include abdominal surgery, intraperitoneal (appendicitis, cholecystitis, diverticulitis, infected ascites) or extraperitoneal (urinary tract infection, pneumonia) infections, hypercoagulable states, pancreatitis, and portal hypertension.

Multiple imaging modalities (ultrasound, multidetector computed tomography [MDCT], magnetic resonance imaging, angiography) are available to image patients with this uncommon but potentially lethal disease. Color Doppler ultrasound examination with duplex scanning, although operator dependent, can be an inexpensive, quick means to demonstrate the thrombus and provide semiquantitative measurements of the portomesenteric blood flow. Ultrasound may also demonstrate associated free intraperitoneal fluid and bowel wall thickening, which suggest bowel ischemia.

MDCT or MDCT angiography is considered the imaging modality of choice in many centers in demonstrating acute mesenteric vein thrombosis. Performed during peak splanchnic venous enhancement, usually at 55 to 70 seconds from the start of intravenous contrast administration, MDCT can demonstrate thrombus within the central veins of the portomesenteric circulation. Acute thrombosis is typically seen as a completely unopacified vein or a well-defined central filling defect surrounded by a rim of intravenous contrast in a normal caliber or enlarged superior mesenteric vein. Other important accompanying CT findings include congestive changes in the mesentery, such as venous engorgement or edema, and hyperattenuating thickening bowel wall that result from venous stasis. Signs of bowel ischemia include the "target" sign, with alternating high- and low-attenuation areas in the bowel wall from edema or hemorrhage, dilatation of bowel loops, and asymmetric bowel wall enhancement. Pneumatosis may be seen with both ischemia and infarct. Ascites can also be seen. A greater volume of ascites reflects the severity of mesenteric congestion, and these patients are at greater risk of developing bowel ischemia. The triad of findings that includes low attenuation within the superior mesenteric vein, small bowel wall edema, and ascites strongly suggests bowel infarction.

Treatment options available to treat patients with superior mesenteric vein thrombosis are anticoagulation, thrombectomy, and mechanical or pharmacological transcatheter thrombolysis. Surgery is the treatment of choice when bowel infarction or clinical signs of peritonitis are present. Patients with mesenteric venous thrombosis with no signs of ischemia or peritonitis may be managed with simple anticoagulation.

Notes

CASE 149

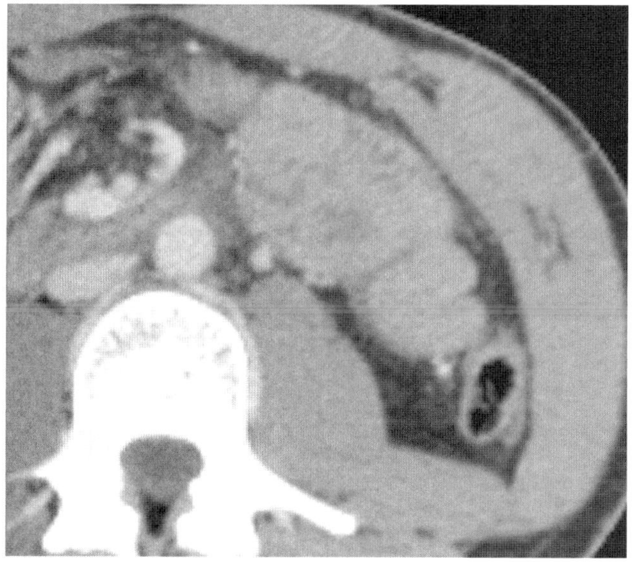

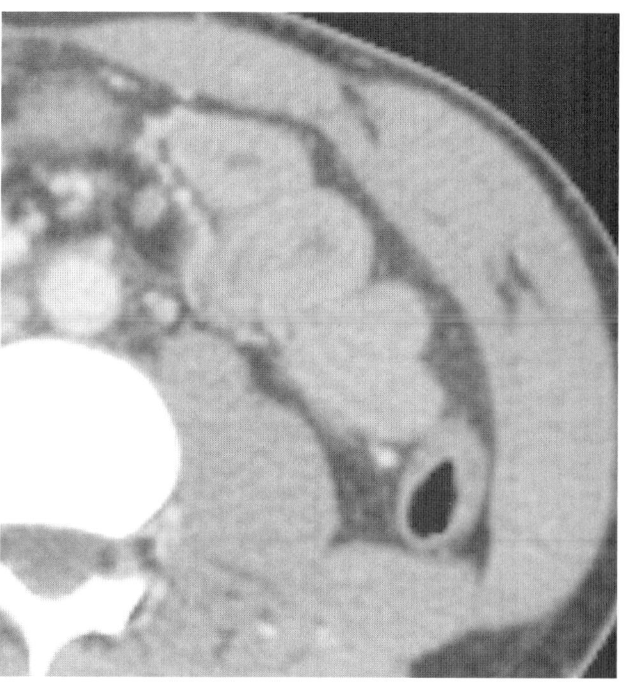

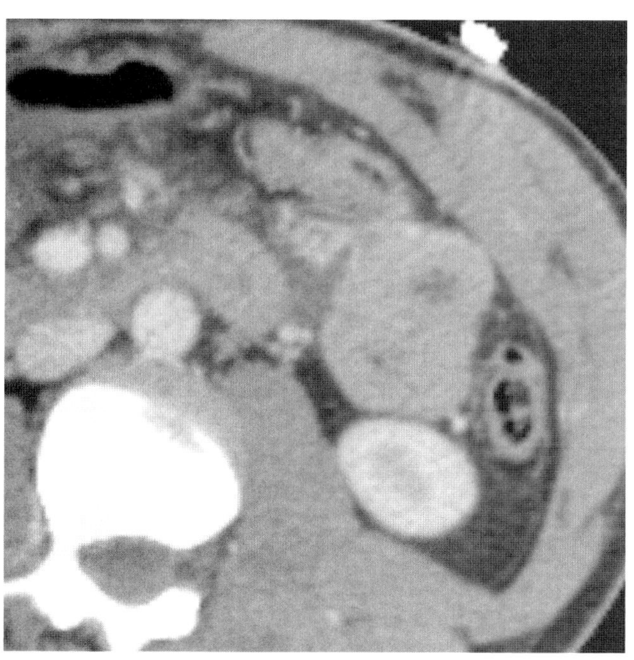

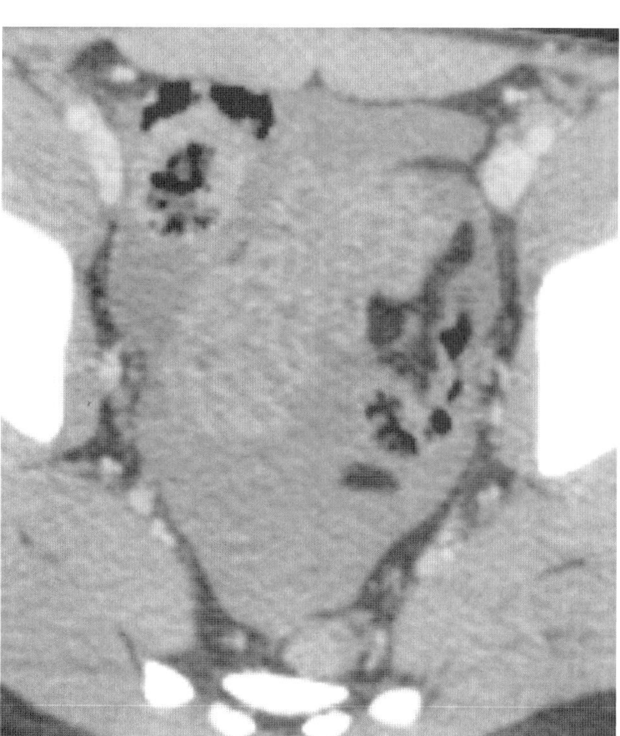

You are shown images of a patient who complained of abdominal pain after a motor vehicle collision.

1. What are the multidetector computed tomography findings?
2. What is the best diagnosis?
3. Name three specific computed tomography findings of blunt bowel injury.
4. What is the next best management option?

CASE 149

Bowel Wall Contusion

1. Small bowel wall thickening, moderate amount of free intraperitoneal fluid, and intermesenteric fluid.
2. Bowel wall contusion.
3. Pneumoperitoneum, oral contrast material extravasation, and discontinuity of the bowel wall.
4. The radiologist and trauma surgeon should discuss the radiological and clinical findings to plan optimal management.

References

Fakhry SM, Watts DD, Luchette FA: Current diagnostic approaches lack sensitivity in the diagnosis of perforated blunt small bowel injury: analysis from 275,557 trauma admissions from the EAST multi-institutional HVI trial, *J Trauma* 54:295–306, 2003.

Watts DD, Fakhry SM: Incidence of hollow viscus injury in blunt trauma: an analysis from 275,557 trauma admissions from the EAST multi-institutional trial, *J Trauma* 54:289–294, 2003.

Cross-Reference

Emergency Radiology: THE REQUISITES, p 95.

Comment

Blunt bowel injury is an uncommon injury seen only in 1% of all patients admitted to level one trauma centers in the United States following blunt trauma. Most trauma surgeons and radiologists are sporadically exposed to this entity. Gaining widespread experience is limited mainly by the infrequent incidence. The workup of patients with potential bowel injury may vary with different institutions.

Prior to the acceptance of computed tomography (CT) as the imaging modality of choice to evaluate stable patients with blunt trauma and to select those who are candidates for nonoperative management, diagnostic peritoneal lavage (DPL) was the most commonly performed diagnostic technique for intraperitoneal injuries. Based on DPL results, laparotomies were frequently performed on hemodynamically stable patients for solid organ injury, while bowel and mesenteric injuries were usually diagnosed incidentally during the surgery.

With the widespread use of CT to evaluate acutely injured blunt trauma patients, blunt bowel injury is more commonly diagnosed without surgery. Extraluminal air, extraluminal gastrointestinal contrast material or intestinal content, discontinuity of bowel wall, and moderate to large amount of isolated free fluid are CT findings of full thickness intestinal injury. Without other specific signs of bowel injury, focal bowel wall thickening (>4 mm) generally indicates bowel wall contusion without a transmural injury. Free intraperitoneal fluid is a nonspecific sign, and when seen without solid organ injury, it can be due to an occult bowel or mesenteric injury. It is imperative to carefully scrutinize the CT scans of patients with nonspecific CT signs for subtle specific signs of a full thickness bowel injury, including those listed above. No clear consensus has been reported in the radiologic or surgical literature on how to optimally manage patients with nonspecific CT findings of bowel injury. Multiple options are available to manage these patients based on the CT findings, physical examination, and presence of injuries. The options include serial physical examinations to assess for signs of peritonitis, a repeat abdominal and pelvic CT at 4 to 6 hours, DPL, laparoscopy, or laparotomies. It is important for the radiologist and trauma surgeon to discuss these findings on an individual basis to select the best option. In patients who cannot be carefully observed with serial physical examination for development of peritonitis, such as those who are anaesthetized or are suffering from severe brain injury, but who have no specific indication for laparotomies, a follow-up CT in 4 to 6 hours' time should be obtained. Follow-up CT should be carefully scrutinized for either increase or decrease in the amount of free intraperitoneal fluid, progressive bowel wall thickening, and interval development of the specific signs of full-thickness bowel injury.

Notes

CASE 150

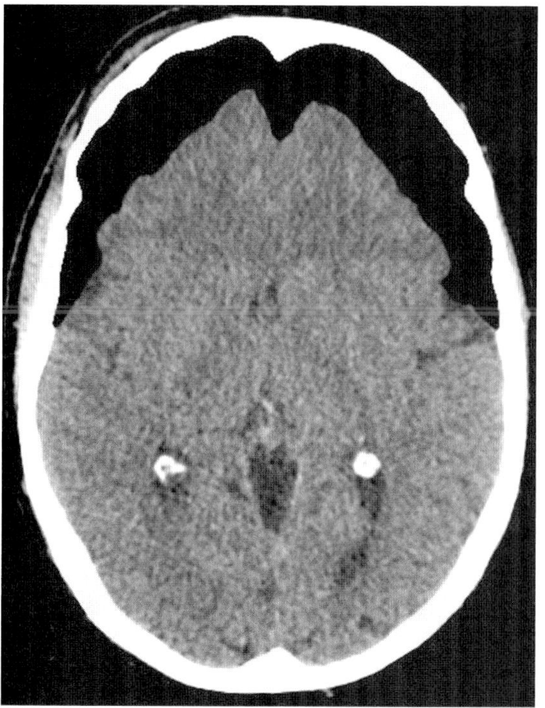

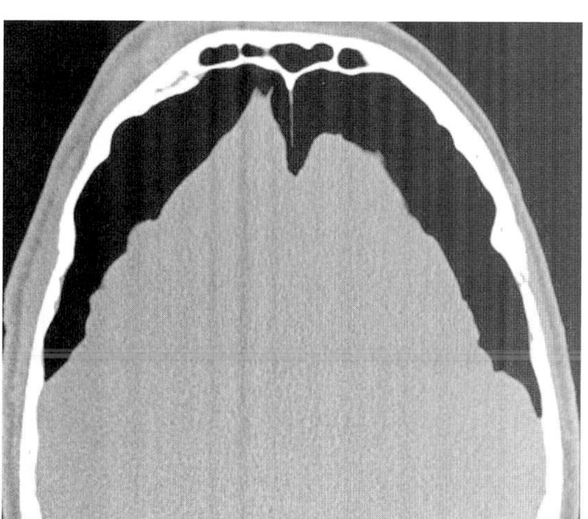

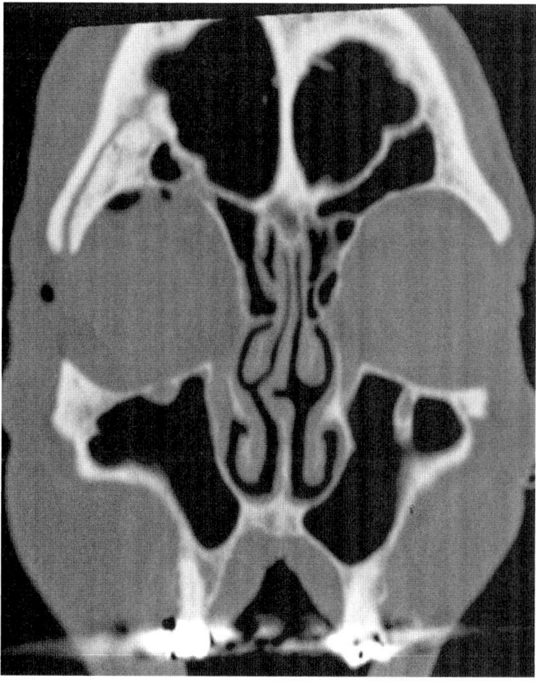

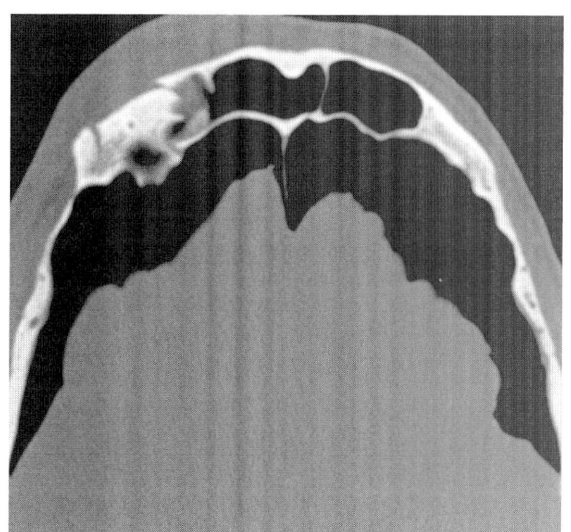

You are shown images of a patient who was scanned after trauma to the head.

1. What radiologic sign can be used to summarize the appearance of the pneumocephalus observed on the axial images?
2. What are the findings that indicate a tension pneumocephalus?
3. What is the source of the tension pneumocephalus?
4. List treatment options for the tension pneumocephalus.

CASE 150

Tension Pneumocephalus

1. "Mount Fuji" sign.
2. Bilateral compression and separation of the frontal lobes.
3. An open right frontal sinus fracture.
4. Treatment options include drilling of burr holes, needle aspiration, craniotomy, ventriculostomy placement, administration of 100% oxygen, and repair of the dural defect.

References

Ishiwata Y, Fujitsu K, Sekino T, et al: Subdural tension pneumocephalus following surgery for chronic subdural hematoma, *J Neurosurg* 68:58–61, 1988.

Michel SJ: The Mount Fuji sign, *Radiology* 232:449–450, 2004.

Comment

The "Mt. Fuji" sign helps differentiate tension pneumocephalus from nontension pneumocephalus. It was initially observed on head computed tomography (CT) images in elderly patients following irrigation of bilateral chronic subdural hematoma. The air collects in the subdural space, causing mass effect on the frontal lobes. The anterior compression and separation of the tips of the frontal lobes observed on axial CT images of the head has the appearance of the silhouette of Mount Fuji.

The volume of intracranial air may not be dissimilar in patients with tension and nontension pneumocephalus. However, in tension pneumocephalus, air enters into the subdural space through a defect in the skull and dura where a ball valve mechanism prevents the egression of air. This allows the intracranial air to accumulate under tension. The resulting pneumocephalus between the frontal lobes and the falx tentorium causes widening of the anterior interhemispheric fissure since the pressure of the air is greater than that of the cerebrospinal fluid normally filling this space.

Bilateral compression of the frontal lobes by subdural air (i.e., "peaking" sign) without separation of the tips of the frontal lobes is also considered a CT sign of tension pneumocephalus. It is postulated that the subdural air under tension may decompress into the subarachnoid space and scatter throughout several cisterns.

The most common cause for tension pneumocephalus is surgical evacuation of chronic subdural hematomas with an incidence between 2% and 16%. Other causes include surgery to the skull base or paranasal sinuses, posterior fossa surgery with the patient in the seated position, and open frontal sinus fractures. A transient rise in pressure within the sinus during coughing or other forms of straining allows air to flow into the low-pressure intracranial space through the osseous and dural defects in the wall of the sinus.

Tension pneumocephalus can lead to rapid neurological deterioration. When the clinical and imaging findings indicate the presence of intracranial air under pressure, emergent decompression is performed to relieve the raised intracranial pressure. Treatment options include drilling of burr holes, needle aspiration, craniotomy, ventriculostomy placement, administration of 100% oxygen, and closure of the dural rent.

Notes

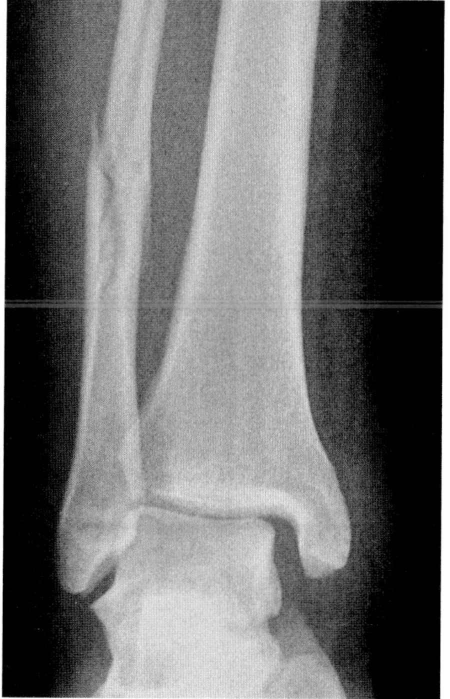

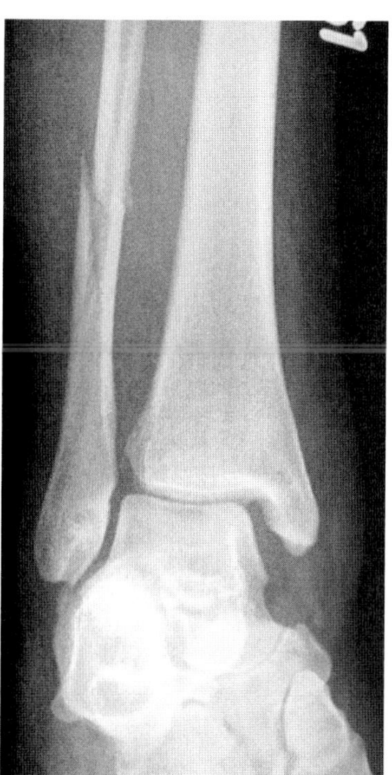

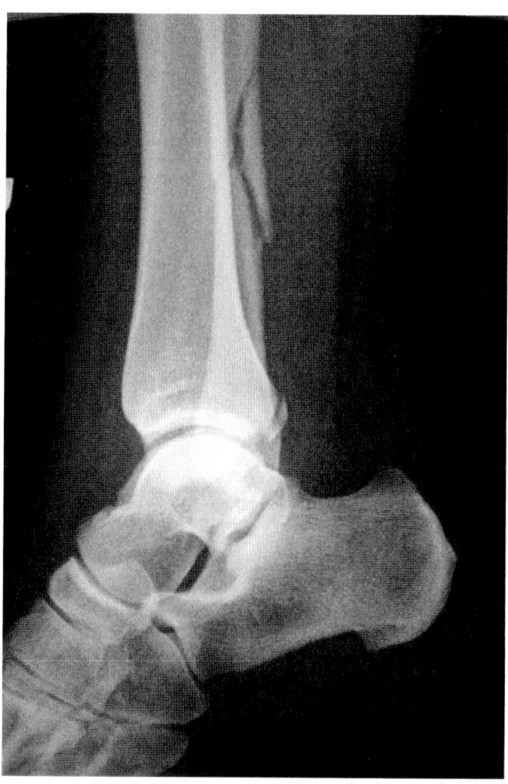

1. What is the mechanism of this injury?
2. What fails in the first stage of this injury?
3. On what injury feature is the Danis-Weber classification system of classifying ankle fractures based?
4. What type of Danis-Weber malleolar injury is this?

CASE 151

Danis-Weber Type C Ankle Injury

1. Pronation with external rotation.
2. Either the deltoid ligament ruptures or the medial malleolus fractures.
3. The classification is based on the level of the fibula fracture.
4. Danis-Weber type C.

References

Carr JB, Trafton PG: Malleolar fractures and soft tissue injury of the ankle. In Browner BD, Jupiter JB, Levine A, Trafton PG, eds: *Skeletal Trauma*, 2nd ed, Philadelphia, WB Saunders, 1998, pp 2327–2404.

Wilson AJ: The ankle. In Rogers LF, ed: *Radiology of Skeletal Trauma*, New York, Churchill Livingstone, 2002, pp 1222–1318.

Cross-Reference

Emergency Radiology: THE REQUISITES, pp 151–155.

Comment

Pronation-external rotation injuries account for 7% to 19% of all ankle malleolar fractures. The initial failure occurs at the medial aspect of the ankle with external rotation of a pronated foot. Rupture of the deltoid ligament or an avulsion fracture of the medial malleolus occurs in stage one. In the second stage, the anterior inferior tibiofibula ligament fails. The third stage produces the characteristic spiral or oblique fracture seen above the tibial plafond. Typically the fibula fracture runs from anterior proximally to posterior distally. In the final stage, the posterior inferior tibiofibular ligament fails, which can be seen on radiographs as a small avulsion fracture of the posterior malleolus (i.e., posterior rim of the distal tibia).

The Danis-Weber classification of ankle fractures is based on the level of the fibula fracture in relation to the tibiofibular syndesmosis or tibial plafond. This classification serves as a basis for surgical treatment. It consists of three basic types: A, B, and C. Type A fractures result from supination-adduction with resulting lateral tensile failure and either disruption of the lateral collateral ligament or a transverse distal fracture of the lateral malleolus. Type B fractures are caused by either supination external rotation or pronation adduction mechanism. The resulting fibula fracture is typically located at or below the plafond, and it is either spiral or laterally comminuted. Type C fractures are caused by a pronation external rotation with the fibula fracture demonstrated at variable levels above the plafond.

The majority of type C malleolar fractures are displaced with syndesmosis instability and will require surgical fixation. Rarely, a nondisplaced type C fracture is successfully treated with nonoperative management. The majority of the undisplaced types A and B fractures are treated nonsurgically.

Notes

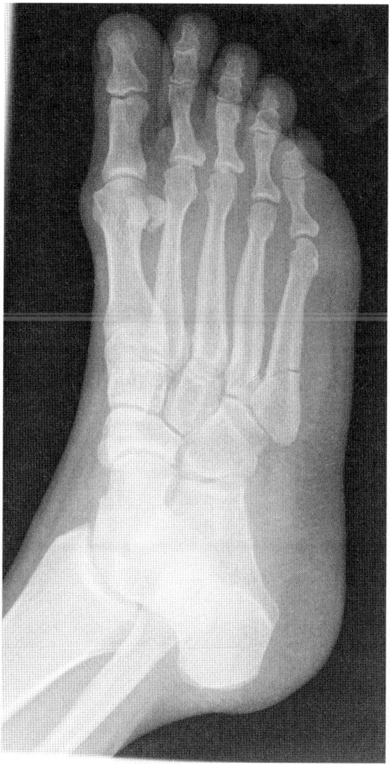

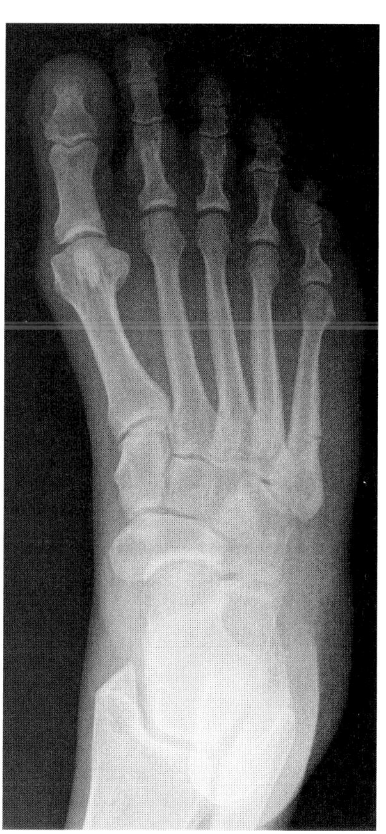

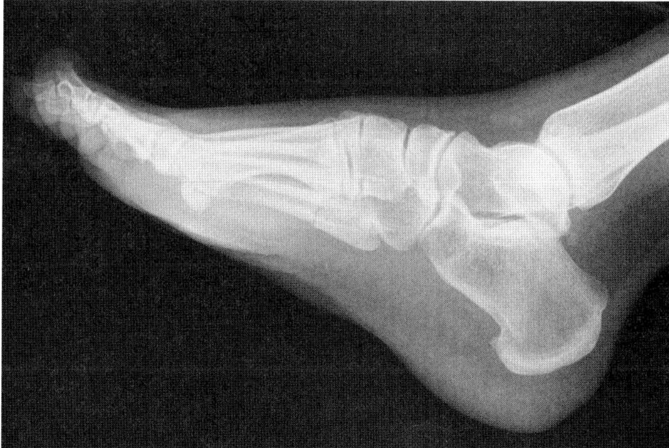

1. What is the specific diagnosis?
2. How does this injury differ from an avulsion of the tuberosity of the fifth metatarsal bone?
3. What other fractures may be seen at the proximal fifth metatarsal?
4. Why do healing complications occur with this fracture?

CASE 152

Jones Fracture

1. Jones fracture.
2. The fracture occurs distal to the metatarsal tubercle and does not involve the fourth and fifth intermetatarsal joint.
3. Diaphyseal stress fractures and proximal tuberosity avulsion fractures.
4. Delayed union or nonunion of fractures is attributed to an inherent poor blood supply to the proximal metadiaphyseal region.

References

Stevens MA, El-Khoury GY, Kathol MH, et al: Imaging features of avulsion injuries, *Radiographics* 19: 655–672, 1999.

Theodorou DJ, Theodorou SJ, Kakitsubata Y, et al: Fractures of proximal portion of fifth metatarsal bone: anatomic and imaging evidence of a pathogenesis of avulsion of the plantar aponeurosis and the short peroneal muscle tendon, *Radiology* 226:857, 2003.

Cross-Reference

Emergency Radiology: THE REQUISITES, pp 158, 159.

Comment

Fractures of the base of the fifth metatarsal bone are common injuries of the foot. They cause pain in the dorsolateral aspect of the proximal forefoot. Three fracture types occur at the proximal fifth metatarsal bone: an avulsion fracture of the tuberosity, Jones fracture, and diaphyseal stress fracture. In the literature there is a considerable amount of confusion on the pathogenesis, diagnosis, and treatment of such fractures. Differentiation of these three types of fractures is important to render the optimal treatment.

The most common fracture is the tuberosity avulsion fracture seen in up to 85% of patients. Typically, the fracture is transverse or oblique, extra-articular, and involves the proximal tuberosity of the metatarsal bone. The mechanism of injury is inversion of a plantarflexed foot. The avulsion fracture occurs at the attachment of the lateral portion of the plantar aponeurosis or the peroneus brevis. The majority of fractures are treated conservatively.

The Jones fracture was originally described in 1902 as a transverse fracture at the junction of the fifth metatarsal proximal metaphysis and diaphysis. It is often comminuted medially and typically with no intra-articular involvement. The mechanism of injury is application of a large adduction force to the plantarflexed foot.

The diaphyseal stress fracture is the least common of the fractures that involve the proximal fifth metatarsal bone. Fractures occur within the proximal 1.5 cm of the diaphysis. They begin as a microfracture and if left untreated progress to complete fractures. Patients with a metatarsus adductus foot deformity are more prone to develop stress fractures.

Due to the poor inherent blood supply to the metadiaphyseal region, patients with Jones fractures and diaphyseal stress fractures have a high prevalence of delayed union, nonunion, and refracture. These fractures are associated with increased disability and require more aggressive treatment than do proximal tuberosity fractures, which usually heal well with closed reduction and casting.

Notes

Challenge

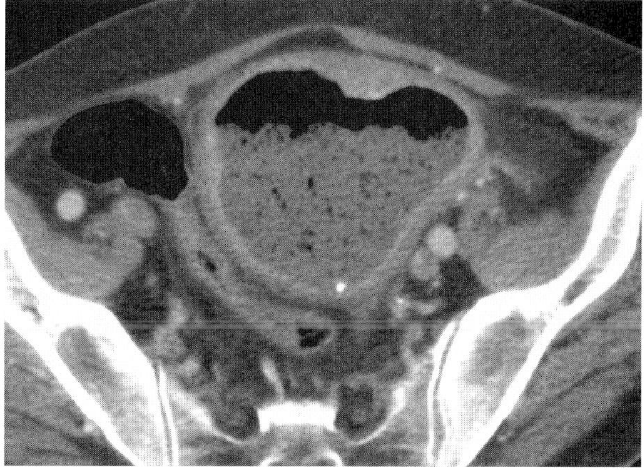

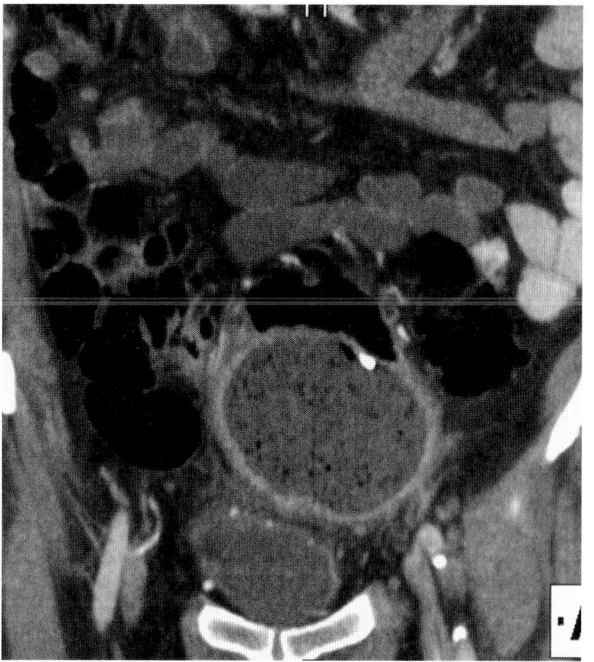

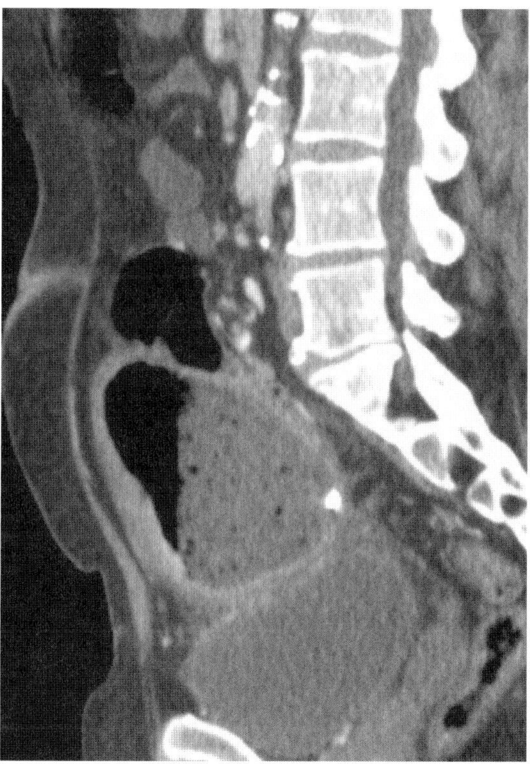

You are shown images of a patient with lower abdominal pain.

1. What is the diagnosis?
2. What other pathologies should be considered in the differential diagnosis?
3. What are two potential complications of this entity?
4. What is the usual treatment?

CASE 153

Giant Sigmoid Diverticulum

1. Giant sigmoid diverticulum.
2. Volvulus, bowel duplication, Meckel's diverticulum, infected pancreatic pseudocyst, abscess, vesicoenteric fistula, or emphysematous cystitis.
3. Torsion and perforation (both require emergency surgery).
4. Surgical removal of the lesion and resection of the sigmoid colon to which it is attached.

References

Mainzer F, Minagi H: Giant sigmoid diverticulum, *Am J Roentgenol Radium Ther Nucl Med* 113:352–354, 1971.

Thomas S, Peel RL, Evans LE, Haarer KA: Best cases from AFIP: giant colonic diverticulum, *Radiographics* 26:1869–1872, 2006.

Cross-Reference

Emergency Radiology: THE REQUISITES, p 285.

Comment

Giant sigmoid diverticula are rare, usually presenting in the sixth decade (50% over 60 years of age). The diverticulum arises along the mesenteric border at the site of vascular penetration. Three subtypes are recognized: the inflammatory (66%) with no lining mucosa; the pseudodiverticulum, partially lined by mucosa and muscularis (22%); and true diverticulum, a communicating duplication with all three colonic layers (11%). The etiology is thought to be related to a ball-valve mechanism leading to expansion of the diverticulum or gas-producing organisms within a noncommunicating diverticulum. Patients typically present with abdominal pain and a mass. Other symptoms can include constipation, diarrhea, nausea, vomiting, and fever.

The diagnosis is suggested by an abdominal radiograph showing a large smooth-walled air-containing lower mid-abdominal cystic mass with smooth walls containing an air-fluid level and/or stool. The diagnosis is verified by barium enema demonstrating sigmoid luminal communication with the diverticulum in 60% of cases or by computed tomography (CT). CT is the diagnostic method of choice to demonstrate the extent of the lesion, associated diverticulitis, or abscess formation. Thickening of the diverticulum wall indicates inflammation, and an irregular wall raises the possibility of perforated neoplasm or tumor within a diverticulum. Among differential diagnoses, Meckel's diverticulum is distinguished by origin from the distal ileum, abscess by immobility and surrounding inflammatory changes, duplication cyst by an elongated mesenteric mass paralleling the colon, and pneumatosis cystoides intestinalis by more diffuse extent. Most cases are treated by surgical resection of the diverticulum and sigmoid colon to which it is attached, although nonoperative management can be attempted.

Notes

CASE 154

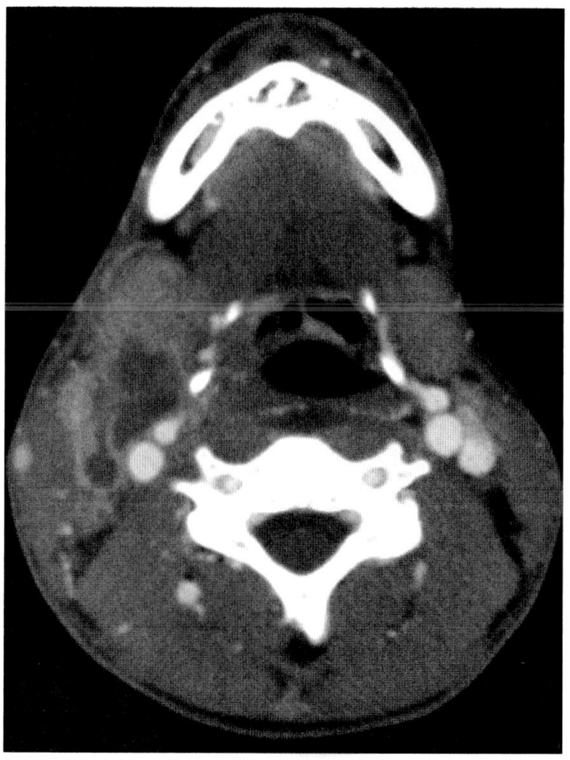

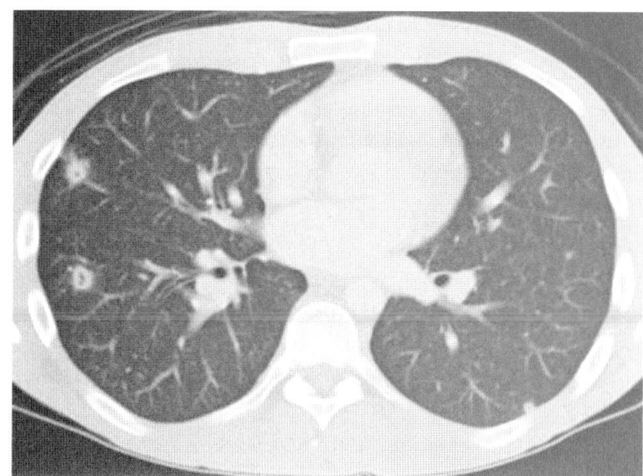

You are shown images of a patient with right neck pain and swelling.

1. What is the diagnosis?
2. What is the major secondary complication of this condition?
3. What is the likely initial clinical presentation?
4. What radiologic finding(s) might be present on the chest radiograph of the patient?

CASE 154

Lemierre Syndrome

1. Lemierre syndrome.
2. Septic emboli, most commonly the lungs, septic arthritis. Hepatic and splenic abscesses, osteomyelitis, meningitis, epidural abscess, and diffuse encephalopathy have also been described.
3. Acute pharyngotonsillitis.
4. Peripheral lung nodules, some with cavitation; possible pleural effusion.

Reference

Screaton NJ, Ravenel JG, Lehner PJ, et al: Lemierre syndrome: forgotten but not extinct—report of four cases, *Radiology* 213:369–374, 1999.

Cross-Reference

Emergency Radiology: THE REQUISITES, pp 45, 208.

Comment

Lemierre syndrome, also known as postanginal sepsis or necrobacillosis, is an uncommon but potentially life-threatening complication of acute pharyngotonsillitis first described in 1936. Anaerobic oropharyngeal infection may result in septic thrombophlebitis of the ipsilateral internal jugular vein (IJV) with subsequent septicemia and septic embolization, which cause metastatic abscesses, commonly in the lungs and less commonly in the large joints. The IJV thrombosis results from an adjacent inflammatory process or extension from the tonsillar veins. Patients typically present with acute pharyngitis followed in 3 to 10 days by development of fever (temperature > 38.5° C), rigors, and malaise with the onset of septicemia. Many patients present with an array of nonspecific symptoms and clinical findings. Infection is caused by *F. necrophorum* in 81% of cases and by other Fusobacterium species in about 11%. IJV thrombosis typically causes pain, tenderness, swelling along the line of the vein, and trismus; involvement of the lower cranial nerves may result in hoarseness and dysphagia.

Noninvasive cross-sectional imaging has superseded contrast-enhanced venography for identification of the presence and the cause of venous obstruction. Ultrasound findings include the presence of noncompressible thrombus, frequently associated with venous distention, and absence of flow. Contrast-enhanced computed tomography (CT) characteristically demonstrates jugular venous distention with a thickened enhancing wall and a hypoattenuating filling defect. Edema of the surrounding soft tissues is often present. If the diagnosis of Lemierre syndrome is suspected clinically or on the basis of chest CT findings, CT of the neck vessels should be performed at the same time as CT of the chest. Magnetic resonance imaging, with its flow sensitivity and excellent soft tissue contrast, has been shown to be an effective modality for the identification and characterization of thrombi.

Notes

CASE 155

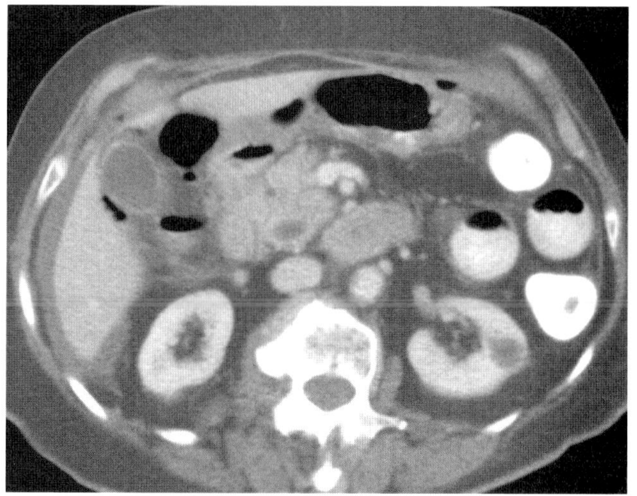

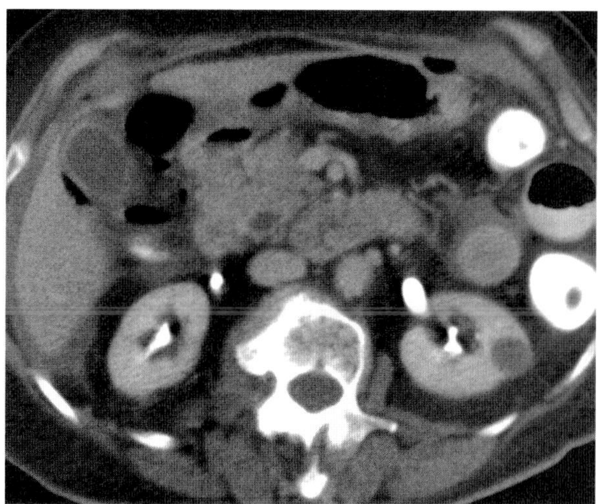

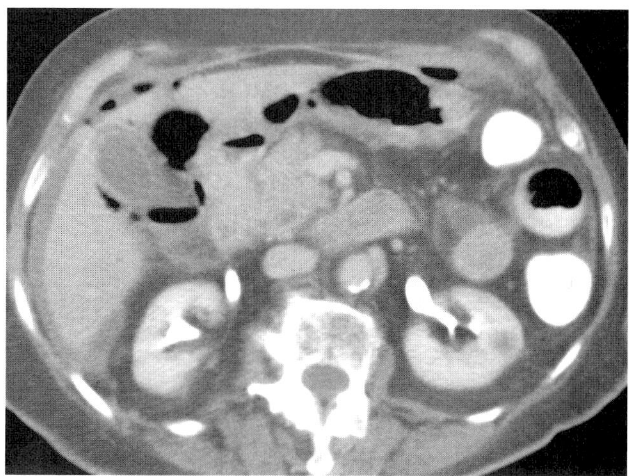

You are shown images of a nontrauma patient with upper abdominal pain.

1. What findings are present in this case?
2. What new finding is seen on the delayed (pyelogram) images?
3. Differential diagnosis considerations should include what?
4. Name an infectious agent and a neoplastic process that predispose to the underlying condition shown by this case.

CASE 155

Perforated Duodenal Ulcer

1. Intra- and extraperitoneal free air, intraperitoneal free fluid, contrast and air collection adjacent to second part of duodenum.
2. There is more oral contrast accumulated at the site of ulcer perforation.
3. Perforated duodenal diverticulitis, ruptured retrocecal appendicitis, traumatic duodenal rupture such as that associated with the ingestion of a foreign body, perforated duodenal malignancy, erosion of gallstone into duodenum.
4. *Helicobacter pylori*, as a significant agent in the development of chronic gastritis and benign gastric and duodenal ulcers. Zollinger-Ellison syndrome (non-beta islet cell tumor) can cause multiple, recurrent, and postbulbar duodenal ulcers due to excessive gastrin secretion.

Reference

Jacobs JM, Hill MC, Steinberg WM: Peptic ulcer disease: CT evaluation, *Radiology* 178:745–748, 1991.

Cross-Reference

Emergency Radiology: THE REQUISITES, p 276.

Comment

Peptic ulcer disease (PUD) involves the mucosa of the esophagus, stomach, and duodenum secondary to gastric acid. Acute perforation occurs in 5% to 10% of patients with PUD when the ulcer extends through the muscularis and serosal layers. Perforations may be into the peritoneal cavity or lesser sac, such as those of the anterior gastric wall, curvatures, and posterior gastric wall, or confined by adjacent structures such as the pancreas, liver, or extraperitoneal soft tissues. Usually PUD is diagnosed by upper endoscopy or, less commonly now, by an upper gastrointestinal contrast study. Computed tomography (CT) can also be useful, especially to establish alternative diagnoses and complications. Distention of the bowel lumen with gas is helpful in determining wall thickening and perforation.

CT findings of perforated duodenal ulcer include focal or diffuse wall thickening, air and/or oral contrast extravasation, inflammatory stranding of adjacent fat, and inflammatory changes of adjacent organs such as the pancreas. It is quite rare to be able to visualize the ulcer crater specifically.

Notes

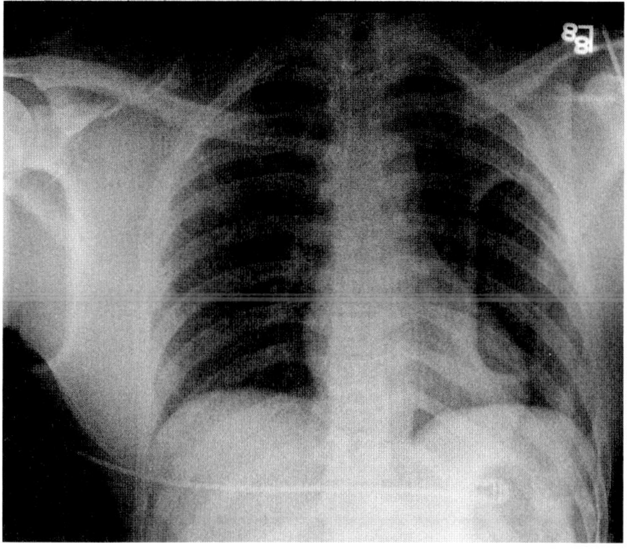

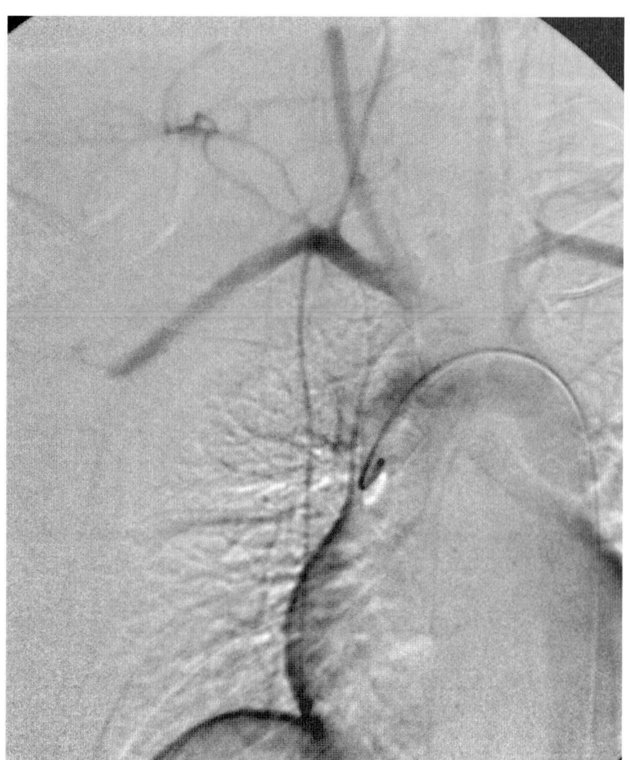

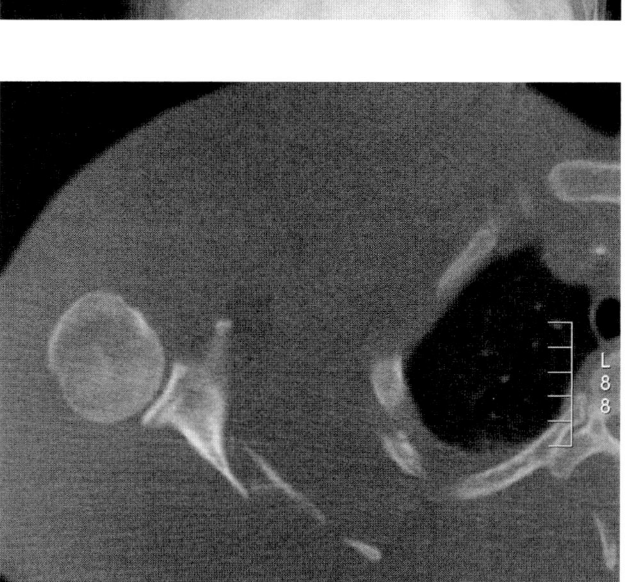

You are shown images of a blunt trauma patient.

1. What is the imaging diagnosis?
2. What associated injuries are expected?
3. What measurement made on the chest radiograph can assist in making the diagnosis?
4. What are the expected physical findings?

CASE 156

Scapulothoracic Dissociation

1. Scapulothoracic dissociation.
2. Subclavian artery and brachial plexus injuries, multiple upper extremity fractures, and/or acromioclavicular separation.
3. The ratio of the lateral displacement of the injured scapula (medial border) from the midline to the medial border of the uninjured scapula exceeds 1.54 (standard deviation = 0.36).
4. Soft tissue swelling over shoulder and chest, decreased pulse pressure, and motor and sensory deficit in involved extremity.

Reference

Sheafor DH, Mirvis SE: Scapulothoracic dissociation: report of five cases and review of the literature, *Emerg Radiol* 2:279–284, 1995.

Comment

Scapulothoracic dissociation is a closed forequarter amputation of the upper extremity with intact overlying skin. The mechanism is a high-energy distraction as may occur with the upper extremity struck while outside a car window or with impact of the shoulder into an immovable object, possibly upon ejection from a motor vehicle. Usually bruising and hematoma is evident over the upper chest and shoulder girdle. The pulse in the involved extremity may be diminished, although collateral arterial supply may make this finding subtle. The arm is insensate and immobile due to stretching and tearing of the brachial plexus.

Chest radiograph shows a lateral displaced and often tilted scapula typically with associated fractures of the scapula and humerus, as well as acromioclavicular separation and distracted clavicular fractures. The ratio of the lateral displacement of the injured scapula (medial border) from the midline to the medial border of the uninjured scapula exceeds 1.54 (standard deviation = 0.36).

Subclavian arteriography should be performed to assess arterial supply and the potential for repair of an injured arterial supply, and to exclude ongoing hemorrhage. A careful inspection of the adjacent chest and thoracic spine is required to assess likely adjacent injuries. Limited functional recovery of the involved extremity occurs in only 17% of patients. In patients with complete brachial plexus disruption and a flail upper extremity, above-elbow amputation and prosthesis fitting is indicated.

Notes

CASE 157

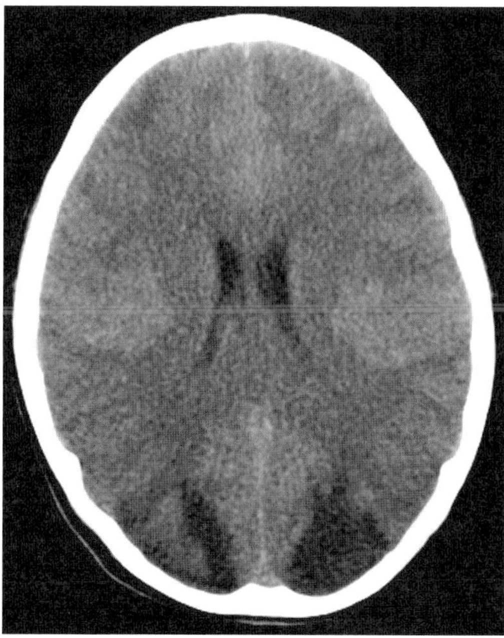

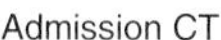

Admission CT

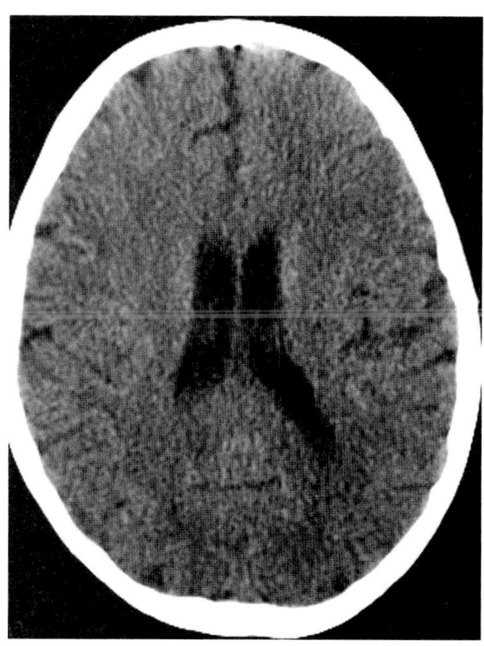

Follow up CT at 7 weeks

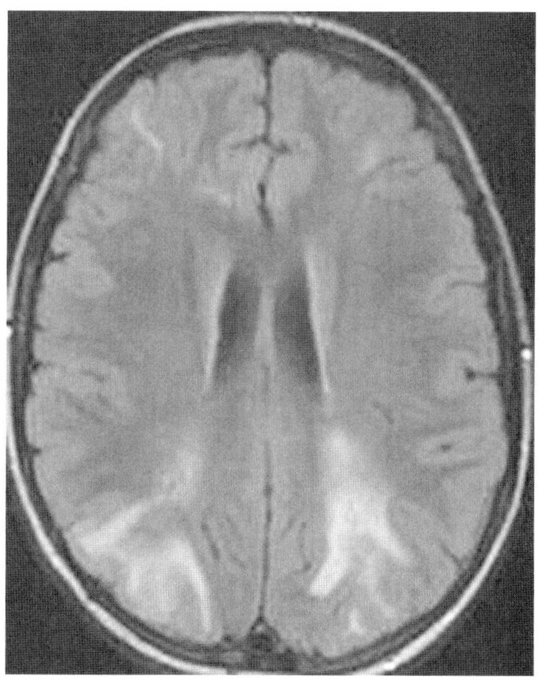

Admission MRI

You are shown images of a patient with encephalopathy syndrome.

1. What is the condition shown?
2. Name several underlying clinical entities that have been associated with this condition.
3. Is the edema seen on computed tomography and magnetic resonance imaging in this condition cytotoxic or vasogenic?
4. What are some typical presenting clinical symptoms?

CASE 157

Posterior Reversible Encephalopathy Syndrome

1. Posterior reversible encephalopathy syndrome.
2. Glomerulonephritis, preeclampsia and eclampsia, systemic lupus erythematosus, thrombotic thrombocytopenic purpura, hemolytic-uremic syndrome, drug toxicity from agents such as cyclosporine, tacrolimus, cisplatin, and erythropoietin.
3. Vasogenic.
4. Headaches, confusion, visual disturbances, elevated blood pressure, and seizures.

References

Brubaker LM, Keith J, Smith JK, et al: Hemodynamic and permeability changes in posterior reversible syndrome measured by dynamic susceptibility perfusion-weighted MR imaging, *Am J Neuroradiol* 26:825–830, 2005.

Hinchey J, Chaves C, Appignani B, et al: A reversible posterior leukoencephalopathy syndrome, *N Engl J Med* 334:494–500, 1996.

Cross-Reference

Emergency Radiology: THE REQUISITES, pp 33–35.

Comment

Posterior reversible encephalopathy syndrome (PRES) is an increasingly recognized neurologic disorder with characteristic computed tomography (CT) and magnetic resonance imaging (MRI) findings. It is associated with a multitude of diverse clinical entities including acute glomerulonephritis, preeclampsia and eclampsia, systemic lupus erythematosus, thrombotic thrombocytopenic purpura, and hemolytic-uremic syndrome, as well as drug toxicity from agents such as cyclosporine, tacrolimus, cisplatin, and erythropoietin. Clinically, patients with PRES have seizures, visual disturbances, altered mental status, and headaches. Most, but not all, cases have acute to subacute hypertension. Classic CT findings include bilaterally symmetric low attenuation in the posterior parietal and occipital lobes. MRI demonstrates hyperintensity on T2-weighted images in the same distribution.

The etiology of PRES is unknown, and hypotheses include hypertension-induced autoregulatory failure resulting in vasodilation and increased capillary hydrostatic pressure with subsequent vasogenic edema. Alternately, excessive arteriolar vasoconstriction could result in decreased blood flow, ischemia, and cytotoxic edema. Studies of cerebral perfusion in PRES have shown decreased cerebral blood volume and cerebral blood flow with associated edema. Given this finding, an alternative suggested etiology is venous vasoconstriction producing increased hydrostatic pressure and vasogenic edema. In most cases of PRES areas of abnormal T2 signal are normal on diffusion-weighted imaging but have increased apparent diffusion coefficient values indicating vasogenic rather than cytotoxic edema. When recognized promptly, the symptoms and radiologic abnormalities can be reversed by rapid control of blood pressure or withdrawal of the offending drug. When the condition is undiagnosed the patient can progress to ischemia, massive infarction, and death.

Notes

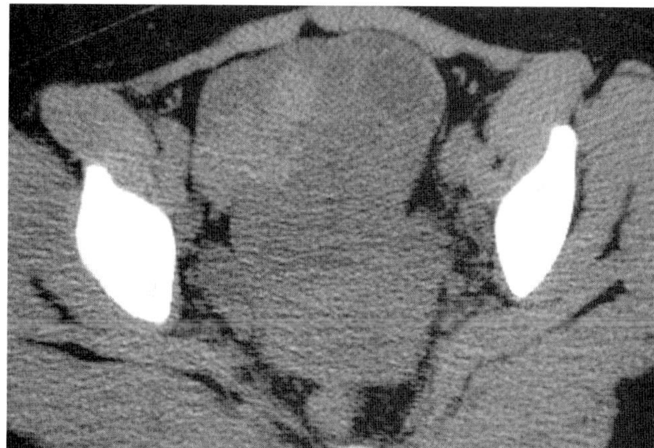

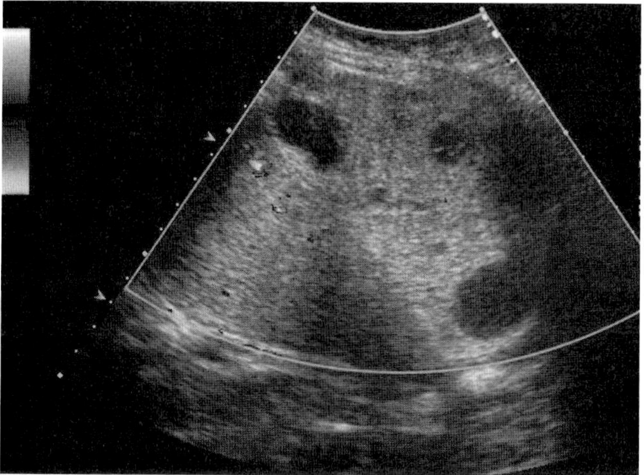

See also Color Plate

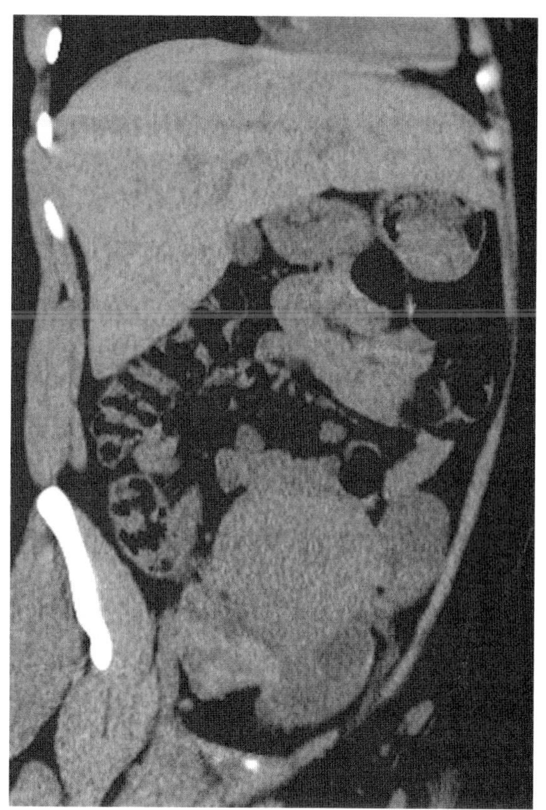

You are shown images of a nontrauma patient with lower abdominal pain.

1. What is the diagnosis?
2. Name four predisposing factors that increase risk likelihood of this condition.
3. Name four other pathologic processes that can mimic this diagnosis clinically.
4. What is the best treatment for prepubertal patients?

CASE 158

Ovarian Torsion

1. Right ovarian torsion.
2. A long mesosalpinx, hypermobility of ovary in prepubertal girls and during pregnancy, previous surgery and adhesions, and ovarian masses.
3. Endometriosis, pelvic inflammatory disease, appendicitis, and hemorrhagic ovarian cyst.
4. Prompt diagnostic laparoscopy and detorsion of the adnexa (ovarian function preserved in majority of patients).

References

Chiou SY, Lev-Toaff AS, Masuda E, et al: Adnexal torsion: new clinical and imaging observations by sonography, computed tomography, and magnetic resonance imaging, *J Ultrasound Med* 26:1289–1301, 2007.

Kimura I, Togashi K, Kawakami S, et al: Ovarian torsion: CT and MR imaging appearances, *Radiology* 190:337–341, 1994.

Cross-Reference

Emergency Radiology: THE REQUISITES, pp 199–200, 314–315.

Comment

Ovarian torsion is most common when ovarian tumors are present but can occur with normal adnexa. Hypermobility of the ovary, often seen in prepubertal girls and during pregnancy, or an excessively long mesosalpinx predisposes to the condition. Previous surgery and adhesions may be predisposing factors for adnexal torsion. Torsion may or may not include the Fallopian tube. Symptoms include gradual or sudden onset of pain consistent with an acute abdomen. It is difficult on clinical grounds to distinguish it from conditions such as appendicitis, internal hemorrhage, salpingitis, and ruptured ectopic pregnancy. When ovarian torsion presents in a subacute or intermittent fashion, the diagnosis is more difficult. Torsion of the ovarian pedicle causes circulatory stasis initially involving venous flow, but ultimately arterial flow. With complete torsion there is hemorrhagic necrosis.

Computed tomography (CT), magnetic resonance imaging (MRI), and sonography with Doppler can be diagnostically valuable. On ultrasound there is a cystic, solid, or complex mass with or without fluid in the Douglas pouch. Peripheral cysts and follicles substantiate identification of the ovary within the mass. Transvaginal sonography with Doppler can help establish the diagnosis by demonstrating an enlarged ovary with no vascular waveforms. CT and MRI typically show a large adnexal mass with smooth wall thickening and no enhancement. A torsed Fallopian tube may appear thickened and fluid-filled. The torsed ovarian pedicle may appear as a whirled structure adjacent to the ovarian mass. Other findings may include deviation of the uterus to the side of the torsion, engorgement of vessels on the twisted side, and obliteration of the normal surrounding fat. Contrast-enhanced CT can better demonstrate the enhancing engorged ovarian vessels. A CT attenuation of greater than 50 Hounsfield units in the nonenhancing mass indicates hemorrhage.

Notes

CASE 159

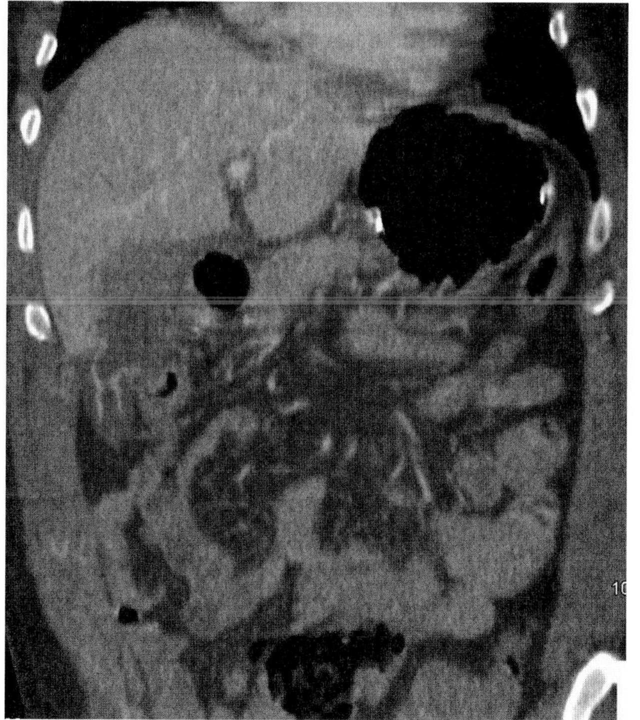

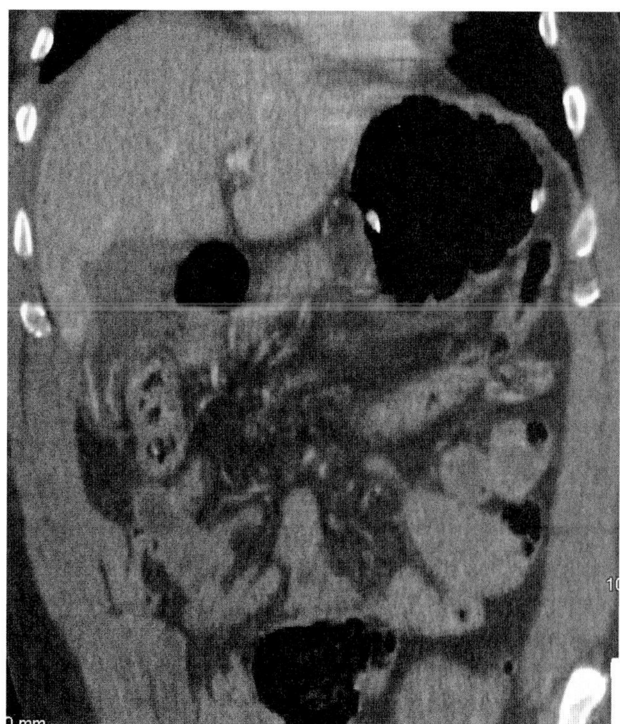

You are shown images of a blunt trauma patient.

1. What is the diagnosis?
2. What factors increase the risk for this injury in trauma?
3. What is the treatment for this lesion?
4. Name two conditions that might simulate injury to this structure.

CASE 159

Traumatic Gallbladder Avulsion and Rupture

1. Traumatic gallbladder avulsion and rupture.
2. Distended gallbladder (fasting) and contraction of the sphincter of Oddi (alcohol) elevating biliary system pressure.
3. Cholecystectomy.
4. Milk of calcium or vicarious excretion of intravenous contrast media from prior computed tomography studies simulates hemorrhage in the gallbladder lumen.

References

Gupta A, Joshua W, Stuhlfaut JW, et al: Blunt trauma of the pancreas and biliary tract: a multimodality imaging approach to diagnosis, *Radiographics* 24: 1381–1395, 2004.

Wittenberg A, Minotti AJ: CT diagnosis of traumatic gallbladder injury, *AJR Am J Roentgenol* 185:1573–1574, 2005.

Cross-Reference

Emergency Radiology: THE REQUISITES, pp 85–88.

Comment

Isolated traumatic gallbladder injuries are uncommon and difficult to diagnose. Motor vehicle collision is the most common cause of gallbladder injury, and about 2% to 3% of patients who undergo laparotomy for traumatic injury have a gallbladder injury. Usually a patient with traumatic gallbladder injury has slowly progressive abdominal complaints, but occasionally, the injury presents as an acute abdomen. The spectrum of gallbladder injuries includes wall contusion, laceration, perforation, and avulsion. A distended preprandial gallbladder is at increased risk for avulsion in acceleration/deceleration mechanisms of injury, as an increased shearing force is generated between the fluid-filled gallbladder and the hepatic parenchyma. Paradoxically, a chronically diseased gallbladder with a thickened wall has a protective effect against gallbladder injury. Elevated serum ethanol can increase the risk of gallbladder injury in trauma. Alcohol increases sphincter of Oddi tone, which causes subsequent gallbladder distention.

The diagnosis can be made most effectively with computed tomography (CT). Sonography may be useful in the diagnosis. Echogenic fluid will be detected within the gallbladder. CT most confidently establishes the diagnosis. Blood in the gallbladder most presents as high-density fluid within the gallbladder lumen. Vicarious contrast excretion, cholelithiasis, and milk-of-calcium bile also appear as hyperdense material within the gallbladder lumen on CT and can be confused with gallbladder injury. Other CT findings that are suggestive of gallbladder injury include thickening or indistinctness of the gallbladder wall and active arterial extravasation into the lumen. Complete avulsion of the gallbladder results in displacement of the gallbladder from its fossa. Pericholecystic fluid and a collapsed gallbladder lumen are less specific indicators of gallbladder trauma. Associated intra-abdominal injuries include liver laceration and duodenal hematoma. If nonoperative management is contemplated, assessment of the biliary system by nuclear scintigraphy may be useful if pericholecystic fluid is present.

Notes

CASE 160

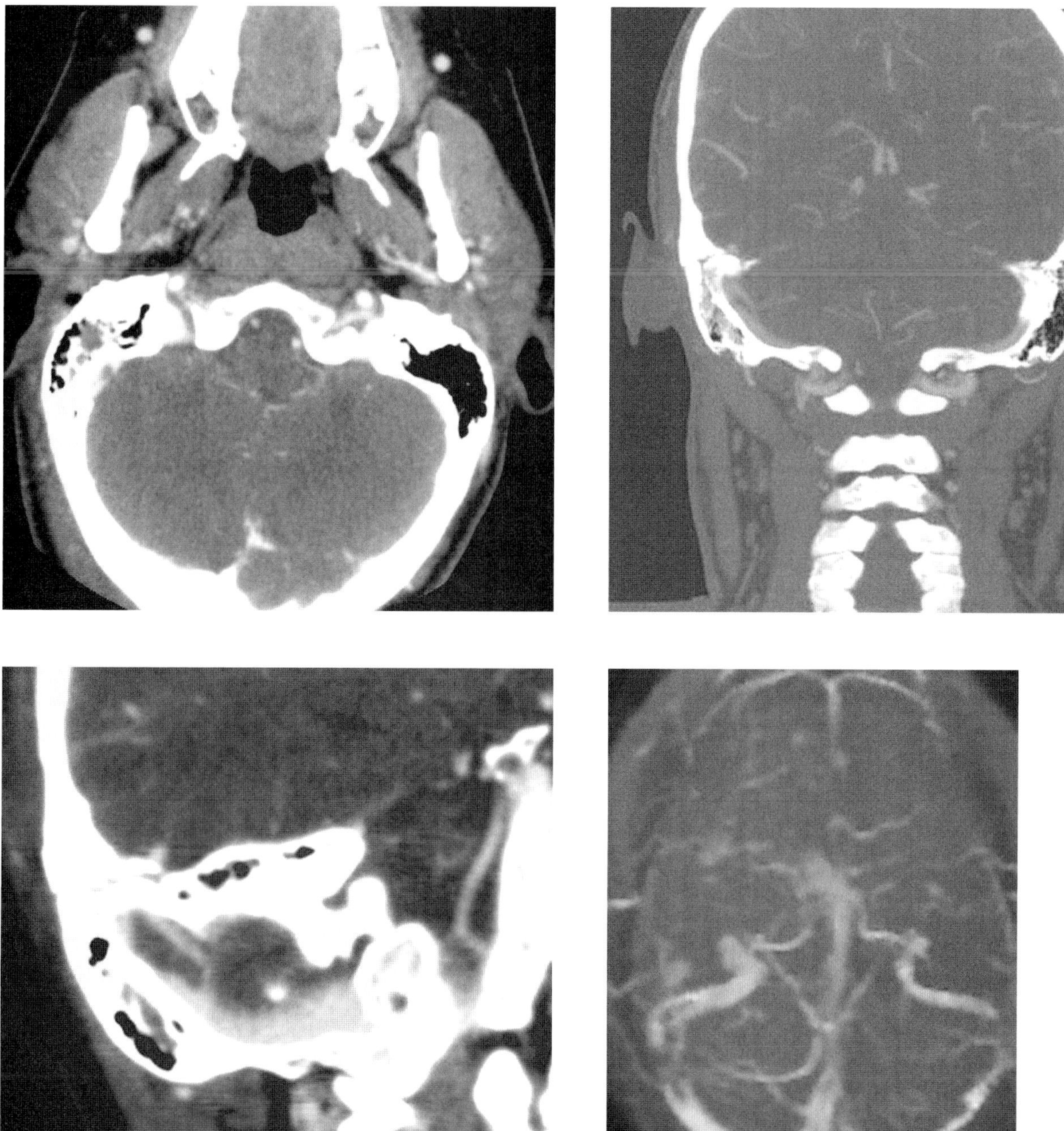

You are shown images of a blunt trauma patient.

1. What is the diagnosis?
2. What is the major complication?
3. Name four nontraumatic causes of this pathology.
4. What is the most common cause of a false positive diagnosis by magnetic resonance imaging?

CASE 160

Traumatic Dural Venous Sinus Thrombosis

1. Traumatic dural sinus thrombosis.
2. Venous occlusion with hemorrhagic cerebral infarct.
3. Dehydration, hypercoagulable states, infection, tumor invasion.
4. Signal gaps resulting from slow intravascular blood flow, in-plane flow, and complex blood flow patterns mimicking thrombosis.

References

Ayanzen RH, Bird CR, Keller PJ, et al: Cerebral MR venography: normal anatomy and potential diagnostic pitfalls, *AJNR Am J Neuroradiol* 21:74–78, 2000.

Rodallec MH, Krainik A, Feydy A, et al: Cerebral venous thrombosis and multidetector CT angiography: tips and tricks, *Radiographics* 26(Suppl):S5–S18, 2006.

Cross-Reference

Emergency Radiology: THE REQUISITES, pp 17–20.

Comment

Dural venous sinus thrombosis is seen in a number of conditions, including dehydration, hypercoagulable states, infection, tumor invasion, trauma, and in conjunction with oral contraception, and may be a cause of neurologic deterioration. This diagnosis has traditionally been made during the venous phase of conventional catheter angiography, which has been considered the standard of reference. Recently, both multidetector computed tomography (MDCT) with CT angiography/venography and magnetic resonance imaging (MRI) and MR angiography/venography have been used in place of conventional angiography. There is a great diversity of clinical features that may result from dural sinus thrombosis and its complications. The evolution of symptoms is unforeseeable, and a small proportion of cases will worsen in the acute phase. Cerebral venous thrombosis must be diagnosed as early as possible so that specific treatment can be started, typically transcatheter thrombolysis or systemic anticoagulation.

Traumatic dural sinus thrombosis most commonly involves the transverse and sigmoid sinus with variable extension into the internal jugular vein. Typically, there is a skull fracture near the site of thrombosis. Unenhanced CT is usually the initial cerebral imaging study in trauma patients. Unenhanced CT allows detection of ischemic changes related to venous insufficiency and sometimes demonstrates a hyperattenuating thrombosed dural sinus or vein. Helical MDCT venography with bolus power injection of contrast material and use of two-dimensional and three-dimensional reformations provides exquisite anatomic detail of the deep and superficial intracranial venous system and can demonstrate filling defects. Common variants of the sinovenous system should not be mistaken for sinus thrombosis. The hyperdense transverse dural sinus can be mistaken for the somewhat normally dense transverse sinus, or an adjacent extra-axial hematoma.

MRI is probably the most accurate method to establish the diagnosis. The signal of the thrombus varies with the age and chemical state of the clotted blood and thus can be confusing. MR venography best shows the filling defect or occlusion of the involved dural sinus. However, transverse sinus flow gaps can be observed in 31% of patients in the nondominant transverse sinuses, mimicking thrombosis. These gaps are most likely artifactual in nature, mainly resulting from slow intravascular blood flow, in-plane flow, and complex blood flow patterns, added to problems with the MR angiographic post-processing method used. Use of Gadolineum contrast enhancement, thin-slice thickness, and perpendicular plane imaging to the sinus to prevent spin saturation helps to lessen signal gaps and false positive diagnosis.

Notes

CASE 161

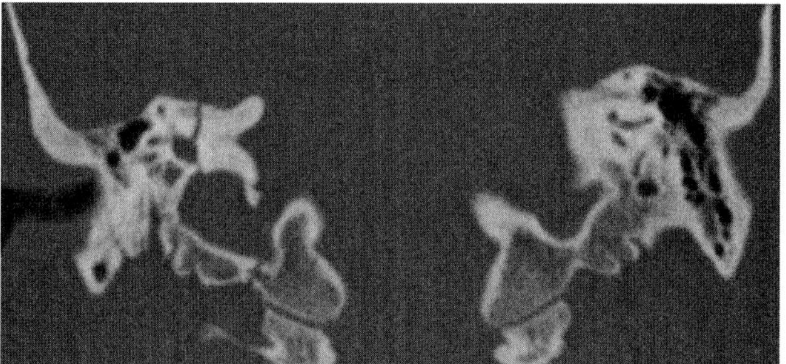

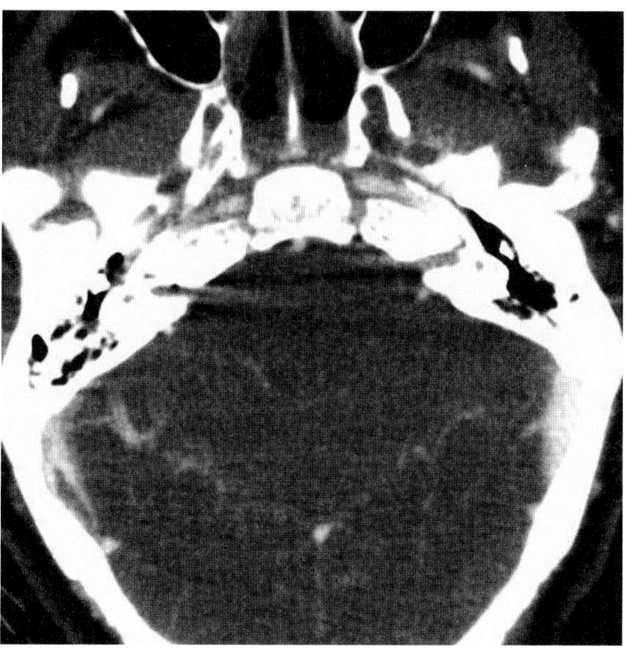

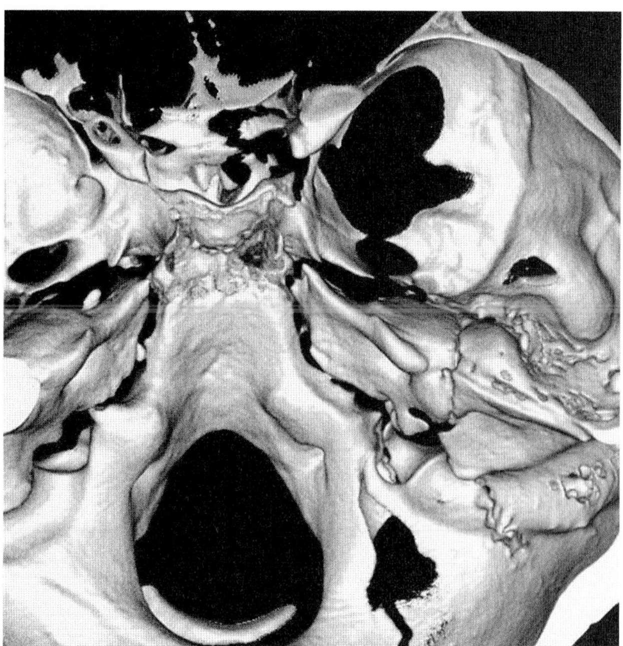

1. What is the diagnosis?
2. What structures are typically involved in this injury pattern?
3. Name three computed tomography (CT) findings often seen on cranial CT (non–thin section) that may indicate injury to this region.
4. What complication of this injury is shown on the contrast-enhanced image?

CASE 161

Transverse Temporal Bone Fracture

1. Transverse temporal bone fracture crossing vestibule.
2. The otic capsule, the vestibular system, and the facial nerve.
3. Mastoid sinus opacification, air in the temporomandibular joint, and pneumocephalus adjacent to petrousmastoid temporal bone.
4. Injury to adjacent transverse dural sinus with thrombus.

Reference

Smirniotopoulos JG, Mirvis SE, Lefkowitz DM: Imaging of craniocerebral trauma, In Mirvis SE, Shanmuganathan K, eds: *Imaging in Trauma and Critical Care*, 2nd ed, Philadelphia, WB Saunders, 2003, pp 133–183.

Cross-Reference

Emergency Radiology: THE REQUISITES, pp 37, 41–43.

Comment

Fractures of the petrous portion of the temporal bone have the potential to injure cranial nerves, ossicular chain, otic capsule, and vestibular system. Fracture planes through the temporal petrous bone can also injure the adjacent dural sinus and carotid/jugular foramina. Computed tomography (CT) is the study of choice to define temporal bone injuries. Imaging should be obtained using overlapping 1-mm images or smaller and reviewed in axial and coronal planes at least. A force applied laterally to the temporoparietal region usually produces a longitudinally oriented fracture paralleling the petrous ridge. An impact to the occipital area may induce a transversely oriented fracture by continuing anterolaterally across the temporal petrous bone. Many fractures, however, are combinations of fracture planes without a distinct pattern.

Longitudinal fractures are most common, have a high incidence of oto- and rhinorrhea, and typically lead to disruption of the otic chain and immediate conductive hearing loss. Fluid accumulated in the middle ear also contributes to conductive loss. Facial nerve injury occurs in 10% to 20% of cases and is often delayed in clinical onset and incomplete. The transversely oriented fracture is complicated by extension into the inner ear, with the potential to cause sensorineural hearing loss by disruption of the cochlea and its innervation, vestibular dysfunction, and facial nerve paralysis in 40% to 50% of cases. Some fractures, particularly non- or minimally displaced ones, may be impossible to detect even with high-resolution targeted temporal bone CT. Clues to the presence of subtle fractures include fluid in the mastoid air cells, air in the temporomandibular fossa, and pneumocephalus adjacent to the temporal bone.

Notes

CASE 162

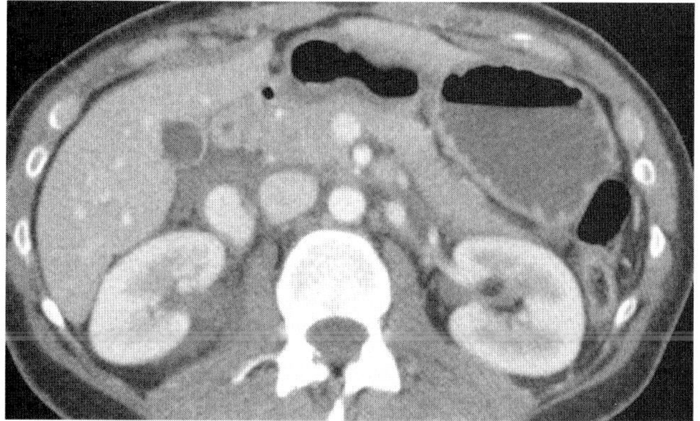

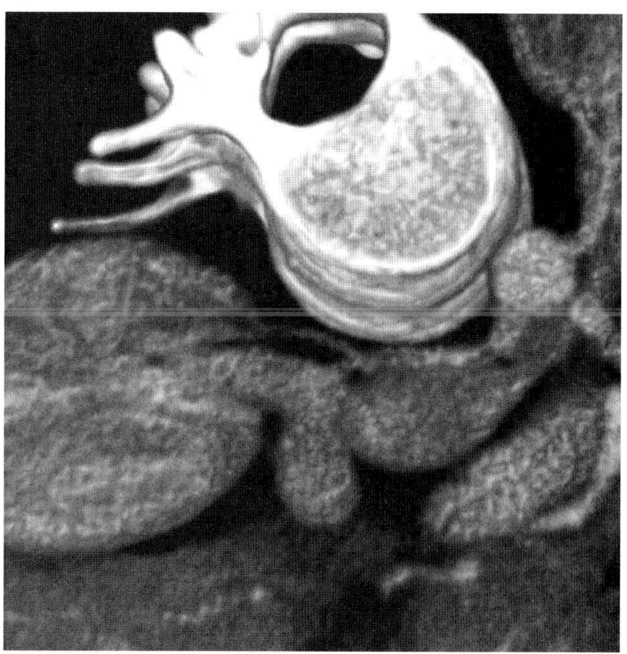

See also Color Plate

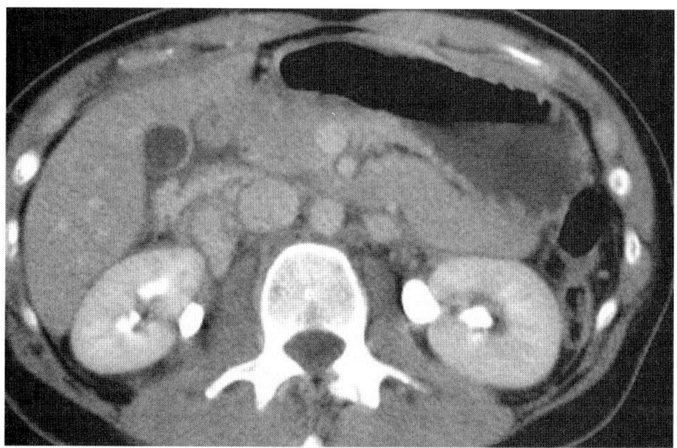

You are shown images of a blunt trauma patient.

1. What is the diagnosis?
2. What are two possible mechanisms of injury in blunt trauma?
3. Does this patient need invasive treatment?
4. Is there computed tomography evidence of urine extravasation?

CASE 162

Bleeding Renal Venous Pseudoaneurysm

1. Bleeding renal venous pseudoaneurysm.
2. Anteroposterior compression and lateral stretching of the renal vein, or direct impact of vein against the spine by compression.
3. Yes. There is active bleeding so angiography or surgery is required.
4. No. Delayed imaging (pyelogram phase) shows an intact collecting system.

References

Kawashima A, Sandler CM, Corl FM, et al: Imaging of renal trauma: a comprehensive review, *Radiographics* 21:557–574, 2001.

Mejia JC, Myers JG, Stewart RM, et al: A right renal vein pseudoaneurysm secondary to blunt abdominal trauma: a case report and review of the literature, *J Trauma* 60:1124–1128, 2006.

Comment

Renal trauma occurs in 8% to 10% of cases of abdominal trauma and, of these, the incidence of renal vascular injury is from 6% to 14%. The incidence of major renal vascular injury is less than 3%. Renal vascular injury may result from blunt or penetrating trauma. Among reported cases, 70% involve renal arteries, 20% renal veins, and 10% both vessels. There are two accepted mechanisms of renal vascular injury in blunt trauma. The acute deceleration of the kidney in a posterior to anterior direction, relative to the fixed position of the aorta, leads to stretching of the vessels. The second mechanism relates to renal vessel compression against the vertebral bodies also causing intimal damage to the endothelium. Because of anatomic configuration and characteristics of the renal vessels, the left renal artery is more commonly injured.

Pseudoaneurysms are disruptions of the vessel walls and comprise blood-containing adventitial sacs and surrounding soft tissues. Pseudoaneurysms of the venous systems, rarely secondary to blunt trauma, can potentially expand and progress to a complete rupture, or decrease in size and eventually calcify.

Computed tomography (CT) is the diagnostic test of choice in the bluntly injured patient with hematuria and has a diagnostic accuracy of as high as 98%. CT can usually characterize renal venous injuries including thrombosis, arteriovenous fistula, pseudoaneurysm, and/or active bleeding. Extravasation of vascular contrast appears on the arterial phase CT with attenuation values of 80 to 370 Hounsfield units (HU), typically within 10 to 15 HU of the aorta or adjacent major artery, and is generally surrounded by lower-attenuation clotted blood. This finding is an important indicator that a patient may be about to pass from hemodynamic stability to decompensation. Delayed scanning is to assess for bleeding with contrast moving away from the injury site and decreasing in attenuation. For more precise evaluation of the renal vascular system, angiography must be employed. Angiography facilitates the use of therapeutic interventions such as stenting and embolization. Depending on the overall clinical picture, surgical exploration may be indicated.

Notes

CASE 163

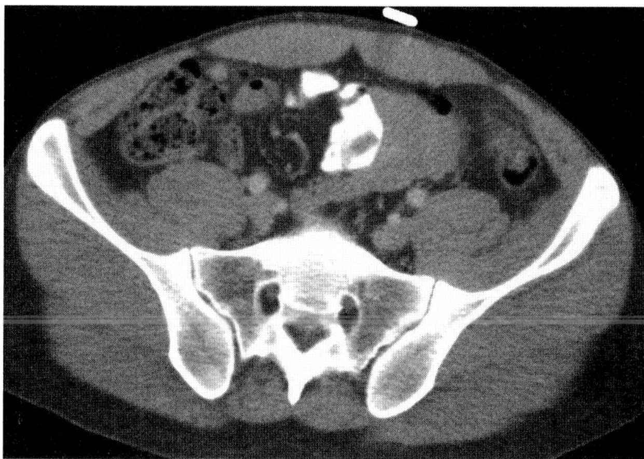

1. What are the findings on this computed tomography (CT) image of a 44-year-old male patient with acute onset of left-sided abdominal pain but no fever or leukocytosis?
2. True or false: The condition shown is most common in teenagers.
3. Name three CT features that can distinguish this entity from segmental omental infarction.
4. True or false: The vast majority of patients with this condition will ultimately require surgery.

CASE 163

Epiploic Appendagitis

1. There is an ovoid fat and soft tissue density along the medial aspect of the proximal sigmoid colon with a hyperdense peripheral ring. There is mild thickening of the adjacent sigmoid wall.
2. False. Epiploic appendagitis is most frequently seen in the fourth to fifth decade of life and is rarely seen in children.
3. Epiploic appendagitis often has a smaller size, has an enhancing peripheral ring, and is typically seen adjacent to the left colon.
4. False. Epiploic appendagitis is a self-limited condition. Symptoms typically resolve within 2 weeks without treatment.

Reference

Singh AK, Gervais DA, Hahn PF, et al: Acute epiploic appendagitis and its mimics, *Radiographics* 25: 1521–1534, 2005.

Cross-Reference

Emergency Radiology: THE REQUISITES, p 284.

Comment

Epiploic appendages are small fatty peritoneal outpouchings along the serosal surface of the colon, extending from the cecum to the distal sigmoid. They are usually 1 to 2 cm in width and are attached to the colon by a vascular stalk. Unless inflamed, they are not seen on computed tomography (CT).

Epiploic appendagitis (EA) occurs when an epiploic appendage becomes inflamed and infarcts, usually due to torsion and ischemia or from spontaneous venous thrombosis. Patients present with acute abdominal pain, often left sided. Nausea, fever, and leukocytosis are uncommon. EA is most frequently seen in the fourth to fifth decade of life and is rarely seen in children. Predisposing factors include obesity and unaccustomed exercise. Symptoms can mimic those of acute appendicitis, diverticulitis, or subacute omental infarction (SOI). Abdominal-pelvic CT is often used to differentiate between these different entities.

The typical appearance of EA on CT is an ovoid fatty lesion with a hyperdense peripheral ring located adjacent to the serosal surface of the colon. There may also be a small hyperdense central focus, thought to be a thrombosed vessel. Mild surrounding fat stranding is common. Subtle thickening of the nearby parietal peritoneum or colonic wall may be seen. EA can occur anywhere along the colon but is most often seen adjacent to the sigmoid colon.

EA can have a CT appearance similar to SOI. Distinguishing features of EA include a smaller size, a typical left-sided location, and presence of an enhancing peripheral ring.

Symptoms generally resolve in most patients within 2 weeks without treatment. CT findings may take up to 6 months to fully resolve.

Notes

CASE 164

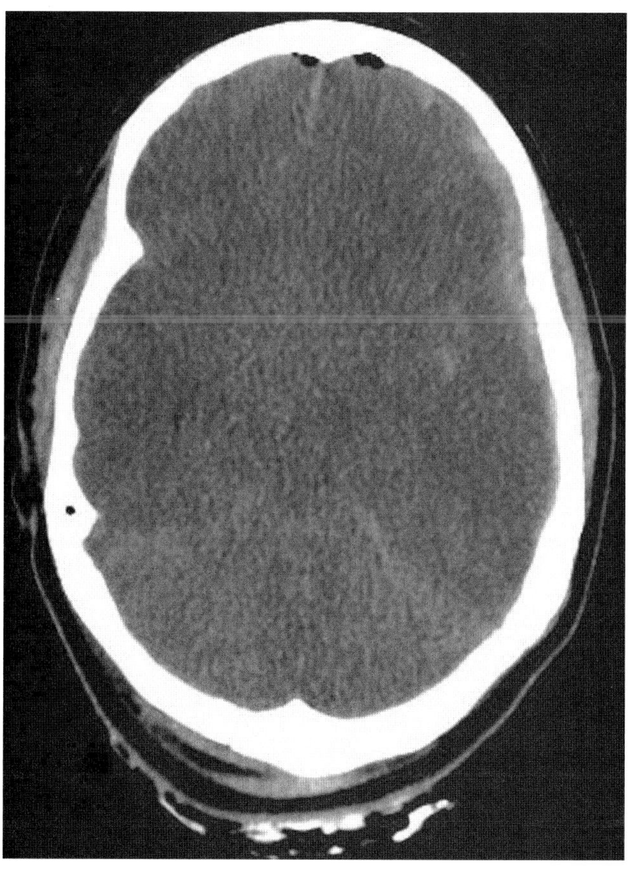

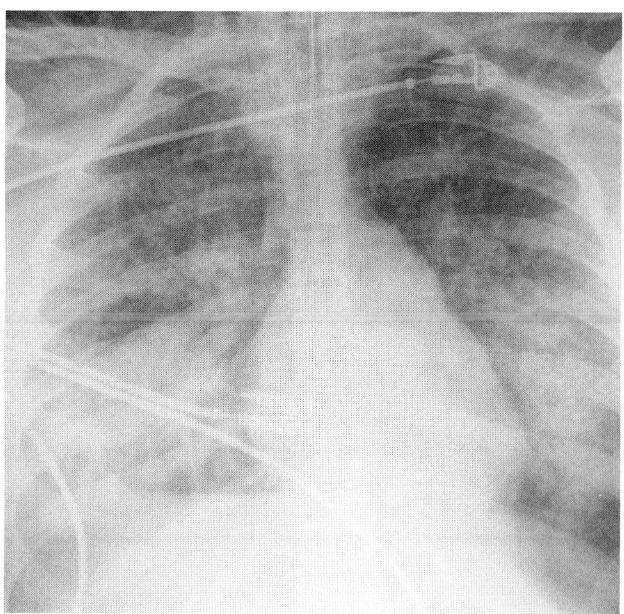

1. What is the best diagnosis for the chest radiograph findings in this patient with severe head trauma?
2. Name three etiologies of this condition.
3. What is the most common chest radiograph finding in a patient seen with this condition?
4. True or false: Respiratory signs and symptoms associated with this process are usually seen within 4 hours of the inciting neurologic event.

CASE 164

Neurogenic Pulmonary Edema

1. Neurogenic pulmonary edema (NPE). The chest radiograph demonstrates pulmonary edema and the computed tomographic image of the head shows severe cerebral edema.
2. NPE can result from trauma, tumor, infection, status epilepticus, stroke, and following neurosurgical procedures.
3. Bilateral diffuse infiltrates, with an upper lobe predilection.
4. True.

References

Bahloul M, Chaari AN, Kallel H, et al: Neurogenic pulmonary edema due to traumatic brain injury: evidence of cardiac dysfunction, *Am J Crit Care* 15: 462–470, 2006.

Fontes RB, Aguiar PH, Zanetti MV, et al: Acute neurogenic pulmonary edema: case reports and literature review, *J Neurosurg Anesthesiol* 15:144–150, 2003.

Gluecker T, Capasso P, Schnyder P, et al: Clinical and radiologic features of pulmonary edema, *Radiographics* 19:1507–1531, 1999.

Cross-Reference

Emergency Radiology: THE REQUISITES, pp 235–236.

Comment

Neurogenic pulmonary edema (NPE) can result from a host of central nervous system insults including trauma, tumor, infection, status epilepticus, stroke, and neurosurgical procedures. The pathogenesis is poorly understood. Elevated intracranial pressure is thought to trigger an abrupt centrally mediated discharge of catecholamines, which causes a shift of blood from the periphery of the pulmonary circulation and alteration in capillary permeability. Capillary permeability may also be altered by stimulation of sympathetic nerve fibers in the pulmonary vasculature, resulting in changes in the size and number of the endothelial pores, leading to pulmonary edema. Although traditionally thought to be a form of noncardiogenic pulmonary edema, Bahloul and colleagues recently described myocardial dysfunction in their series of seven patients with NPE due to subarachnoid hemorrhage.

NPE is often underdiagnosed. Symptoms such as dyspnea, tachypnea, tachycardia, and hypoxemia are similar to those seen in simple fluid overload or aspiration pneumonia. A recent review of 21 cases by Fontes and colleagues (2003) showed that the mean age of patients with NPE was 31.6 years, subarachnoid hemorrhage was the most common head injury (42.9%), and the onset of symptoms occurred less than 4 hours after the neurologic event in most patients.

The most common finding on chest radiograph is bilateral diffuse infiltrates, often with an upper lobe predilection. Radiographic findings usually clear within 48 hours.

Notes

CASE 165

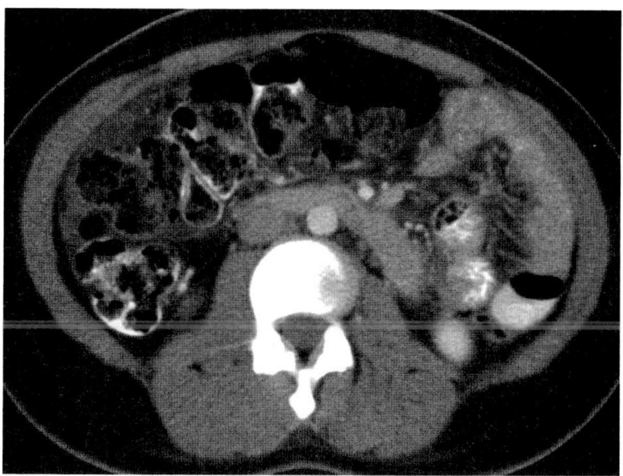

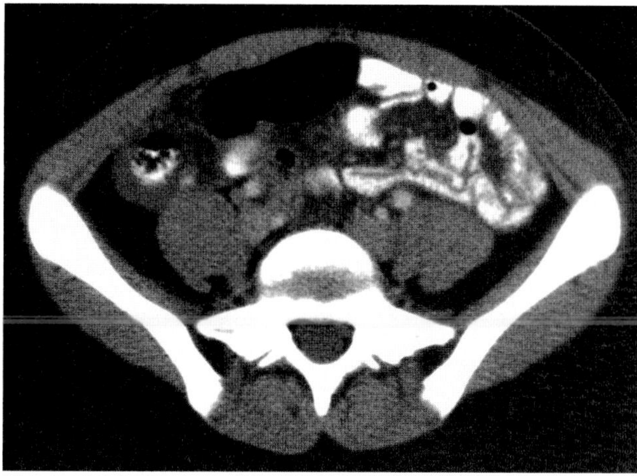

1. What is the most likely diagnosis in this patient with acute onset of right lower quadrant pain?
2. Name three computed tomography findings that can help distinguish this abnormality from epiploic appendagitis.
3. Name two factors that predispose a patient to the development of this condition.
4. True or false: Segmental omental infarction is a surgical emergency.

CASE 165

Segmental Omental Infarction

1. Segmental omental infarction (SOI).
2. Location: SOI is almost always right sided; epiploic appendagitis (EA) is typically left sided. Size of abnormality on CT: SOI is often greater than 5 cm, whereas EA is typically 1.5 to 3.5 cm in diameter. Enhancement pattern: EA often demonstrates ring enhancement; SOI does not.
3. Obesity and unaccustomed exercise.
4. False. SOI is self-limiting and resolves without treatment.

References

Abadir JS, Cohen AJ, Wilson SE: Accurate diagnosis of infarction of omentum and appendices epiploicae by computed tomography, *Am J Surg* 70:854–857, 2004.

Pickhardt PJ, Bhalla S: Unusual neoplastic peritoneal and subperitoneal conditions: CT findings, *Radiographics* 25:719–730, 2005.

Cross-Reference

Emergency Radiology: THE REQUISITES, pp 284–285.

Comment

SOI is caused by thrombosis of omental vessels with resultant infarction of a small section of omentum. The etiology is unknown but is likely related to anomalous arterial supply, adhesions, or torsion. Previously thought to be a rare entity, SOI is being diagnosed with increased frequency, likely due to the increased use of computed tomography (CT) for evaluation of patients with acute abdominal pain.

In addition to right-sided abdominal pain, patients with SOI may present with peritoneal findings, fever, or mild leukocytosis. Obesity and unaccustomed exercise are predisposing factors.

CT is useful to differentiate between SOI and conditions such as cholecystitis, right-sided diverticulitis, and appendicitis. Typical CT findings of SOI include a heterogeneous omental fatty mass greater than 5 cm in diameter anterior to the transverse colon or anteromedial to the ascending colon. There may be fat stranding around the mass, thickening of the parietal peritoneum, or mild bowel wall thickening. Less severe cases may show only focal fat infiltration.

Epiploic appendagitis (EA) is often included in the differential diagnosis of SOI. Several features distinguish EA from SOI: size, location, age of patient, and presence of ring enhancement. EA is usually less than 3.5 cm in diameter and is located adjacent to the anterior sigmoid colon wall. EA is rarely seen in patients less than 19 years of age, while approximately 15% of cases of SOI occur in children. EA also typically appears as an ovoid fatty lesion with a rim of enhancement, a feature not seen in SOI.

SOI is a self-limiting condition that uniformly resolves without surgery or antibiotics. Distinguishing SOI from other surgical causes of acute right-sided abdominal pain is important in order to avoid unnecessary laparotomy.

Notes

CASE 166

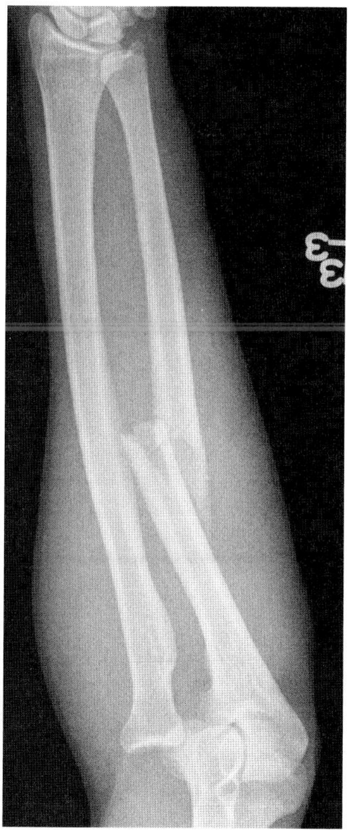

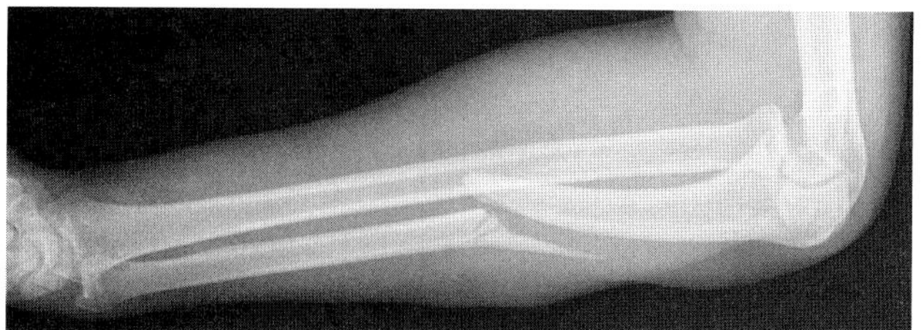

1. By what eponym is this injury known?
2. What is the significance of the radiocapitellar line?
3. The Bado classification divides these fractures into four different fracture types based on what two variables?
4. What is the mechanism of injury?

CASE 166

Monteggia Fracture-Dislocation

1. Monteggia fracture-dislocation.
2. A line drawn through the proximal radial shaft and radial head should bisect the capitellum. Absence of this normal relationship may indicate a radial head dislocation.
3. The Bado classification divides these fractures into types I through IV, based on the location of the ulnar fracture and the direction of the radial head dislocation.
4. The fracture typically occurs when the forearm is in forced pronation during a fall or as the result of a direct blow to the ulna.

References

Perron AD, Hersh RE, Brady WJ, et al: Orthopedic pitfalls in the ED: Galeazzi and Monteggia fracture-dislocation, *Am J Emerg Med* 19:225–228, 2001.

Ring D, Jupiter JB, Simpson NS: Monteggia fractures in adults, *J Bone Joint Surg Am* 80:1733–1744, 1998.

Cross-Reference

Emergency Radiology: THE REQUISITES, pp 124–126.

Comment

The Monteggia fracture-dislocation consists of a fracture of the proximal one third of the ulna with an anterior dislocation of the radial head. The fracture often occurs when the forearm is in forced pronation during a fall or as the result of a direct blow to the ulna. Patients typically have significant pain and swelling at the elbow with extremely limited range of motion. A branch of the radial nerve may be injured by the radial head dislocation, which can result in weakness of extension of the digits. Whenever an ulnar fracture is seen routine radiographs of the elbow should be obtained to evaluate for radial head dislocation. The radiocapitellar line is a line drawn through the proximal radial shaft and radial head. On an elbow radiograph, this line should normally bisect the capitellum. Evaluation of this relationship can be useful in detection of subtle radial head dislocations.

Monteggia fracture-dislocations are frequently classified using the Bado system, which divides these fractures into four different types depending on the location of the ulnar fracture and the direction of the radial head dislocation. Type I is a fracture of the proximal one third of the ulna with anterior dislocation of the radial head. Type I is the most common, accounting for approximately 60% of cases. Type II also involves a fracture of the proximal one third of the ulna, but with a posterior radial head dislocation. Type III is a fracture of the ulna just distal to the coronoid process with a lateral dislocation of the radial head. Type IV is the most complex and involves a fracture of the upper or middle one third of the ulna with anterior dislocation of the radial head. Fractures of the upper one third of the radius are also seen. The treatment of Monteggia fracture-dislocations in adults requires surgical open reduction and internal fixation.

Notes

CASE 167

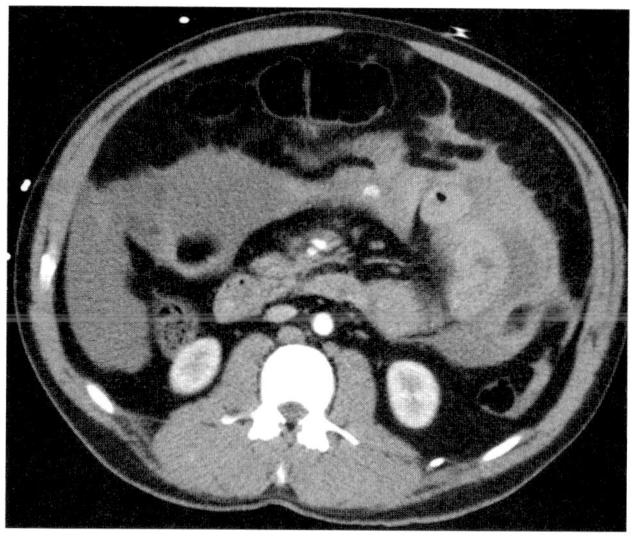

Initial

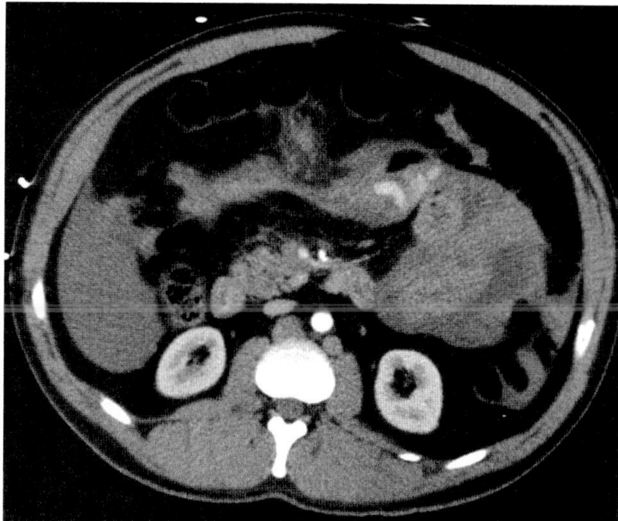

Delays

You are shown images of a blunt trauma patient.

1. What is the diagnosis?
2. How often are peritoneal signs elicited in patients with mesenteric injury?
3. What are the most specific computed tomography signs of a mesenteric injury requiring surgical intervention?
4. What are potential complications of this injury?

CASE 167

Mesenteric Hematoma with Active Bleeding

1. Mesenteric hematoma with active bleeding.
2. Peritoneal signs are absent in one third of patients with mesenteric injury.
3. Active bleeding within the mesentery and bowel wall thickening.
4. Ongoing blood loss; bowel ischemia with necrosis, rupture, or bowel stricture formation; peritonitis; and sepsis.

Reference

Ngheim HV, Jeffrey RB Jr, Mindelzun RE: CT of blunt trauma to the bowel and mesentery, *AJR Am J Roentgenol* 160:53–58, 1993.

Cross-Reference

Emergency Radiology: THE REQUISITES, pp 93–98.

Comment

Bowel and/or mesenteric injuries are seen in 5% of blunt abdominal trauma patients. Early and accurate diagnosis of mesenteric injuries prevents ongoing blood loss and complications such as bowel ischemia with necrosis, rupture, or bowel stricture formation, peritonitis, and sepsis. A delay in the diagnosis of a bowel or mesenteric injury of only 8 hours is associated with increased morbidity and mortality.

The physical exam is often limited in a patient with a mesenteric injury. Peritoneal signs are absent in one third of these patients. Diagnostic peritoneal lavage can be used but is invasive, is nonspecific to the site of injury, and is unable to detect a retroperitoneal bowel injury. Abdominopelvic computed tomography (CT) with intravenous and oral contrast has 54% to 75% accuracy in determining the need for surgical intervention for mesenteric injuries. The most specific CT sign of a mesenteric injury requiring surgery is active mesenteric bleeding with bowel wall thickening. Blood surrounding the site of active bleeding will typically dissect in between the leaves and folds of the mesenteric fat, forming "mesenteric triangles" of blood. Isolated mesenteric hematoma and mesenteric infiltration indicating contusion are CT findings that do not typically require urgent surgery.

The ideal management of mesenteric injuries not requiring urgent surgery is not known. Typically, patients will be admitted to the hospital and serial abdominal physical exams will be performed. An abdominopelvic CT is often repeated in 4 to 6 hours to evaluate for progression of the mesenteric injury.

Notes

CASE 168

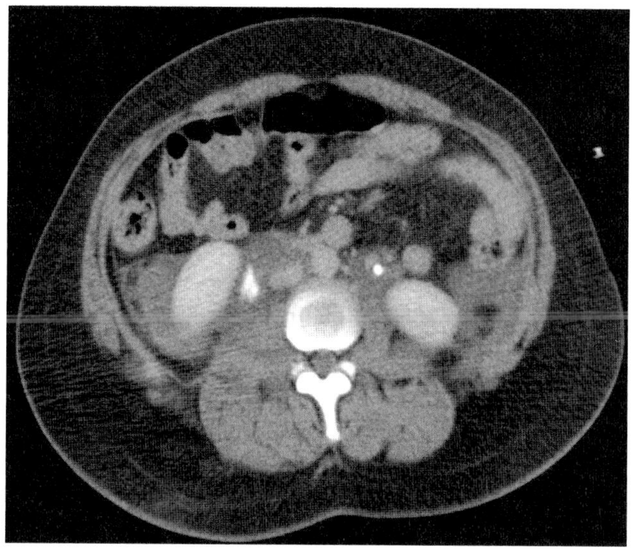

Initial

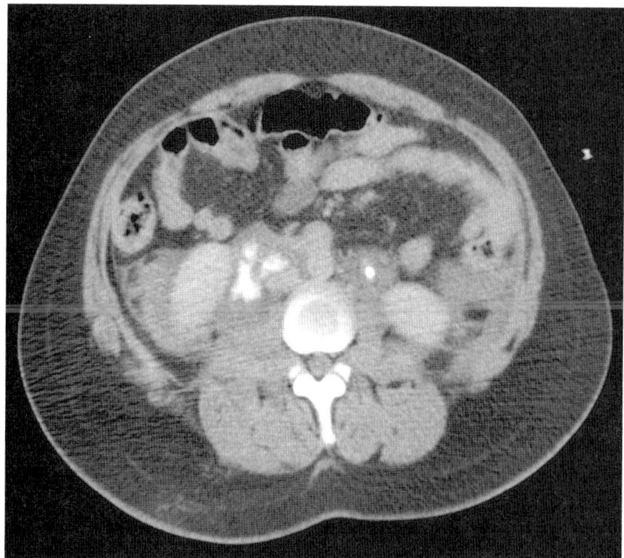

Delays

You are shown images of a trauma patient.

1. What are the findings on the initial and delayed images of this trauma patient with flank trauma and hematuria?
2. What is the diagnosis?
3. Name three imaging modalities other than computed tomography that could be used to make this diagnosis.
4. Name three ways in which these injuries may be treated.

CASE 168

Right Ureteral Injury with Extravasation of Intravenous Contrast

1. Foci of high density along the proximal ureter on the initial image, which increases in size on the delayed image. There is also right perinephric and left periureteral hemorrhage and blood within the left paracolic gutter.
2. Proximal right ureteral tear.
3. Retrograde or antegrade pyelography, scintigraphy, and intravenous pyelography.
4. Placement of nephroureteral catheter across the site of injury, percutaneous nephrostomy tube placement with or without ureteral stent placement, and, in cases of complete ureteral transection, surgical repair.

Reference

Tilton RL, Gervais DA, Hahn PF, et al: Urine leaks and urinomas: diagnosis and imaging-guided interventions, *Radiographics* 23:1133–1147, 2003.

Cross-Reference

Emergency Radiology: THE REQUISITES, p 102.

Comment

Blunt ureteral injury is uncommon, due to the relatively protected status of the ureter in the retroperitoneum. The most common site of blunt ureteral injury is the ureteropelvic junction, likely due to either hyperextension and stretching of the ureter or compression of the ureter against the spine.

Penetrating injury, such as a stab wound to the flank, accounts for 84% of all ureteral injuries. In the nontraumatic setting, iatrogenic injury after gynecological surgery or endourologic procedures may also cause ureteral injury.

Optimal evaluation with computed tomography (CT) includes unenhanced, corticomedullary, and delayed (5 to 15 minutes after injection of intravenous contrast) phases of imaging. Additional delayed images may be necessary if initial images fail to reveal an injury but there is a high suspicion for one. CT findings demonstrated in the excretory and delayed images include collection of high-density intravenous contrast material in the inferomedial perinephric space or along the expected course of the ureter. Abnormal high density seen in the region of the kidney or ureter during the corticomedullary phase, before contrast has reached the collecting system, cannot represent ureteral injury. More subtle signs of ureteral injury include periureteral fluid, ureteral wall thickening, and a wound tract near the ureter in the setting of penetrating injury. Visualization of contrast material within the ureter distal to the site of injury indicates a partial rather than complete ureteral tear.

Notes

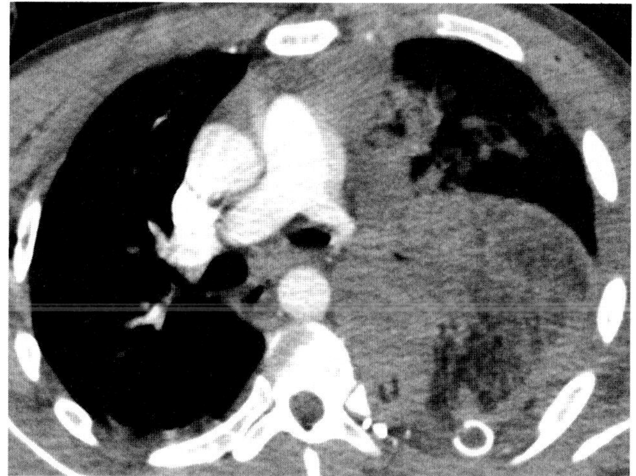

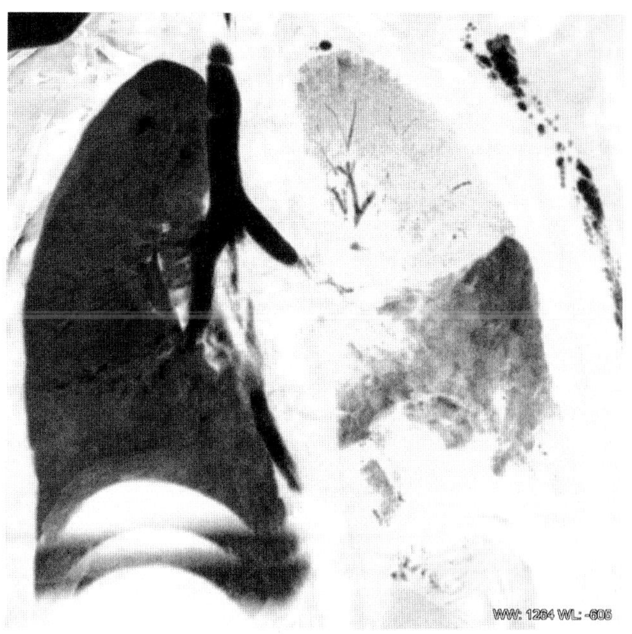

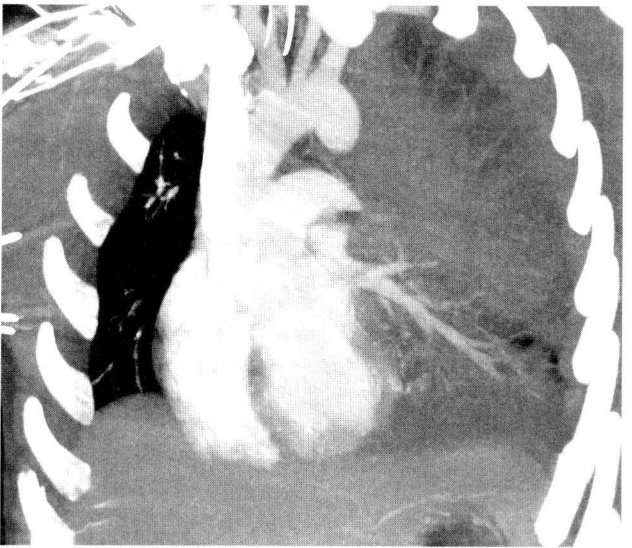

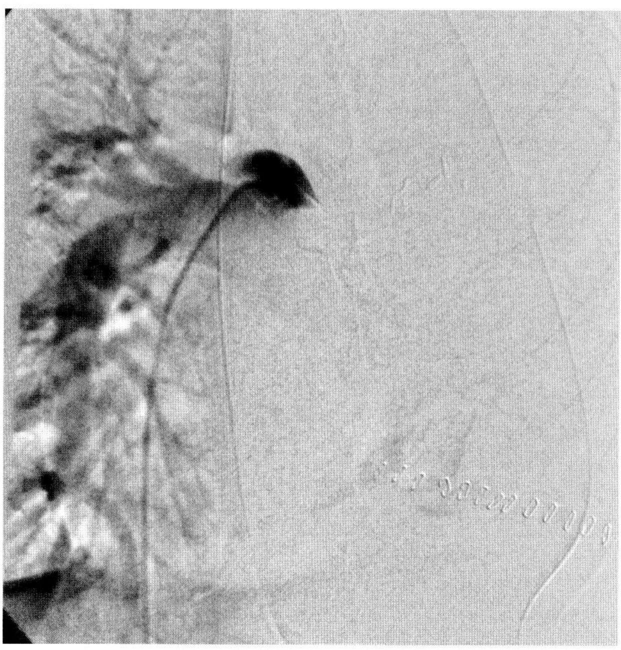

You are shown images of a 24-year-old man with respiratory distress following left thoracotomy for a stab wound to the left chest.

1. What are the imaging findings?
2. What is the best diagnosis?
3. What are the predisposing factors for this entity?
4. What are the common anatomical sites for this lesion?

CASE 169

Torsion of the Left Upper Lobe

1. Consolidation in the left upper lobe, normal venous return from the left lower lobe, abrupt termination of the left pulmonary artery and main bronchus.
2. Torsion of the left upper lobe.
3. Lobectomy, lobar atelectasis or consolidation, pneumothorax, pleural effusion, and transection of the pulmonary ligament.
4. Right middle lobe followed by the left upper lobe.

Reference

Banki F, Velmahos G: Partial pulmonary torsion after thoracotomy without pulmonary resection, *J Trauma Injury Infect Crit Care* 59:476–479, 2005.

Kim EA, Lee KS, Shim YM, et al: Radiographic and CT findings in complications following pulmonary resection, *Radiographics* 22:67–86, 2002.

Comments

Lung torsion is an uncommon entity, with fewer than 60 reported cases. The etiology is poorly understood. It is speculated that the twisting around the pedicle occurs during the expansion of the remaining normal lung to occupy the entire thoracic cavity. It is more common for the entire lung to undergo torsion than just a lobe. When there is isolated lobar torsion, the middle lobe is likely to be involved due to its small size and relative mobility compared to the other lobes. The degree of torsion may vary between 90 degrees and 1080 degrees. The term *complete torsion* is used when the twisting is greater than 180 degrees.

Immediately following torsion, the clinical symptoms are unimpressive, but rapid progressive clinical effects from the obstruction of the respective bronchus, pulmonary artery, and pulmonary vein may develop. Obstruction of the venous circulation is the earliest event and leads to alveolar congestion, exudation, and finally hemorrhagic infarction. Predisposing factors include lobectomy, pneumothorax, lobar atelectasis or consolidation, long lobar pedicle, transaction of the pulmonary ligament, and complete interlobar fissure.

Chest radiographs may demonstrate complete consolidation without any volume loss of the involved lobe or lung. CT may also demonstrate the site of torsion, which is typically seen as abrupt tapering and obliteration of the proximal pulmonary artery and accompanying bronchus. Other findings include increased soft tissue attenuation at the hilum, poorly enhancing consolidation of the torsed lobe, ground glass opacity, interlobular septal thickening, and either normal or increased pulmonary volume. Pulmonary arteriography is the reference standard study and typically demonstrates occlusion of the affected pulmonary artery or lobar arterial branch. The typical findings on bronchoscopy are smooth bronchial obstruction without any obvious mucosal abnormalities.

Awareness of this entity is important because early diagnosis and expeditious treatment help to limit the significant risk of morbidity and mortality. It takes up to 24 hours for severe pulmonary hemorrhage and necrosis to occur. Expeditious use of CT may promote early confirmatory diagnosis. In the majority of cases, complete resection of the involved lobe or lung is required.

Notes

CASE 170

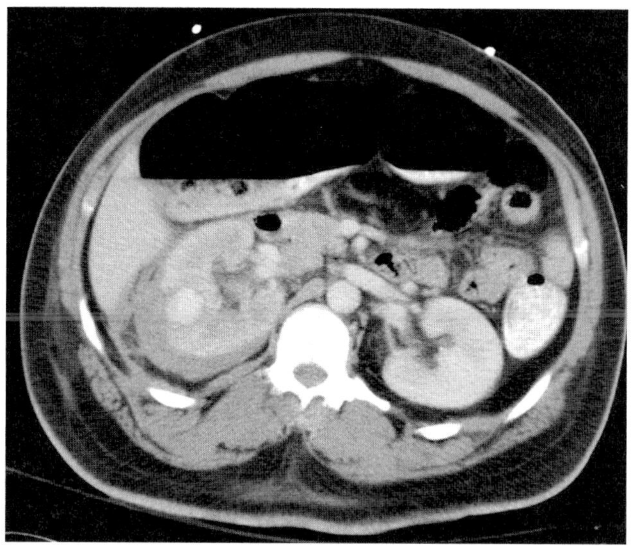

Initial

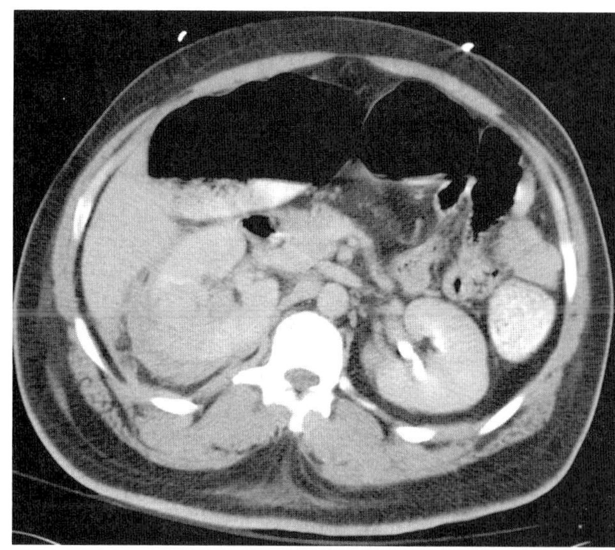

Delays

You are shown images of a blunt trauma patient.

1. What are the findings?
2. Why does this lesion form?
3. What is the significance of this lesion?
4. True or false: All patients with a renal pseudoaneurysm will have hematuria.

CASE 170

Renal Pseudoaneurysm

1. On the initial corticomedullary phase images, there is a round focus of high density that decreases in attenuation on the excretory phase images. These findings are consistent with a traumatic renal pseudoaneurysm. There is also a small amount of right perinephric hematoma and a right lateral renal laceration.
2. A pseudoaneurysm is formed when a small amount of blood escapes from an injured vessel but is contained by the adventitia or surrounding tissues.
3. Untreated pseudoaneurysms have a significant risk of rupture and therefore require urgent treatment.
4. False. Hematuria may or may not be present. Many patients have no symptoms or signs associated with a renal pseudoaneurysm.

References

Miller LA, Shanmuganathan K: Multidetector CT evaluation of abdominal trauma, *Radiol Clin North Am* 43:1079–1095, 2005.

Cross-Reference

Emergency Radiology: THE REQUISITES, p 343.

Comment

Renal trauma is seen in 10% of blunt abdominal trauma patients. Patients with a renal injury may be asymptomatic, have flank pain or tenderness, or have hematuria, either microscopic or gross. Intravenous contrast-enhanced computed tomography (CT) is the test of choice in the evaluation of renal trauma.

Vascular injuries of the kidney, such as pseudoaneurysms and active bleeding, are considered major renal injuries. It is important to distinguish renal pseudoaneurysm, active bleeding, and collecting system injury on CT. A collecting system injury will not be detected on the initial corticomedullary images. This injury can only be seen on the delayed, renal excretory phase images. Additional 5 to 15 minute delayed images can be useful if there are suspicious findings on the initial images. Active bleeding and pseudoaneurysms are both seen on the initial, corticomedullary images. A pseudoaneurysm will appear as a high-density, well-circumscribed round lesion on initial images and will wash out, or become less dense, on delayed images. Active bleeding is seen as an irregular or linear focus of high-density intravenous contrast extravasation. On excretory phase images, the focus remains high in density and will increase in size as contrast-enhanced blood continues to extravasate from the injured vessel.

Renal pseudoaneurysms may rupture and cause hemodynamically significant hemorrhage. They are typically treated with urgent renal angiography with endovascular embolization and occlusion of the affected branch vessel.

Notes

CASE 171

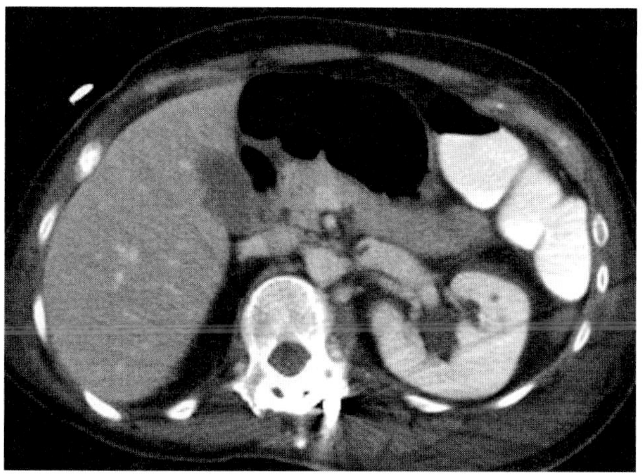

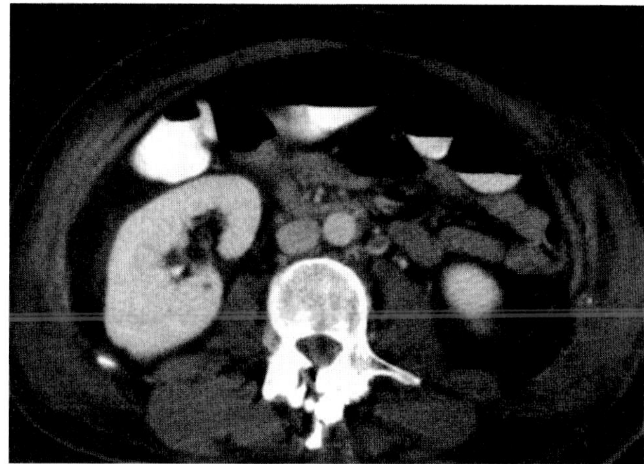

1. What is the finding on this contrast-enhanced computed tomography of the abdomen in this patient with a fever postoperative day 2 after a hysterectomy?
2. What is Virchow's triad?
3. In what patient population is this condition most commonly seen?
4. What are two other imaging modalities that can be used to diagnose this condition?

CASE 171

Left Ovarian Vein Thrombosis with Extension into the Left Renal Vein

1. There is a filling defect consistent with thrombus within the left ovarian vein with extension into the left renal vein.
2. Venous stasis, hypercoagulability, and vessel wall injury, the three classic factors that predispose to venous thrombosis.
3. The postpartum patient. Gonadal vein thrombosis complicates 0.2% of all deliveries.
4. Ultrasound and magnetic resonance imaging.

References

Kominiarek MA, Hibbard JU: Postpartum ovarian vein thrombosis: an update, *Obstet Gynecol Surv* 61: 337–342, 2006.

Twickler DM, Setiawan AT, Evans RS: Imaging of puerperal septic thrombophlebitis: prospective comparison of MR imaging, CT and sonography, *AJR Am J Roentgenol* 169:1039–1043, 1997.

Cross-Reference

Emergency Radiology: THE REQUISITES, pp 317–318.

Comment

Septic ovarian vein thrombosis is an uncommon condition associated with childbirth, pelvic inflammatory disease, malignancy, or gynecologic surgery. All of these conditions predispose the patient to venous thrombosis. Gonadal vein thrombosis is rarely seen in males and is usually associated with hypercoagulable states.

Symptoms of gonadal vein thrombosis include fever unresponsive to antibiotics, abdominal pain and tenderness, and a lower abdominal mass representing the thrombosed vein. Nausea, vomiting, malaise, and tachycardia may be present. The condition can be difficult to differentiate on physical examination from more common conditions such as appendicitis, pyelonephritis, tubo-ovarian abscess, or adnexal torsion.

On sonography, the thrombosed gonadal vein appears as an anechoic to hypoechoic mass extending between the adnexa and IVC with absence of normal blood flow. Ultrasound is often limited due to overlying bowel gas. Computed tomography (CT) or magnetic resonance imaging (MRI) should follow a negative or equivocal ultrasound. On CT, a tubular mass between the adnexa and renal hilum is seen. Intravenous contrast administration is needed to see the low-density thrombus within the vessel lumen. On MRI, a gonadal vein thrombosis will appear as a tubular mass that is low signal on T1-weighted images and variable signal on T2-weighted images.

Treatment consists of antibiotics and anticoagulation. The mortality of this condition is less than 5% and is usually attributable to pulmonary embolus occurring after thrombus extension into the renal veins and inferior vena cava.

Notes

CASE 172

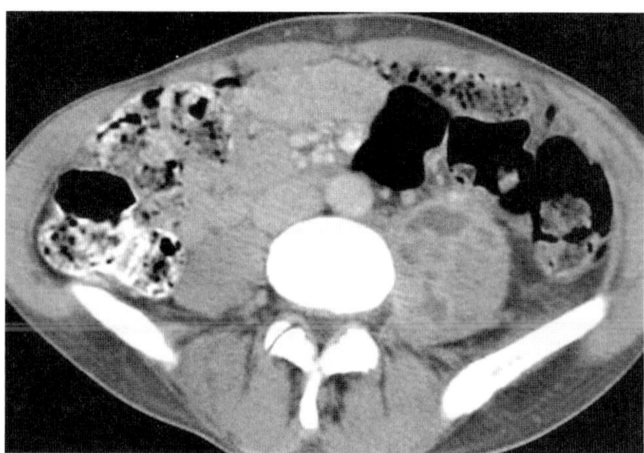

1. What are the findings?
2. What is the differential diagnosis?
3. What computed tomography characteristics can help differentiate between these different diagnoses?
4. What is a risk factor for this condition?

CASE 172

Left Psoas Abscess

1. The left psoas muscle is enlarged and contains a well-defined hypodensity demonstrating rim enhancement.
2. Abscess, tumor, or hemorrhage.
3. The appearance of tumor, infection, and hematoma can be very similar. Gas is more commonly seen in abscess. Acute hemorrhage will be hyperdense. Computed tomography-guided aspiration and drainage may be required for diagnosis.
4. Immunosuppression.

References

Multarak M, Peh WCG: CT of unusual iliopsoas compartment lesions, *Radiographics* 20(Suppl):S53–S66, 2000.

Garner JP, Meiring PD, Ravi K, et al: Psoas abscess—not as rare as we think? *Colorectal Dis* 9:269–274, 2007.

Comment

The iliopsoas muscle can be involved by infection, tumor, or hemorrhage. All of these conditions have a similar appearance on contrast-enhanced computed tomography (CT). CT-guided aspiration and drainage may be needed to make the diagnosis.

Primary abscesses of the iliopsoas muscle are rare, with a reported worldwide incidence of 12 cases per year. These are usually idiopathic and arise in immunocompromised patients. Secondary infection of the iliopsoas is much more common and is usually due to spread to the muscle from an adjacent bowel, kidney, or bone infection. Symptoms of an iliopsoas abscess include vague or chronic pain, fever, limp, general malaise, and weight loss. On CT an abscess will appear as a low attenuation fluid collection with rim enhancement. Gas may be seen in the abscess lumen.

Primary iliopsoas muscle tumors such as a leiomyosarcoma are rare. Secondary psoas involvement due to direct extension of a tumor within the peritoneum or retroperitoneum is more common.

Hemorrhage within the iliopsoas is usually seen in patients with a bleeding diathesis or who are on anticoagulant therapy. Acute hemorrhage on CT will be high density. A fluid-fluid level may be seen within the hematoma due to the hematocrit effect. A chronic hematoma shares many of the same imaging characteristics as tumor and infection.

Notes

CASE 173

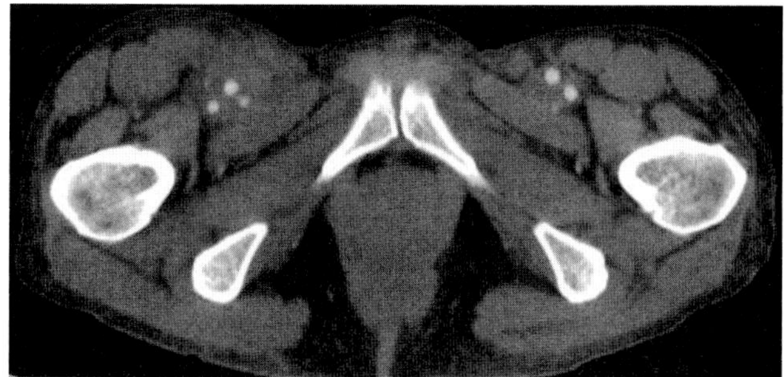

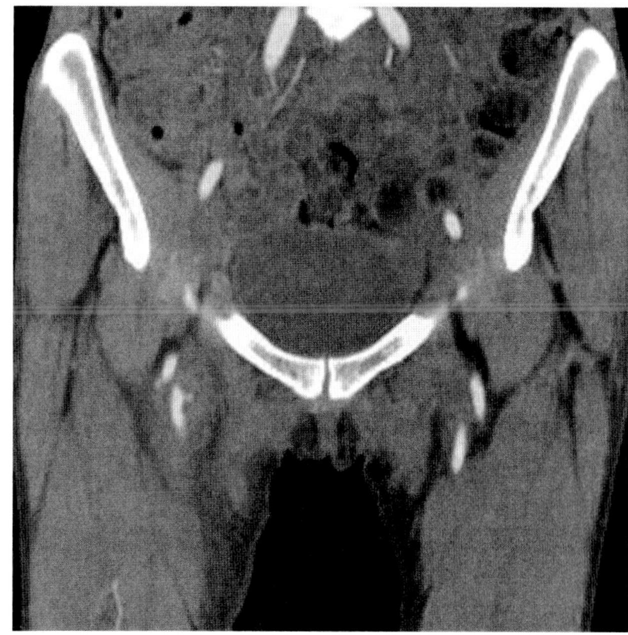

1. What is the finding on this contrast-enhanced computed tomography of a patient with a history of intravenous drug abuse and 3 weeks of right groin pain?
2. What is the diagnosis?
3. What other imaging modality could be used to diagnose this condition?
4. How is this condition treated?

CASE 173

Right Common Femoral Artery Pseudoaneurysm

1. Axial contrast-enhanced image of the lower pelvis shows soft tissue swelling in the right groin. There is a small round focus of hyperdensity medial to the common femoral vessels. Coronal reformatted images demonstrate a focal bulge in the medial wall of the right common femoral artery.
2. Right common femoral artery pseudoaneurysm.
3. Doppler ultrasound.
4. Surgically. Optimal surgical treatment is not known, but may include débridement with arterial ligation and excision of the pseudoaneurysm with revascularization.

References

Klonaris C, Katsargyris A, Papapetrou A, et al: Infected femoral artery pseudoaneurysm in drug addicts: the beneficial use of the internal iliac artery for arterial reconstruction, *J Vasc Surg* 45:498–504, 2007.

Ting AC, Cheng SW: Femoral artery pseudoaneurysms in drug addicts, *World J Surg* 21:783–786, 1997.

Cross-Reference

Emergency Radiology: THE REQUISITES, p 351.

Comments

Infected femoral artery pseudoaneurysms are the most common arterial complication seen in intravenous drug abuse. This can be a serious, potentially fatal condition. The untreated patient is at risk for pseudoaneurysm rupture and life-threatening hemorrhage or arterial compromise of the lower extremity. The condition arises due to inadvertent intra-arterial puncture with a needle. Focal extravasation of blood and contamination of the hematoma lead to local infection and pseudoaneurysm formation.

Patients will typically have a history of recent injection into the groin, groin pain and swelling, and fever. On physical examination a painful pulsatile groin mass is often appreciated. Diagnosis can be made with either Doppler ultrasound or contrast-enhanced computed tomography (CT). Sonography will show a fluid collection adjacent to the femoral artery that demonstrates arterial flow. On intravenous contrast-enhanced CT, the enhancing pseudoaneurysm will be seen arising off the femoral artery. A surrounding abscess or phlegmon may also be seen.

Treatment of this condition is surgical. There is controversy as to the optimal surgical treatment of the pseudoaneurysm but may include débridement with arterial ligation and excision of the pseudoaneurysm with arterial revascularization.

Notes

CASE 174

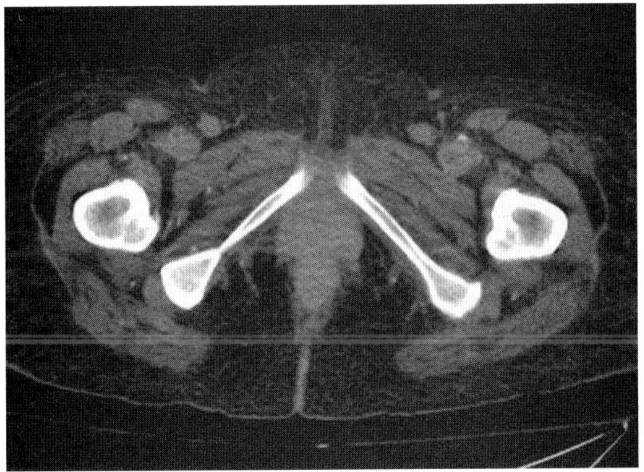

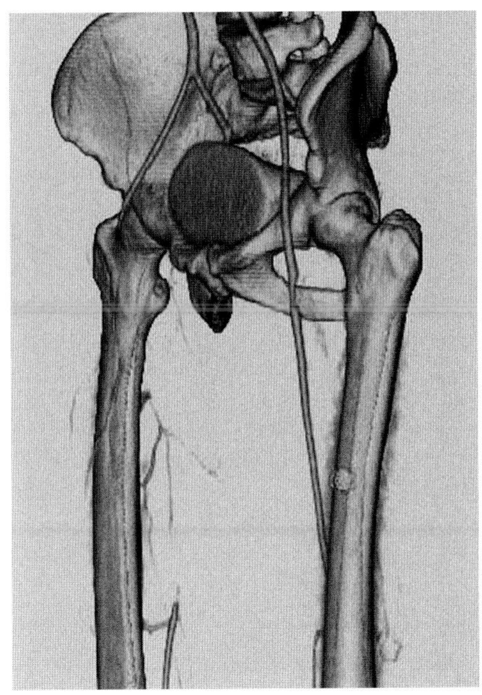

See also Color Plate

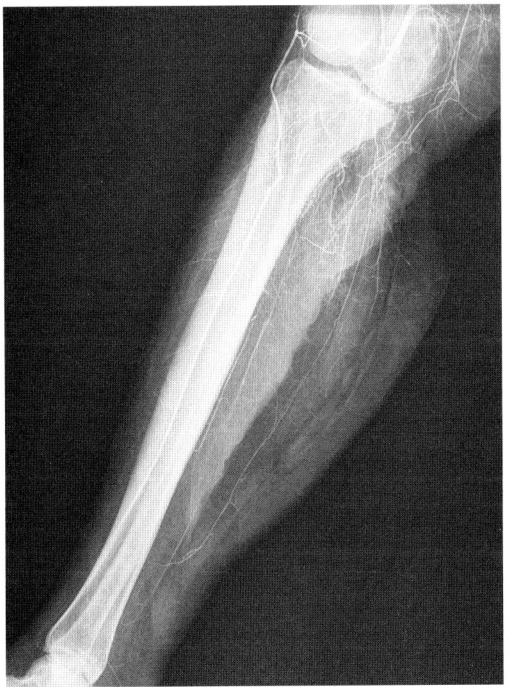

1. This 30-year-old female with a history of endocarditis presented with acute bilateral lower extremity pain and diminished distal pulses. What is the diagnosis?
2. What is the most common cause of embolic lower extremity arterial occlusion?
3. Where do in situ thrombotic lower extremity arterial occlusions usually occur?
4. What can reduce the sensitivity of multidetector computed tomographic angiography for significant lower extremity arterial stenoses or occlusions?

CASE 174

Acute Lower Extremity Arterial Occlusion

1. Embolic arterial occlusion.
2. Cardiac thrombi secondary to cardiac arrhythmias.
3. Preexisting arterial stenoses and arterial bypass grafts.
4. Arterial spasm, suboptimal bolus timing, and sluggish arterial flow from decreased cardiac output and/or extensive arterio-occlusive disease.

References

Hiatt MD, Fleischmann D, Hellinger JC, Rubin GD: Angiographic imaging of the lower extremities with multidetector CT, *Radiol Clin North Am* 43: 1119–1127, 2005.

Klonaris C, Georgopoulos S, Katsargyris A, et al: Changing patterns in the etiology of acute lower limb ischemia, *Int Angiol* 26:49–52, 2007.

Cross-Reference

Emergency Radiology: THE REQUISITES, pp 350–353.

Comment

Acute extremity ischemia is relatively common and occurs when there is a sudden decrease in limb perfusion that poses a threat to limb viability. Limb ischemia typically results from embolism or thrombosis, although there are other causes that include trauma, vasculitis, and spontaneous dissection. Embolism from cardiac valvular heart disease had been the most common cause of acute lower extremity ischemia. However, with the decrease in valvular heart disease seen in Western countries over recent decades, peripheral embolism now more commonly occurs as a consequence of cardiac arrhythmias. Moreover, the frequency of in situ arterial thrombosis at sites of preexisting arterial stenosis or within arterial bypass grafts has increased. Some studies have shown that acute lower extremity ischemia secondary to arterial thrombosis now occurs with a frequency comparable to, or greater than, that of peripheral arterial embolism. Others have shown that patients with thrombotic occlusion tend to experience repeat episodes of ischemia due to higher frequency of bypass graft thrombosis in this subpopulation.

Angiography is the diagnostic reference standard for evaluating the lower extremity arterial system. However, multidetector computed tomographic angiography (MD-CTA) has become a viable, noninvasive alternative to angiography in many clinical settings. In young patients with clinically suspected lower limb ischemia, it may assess the arterial system with less radiation than angiography. If catheter-based intervention is not anticipated, in the emergency department, MD-CTA can frequently be obtained more quickly, and at a lesser expense, than angiography. With a four-channel scanner, the sensitivities of MD-CTA for severe stenoses (>75% luminal compromise) and occlusions are 92% and 89%, respectively, while the respective specificities are 97% and 98%. Arterial spasm, suboptimal bolus timing, and sluggish arterial flow from decreased cardiac output and/or extensive arterio-occlusive disease can reduce the accuracy of MD-CTA for severe stenoses and occlusions.

Notes

CASE 175

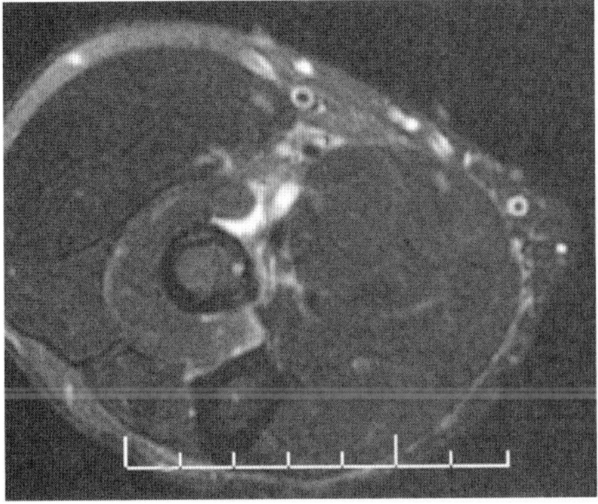
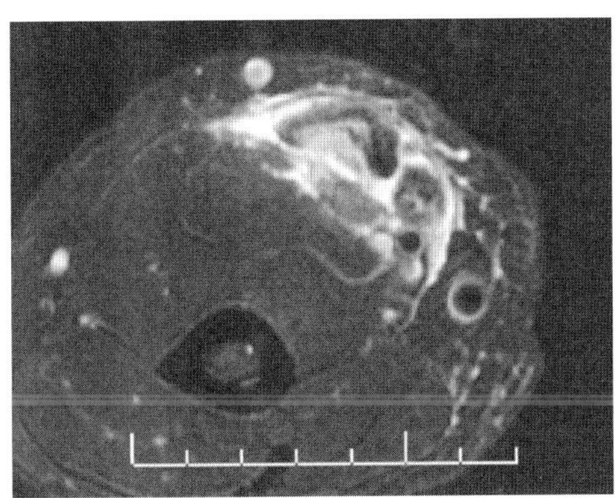
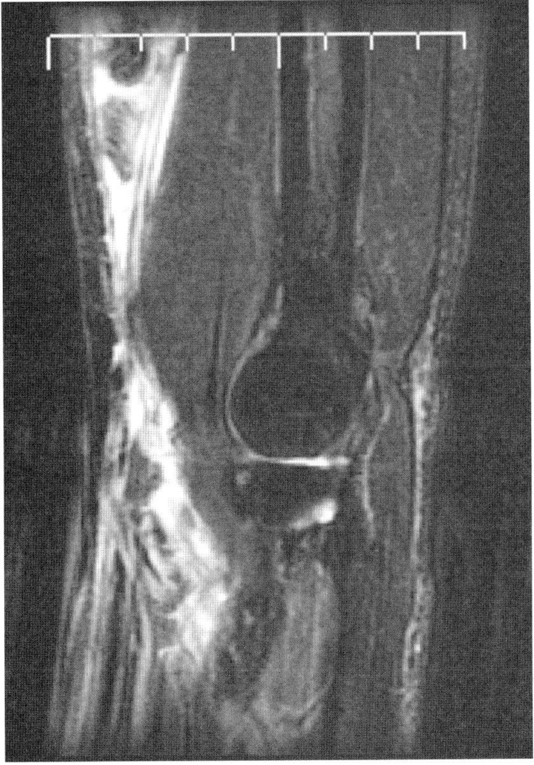
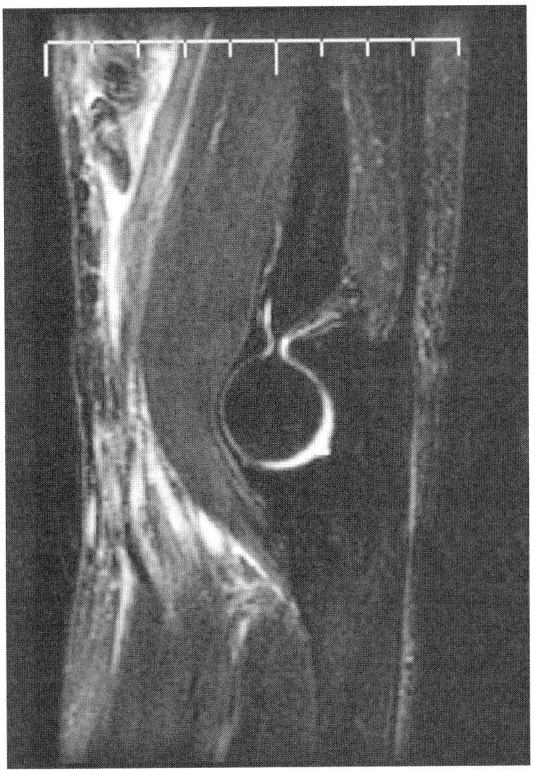

1. What is ruptured?
2. What is the mechanism of injury?
3. Where do most ruptures of this structure occur?
4. When magnetic resonance imaging is used to diagnosis this injury, what information should be reported?

CASE 175

Acute Rupture of Distal Biceps Brachii Tendon

1. Distal biceps brachii tendon.
2. Sudden forceful overload of the flexed elbow.
3. Tendon insertion on the radial tuberosity.
4. Integrity of the tendon, location of injury within the tendon, tendon retraction and size of tendon gap, and integrity of bicipital aponeurosis.

References

Chew ML, Giuffrè BM: Disorders of the distal biceps brachii tendon, *Radiographics* 25:1227–1237, 2005.

Fitzgerald SW, Curry DR, Erickson SJ, et al: Distal biceps tendon injury: MR imaging diagnosis, *Radiology* 191:203–206, 1994.

Comment

Complete rupture of the distal biceps brachii tendon is uncommon. In contrast to partial tears, which are frequently due to repetitive microtrauma, complete tendon rupture is usually the result of a single, sudden forceful overload of the flexed elbow. Rupture may occur over the length of the tendon, but most occur at the tendon insertion on the radial tuberosity. Clinical diagnosis is usually straightforward with most patients exhibiting weakened flexion and supination at the elbow, in addition to a painful mass corresponding to hematoma and retracted tendon. However, clinical diagnosis can be challenging when the bicipital aponeurosis and flexion at the elbow is relatively preserved. In addition, an intact distal biceps tendon sheath may mask a torn, retracted tendon on clinical examination. Early primary surgical repair minimizes permanent loss of strength.

In clinically equivocal cases, magnetic resonance imaging can be used to assess the integrity of the biceps tendon and bicipital aponeurosis and the site of tendon injury. Since injuries can occur along the entire length of the tendon and the torn tendon may retract, both axial and sagittal images should include the region between the bicipital tuberosity and distal biceps myotendinous junction. Localization of the free tendon ends and quantification of the intervening gap facilitate surgical planning.

Notes

CASE 176

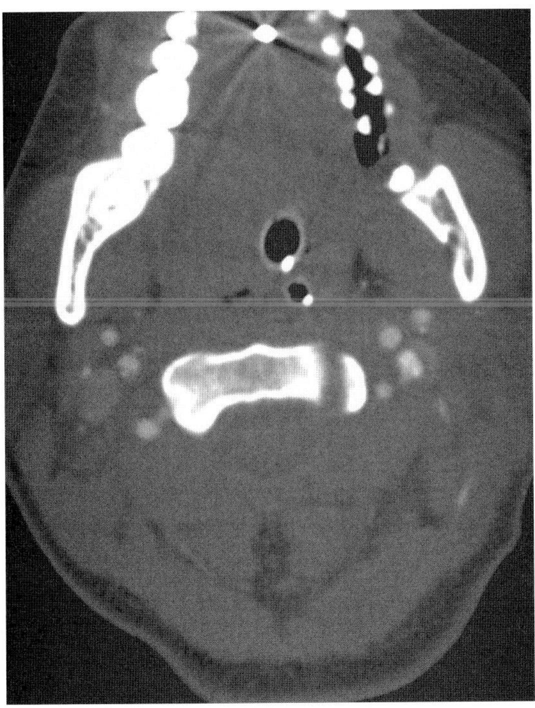

1. This image is from a computed tomographic angiography used to evaluate a 21-year-old female pedestrian who was struck by a motor vehicle. What is the diagnosis?
2. What is the incidence of this injury?
3. What are the potential consequences of this injury?
4. What is the reported value of screening blunt trauma patients for this injury?

CASE 176

Blunt Internal Carotid Artery Injury

1. Blunt right internal carotid artery injury (i.e., blunt cerebrovascular injury) with possible left-sided internal carotid artery injury.
2. Blunt cerebrovascular injuries are encountered in 1% of all blunt trauma patients.
3. Stroke and death.
4. Identification and treatment of asymptomatic injuries can reduce mortality.

References

Schneidereit NP, Simons R, Nicolaou S, et al: Utility of screening for blunt vascular neck injuries with computed tomographic angiography, *J Trauma* 60: 209–215, 2006.

Sliker CW, Mirvis SE: Imaging of blunt cerebrovascular injuries, *Eur J Radiol* 64:3–14, 2007.

Cross-Reference

Emergency Radiology: THE REQUISITES, pp 21–23, 321–322.

Comment

Blunt cerebrovascular injuries (BCVI) (i.e., injuries of the carotid arteries and vertebral arteries) affect only approximately 1% of blunt trauma patients. Injuries most commonly occur in the cervical segments of the internal carotid and vertebral arteries. More than one major cervical artery is injured in 18% to 38% of patients with BCVI. Untreated blunt carotid artery and vertebral artery injuries are associated with mortality rates of up to 17% to 38% and 8% to 18%, respectively. Death is usually caused by stroke related to either hypoperfusion or thromboembolism.

Patients at high risk for harboring a BCVI include those with LeFort II or III facial fractures, basilar skull fractures, diffuse axonal injury with Glasgow coma scale score less than 8, cervical spinal fractures that involve C1 through C3 or a foramen transversarium, cervical subluxation, seatbelt contusions on the neck, or a history of near-hanging with anoxic brain injury. Specific clinical and imaging signs of BCVI include arterial hemorrhage, expanding neck hematoma, massive epistaxis, cervical bruit, Horner syndrome, focal neurologic deficit unexplained by neuroimaging, and infarct depicted on diagnostic brain imaging. In many patients, clinically significant BCVIs can be silent for over 12 hours. Since treatment with either anticoagulation or antiplatelet therapy can prevent or limit injury-related stroke and reduce mortality, some institutions screen asymptomatic high-risk blunt trauma patients for BCVI in order to promote initiation of treatment while the injury is clinically silent.

In the study of Schneidereit and colleagues (2006), the authors initiated a screening program that utilized defined screening criteria to identify high-risk patients and multidetector computed tomographic angiography to identify BCVI, and subsequently lowered the injury-specific mortality at their institution from 38% to zero. Despite its ability to positively impact patient outcomes, screening still fails to identify approximately 25% of patients harboring clinically significant BCVIs as these patients may not exhibit any of the commonly reported risk factors.

Notes

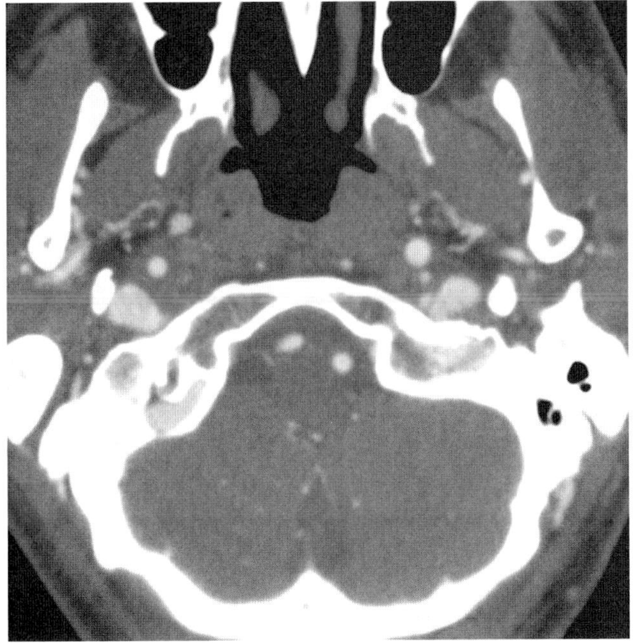

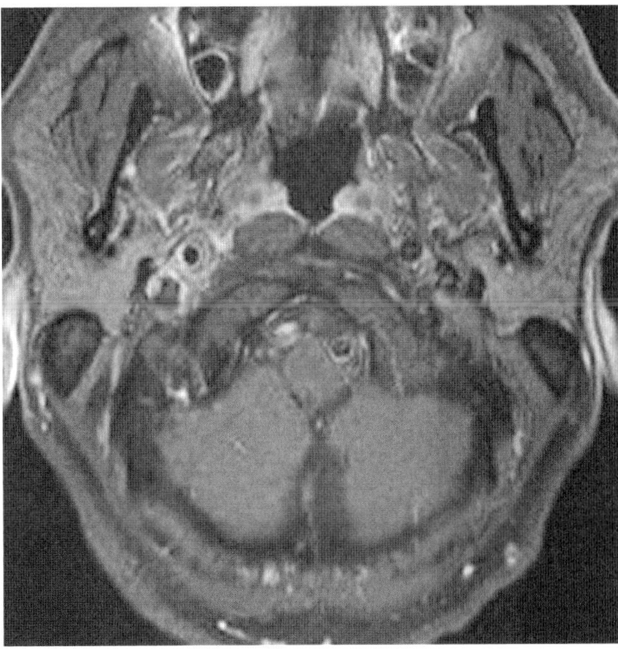

1. This patient presented with right neck and face pain with ptosis after straining to move heavy machinery. Is this a typical history associated with the correct diagnosis?
2. What imaging abnormalities typical of the diagnosis are demonstrated in this patient?
3. Are similar abnormalities common elsewhere in the neck?
4. What is the risk to the patient if this abnormality is not treated?

CASE 177

Spontaneous Internal Carotid Artery Dissection

1. Yes.
2. Right internal carotid artery mural thickening, increased arterial caliber, eccentric luminal narrowing, and minimally hyperintense T1-weighted signal.
3. Yes.
4. Stroke.

References

Ozdoba C, Sturzenegger M, Schroth G: Internal carotid artery dissection: MR imaging features and clinical-radiologic correlation, *Radiology* 199:191–198, 1996.

Schievink WI: Spontaneous dissection of the carotid and vertebral arteries, *N Engl J Med* 344:898–906, 2001.

Cross-Reference

Emergency Radiology: THE REQUISITES, pp 321–322.

Comment

Spontaneous internal carotid artery (ICA) and vertebral artery dissections occur when there is intramural arterial hemorrhage without preceding major blunt or penetrating trauma. Although it may be truly spontaneous, without clearly preceding significant trauma, there is frequently "trivial trauma" that may include sudden, rapid turning of the head or either neck flexion or extension. Strenuous physical exercise or strain may also induce ICA or vertebral artery dissection. While responsible for only 2% of ischemic strokes, they cause 5% to 20% of strokes in young or middle-aged patients. Spontaneous ICA dissections are more common than vertebral artery dissections. Up to 20% of symptomatic dissections may be associated with a dissection in another ICA or vertebral artery. Diagnosis of both types of dissection usually warrants immediate anticoagulation therapy.

Patients with ICA dissection frequently present with ipisilateral headache, especially retro-orbital, face pain, or upper neck pain. Miosis and ptosis may also be present, but associated anhidrosis is characteristically absent. Patients may also present with lower cranial nerve palsies and pulsatile tinnitus. Auscultation may reveal a bruit. Fifty percent to 95% of ICA dissections may lead to ischemia.

Both computed tomographic (CT) angiography and magnetic resonance (MR) angiography supplemented by cross-sectional MR imaging are used to diagnose cervical arterial dissections in current clinical practice. CT-angiography and MR-angiography/imaging typically demonstrate an eccentric, narrowed arterial lumen associated with crescentic, sometimes circumferential, mural thickening. Characteristically, the mural thickening causes an overall increased arterial diameter relative to the contralateral artery. Either arterial occlusion or luminal distention (i.e., pseudoaneurysm) can be encountered. With MR imaging, the intramural hematoma may isointense or minimally hyperintense on fat-suppressed T1-weighted images, but after several days, signal is characteristically hyperintense.

Notes

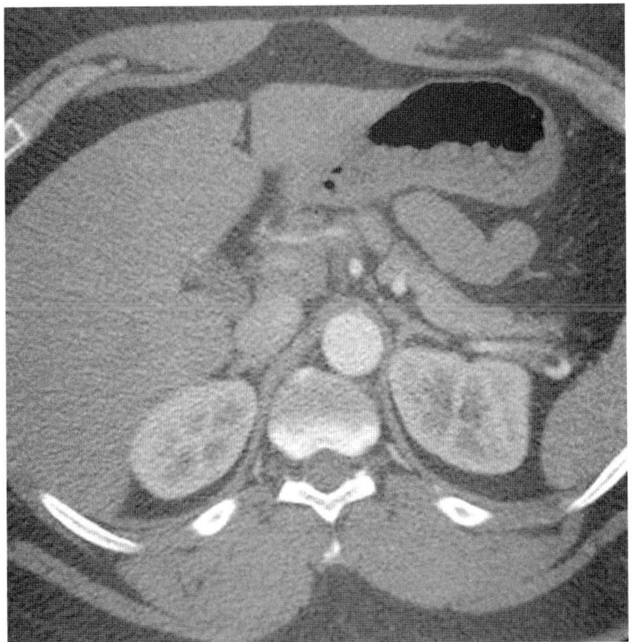

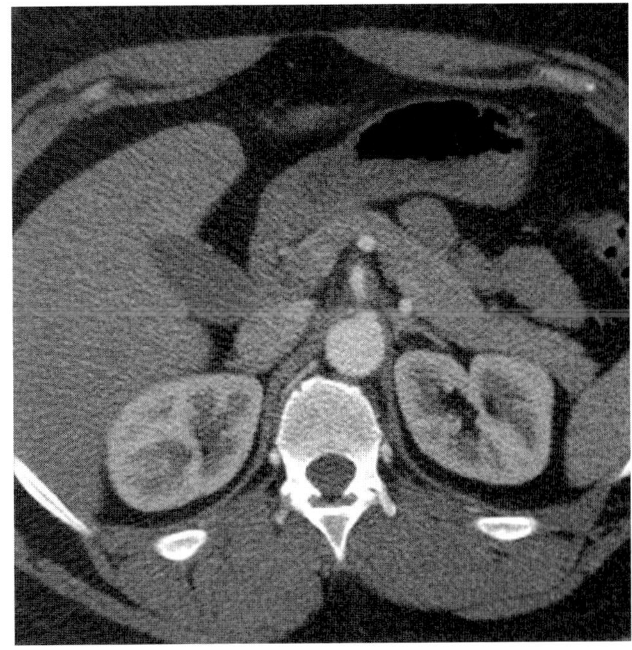

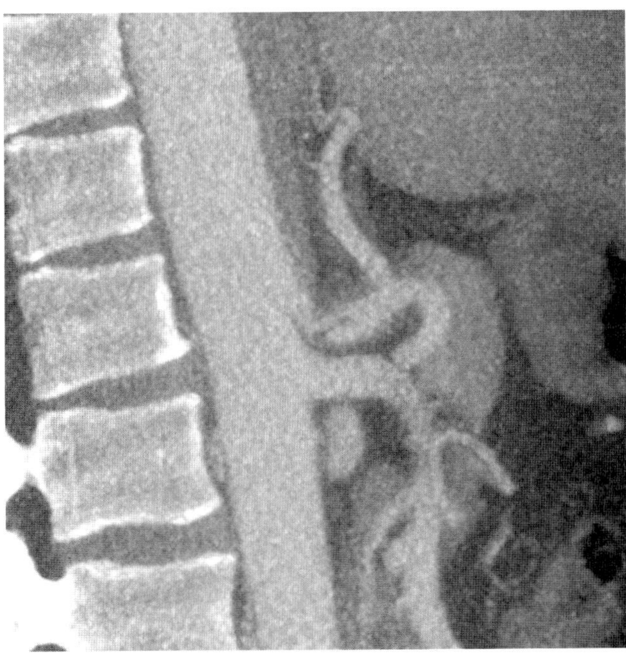

1. There is no history of trauma or instrumentation. What is the diagnosis?
2. What is the most common symptom at presentation?
3. Is this a common abnormality?
4. What are poor prognostic indicators associated with this diagnosis?

CASE 178

Spontaneous Celiac Artery Dissection

1. Spontaneous celiac artery dissection.
2. Epigastric pain.
3. No. It is rare.
4. Hemorrhage and liver ischemia.

Reference

D'Ambrosio N, Friedman B, Siegel D, et al: Spontaneous isolated dissection of the celiac artery: CT findings in adults, *AJR Am J Roentgenol* 188: W506–W511, 2007.

Comment

Spontaneous dissections of visceral arteries are rare, and superior mesenteric artery dissections occur more frequently than celiac artery dissections. Risk factors include hypertension, cystic medial necrosis, abdominal aortic aneurysm, fibromuscular dysplasia, pregnancy, and connective tissue disease. Patients can present with acute epigastric pain or intestinal angina. Celiac artery dissections may also be incidental findings discovered on scans performed for unrelated reasons.

Some, if not most, celiac artery dissections spontaneously heal. However, others may lead to aneurysm formation and/or rupture with hemorrhage. Vascular compromise can lead to hepatic or splenic ischemia. Hemorrhage and liver ischemia are poor prognostic indicators that are seen in 40% of fatal cases.

On computed tomography, an intimal flap is pathognomonic. Other signs include a celiac artery aneurysm and celiac perivascular fat infiltration. An eccentric celiac artery mural thrombus should lead one to consider the diagnosis. Dissection can propagate into the branches of the celiac artery where it may lead to aneurysm formation.

Notes

CASE 179

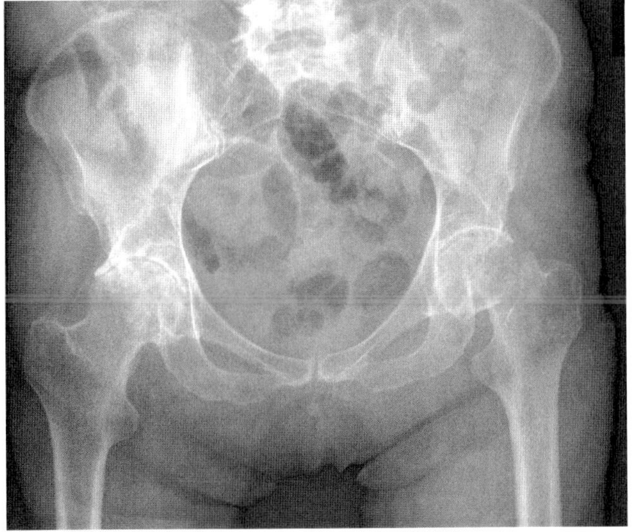

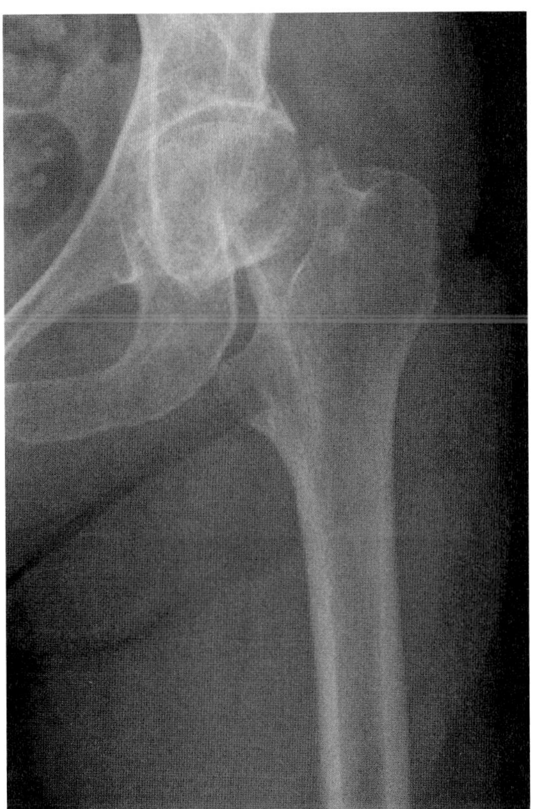

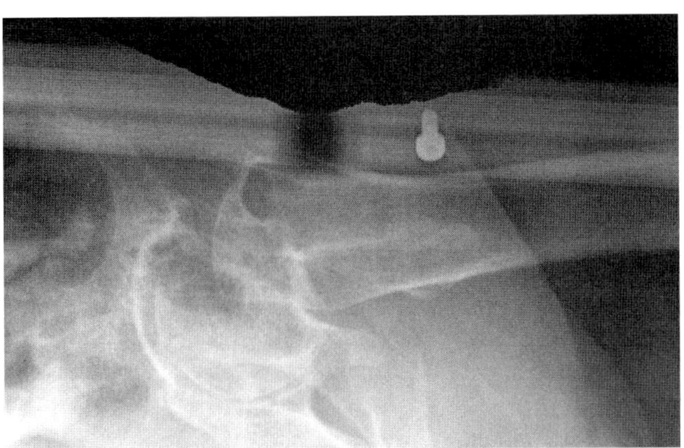

1. Where is the exact site of fracture?
2. What is the long-term significance of this type of fracture when encountered in the elderly (>65 years old)?
3. When displacement is more than minimal, what are potential complications of this fracture?
4. How does treatment of minimally displaced forms of this fracture differ from more displaced ones?

CASE 179

Subcapital Femoral Neck (Hip) Fracture

1. Subcapital femoral neck.
2. High mortality rates within 1 year after injury. Mortality is 12 to 16 times higher than in the general population, when corrected for age.
3. Osteonecrosis and nonunion.
4. Minimally displaced fractures can be treated with percutaneous screws or pins. More displaced fractures are treated with either open reduction with internal fixation or hip arthroplasty.

References

Ashman CJ, Yu JS: The hip and femoral shaft. In Rogers LF, ed: *Radiology of Skeletal Trauma*, 3rd ed, Philadelphia, Churchill Livingstone, 2002, pp 1038–1052.

Bottle A, Aylin P: Mortality associated with delay in operation after hip fracture: observational study, *BMJ* 332:947–951, 2006.

Roberts SE, Goldacre MJ: Time trends and demography of mortality after fractured neck of femur in an English population, 1968–98: database study, *BMJ* 327:771–775, 2003.

Cross-Reference

Emergency Radiology: THE REQUISITES, pp 142–144.

Comment

Femoral neck and intertrochanter fractures (i.e., "hip" fractures) are injuries typically encountered in the elderly. Unusual in patients younger than 45 years, they are encountered with increasing frequency with increasing patient age. The age distribution can be best explained by the increased frequency of osteoporosis and fall in the elderly. Women are more prone to hip fractures than men. Within 1 year of the injury, patients with hip fracture exhibit mortality rates 12 to 16 times higher than the general population of similar age, with overall mortality rates reaching as high as 18% at 90 days following injury. Most injuries occur as a consequence of a relatively minor fall with a direct blow to the greater trochanter or lateral rotation of the distal leg relative to the proximal femur.

Nearly two thirds of hip fractures are intracapsular (femoral neck) while the remainder are extracapsular (intertrochanteric). Most intracapsular fractures are subcapital (i.e., at the junction of the femoral head and neck), while the remainder are either midcervical (i.e., at mid femoral neck), or basicervical (i.e., at the junction of the femoral neck and trochanters). Because the blood supply to the femoral neck is tenuous and there is no periosteal healing in the region, patients with intracapsular fractures are prone to femoral head osteonecrosis and/or fracture nonunion.

With minimal displaced or impacted fractures, there is relatively little compromise of blood supply to the femoral head, with accordingly low rates of complication. In contrast, displaced fractures tend to have more compromise of blood supply with higher rates of complications. For example, 8% of fractures with minor displacement may lead to osteonecrosis, while 30% of severely displaced fractures can result in osteonecrosis. Up to 25% of displaced fractures are complicated by nonunion.

To limit the risk of fracture motion and displacement, thereby preserving local blood supply and reducing the risk of osteonecrosis and nonunion, minimally displaced fractures are frequently treated with percutaneous screws or pins. Because of their higher likelihood of vascular compromise, displaced fractures are usually treated with open reduction and some form of plate-and-screw fixation. In some cases, severely displaced fractures are treated with primary hip arthroplasty.

Standard radiographic assessment of patients with suspected hip fractures includes an anteroposterior (AP) view and either a frog-leg view or a groin lateral view. An AP view of the pelvis facilitates identification of subtle abnormalities best demonstrated by bilateral asymmetry. Radiographic signs of a subcapital fracture include discrete cortical or trabecular disruption, a sclerotic line secondary to impaction, angulation of the cortex or trabeculae, and rotation of the femoral head. When there is a minimally displaced fracture in the presence of severe osteoporosis, the fracture can be radiographically occult.

If a radiographically occult fracture is suspected in the setting of osteopenia, magnetic resonance imaging (MRI) can be performed to facilitate rapid diagnosis and limit the risk of fracture fragment displacement. Because MRI identifies the bone marrow edema and hemorrhage associated with the acute fracture, it diagnoses nondisplaced fractures sooner after injury and with greater sensitivity than both computed tomography (CT) and bone scanning. Compared with MRI, CT can be relatively insensitive to nondisplaced fractures, like radiography, while bone scans may be falsely negative for fractures within the first 72 hours after an injury. MRI can also diagnose or exclude alternative causes of hip pain and reduced range of motion, such as muscle strain.

Notes

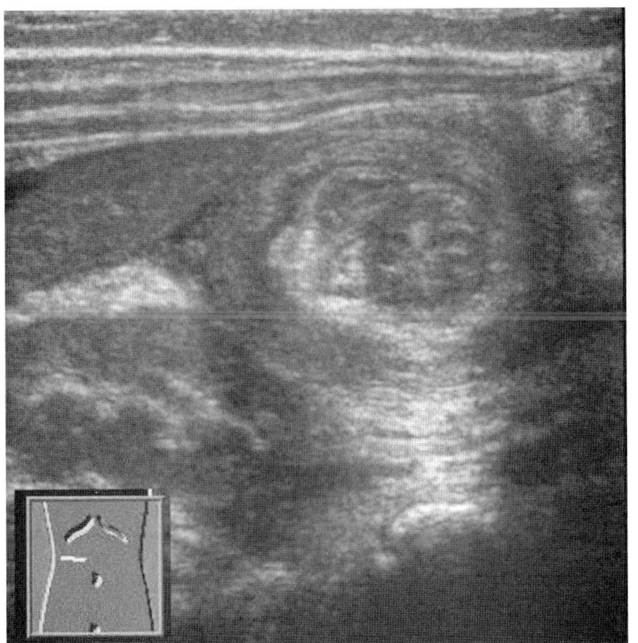

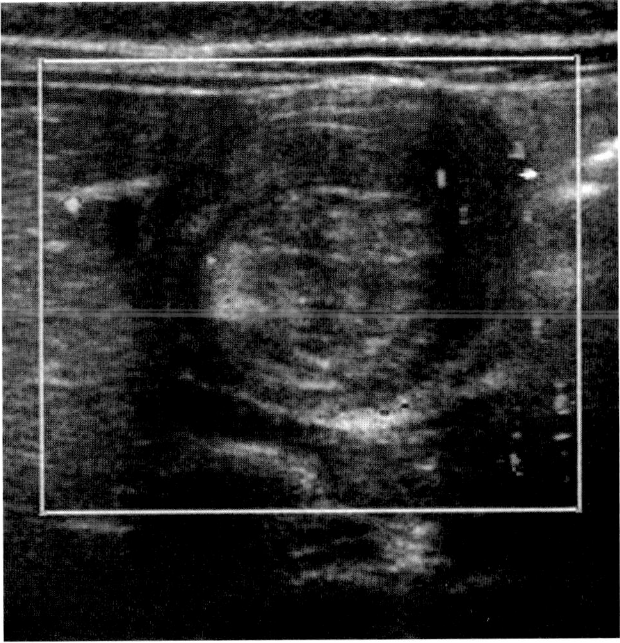

See also Color Plate

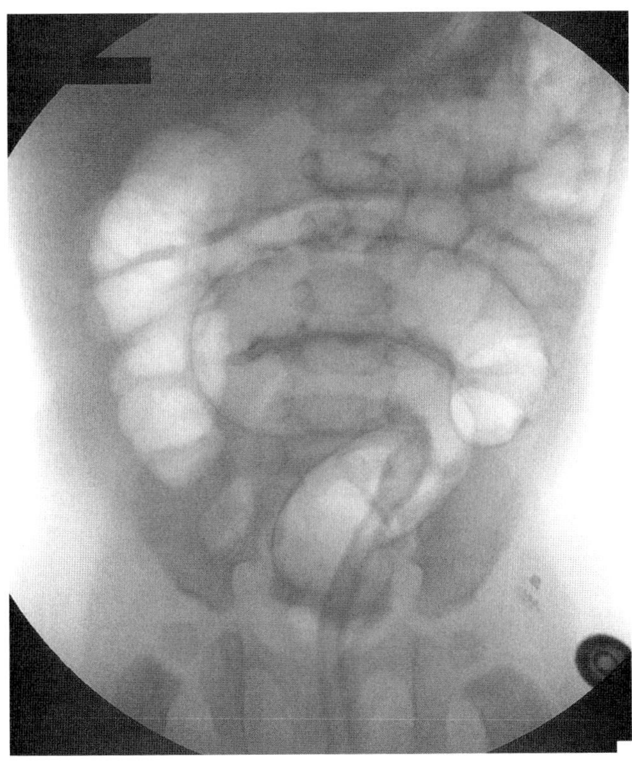

1. What is the diagnosis?
2. What is the classic clinical triad for patients presenting with this condition?
3. What two sonographic signs of this diagnosis are illustrated?
4. What is the primary role of imaging-observed enema in the management of children with this condition?

CASE 180

Intussusception—Pediatric

1. Intussusception.
2. Abdominal colic, red currant–jelly stools, palpable abdominal mass.
3. "Target" sign and "crescent-in-doughnut" sign.
4. Reduction of intussusception.

References

del-Pozo G, Albillos JC, Tejedor D, et al: Intussusception in children: current concepts in diagnosis and enema reduction, *Radiographics* 19:299–319, 1999.

Ko HS, Schenk JP, Troger J, Rohrschneider WK: Current radiological management of intussusception in children, *Eur Radiol* 17:2411–2421, 2007.

Cross-Reference

Emergency Radiology: THE REQUISITES, pp 192–193.

Comment

Intussusception is the most common cause of acute bowel obstruction in infants, and most cases occur in the first 3 years of life. The clinical presentation can be varied, and clinical findings include irritability, intermittent crying, abdominal colic, vomiting, hematochezia or currant-jelly stools, and a right upper quadrant abdominal mass. The classic clinical findings of abdominal colic, red currant–jelly stools, and palpable abdominal mass are exhibited by less than 50% of children with intussusception, but, when they are seen in conjunction with vomiting, the positive predictive value for intussusception is nearly 100%. Untreated intussusceptions generally lead to bowel obstruction, bowel ischemia, perforation, and, possibly, death.

Most pediatric intussusceptions are encountered in the right upper quadrant at the hepatic flexure, and they are usually ileocolic. Less common intussusceptions are ileo-ileal and ileo-ileocolic. In young children, approximately 95% of intussusceptions do not occur as a consequence of a pathologic lead point. However, some idiopathic intussusceptions may be associated with hyperplastic lymphoid tissue.

Although radiographs can be used to diagnose intussusception when clinical suspicion is high, their sensitivity is only 45%. The greatest value of radiographs may be in demonstrating the complications of intussusception, which include bowel obstruction and perforation.

The sensitivity of ultrasound (US) for detecting is 98% to 100%. The relatively large size of the intussusception, small size of the patients, and characteristic subhepatic location facilitate diagnosis. The US-appearances of the intussusception result from the alternating bands of the wall of the receiving bowel (i.e., intussuscipiens), invaginated mesentery, and both the entering and exiting walls of the invaginated bowel (i.e., intussusceptum). When viewed in axial cross-section, US may demonstrate multiple crescentic rings of bowel wall and mesentery (the "target" sign). When imaged near the base of the intussusception, axial US may demonstrate more eccentric and thicker invaginated mesentery that results in the "crescent-in-doughnut" sign.

While they are the reference standard for diagnosis, contrast enema examinations are not a primary means for diagnosing intussusception at many centers. However, enema reduction under imaging observation is the first-line means for treating pediatric intussusception. Techniques include fluoroscopically observed air enema, positive-contrast enema reduction, and US-observed water/saline reduction. Enema reduction can be successful in over 80% of cases. Contraindications to enema reduction include radiographic signs of perforation, clinical signs of peritonitis, and shock refractory to intravenous hydration. US findings that indicate a lower likelihood of successful enema reduction, due to bowel wall edema and/or ischemia, respectively, include a thick (>10 mm) rim of the intussusception and fluid trapped within the invaginated mesentery. Regardless of the presence of the aforementioned US signs of poor reducibility, enema reduction should be considered in all patients without clear contraindications to the procedure.

Notes

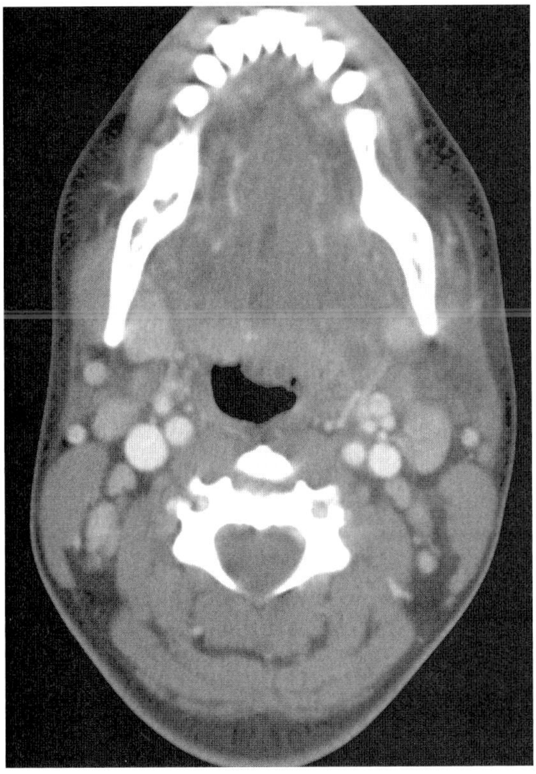

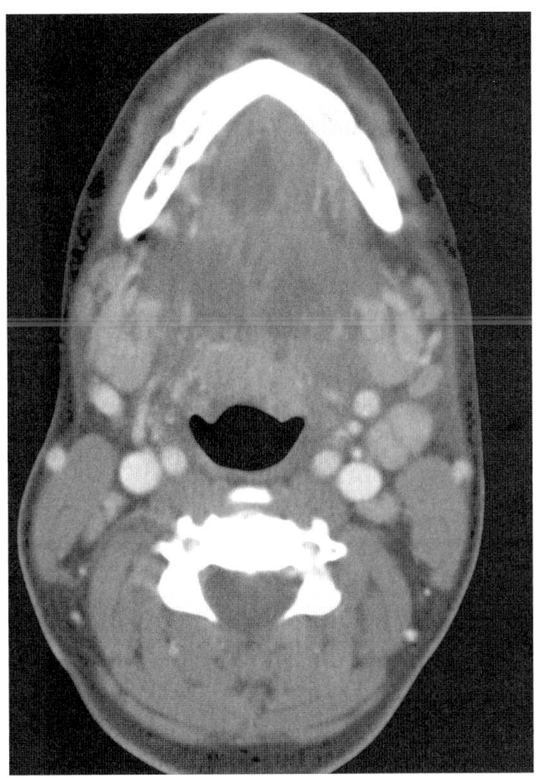

1. What is the diagnosis?
2. What anatomic spaces are involved?
3. When this disease is suspected, what is the risk that imaging with computed tomography poses to the patient?
4. What is the usual source of this infectious process?

CASE 181

Ludwig's Angina

1. Ludwig's angina.
2. Sublingual and submandibular.
3. Supine positioning for the scan may elicit rapid airway compromise.
4. Odontogenic disease.

Reference

Nguyen VD, Potter JL, Hersh-Schick MR: Ludwig angina: an uncommon and potentially lethal neck infection, *AJNR Am J Neuroradiol* 13:215–219, 1992.

Cross-Reference

Emergency Radiology: THE REQUISITES, p 57.

Comment

Ludwig's angina is a rare, rapidly progressive, and potentially lethal gangrenous soft tissue infection that involves both the sublingual and submandibular spaces. An odontogenic infection of one of the lower molars is the typical source. While there may be focal areas of phlegmon or serosanguinous fluid, discrete abscesses are uncommon. Spread is by continuous extension, and both lymphatic spread and salivary gland involvement are atypical. Extension into the deep neck soft tissue can occur, and necrotizing mediastinitis may result from spread through the retropharyngeal space or carotid sheath.

Although predisposing factors include diabetes mellitus and immunosuppression, most patients are otherwise healthy. Patients typically present with brawny submandibular edema and induration. Sublingual edema causes elevation or protrusion of the tongue. Symptoms include pain, reduced neck mobility, dysphagia, odynophagia, dysphonia, and trismus. Fever and tachycardia can be seen. There may be stridor, although signs of airway compromise may be subtle. Classically, breathing difficulties are exacerbated by supine positioning which can elicit airway spasm with the potential for rapid, complete, and fatal airway compromise.

Radiographs can be used to assess the degree of airway compromise. Given the risk of sudden airway compromise, portable neck radiographs with the patient positioned erect should be obtained within the emergency department. Since supine positioning can induce airway compromise, computed tomography (CT) should be avoided as a first-line examination unless the airway is maintained with intubation. However, in clinically unexpected cases, CT may demonstrate the characteristic inflammatory changes in the sublingual and submandibular spaces, in addition to any focal pockets of fluid or deep neck extension. Imaging may also reveal odontogenic disease as the source of infection or soft tissue gas related to infection with gas-forming organisms.

Notes

CASE 182

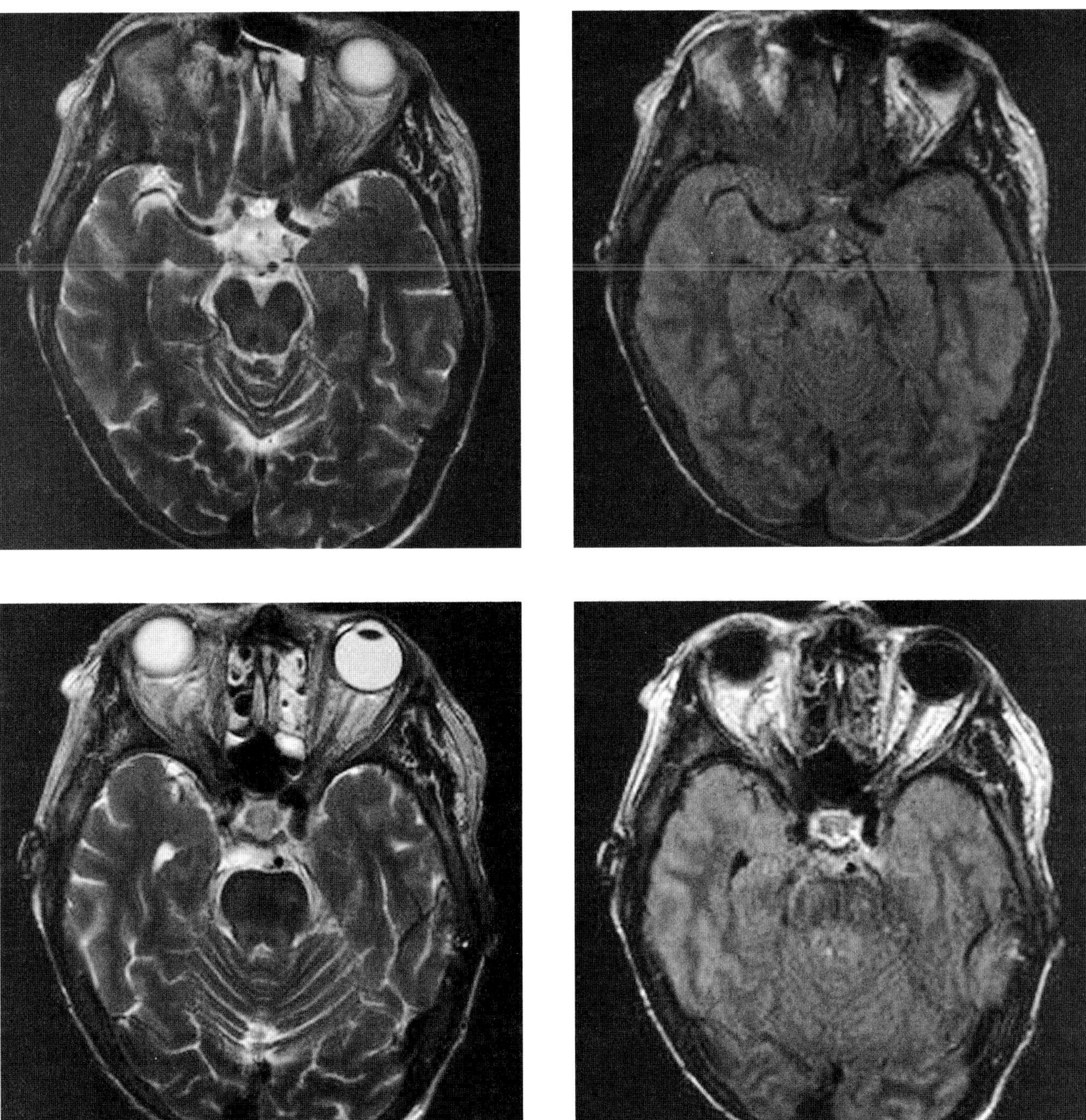

1. What are the abnormalities?
2. What is the usual cause of mesenrhombencephalitis?
3. What are two frequently implicated infectious causes of mesenrhombencephalitis?
4. Do normal antibody titers preclude the diagnosis of infectious mesenrhombencephalitis?

CASE 182

Mesenrhombencephalitis

1. Faint areas of T2- and FLAIR-signal hyperintensity in the mid-brain and pons.
2. Often unidentified but frequently infectious.
3. Herpes simplex and *Listeria monocytogenes.*
4. No.

References

Soo MS, Tien RD, Gray L, et al: Mesenrhombencephalitis: MR findings in nine patients, *AJR Am J Roentgenol* 160:1089–1093, 1993.

Wasenko JJ, Park BJ, Jubelt B, et al: Magnetic resonance imaging of mesenrhombencephalitis, *Clin Imaging* 26:237–242, 2002.

Comment

Mesenrhombencephalitis is a rare inflammatory disorder involving the mid-brain, pons, and medulla. The cerebellum is frequently involved, and concurrent supratentorial inflammation may be demonstrated as well. Often, the source of the inflammation is not identified. Viruses are the most frequently suspected causes, although parasitic and bacterial infections are also possible. Two frequently implicated infectious causes of mesenrhombencephalitis include herpes simplex and *Listeria monocytogenes.* Paraneoplastic syndromes and postinfectious immune-mediated encephalomyelitis are other reported causes.

The clinical diagnosis can be difficult. While the typical clinical presentation usually includes areflexia, ataxia, and ophthalmoplegia, the signs and symptoms may be nonspecific and include: headache, fever, lethargy, seizures, nausea and vomiting, cranial nerve palsies, nystagmus, amnesia, and coma. Cerebrospinal fluid (CSF) analysis may be normal, or it may show a few nonspecific abnormalities. Both blood and CSF cultures may be negative for infectious agents. Antibody titers may be normal initially, and they may not become elevated until weeks after initial clinical presentation.

Magnetic resonance imaging (MRI) is the imaging method of choice, and it may provide the first clues to the correct diagnosis. MRI may demonstrate hyperintense T2-weighted abnormalities in the pons, medulla, and mid-brain. Areas of patchy enhancement may be seen, but enhancement is not universal. The cerebellar peduncles and cerebellum are frequently involved. Other sites of involvement include the temporal and frontal lobes, internal capsules, thalami, and basal ganglia. Occasionally, the brainstem may be enlarged, although this finding should elicit close inspection for an underlying mass.

Notes

CASE 183

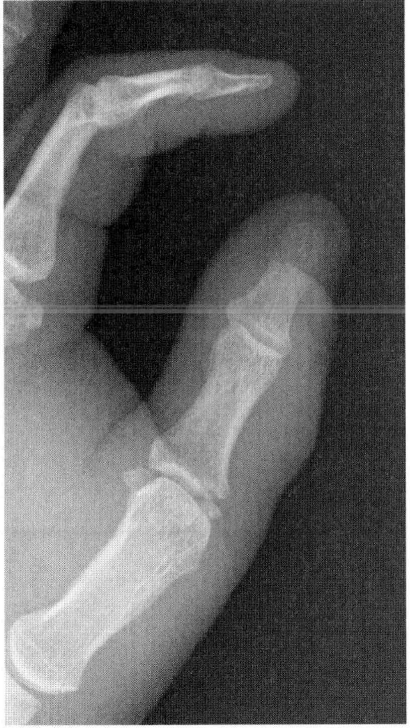

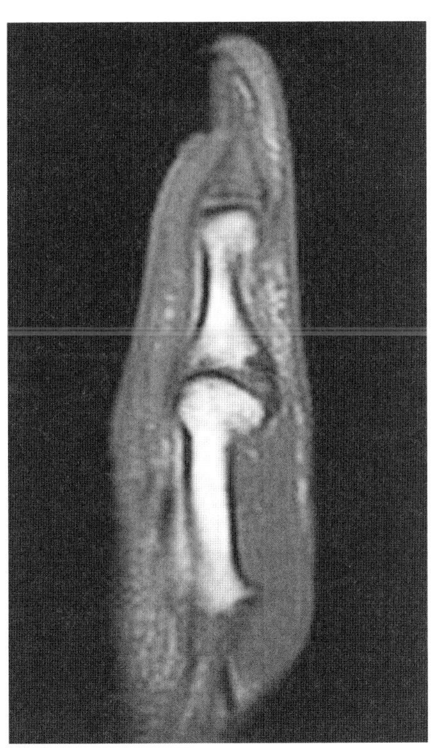

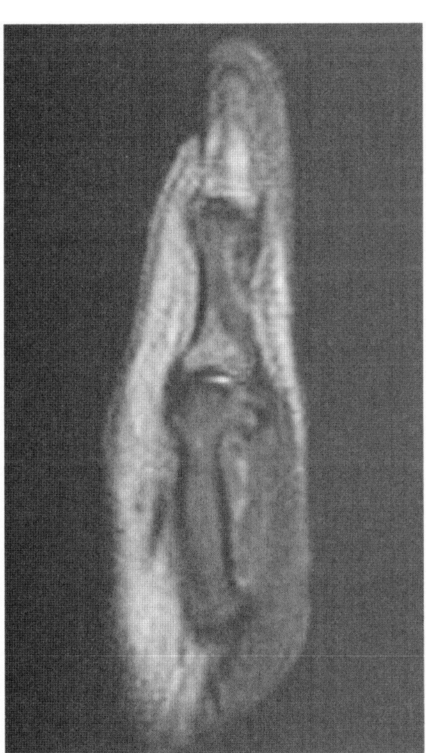

1. How long may it take for radiographs to exhibit signs of this disease?
2. What is the sensitivity of magnetic resonance imaging (MRI) for this disease?
3. Are the MRI manifestations of this disease specific?
4. Is intravenous gadolinium required to diagnose this disease with MRI?

CASE 183

Acute Osteomyelitis

1. 7 to 14 days.
2. 82% to 100%.
3. No.
4. No.

Reference

Restrepo CS, Lemos DF, Gordillo H, et al: Imaging findings in musculoskeletal complications of AIDS, *Radiographics* 24:1029–1049, 2004.

Cross-Reference

Emergency Radiology: THE REQUISITES, pp 177–180, 376–377.

Comment

Osteomyelitis, or bone infection, may result from hematogenous spread of infection, direct spread from an adjacent infection, or direct inoculation of microorganisms. Patients typically present with pain with local soft tissue erythema and swelling. There may be a fever. The erythrocyte sedimentation rate is usually elevated, while the serum white blood cell count is frequently normal.

For the first 7 to 14 days, acute osteomyelitis may not show radiographic abnormalities other than soft tissue swelling. Subsequently, radiographs may demonstrate periosteal elevation and osteolysis. In cases of suspected direct implantation of microorganisms, radiographs can be used to search for retained foreign bodies.

Magnetic resonance imaging (MRI) is highly sensitive, 82% to 100%, for detecting acute osteomyelitis. With a negative predictive value of nearly 100%, MRI is a useful means to exclude acute osteomyelitis. However, since the early manifestations of osteomyelitis detected by MRI are nonspecific, they cannot be interpreted out of clinical context. Mirroring the radiographic manifestations of disease, as the osteomyelitis progress, MRI may demonstrate destruction of cortical bone and subperiosteal fluid. While not necessary to detect osteomyelitis, intravenous gadolinium may help identify the full extent of bone and soft tissue infection, distinguish abscesses from focal inflammation, and distinguish devitalized tissue from viable tissue.

Notes

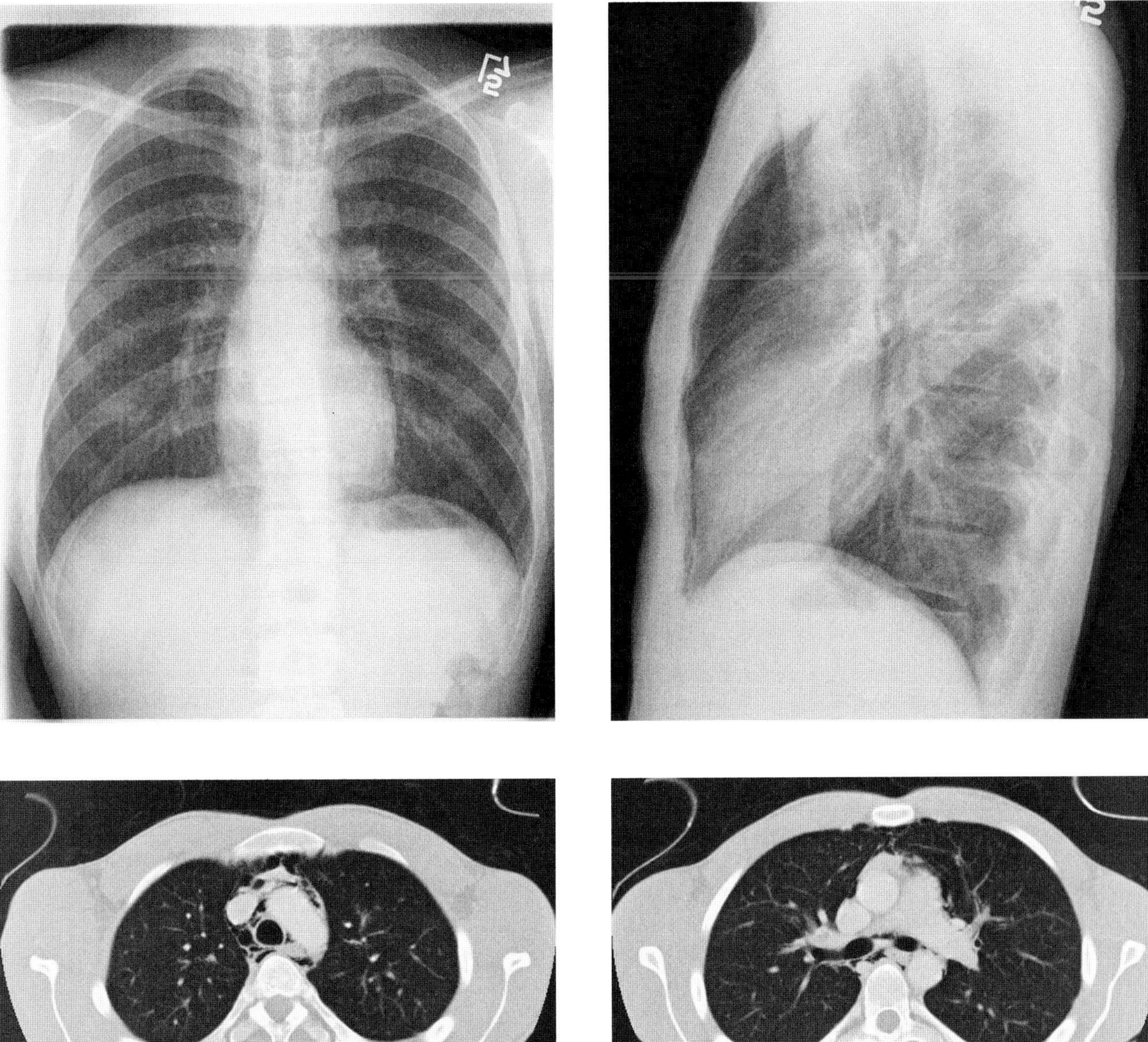

1. What was the most likely clinical presentation of this patient?
2. What is the source of the mediastinal gas in spontaneous pneumomediastinum?
3. Where is pneumomediastinum commonly seen on chest radiographs?
4. What is the clinical management of spontaneous pneumomediastinum?

CASE 184

Spontaneous Pneumomediastinum

1. Chest pain and dyspnea.
2. Increased alveolar pressure causes rupture of alveolar walls and dissection of air through the pulmonary interstitium and into the mediastinum.
3. On posteroanterior chest radiographs, in the region of the aortopulmonary window. On lateral chest radiographs, it is frequently retrosternal.
4. Conservative.

References

Bejvan SM, Godwin JD: Pneumomediastinum: old signs and new signs, *AJR Am J Roentgenol* 166:1041–1048, 1996.

Zylak CM, Standen JR, Barnes GR, Zylak CJ: Pneumomediastinum revisited, *Radiographics* 20:1043–1057, 2000.

Cross-Reference

Emergency Radiology: THE REQUISITES, p 245.

Comment

Pneumomediastinum refers to gas within the mediastinal soft tissues. Typically, the gas results from alveolar, airway, or esophageal injury within the thorax. However, injury to structures in the head, neck, peritoneum, and retroperitoneum may result in gas dissecting into the mediastinum. Pneumomediastinum caused by mediastinal infection with gas-forming organisms is uncommon.

Spontaneous pneumomediastinum results from noniatrogenic and nontraumatic disruption of the alveolar walls secondary to increased alveolar pressure. Air then dissects along the perivascular and peribronchial sheaths into the mediastinum. Causes of spontaneous pneumomediastinum include asthma exacerbation, croup, "crack" cocaine smoking, emesis, parturition, and coughing. Spontaneous pneumomediastinum may also complicate pneumonia, emphysema, and pulmonary fibrosis. It is differentiated from pneumomediastinum that results from esophageal rupture, blunt or penetrating trauma, or iatrogenic injury.

Pneumomediastinum may present with chest pain or dyspnea, although it can be asymptomatic. It may be associated with fever and leukocytosis. Once other sources of pneumomediastinum are excluded, spontaneous pneumomediastinum usually requires little, if any, treatment. Rarely, tension pneumomediastinum (i.e., mediastinal gas under pressure) impairs venous return and results in hypotension that requires mediastinal decompression.

Radiographically, pneumomediastinum is manifested by radiolucent streaks, bubbles, or collections of air that may outline mediastinal structures, such as the diaphragm, aorta, and central pulmonary arteries. Gas may dissect into the lower neck or deep to the parietal pleura at the chest wall or diaphragm. Pneumomediastinum is frequently demonstrated in the region of the aortopulmonary window on posteroanterior chest radiographs. On the lateral chest radiograph, gas is frequently substernal. In children, pneumomediastinum may outline the inferior and medial thymic margins.

Notes

CASE 185

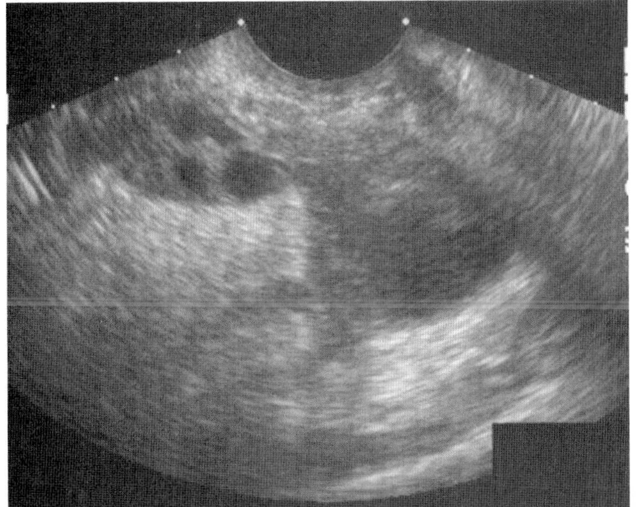

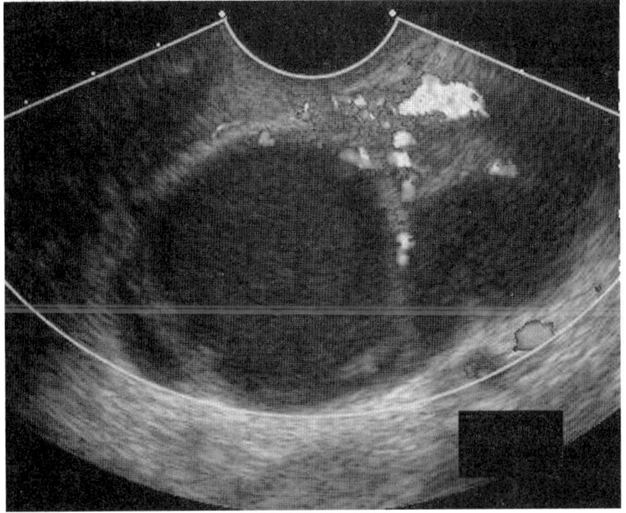

See also Color Plate

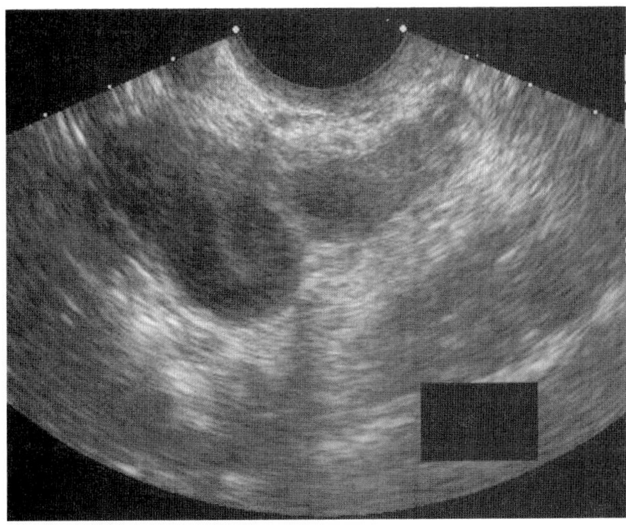

1. What structures are abnormal?
2. What disease causes these abnormalities?
3. Are these abnormalities commonly bilateral?
4. How can these abnormalities be differentiated from a tubo-ovarian abscess with ultrasound?

CASE 185

Pyosalpinx

1. The Fallopian tubes.
2. Pelvic inflammatory disease.
3. Yes.
4. A pyosalpinx typically has a tubular shape, and it is distinct from the ovary.

Reference

Horrow MM: Ultrasound of pelvic inflammatory disease, *Ultrasound Q* 20:171–179, 2004.

Cross-Reference

Emergency Radiology: THE REQUISITES, pp 315–316.

Comment

Pelvic inflammatory disease (PID) is a common cause of acute abdominal and pelvic pain in women. PID is an infection of the upper genital tract secondary to sexually transmitted disease. PID is usually caused by *Chlamydia trachomatis* or *Neisseria gonorrhoeae*, although superinfection with other bacteria is common. The spectrum of disease that makes up PID, encompassed by endometritis, salpingitis, perio-ophoritis, and tubo-ovarian abscess, reflects the ascending spread of the disease. As salpingitis progresses, the Fallopian tubes may occlude and dilate as a consequence of secreted fluid accumulation, thereby leading to pyosalpinx in the acute phase. With disease progression, a tubo-ovarian complex forms as the inflamed ovary and Fallopian tube adhere to one another. More advanced disease results in a tubo-ovarian abscess in which normal ovarian and tubal landmarks are lost. Characteristically, PID is bilateral.

While advanced, severe PID can result in acute morbidity and mortality, the long-term sequelae of severe or untreated disease, including elevated risk of ectopic pregnancy, infertility, and chronic pelvic pain, underscore the importance of early diagnosis and treatment. Clinical features are frequently nonspecific and include fever, abdominal or pelvic pain, vaginal discharge, dyspareunia, nausea, vomiting, adnexal tenderness, and cervical motion tenderness. Occasionally, only vague constitutional symptoms are present. Given the wide clinical spectrum of its presentation, imaging is a frequent adjunct to clinical diagnosis.

Ultrasound is the initial imaging modality used to evaluate suspected cases of PID. Sonographic abnormalities in uncomplicated PID may be subtle. The endometrium and uterus may be indistinct. The Fallopian tubes, rarely seen when normal, may be thickened. Increased echogenicity of pelvic fat reflects inflammatory edema. Free fluid is a frequent, albeit nonspecific, finding, although its absence does not preclude the diagnosis of PID. When there are internal echoes within the fluid, peritoneal pus should be suspected.

On ultrasound, pyosalpinx is characterized by a dilated, thick-walled, fluid-filled Fallopian tube. Characteristically, its shape is tubular. Internal echoes reflect inflammatory debris or pus, and a dependent fluid–debris level may be identified. Superinfection with gas-forming organisms may cause intraluminal gas. Color or power Doppler interrogation may demonstrate increased hyperemia within the Fallopian tube walls. The contralateral Fallopian tube is frequently abnormal as well. Pyosalpinx can be differentiated from tubo-ovarian abscess both through its characteristic shape and by demonstrating it to be distinct from the ovary.

Notes

CASE 186

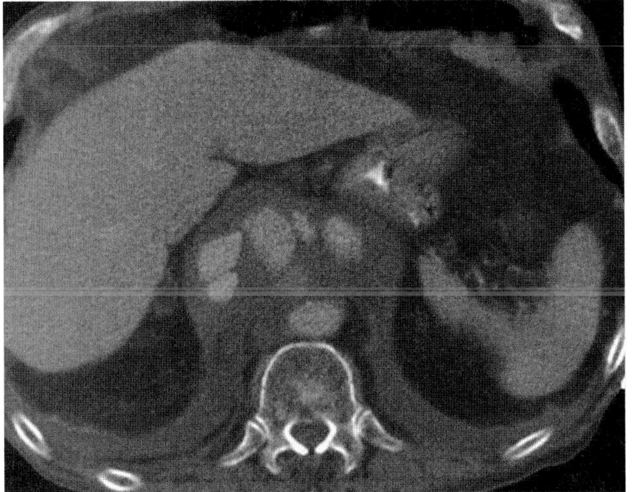

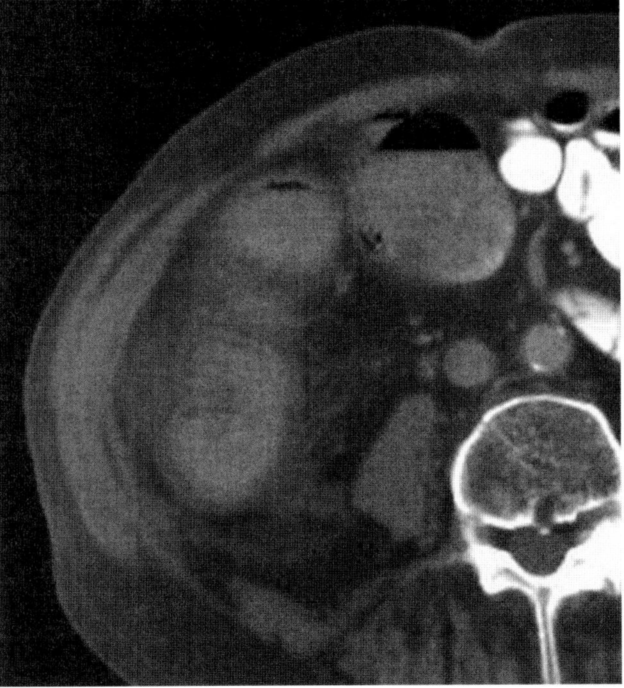

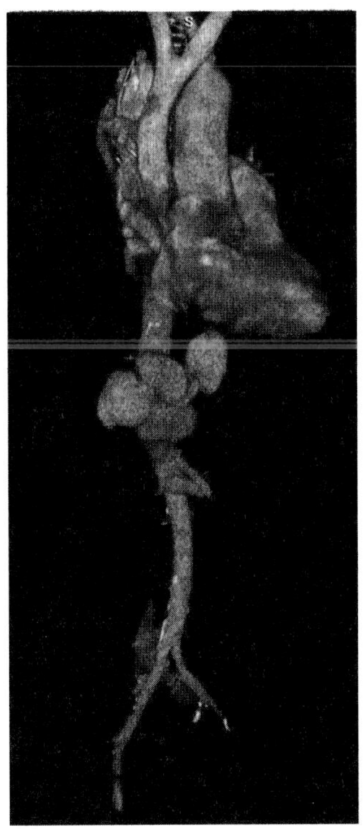

See also Color Plate

1. What is the pathogenesis of this vascular abnormality?
2. What are characteristic imaging features of aortic mycotic aneurysms?
3. What clinical history and laboratory abnormalities may help derive the diagnosis?
4. What is the treatment for aortic mycotic aneurysms?

CASE 186

Ruptured Aortic Mycotic Aneurysm

1. Infection and subsequent weakening of the aortic wall.
2. Saccular morphology with lobulations and periaortic inflammation.
3. Clinical history is frequently noncontributory, although patients may present with fever, abdominal pain, or back pain. There may be an elevated erythrocyte sedimentation rate, leukocytosis, and/or positive blood cultures.
4. Surgery and antibiotics.

Reference

Macedo TA, Stanson AW, Oderich GS, et al: Infected aortic aneurysms: imaging findings, *Radiology* 231: 250–257, 2004. Erratum in *Radiology* 238:1078, 2006.

Cross-Reference

Emergency Radiology: THE REQUISITES, pp 246, 333–334.

Comment

Mycotic aneurysms refer to infected sites of abnormal arterial caliber. Although *mycotic* suggests fungal infection, the term broadly refers to an infected aneurysm resulting from any microorganism. Although rare, the aorta is the most common location for mycotic aneurysms, representing 0.7% to 2.6% of all aortic aneurysms. Pathogenesis includes bacterial seeding of either the vasa vasorum or a damaged artery (e.g., ulcerated atherosclerotic plaque), direct spread from a local infection, or iatrogenic implantation of microorganism during vascular procedures. As the infection and inflammation progress, the arterial wall weakens, and the arterial luminal caliber increases. Mycotic aneurysms rupture with a frequency of 53% to 75%, with ruptured aortic aneurysms carrying a mortality rate of 80% to 90%. The overall mortality rate of aortic mycotic aneurysms is 16% to 67%. Treatment consists of intravenous antibiotics and urgent surgery.

Predisposing factors for development of a mycotic aneurysm include bacterial endocarditis, intravenous drug use, immunocompromise, alcoholism, malignancy, and diabetes mellitus. The diagnosis is frequently delayed due to a nonspecific clinical presentation. Typical symptoms include fever and/or abdominal or back pain, but patients may be asymptomatic. Serum white blood cell count and erythrocyte sedimentation rate can be elevated or normal. Blood cultures may be negative in nearly half of cases.

Computed tomography (CT) may provide the first clues to the appropriate diagnosis. Since vessel caliber may not always be increased based on size, vessel morphology and periarterial inflammatory changes are important clues to the diagnosis. Aortic mycotic aneurysms are saccular in the vast majority of cases, and they are frequently lobulated. CT may demonstrate potentially subtle periaortic inflammatory changes, such as soft tissue mass, fat stranding, or fluid. CT findings indicative of hemorrhage due to rupture may overlap and coexist with those of inflammation, although hemorrhage should show no enhancement if pre- and postintravenous contrast scans are obtained. Rapid enlargement of the aneurysm on serial CT examinations is characteristic of mycotic aortic aneurysms.

Notes

CASE 187

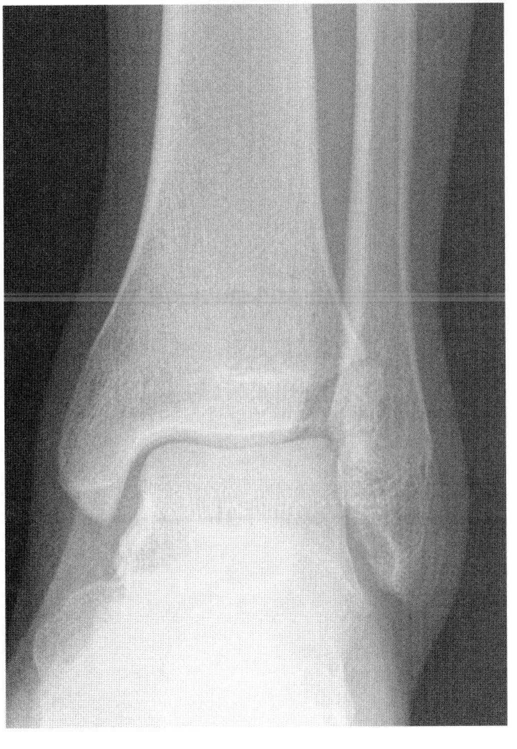

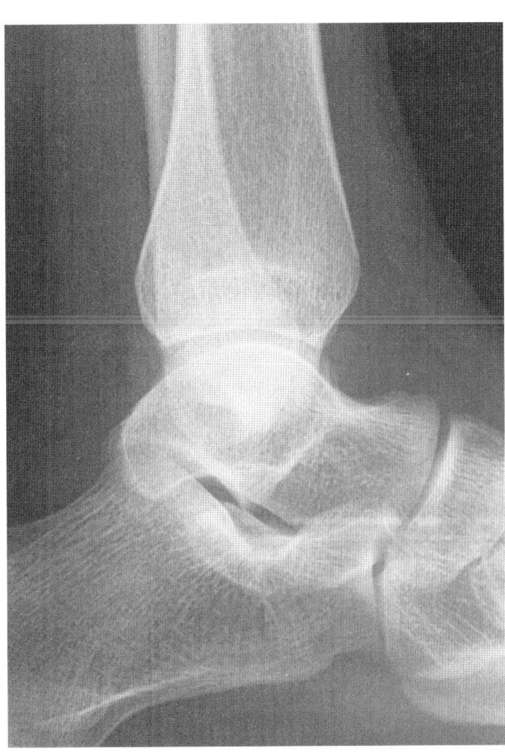

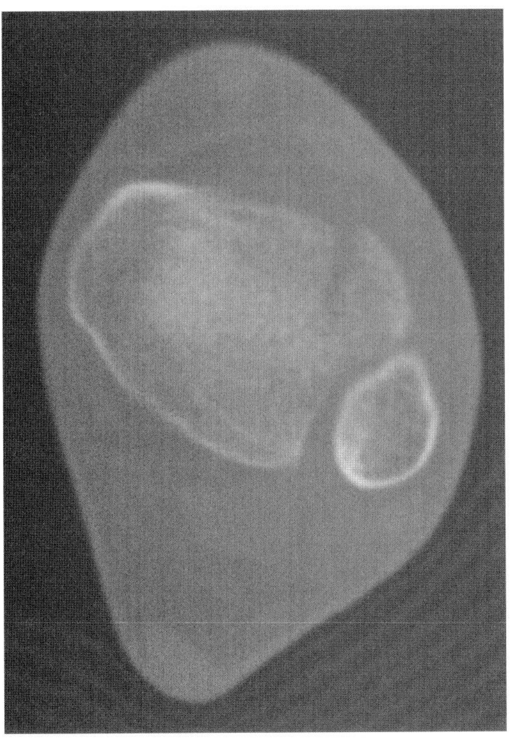

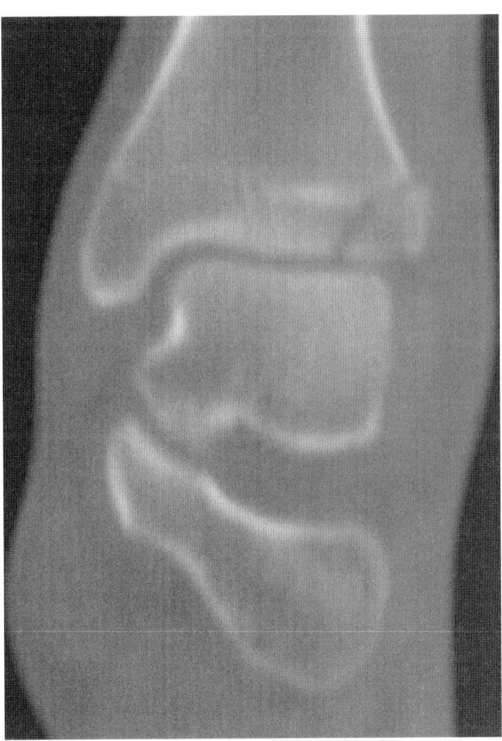

1. What specific anatomic structure is fractured?
2. This injury represents an avulsion fracture of what ligament?
3. Does this injury commonly occur in isolation?
4. What is the role of computed tomography in the management of this fracture?

CASE 187

Tillaux Fracture

1. The tibial anterior tubercle.
2. The anterior inferior tibiofibular ligament insertion.
3. No. A Tillaux fracture is frequently associated with other ankle injuries.
4. Computed tomography better defines the injury, and it differentiates a Tillaux fracture from an avulsion fracture of the tibial posterior tubercle.

References

Protas JM, Kornblatt BA: Fractures of the lateral margin of the distal tibia. The Tillaux fracture, *Radiology* 138:55–57, 1981.

Wilson AJ: The ankle. In Rogers LF, ed: *Radiology of Skeletal Trauma*, 3rd ed, Philadelphia, Churchill Livingstone, 2002, pp 1248–1301.

Comment

An anterior tibial tubercle avulsion at the anterior inferior tibiofibular ligament insertion is known as a Tillaux fracture. Tillaux fractures are caused by external rotation of the foot. While they may occur in isolation, they are frequently associated with more extensive ankle injury. Coexisting ankle injuries generally direct the clinical approach to injury repair, but if they warrant open reduction and internal fixation (ORIF), the Tillaux fracture may require its own fixation screw. In cases of isolated Tillaux fracture, closed reduction is usually adequate. However, if the tibial articular surface is involved or if the fracture fragment is larger than the tibial tubercle, ORIF is generally required.

The fracture is usually identified on anteroposterior and oblique ankle radiographs, although it may not be apparent on a lateral radiograph. As a consequence, differentiation between a Tillaux fracture and an avulsion fracture of the posterior inferior tibiofibular ligament insertion on the posterior tubercle ligament may be difficult or impossible. Computed tomography clearly differentiates the two types of fracture while defining those features of a Tillaux fracture that may indicate surgical fixation.

Notes

CASE 188

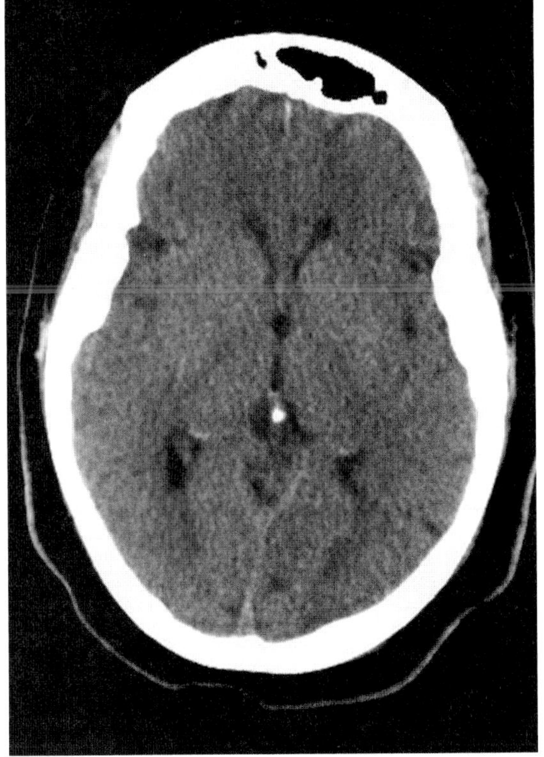

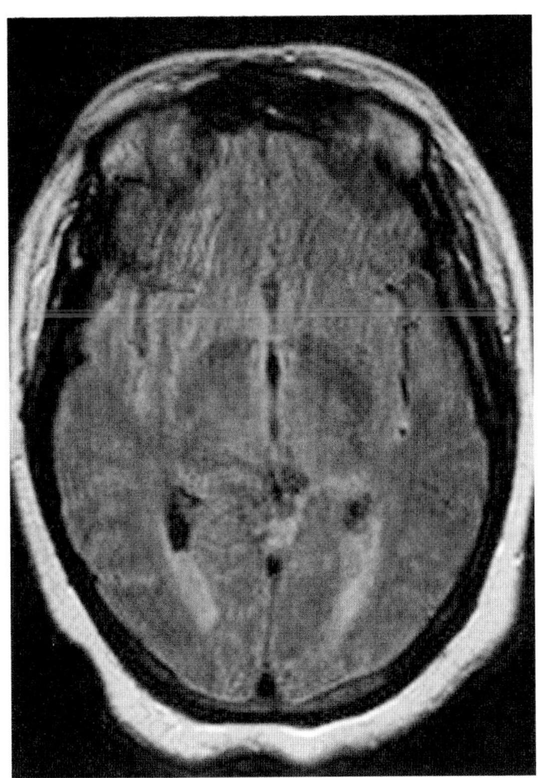

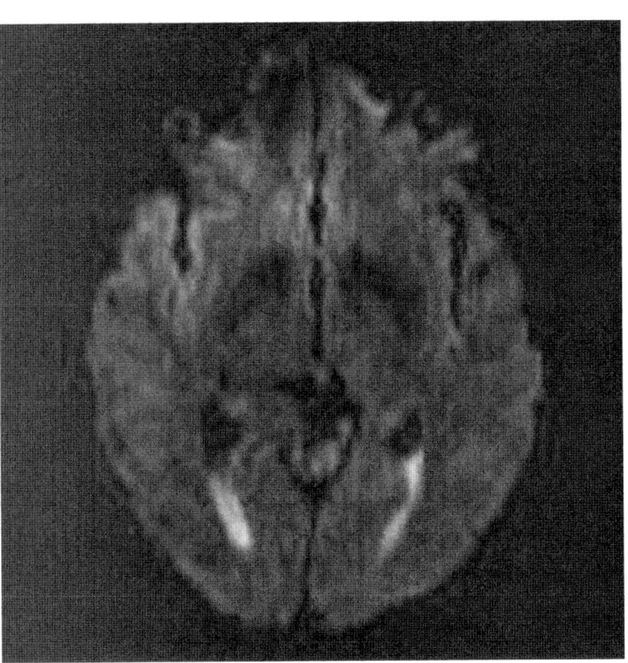

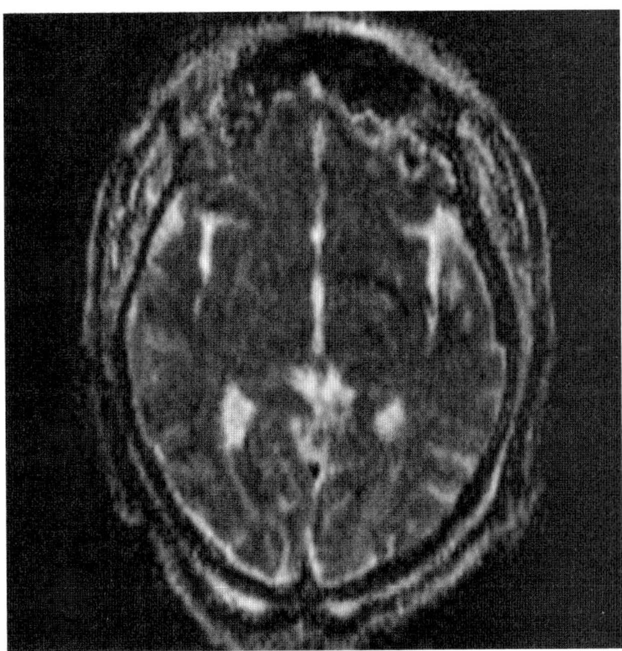

1. What is the diagnosis if this patient presented with a fever and altered level of awareness?
2. What disease does this entity commonly complicate?
3. What magnetic resonance imaging sequences are most sensitive for the intraventricular debris that is characteristic of this disease?
4. What are conditions that predispose to this disease?

CASE 188

Ventriculitis

1. Ventriculitis.
2. Meningitis.
3. Diffusion-weighted and fluid attenuated inversion recovery (FLAIR) sequences.
4. Immunosuppression, alcoholism, cirrhosis, diabetes mellitus, and recent neurosurgical procedure.

References

Fujikawa A, Tsuchiya K, Honya K, Nitatori T: Comparison of MRI sequences to detect ventriculitis, *AJR Am J Roentgenol* 187:1048–1053, 2006.

Fukui MB, Williams RL, Mudigonda S: CT and MR imaging features of pyogenic ventriculitis, *AJNR Am J Neuroradiol* 22:1510–1516, 2001.

Cross-Reference

Emergency Radiology: THE REQUISITES, p 27.

Comment

In adults, ventriculitis is an uncommon intracranial infection, although it is a common complication of meningitis in infants. It is a potential cause of therapeutic failure in the treatment of meningitis. Ventriculitis is commonly caused by gram-negative organisms. Accordingly, the risk factors for ventriculitis include those for gram-negative meningitis: immunosuppression, alcoholism, cirrhosis, diabetes mellitus, and recent neurosurgical procedure. Other risk factors for ventriculitis include cerebrospinal fluid leak and head trauma.

Patients with ventriculitis may present similarly to uncomplicated meningitis with headache, fever, photophobia, and/or nuchal rigidity. However, those with ventriculitis may present with nonspecific neurologic symptoms, and fever may be absent.

Both computed tomography and magnetic resonance imaging (MRI) may demonstrate debris–fluid levels that are usually located in the occipital horns and ventricular atria, although debris can be seen in the fourth ventricle. Debris consists of pus and necrotic ependyma. With MRI, diffusion-weighted images and, to a lesser extent, FLAIR images demonstrate the debris with greatest sensitivity. Occasionally, debris associated with postoperative intraventricular hemorrhage and ventriculitis can be difficult to differentiate, but irregular debris–fluid levels and septations favor ventriculitis.

Hydrocephalus frequently accompanies ventriculitis. FLAIR MRI may demonstrate associated subependymal periventricular high-signal abnormalities, although these may also reflect preexisting abnormalities or transependymal spread of cerebrospinal fluid if there is hydrocephalus. Postcontrast T1-weighted MRI may demonstrate ependymal and/or subependymal enhancement. An infrequent finding with ventriculitis is choroid plexitis, which is manifested by an enlarged, poorly defined, enhancing choroid plexus.

Notes

CASE 189

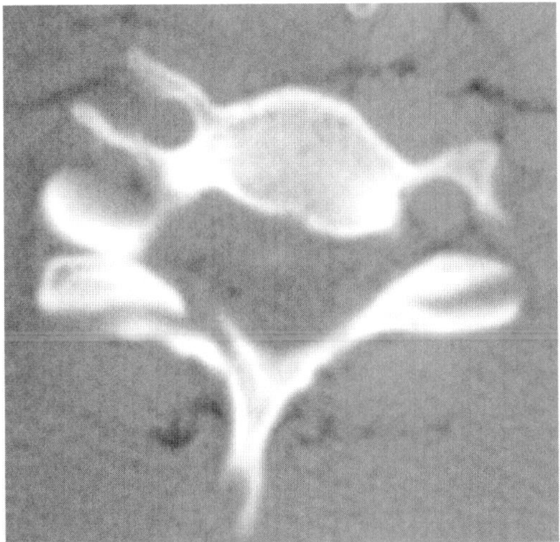

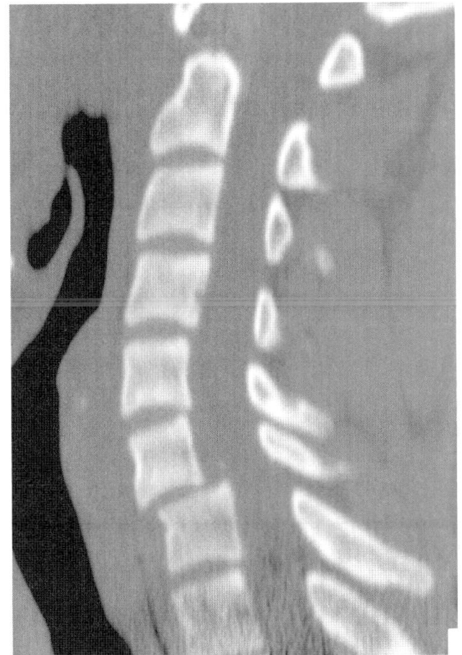

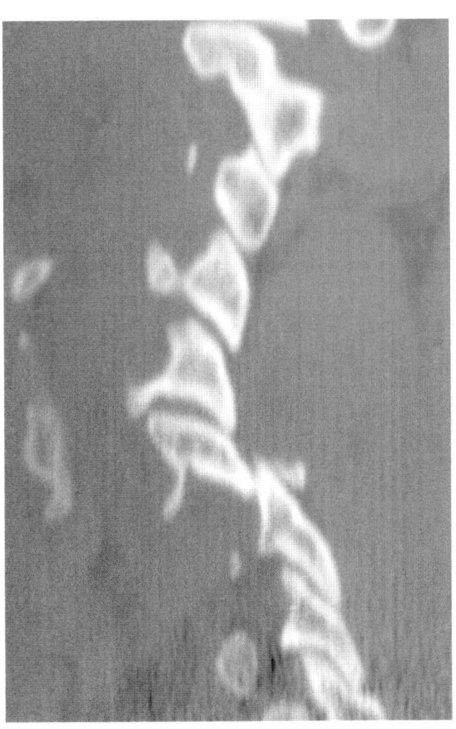

You are shown images of a patient with neck pain following a motor vehicle collision.

1. What is the diagnosis?
2. What are the predominant forces that produce this injury?
3. How does the anterior subluxation of this injury differ from subluxation seen in bilateral facet dislocation?
4. True or false: Facet fractures are commonly seen in this injury.

CASE 189

Unilateral Facet Fracture Dislocation

1. Unilateral facet fracture dislocation.
2. Hyperflexion with simultaneous rotation.
3. The anterior subluxation is less than 50% of the anteroposterior vertebral body width in patients with unilateral facet fracture dislocation and greater than 50% of the anteroposterior vertebral body width in patients with bilateral facet dislocation.
4. True.

References

Lingawi SS: The naked facet sign, *Radiology* 219: 366–367, 2001.

Shanmuganathan K, Mirvis SE, Levine AM: Rotational injury of cervical facets: CT analysis of fracture patterns with implications for management and neurologic outcome, *AJR Am J Roentgenol* 163:1165–1169, 1994.

Cross-Reference

Emergency Radiology: THE REQUISITES, p 220.

Comment

Cervical rotational facet injury (RFI) is a term used to describe unilateral injuries occurring to the facets and articulations. This term encompasses both pure unilateral facet subluxation and dislocation with or without facet fractures. Pure dislocation is seen in 27% of patients with RFI. Simultaneous hyperflexion and rotation produce these injuries.

Radiographic findings include anterior subluxation of less than half the anteroposterior diameter of the vertebral body, abrupt decrease in the laminar space between the posterior surface of the articular masses and spinolaminar line, fracture fragments seen adjacent to the margins of the articular processes, lack of normal alignment of the articular masses and facet joins at the level of injury, and widening of the interspinous and interlaminar distances at the level of injury.

Axial, sagittal, and coronal reformatted computed tomography (CT) images are all valuable to demonstrate the fractures and plan surgical fixation. Facet fractures are seen in 73% of patients with RFI with subluxation or dislocation. Most facet fractures are oriented vertically. Contralateral facet injuries are seen in up to 50% of patients. CT may demonstrate an associated fracture of the posterior inferior aspect of the rotated vertebra. This avulsion fracture occurs adjacent to the intervertebral disc at the site of attachment of the posterior longitudinal ligament to the vertebral body.

Magnetic resonance imaging helps to demonstrate injury to ligaments, intervertebral disc, cord, nerve roots, and carotid and vertebral arteries. Objective neurological deficit related to the RFI may be seen in 73% of patients. Cord injuries are significantly more commonly seen in patients with pure unilateral facet dislocation compared with patients with facet fracture with subluxation or dislocation.

Notes

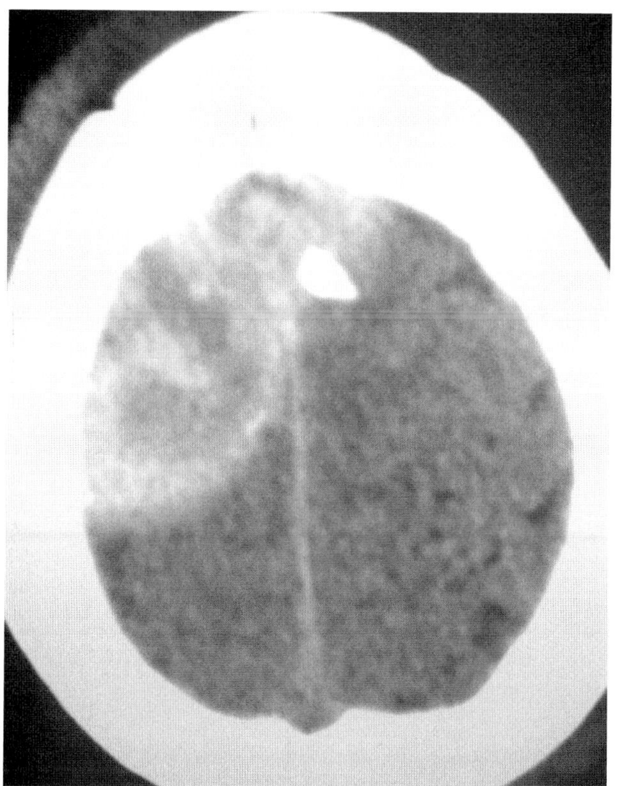

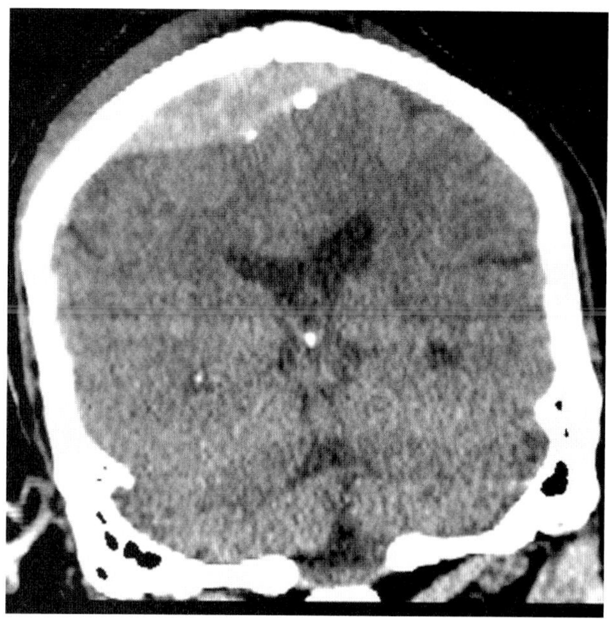

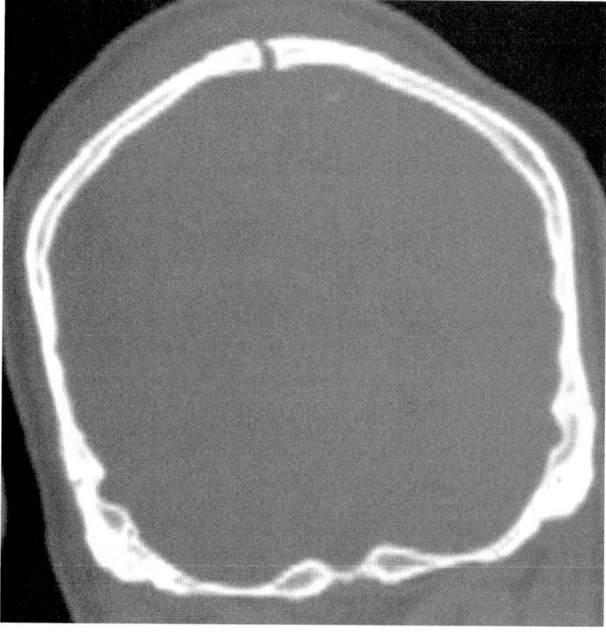

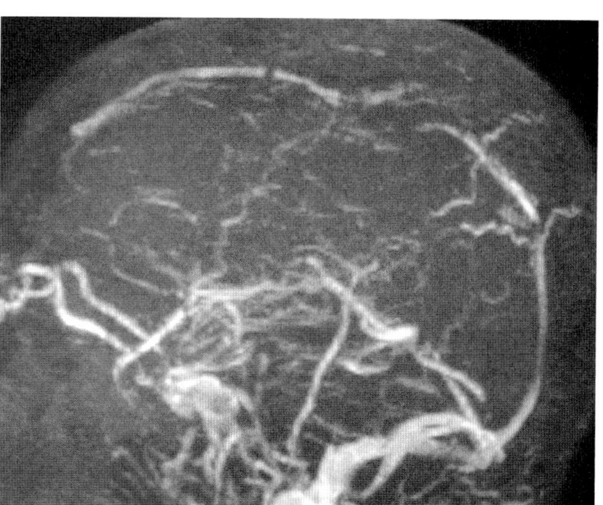

You are shown images of a fall on the vertex of the head.

1. What are the computed tomography and magnetic resonance imaging findings?
2. What is the diagnosis?
3. What is the anatomic location of the bleed?
4. What are three sources of this type of hemorrhage?

CASE 190

Venous Epidural Hematoma

1. A lentiform extra-axial bleed is seen crossing the midline with mass effect on the frontal lobes bilaterally. The calcification in the dura is displaced inferiorly. Diastasis of the sagittal suture is also seen. The magnetic resonance venogram shows loss of high signal in a segment of the superior sagittal sinus in keeping with an injury.
2. Venous epidural hematoma.
3. Bleeding occurs between the inner table of calvarium and periosteal dura.
4. Meningeal vessels, diploic veins, or dural sinus.

References

Gean AD: Extra-axial collections. In Gean AD: *Imaging of Head Trauma*, New York, Raven Press, 1994, pp 75–146.

Han JS, Kaufman B, Alfidi RJ, et al: Head trauma evaluated by magnetic resonance and computed tomography: a comparison, *Radiology* 150:71–77, 1984.

Cross-Reference

Emergency Radiology: THE REQUISITES, p 2.

Comment

Epidural hematoma (EDH) is a relatively uncommon injury, occurring in 0.2% to 5% of patients with head injury. The bleeding occurs between the inner table of the calvarium and the periosteal dura. The two layers of the dura are the outer periosteal dura and the inner meningeal dura. The two layers are tightly adherent to each other and to the calvarium. The EDH forcefully strips the periosteal dura from the inner table of the skull. The source of bleeding may be arterial or venous in origin and result from injury to the meningeal vessels, diploic veins, or dural sinus. Arterial bleeding usually results in rapid expansion of the EDH.

On computed tomography (CT) and magnetic resonance imaging (MRI), EDHs are well-defined, biconvex extra-axial collections, usually confined by the sutures of the skull. Since the anatomical location of the bleeding is outside the outer dura the collections may extend across the midline, displacing the sagittal sinus inferiorly. This also allows the bleeding to extend superiorly from the posterior cranial fossa into the middle cranial fossa. The margins are less well defined on axial CT images when the EDH is seen over the vertex. An overlying fracture is seen on CT in almost all adult cases (85% to 95%). The most common location is the temporoparietal region because the majority of EDHs result from injury to the middle meningeal artery. Other sites include the posterior cranial fossa and the frontal, occipital, and clival regions. The majority of the extra-axial collections seen in the posterior cranial fossa are venous EDHs. The bleeding usually results from an injury to the dural sinus. A common site for supratentorial venous EDH is along the greater wing of the sphenoid bone in the anterior middle cranial fossa. The bleeding occurs from the sphenoparietal sinus with an associated fracture of the greater wing of sphenoid bone.

On CT, differentiation of an EDH from a subdural hematoma (SDH) is not always possible. A combined EDH and SDH may coexist in 20% of patients. The ability to visualize the dura as a thin linear low signal intensity between the bleed and brain parenchyma on MRI helps to differentiate EDH from SDH.

The mortality rate is about 5% to 8% for surgically treated EDH. Immediate evacuation of an EDH causing mass effect on brain parenchyma results in reestablishing the perfusion to the underlying parenchyma and return of the ventricular system to a normal position. The prognosis usually depends on the extent of underlying cerebral injury and size of the EDH.

Notes

CASE 191

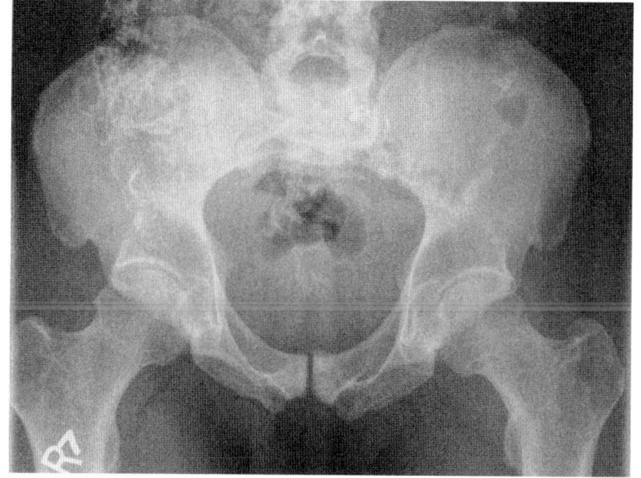

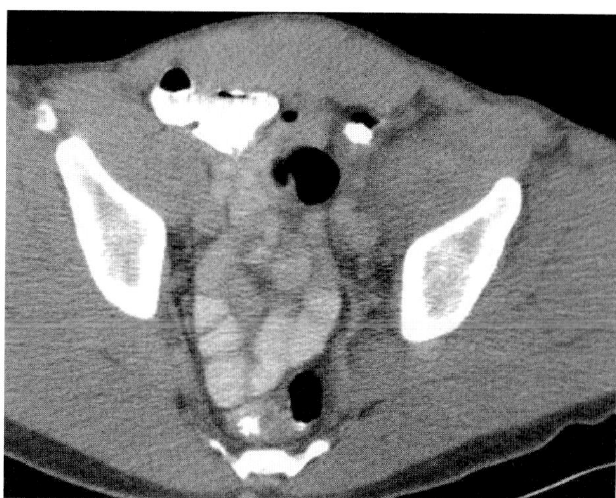

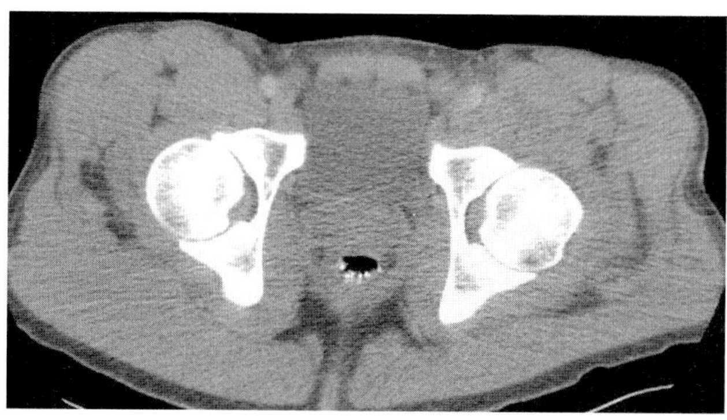

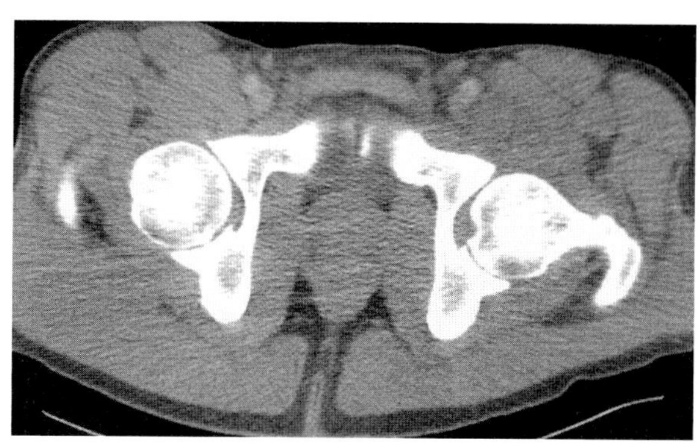

You are shown images of a 49-year-old man who presented with left-sided pelvic pain exacerbated by exercise.

1. What are the computed tomography findings?
2. What is the best diagnosis?
3. What diagnostic procedure should be performed to confirm the diagnosis?
4. Give three contrast-enhanced magnetic resonance findings that have a high correlation with this entity.

CASE 191

Septic Arthritis

1. A small left hip joint effusion; edema in the soft tissues causing infiltration of fat lateral to left hip, left pelvic wall, and groin; and edematous left iliopsoas and obturator internus muscles.
2. Septic arthritis.
3. Arthrocentesis of left hip joint to obtain fluid for culture.
4. Magnetic resonance findings strongly correlated to septic arthritis include edema in the perisynovial soft tissues, synovial enhancement, and joint effusion.

References

Karchevsky M, Schweitzer ME, Morrison WB, et al: MRI findings of septic arthritis and associated osteomyelitis in adults, *AJR Am J Roentgenol* 182:119–122, 2004.

Restrepo CS, Lemos DF, Gordillo H, et al: Imaging findings in musculoskeletal complications of AIDS, *Radiographics* 24:1029–1049, 2004.

Cross-Reference

Emergency Radiology: THE REQUISITES, pp 176, 177.

Comment

Septic arthritis is a common disease most frequently seen in intravenous drug abusers, diabetics, and immunosuppressed patients. Initial clinical findings may be nonspecific. Most patients present with nonspecific signs and symptoms including fever, pain, erythema, soft tissue swelling, and loss of range of motion of the affected joint.

Joint infection may result from hematogenous spread or extend directly from adjacent infected soft tissue or bone. Early diagnosis and treatment are very important for optimal outcome. Delay in diagnosis or treatment may result in complications, including destruction of the articular cartilage and bone, osteonecrosis, osteomyelitis, secondary osteoarthritis, and joint ankylosis. No current imaging option can definitively diagnose or exclude septic arthritis. Aspiration and culture of the joint fluid from the affected joint is mandatory to make a definitive diagnosis while determining the causative microorganism and its sensitivity to antibiotic therapy.

Radiographic and computed tomography (CT) soft tissue and osseous changes may be absent or subtle in early septic arthritis. Nonspecific findings include bone erosion, joint effusion, osteopenia, joint space narrowing, and periarticular soft tissue and muscle edema on both radiographs and CT.

Magnetic resonance imaging (MRI) with intravenous contrast material is sensitive to signs of septic arthritis within the infected joint, as well as the periarticular bone marrow and soft tissues. MRI findings have been reported to be abnormal as early as 24 hours after infection. Frequently observed findings on contrast-enhanced MRI include synovial enhancement, periarticular soft tissue edema, joint effusion, and either synovial or joint fluid outpouching. Less commonly observed findings include synovial thickening and enhancement of the joint fluid. In immunocompromised patients, extension of the infection into adjacent bursa may be demonstrated. Patients with concomitant local extension of infection into the bone will have diffuse marrow edema seen on T1-weighted or fat-suppressed inversion recovery (STIR) images, although edema can also be a reaction to adjacent soft tissue inflammation rather than a consequence of osteomyelitis.

Notes

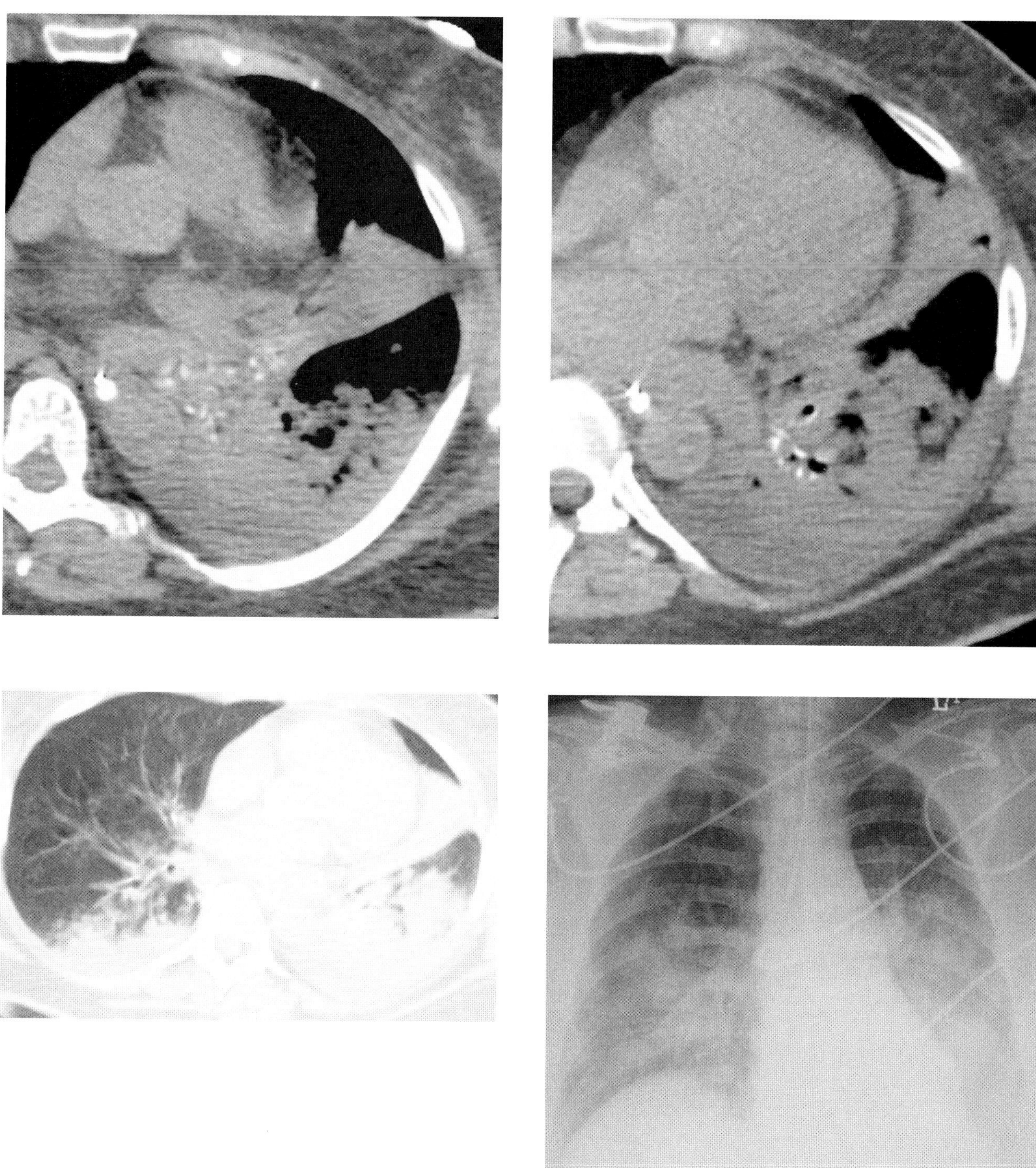

You are shown multidetector computed tomography images obtained after administration of oral contrast material.

1. What is the high attenuation material seen in the left lower lobe?
2. What is the best diagnosis?
3. What are the most common lobes involved by this entity?
4. What is Mendelson's syndrome?

CASE 192

Aspirated Pneumonia

1. Aspirated oral contrast material.
2. Aspiration pneumonia.
3. The superior segments of the lower lobes and posterior segments of the upper lobes.
4. Acute aspiration of massive amount of low pH gastric acid.

References

Franquet T, Giménez A, Rosón N, et al: Aspiration diseases: findings, pitfalls, and differential diagnosis, *Radiographics* 20:673–685, 2000.

Marom EM, McAdams HP, Erasmus JJ, et al: The many faces of pulmonary aspiration, *AJR Am J Roentgenol* 172:121–128, 1999.

Comment

Solid or liquid material may be aspirated into the tracheobronchial tree and lungs in a variety of conditions. The clinical presentation and pathological manifestations seen depend on both the amount and nature of the substance aspirated plus the tonicity of the process. In adults, alcoholism is the most common predisposing factor for pulmonary aspiration. Other conditions that predispose to aspiration include loss of consciousness, general anesthesia in nonfasting patients, swallowing disorders, and structural abnormalities of the pharynx, esophagus, or trachea. Patients with poor oral hygiene, with prolonged hospitalization, or requiring mechanical ventilation are at risk of aspirating infected oral or gastric contents. Aspiration of infected material may cause pneumonia due to anaerobic organisms, lung abscess, or empyema.

Multidetector computed tomography (MDCT) is much more sensitive than radiographs in demonstrating pulmonary manifestations of aspiration pneumonia. Both the radiographic and CT manifestations of aspiration may be often nonspecific, and the diagnosis may be difficult because the patient may not have a known predisposing risk factor. Imaging abnormalities can mimic other conditions, including tuberculosis, pulmonary edema, and lung cancer. The most common finding is patchy pulmonary opacities seen in the dependent aspects of the lungs, most commonly the posterior segments of the upper lobes and superior segments of the lower lobes. These opacities represent areas of atelectasis seen due to obstruction of the distal airways by the aspirated material. The posterior upper lobes and superior segments of the lower lobes are the most frequent sites of these abnormalities. Areas of segmental or lobar hyperinflation or atelectasis may be seen following aspiration of a foreign body.

Mendelson's syndrome results from massive aspiration of low pH gastric fluid throughout the bronchial tree with resulting bronchiolitis, chemical pneumonitis, and hemorrhagic pulmonary edema. Initially described as a complication of pregnancy, it can also be seen following general anesthesia for emergency surgery, alcoholic stupor, and following acute trauma. The classic radiographic findings include bilateral symmetrical homogeneous or heterogeneous airspace disease mimicking pulmonary edema that can progress to acute respiratory distress syndrome.

Aspiration of small quantities of mineral oil occurs over a chronic period of time in patients using nasal drops or ingestion of mineral oil for constipation. Chronic segmental or lobar consolidation, multifocal scattered consolidation, and focal masses resembling a neoplasm may be seen in these patients. Aspiration of large quantities of petroleum or paraffin may lead to the rare form of acute exogenous lipoid pneumonia. This may be seen in children from accidental poisoning or fire eaters. The characteristic postinflammatory thin wall pneumatoceles seen may mimic lesion seen after staphylococcal pneumonia.

Notes

CASE 193

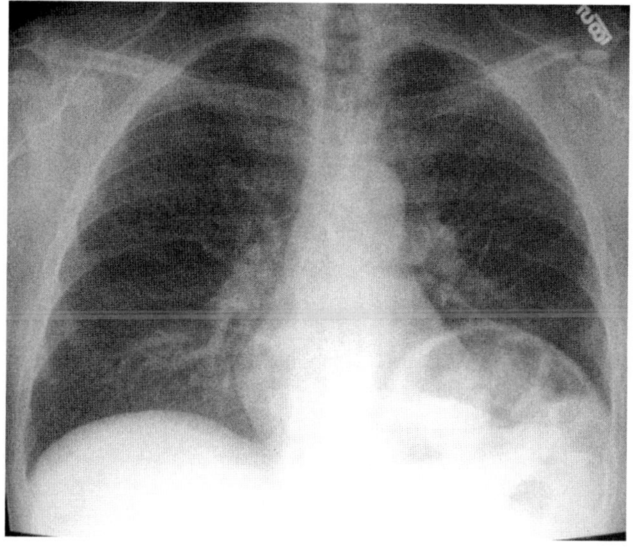

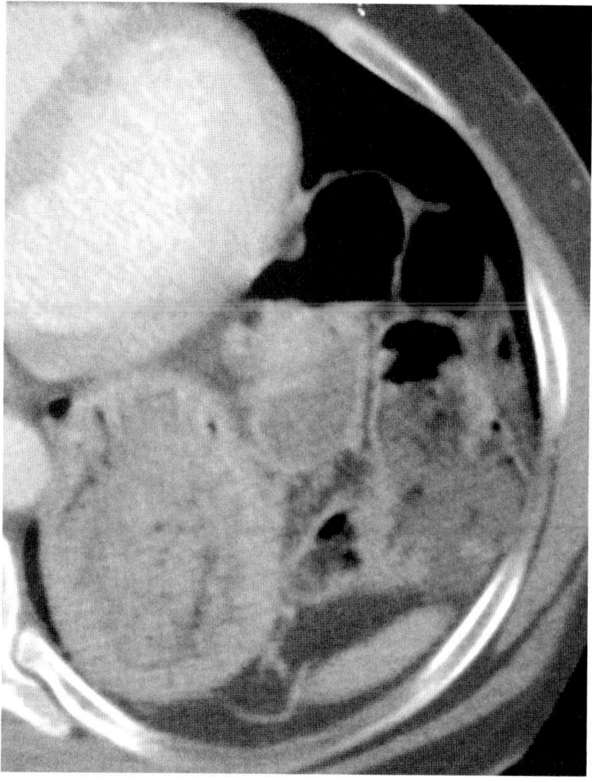

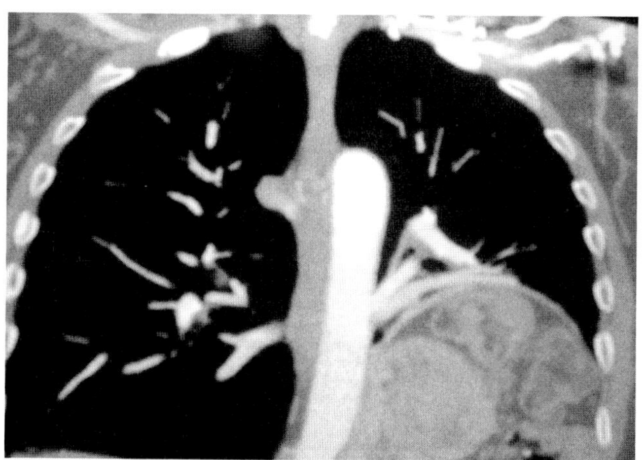

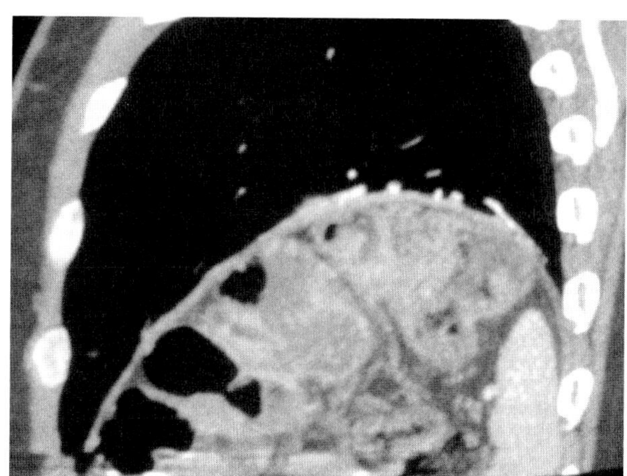

You are shown images of a patient with left-sided chest pain after blunt chest trauma.

1. What are the multidetector computed tomography findings?
2. What is the best diagnosis?
3. What is the differential diagnosis?
4. What is the "sniff" test?

CASE 193

Complete Eventration of the Hemidiaphragm

1. Elevation of the left hemidiaphragm, a thin intact left hemidiaphragm, and abdominal contents confined to the subphrenic space.
2. Complete eventration of left hemidiaphragm.
3. Paralysis of the left hemidiaphragm.
4. Fluoroscopically observe the diaphragm for motion while the patient "sniffs." Paradoxical motion will be seen in patients with paralysis or eventration of the diaphragm.

References

Hesselink JR, Chung KJ, Peters ME, et al: Congenital partial eventration of the left diaphragm, *AJR Am J Roentgenol* 131:417–419, 1978.

Iochum S, Ludig T, Walter F, et al: Imaging of diaphragmatic injury: a diagnostic challenge? *Radiographics* 22(Suppl):S103–S116, 2002.

Comment

The diaphragm is a musculotendinous sheet separating the thoracic and abdominal cavities. It is formed by three groups of muscles arising from the xiphoid process, from the 7th rib to the 12th rib, from the lateral margins of the upper three lumbar vertebral bodies on the right, and from the lateral margins of the upper two lumbar vertebral bodies on the left. The fibers converge centrally and form the central tendon.

Eventration of the diaphragm is a congenital abnormality that may involve part or all of either one or both hemidiaphragms. While failure of proper development of the membranous diaphragm may result in a diaphragmatic hernia, incomplete muscularization of the membranous diaphragm results in eventration. Failure of muscular development leads to a diaphragm consisting of a thin membranous sheet attaching to the points of origin, especially the seventh to twelve ribs. Partial eventration typically involves the anteromedial aspect of the right hemidiaphragm, and total eventration is much more common on the left side. Partial eventration is more common than total eventration.

Eventration of the diaphragm is usually asymptomatic, and it is typically recognized as an incidental finding on chest radiographs or computed tomography scans. In the emergency department, it is usually significant when the radiologist tries to differentiate it from a diaphragmatic rupture or hernia.

On chest radiographs, the dome of the right hemidiaphragm is half an interspace higher than the dome of the left hemidiaphragm. In about 9% of normal subjects the heights may be similar or the left diaphragm dome may be higher than the right.

The dome of the involved hemidiaphragm is noted to be in an abnormally high position. The margins of adjacent mediastinal structures may be obscured in total eventration of the diaphragm. A diminished liver shadow and a transversely oriented stomach may be seen due to the abnormal position of the liver in right-sided total eventrations. Sagittal and coronal reformatted multidetector CT images may demonstrate an intact thin membranous diaphragm seen above the abdominal content that is seen high within the thoracic cavity.

In contrast to patients with diaphragmatic eventration, patients with diaphragmatic paralysis frequently complain of exertional dyspnea, their vital capacity and total lung capacity are decreased by 25% to 50%, and idiopathic paralysis of the diaphragm almost exclusively occurs on the right side. In some cases it may be difficult or impossible to clinically differentiate eventration from a paralysis of the diaphragm. Fluoroscopy may be performed to demonstrate paradoxical motion of the involved hemidiaphragm during normal respiration or following an augmented load (sniffing).

Notes

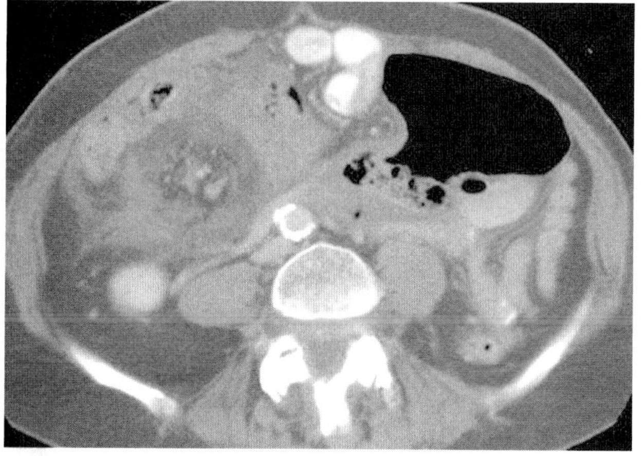

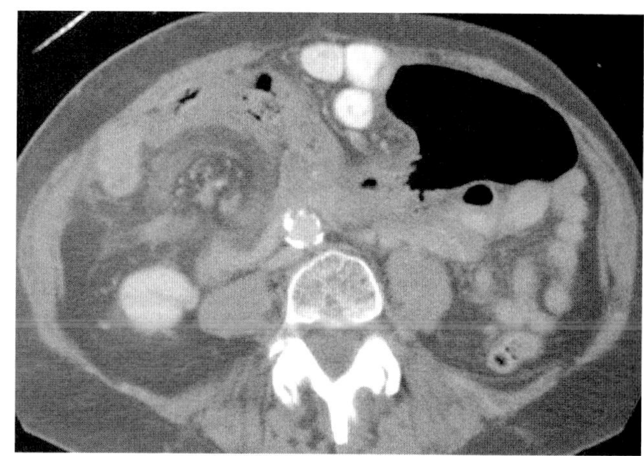

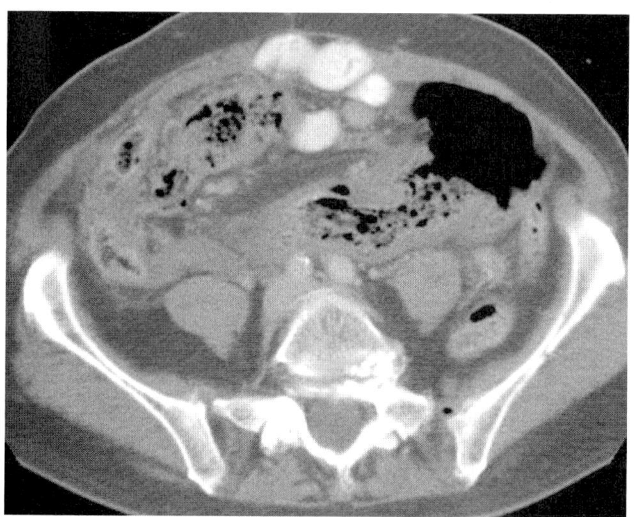

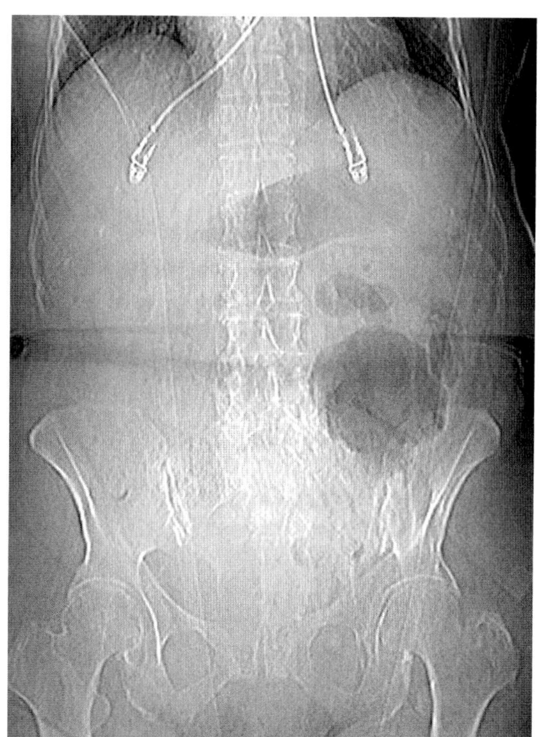

An 83-year-old woman presented with abdominal pain and guarding on clinical examination.

1. What are the multidetector computed tomography findings?
2. What are the three types of cecal volvulus?
3. What type of cecal volvulus is this?
4. Name three types of volvulus in which the computed tomography "whirl" sign can be seen.

CASE 194

Cecal Bascule

1. The cecum is displaced from the right iliac fossa into the mid and left lower abdomen, normal descending colon caliber, a mesenteric "whirl" sign in right mid abdomen, free intraperitoneal fluid, infiltration of the mesenteric fat.
2. Longitudinal cecal volvulus, oblique cecal volvulus, and cecal bascule.
3. Cecal bascule.
4. Midgut, sigmoid, cecal volvulus.

References

Bobroff LM, Messinger NH, Subbarao K, et al: The cecal bascule, *AJR Am J Roentgenol* 115:249–252, 1972.

Moore CJ, Corl FM, Fishman EK: CT of cecal volvulus: unraveling the image, *AJR Am J Roentgenol* 177: 95–98, 2001.

Comment

Cecal volvulus accounts for 11% of all intestinal volvuli. During embryogenesis the cecum assumes its normal anatomic location by rotating and descending caudally from the hepatic flexure into the right iliac fossa. Congenital failure of proper fixation of the cecum to the posterior abdominal wall allows a free and mobile proximal colon. Adhesions, masses, or fibrosis from calcified lymph nodes can act as a point of fixation and serve as an axis of rotation. Predisposing factors for volvulus include prior abdominal surgery, pelvic masses, colonic atonia, visceroptosis, and violent coughing.

Three types of cecal volvulus have been described in the literature. Longitudinal or axial volvulus occurs when the cecum twists clockwise or counterclockwise around its long axis with the distended cecum usually located in the right lower quadrant. In the oblique or loop type of volvulus, both the cecum and terminal ileum twist and invert, and the cecum occupies the left upper quadrant. Cecal bascule occurs when the free cecum folds upon itself without any torsion and forms an inflammatory adhesion to the anterior wall of the ascending colon thereby leading to a "flap valve" obstruction, and presence of a competent ileocecal valve prevents retrograde decompression of the cecum. With cecal bascule, the dilated cecum is usually located in the mid abdomen.

On abdominal radiographs the cecum is disproportionately distended compared with the rest of the colon. With oblique volvulus, the dilated cecum resembles a coffee bean.

Computed tomography (CT) also demonstrates a markedly distended cecum. Where the two limbs of the obstructed cecum converge and taper toward the point of torsion, CT may demonstrate the "beak" sign. The "whirl" sign, a specific CT finding of volvulus that has been described in midgut, cecal, and sigmoid volvulus, is formed by the twisted collapsed loops of bowel. The center of the whirl is formed by mesenteric fat and engorged mesenteric vessels arising from the twisted bowel.

Surgery is the treatment of choice for patients with cecal volvulus. In uncomplicated patients, cecopexy is performed to prevent recurrence of the volvulus. Reduction rates using colonoscopy are low in patients with cecal volvulus in contrast to those with sigmoid volvulus.

Notes

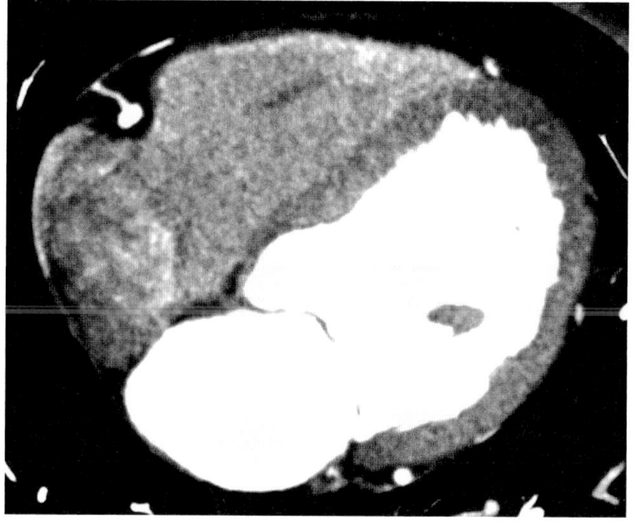

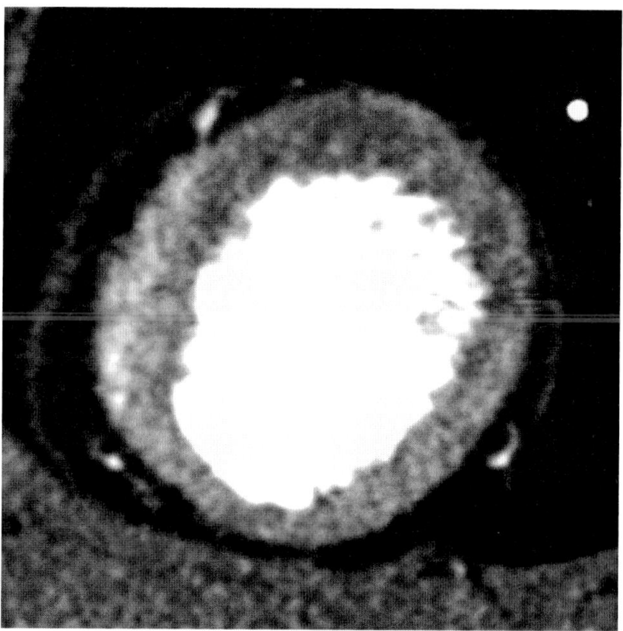

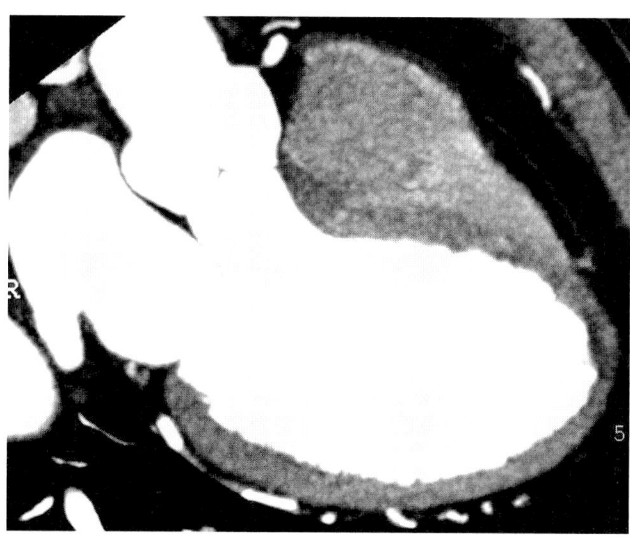

Images provided by Ethan Halprin, MD, Philadelphia, PA.

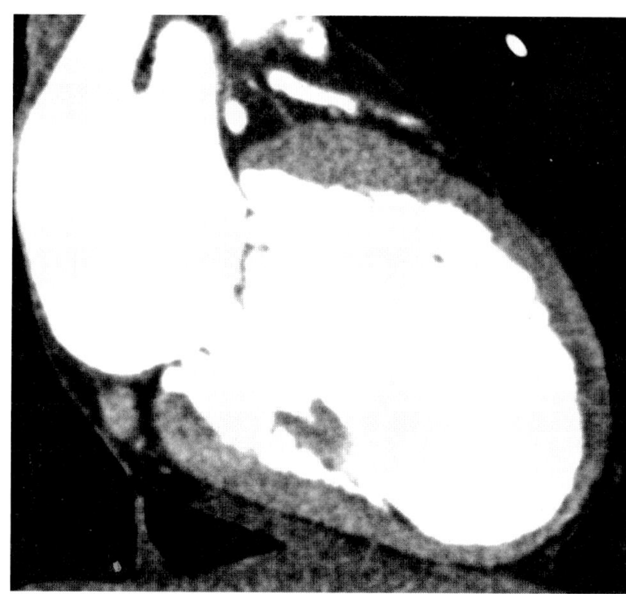

1. What is the best diagnosis in this patient presenting with acute left-sided chest pain?
2. What abnormality suggests the diagnosis?
3. What would be the appearance of this abnormality on delayed (10 minutes post injection of intravenous contrast) imaging?
4. What is the differential diagnosis?

CASE 195

Acute Myocardial Infarction

1. Acute myocardial infarction.
2. A low attenuation area is seen in the apical and inferior septal region.
3. The infarction would appear as an area of hyperenhancement.
4. Fatty degeneration in an old myocardial infarction and left ventricular mural thrombus.

References

Gerber BL, Belge B, Legros GJ, et al: Characterization of acute and chronic myocardial infarcts by multidetector computed tomography comparison with contrast-enhanced magnetic resonance, *Circulation* 113: 823–833, 2006.

White CS, Kuo D: Chest pain in the emergency department: role of multidetector CT, *Radiology* 245: 672–681, 2007.

Cross-Reference

Emergency Radiology: THE REQUISITES, pp 261, 262.

Comment

In the emergency department, acute chest pain is a common (5% of all emergency room visits) and important diagnostic challenge. A small but significant number of patients (2%) with myocardial infarction are discharged inappropriately from the emergency department. To avoid this, a large number of patients with no serious cause for chest pain are admitted to hospital for observation and further workup.

The initial assessment of chest pain in the emergency department should include a history, physical examination, electrocardiography (EKG), and cardiac enzymes. In the initial few hours following onset of chest pain, the EKG and cardiac enzyme levels are frequently normal. In order to both streamline the diagnostic workup and decrease the average cost per patient, some centers use multidetector computed tomography (MDCT) to evaluate patients with low to intermediate risk for acute coronary syndrome (includes acute myocardial infarction, nontransmural infarction, and unstable angina).

Typically two distinct enhancement patterns are seen in acute myocardial infarction on contrast enhanced MDCT. In the early phase (immediately following injection of contrast material), the infarction is seen as an area of hypoattenuation that results from the phenomenon of "no-reflow" whereby the microvascular obstruction reduces the amount of contrast delivered to the infarct. Due to increased redistribution and poor washout of contrast from the infarct, on delayed imaging (10 to 15 minutes after contrast material) both acute and chronic myocardial infarctions are seen as hyperattenuating areas. Using these enhancement patterns, two-phase MDCT can help to assess myocardial viability and characterize acute and chronic infarctions.

Fatty degeneration in an old myocardial infarction and mural thrombus may mimic an acute myocardial infarction on contrast-enhanced MDCT. Obtaining a noncontrast CT can help to avoid this pitfall.

Notes

CASE 196

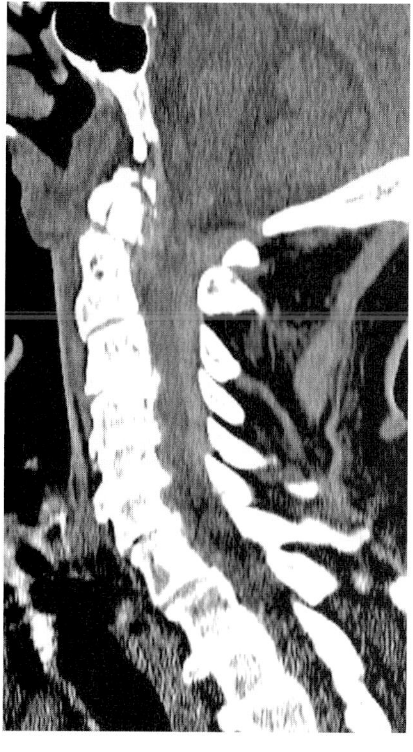

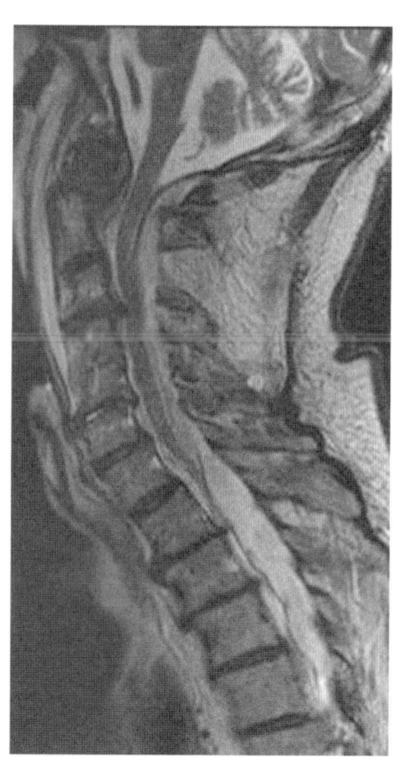

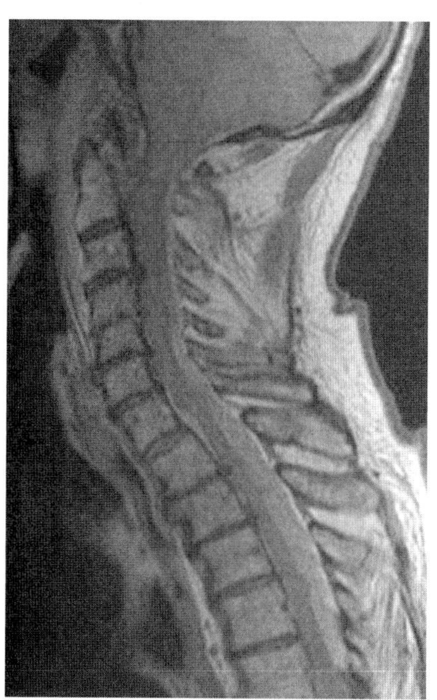

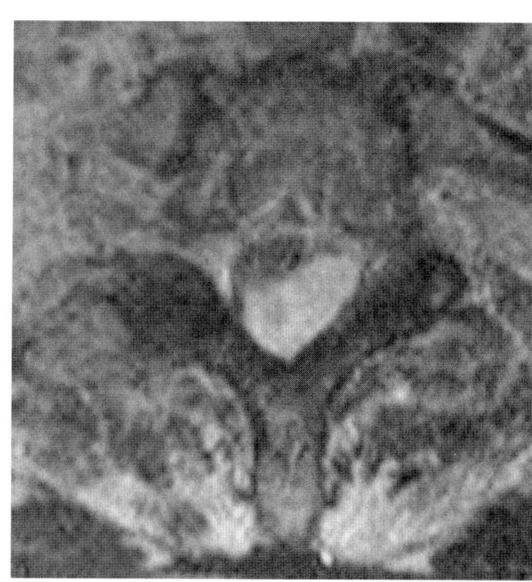

1. Describe the abnormalities seen on both multidetector computed tomography and magnetic resonance imaging other than the type 2 dens fracture.
2. What is the diagnosis?
3. What is the etiology of this lesion?
4. Give three predisposing factors for this lesion.

CASE 196

Spinal Epidural Hematoma

1. Computed tomography shows a high attenuation area posterior to the dens and spinal cord. On T2-weighted and proton density (only sagittal) images the corresponding lesions have a high signal intensity. The abnormality posterior to the cord extends into the upper thoracic spine with a linear low signal intensity within it representing the dura. The cord is displaced anteriorly and to the right side.
2. Spinal epidural hematoma.
3. The bleeding typically originates from the spinal epidural venous plexus.
4. Predisposing factors for this lesion include trauma, anticoagulant therapy, bleeding diatheses, arteriovenous malformations, hemangiomas, and spinal surgery.

References

Gundry CR, Heithoff KB: Epidural hematoma of the lumbar spine: 18 surgically confirmed cases, *Radiology* 187:427–431, 1993.

Holtas S, Heiling M, Lonntoft M: Spontaneous spinal epidural hematoma: findings at MR imaging and clinical correlation, *Radiology* 199:409–413, 1996.

Cross-Reference

Emergency Radiology: THE REQUISITES, pp 225, 226.

Comment

Spinal epidural hematomas are rare extramedullary lesions. The majority of the spinal epidural hematomas are typically seen posterior to the cord in the upper thoracic spine. Bleeding originates from the venous epidural plexus. The typical clinical presentation includes acute spinal pain, motor dysfunction in the extremities, sensory disturbance, bladder dysfunction, and radiculopathy.

Acute intraspinal hematomas are typically high-attenuation extramedullary lesions when demonstrated by computed tomography (CT). Differentiation between subdural and epidural hematomas cannot be made with certainty using CT.

Magnetic resonance imaging (MRI) is the modality of choice for diagnosis of spinal epidural hematomas. MRI can demonstrate the nature and the extent of the hematoma, as well as the amount of associated cord compression. The signal patterns can vary depending on the timing of the examination, the scanner field strength, and the imaging sequences used. Epidural hematomas are isointense to cord on T1-weighted images in the acute period, and they become hyperintense during the subacute period. On T2-weighted sequences, both increased and decreased signal intensity can be seen in relation to the spinal cord during the acute period. The dura can be visualized as a linear low intensity that separates the hematoma from the spinal cord. Transverse MR images can differentiate subdural and epidural hematomas. Subdural hematomas have outer convex and inner concave margins, and the low-intensity dura will not be seen separating the spinal cord from the hematoma. Epidural hematomas are biconvex lesions that cause a variable amount of mass effect on the cord depending on their size.

Spinal epidural hematomas are usually associated with trauma. Other predisposing factors include spinal surgery, anticoagulation, bleeding diatheses, hemangiomas, and arteriovenous malformations. The majority of spinal epidural hematomas can be managed conservatively with good clinical outcomes, especially in young patients.

Notes

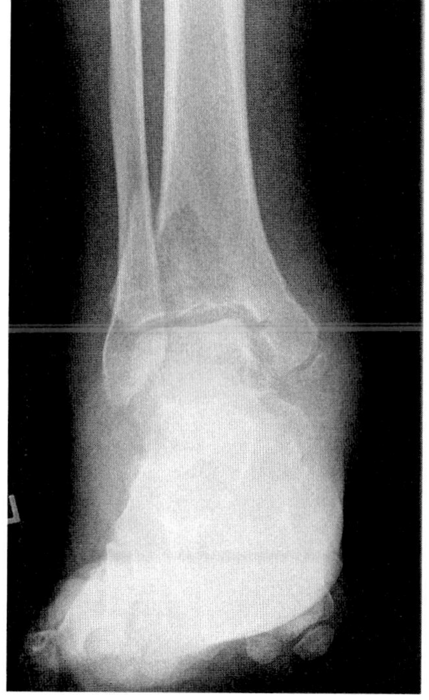

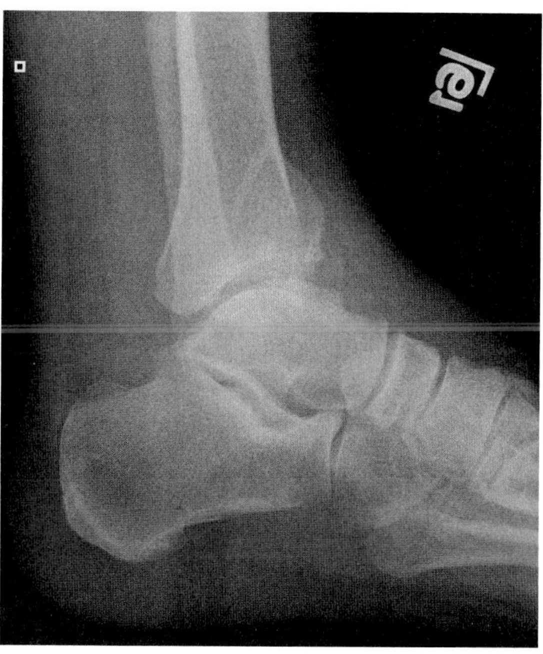

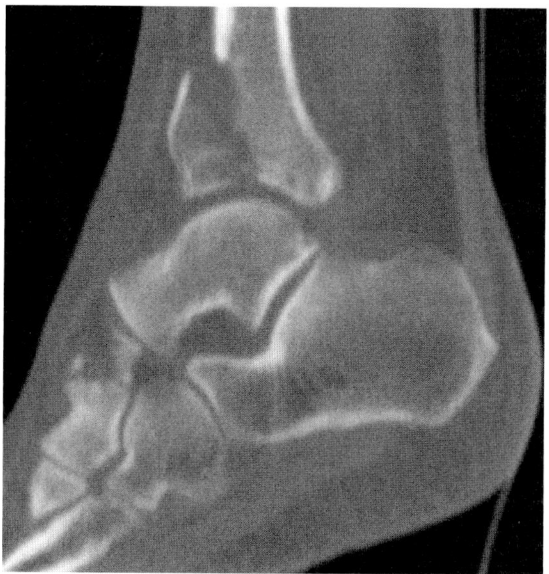

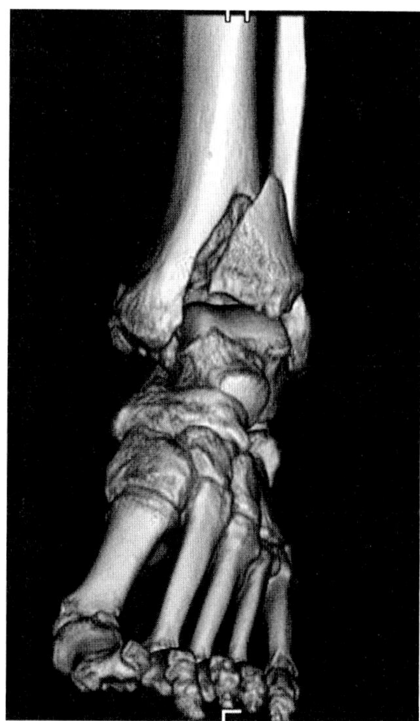

See also Color Plate

You are shown images of a 56-year-old man with pain and swelling after a twisted ankle.

1. What is the diagnosis?
2. What determines the ensuing fracture pattern?
3. In what position was the foot at the time of injury?
4. Name common associated fractures seen with this injury.

CASE 197

Pilon Fracture

1. Pilon fracture of the tibia.
2. The position of the foot, if it is in plantar flexion, neutral, or dorsiflexed at the time of injury, determines the ensuing fracture pattern.
3. The large anterior bone fragment indicates that the foot was dorsiflexed at the time of injury.
4. Fractures of the contralateral calcanium and ipsilateral tibial shaft.

Reference

Bartlett CS III, D'Amato MJ, Weiner LS: Fractures of the tibial pilon. In Browner BD, Jupiter JB, Levine A, Trafton PG, eds: *Skeletal Trauma*, Philadelphia, WB Saunders, 1998, pp 2295–2309.

Cross-Reference

Emergency Radiology: THE REQUISITES, pp 151–156.

Comment

Fractures that involve a significant portion of the articular surface and overlying metaphysis of the distal tibia are called pilon fractures. Pilon fractures commonly occur as a result of high-energy trauma. The talus is usually driven into the tibial weight-bearing articular surface or the plafond. The orthopedic literature emphasizes the importance of how the position of the foot at the time of injury relates to the fracture pattern seen. If the foot is plantar flexed the axial force is directed posteriorly, and results in a large posterior tibial fragment. With a neutral foot, the axial force acts on the entire plafond and a Y-shaped fracture results in large anterior and posterior fragments. A dorsiflexed foot results in a large fracture fragment arising from the anterior margin of the ankle mortis.

Involvement of the supra-articular metaphysis of the lower tibia defines the character of the pilon fracture. Fractures of the medial, lateral, and posterior malleoli may be seen in patients with tibial pilon fractures. The most common associated fractures include a contralateral calcanial fracture and an ipsilateral tibial shaft fracture. Other less-common associated fractures may involve the talus, proximal fibula, femur, and pelvis. Anterior compartment syndrome is a well-recognized complication for the associated soft tissue injuries.

Classification systems are based on the extent of involvement of the articular surface of the distal tibia, the amount of displacement of fracture fragments, metaphyseal impaction, and metaphyseal-diaphyseal dissociation. High-energy injuries typically tend to cause a greater degree of soft tissue injury and articular and metaphyseal comminution. High-resolution multidetector computed tomography images help to demonstrate the fracture pattern and the amount of comminution and displacement. Three-dimensional volume rendered sagittal and coronal reformatted images can provide additional information for the surgeon to specifically plan the surgical approach and the position of the hardware and screws.

Pilon fractures are notoriously difficult to treat. Acceptable results from surgical treatment for severely comminuted and impacted fractures vary from 50% to 69%. More recently, a combined limited internal and external surgical fixation approach has become a popular method of treatment.

Notes

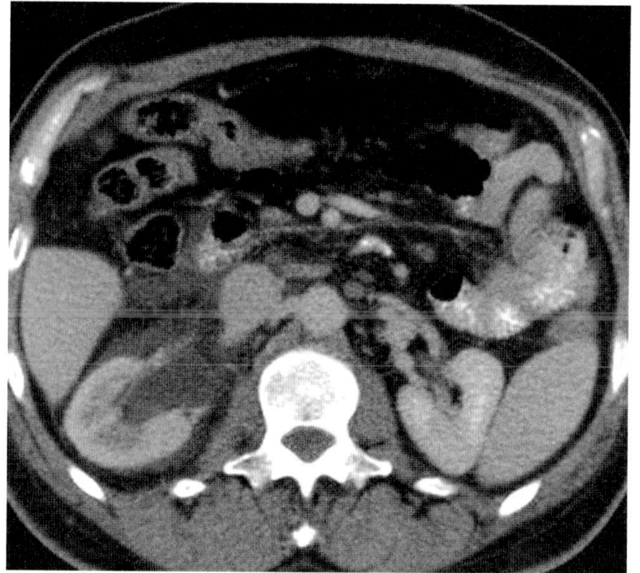

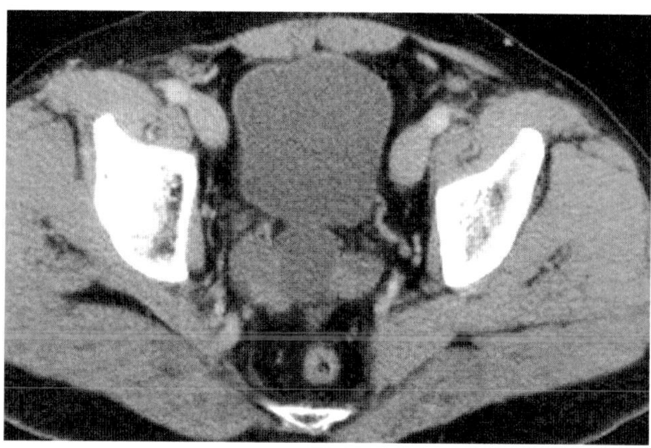

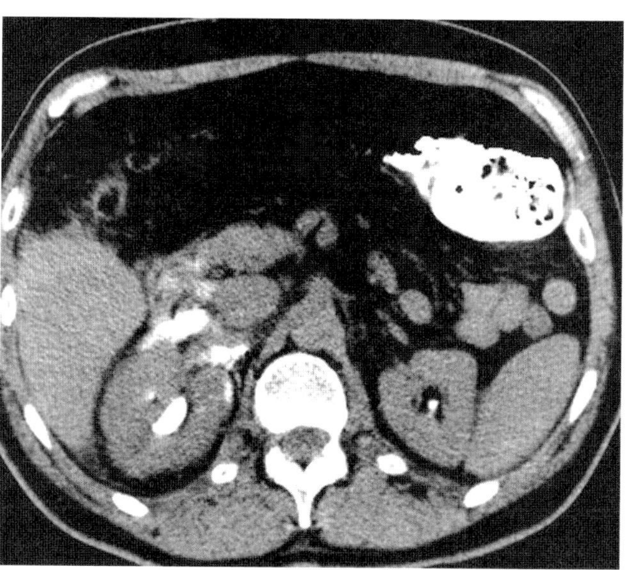

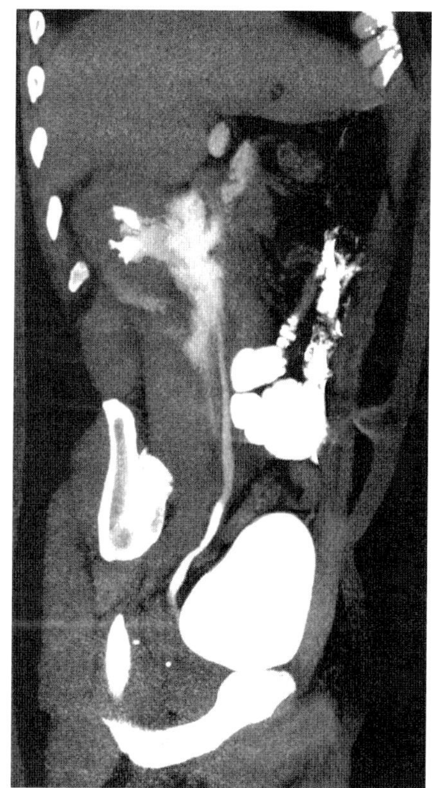

You are shown images of an emergency department patient who is HIV positive.

1. What is the diagnosis?
2. What are two possibilities to explain the findings?
3. What therapy might the patient be receiving that would be associated with this pathology?
4. What treatment is indicated?

CASE 198

Ureteral Obstruction, Calyx Rupture, and Radiolucent Calculus

1. Ureteral obstruction, pelvo-calyceal rupture, and radiolucent calculus.
2. Radiolucent ureteral stone and recently passed stone.
3. Protease inhibitor therapy for AIDS; the drug can crystallize in urine and form calculi.
4. Hydration, analgesia, and acidification of the urine usually lead to a favorable clinical outcome.

References

Dalrymple NC, Casford B, Raiken DP, et al: Pearls and pitfalls in the diagnosis of ureterolithiasis with unenhanced helical CT, *Radiographics* 20:439–447, 2000.

Koh DM, Langroudi B, Padley SPG: Abdominal CT in patients with AIDS, *Imaging* 14:24–34, 2002.

Cross-Reference

Emergency Radiology: THE REQUISITES, pp 299, 308, 309.

Comment

Unenhanced computed tomography (CT) has become the investigation of choice for acute loin pain suggestive of ureteric obstruction, particularly in North America. It has the advantages of being more accurate than intravenous urography in detecting calculi and secondary signs of obstruction, can be quickly performed, and does not require contrast medium or delayed radiographs. Primary signs of acute obstruction seen on CT include dilatation of the pelvicalyceal system and the ureter. Secondary signs of obstruction include enlargement of the kidney, perirenal stranding, urine extravasation, and periureteric edema around the obstructing calculus. Ureteral obstruction may also result in tubular hydronephrosis, decreasing the attenuation of the medullary pyramid on the obstructed side so that the pyramids have high attenuation on only the unobstructed side.

Although virtually all stones previously considered radiolucent on plain radiographs, such as uric acid stones, are readily identified on CT scans, the recent use of protease inhibitors to treat human immunodeficiency viral (HIV) disease has led to an increasing prevalence of urinary tract obstruction caused by deposition of crystals that are nonopaque on CT. HIV patients receiving Indinavir sulfate, a widely used protease inhibitor, have an incidence of crystallization and stone formation within the urinary tract of up to 20%. In patients showing evidence of ureteral obstruction without an obvious cause on nonenhanced CT, a diagnosis of recently passed stone or, in the setting of HIV treatment, a nonopaque obstructing stone should be considered. Indinavir stones are best diagnosed on CT after intravenous contrast medium administration to delineate the presence of a stone as a filling defect in the contrast column.

Notes

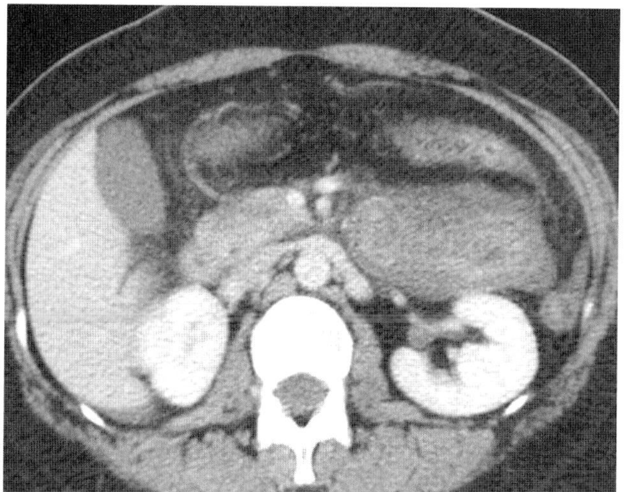

Admission CT

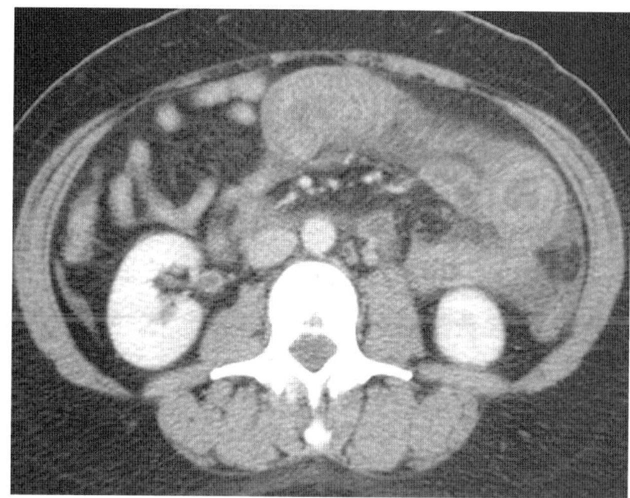

Admission CT

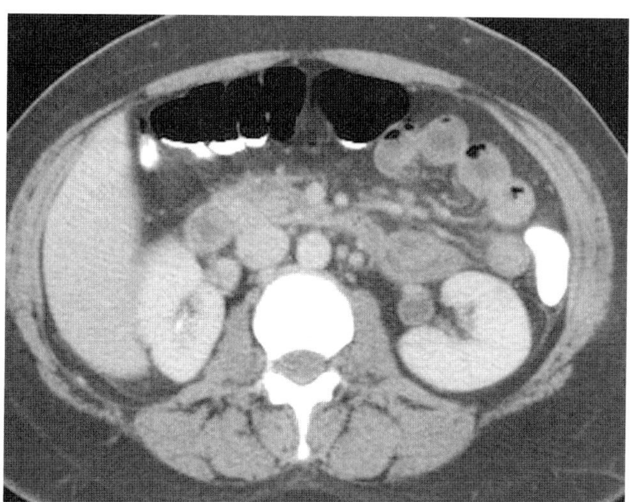

CT 24 hours after therapeutic maneuver

Figures reprinted from Marmery H, Mirvis SE: Angiostensin-converting enzyme inhibitor-induced visceral angioedema, *Clin Radiol* 61:979–982, 2006, with permission from Elsevier.

You are shown images of an emergency admission with abdominal pain and emesis.

1. What are the computed tomography findings on admission?
2. Name three other conditions that have a similar appearance.
3. What medication may produce this appearance?
4. What is the treatment?

CASE 199

Angiotensin-Converting Enzyme Inhibitor–Induced Visceral Angioedema

1. Bowel wall edema localized to duodenum and proximal jejunum, bright mucosal enhancement, and small amount of ascites.
2. Bowel ischemia, bleeding into bowel (e.g., anticoagulants, trauma, hemophilia), and hereditary angioedema.
3. Angiotensive-converting enzyme inhibitors.
4. Withdrawal of medication.

Reference

Marmery H, Mirvis SE: Angiotensin-converting enzyme inhibitor-induced visceral angioedema, *Clin Radiol* 61:979–982, 2006.

Comment

Angiotensin-converting enzyme (ACE) inhibitors are known to cause potentially life-threatening peripheral angioedema in some patients. Much more rarely they can produce visceral angioedema. Gastrointestinal involvement can mimic an acute abdomen. Little is known about this condition, and unless the diagnosis is considered patients often undergo extensive unnecessary further investigation of their abdominal pain. Peripheral angioedema secondary to ACE inhibitors is reported to occur in 0.1% to 0.2% of patients. Visceral angioedema occurs far more rarely. The condition is more common in blacks, women, and smokers. Periorbital edema and airway compromise are more likely than visceral edema.

Angioedema is a noninflammatory disease characterized by increased capillary permeability with extravasation of intravascular fluid and subsequent edema of the mucosa. When this involves the gastrointestinal tract symptoms can mimic an acute abdomen. The most commonly reported symptoms include abdominal pain, vomiting, and watery diarrhea. The diagnosis of ACE-inhibitor induced visceral angioedema is based on the temporal relationship between the symptoms and drug administration, exclusion of other causes, including causes of angioedema, and resolution of symptoms after discontinuation of the ACE inhibitor.

Computed tomography findings consist of circumferential small bowel wall thickening, which may be segmental. Mucosal enhancement is seen with prominence of the mesenteric vessels. There is a striking contrast between the low-attenuation edematous submucosa separating the outer muscular layers and serosa from brightly enhanced thickened mucosa. Ascites is invariably present. The differential diagnosis based on radiological findings is limited because of the transient and segmental nature of the small bowel edema. The differential diagnosis includes ischemia, Henoch-Schönlein purpura, and intramural bleeding from trauma, anticoagulation, or hemophilia. Hereditary angioedema is caused by a deficiency of complement component C1 esterase inhibitor, which is inherited as an autosomal dominant condition. Small bowel angioedema may also rarely be seen secondary to iodinated radiographic contrast medium reaction.

Notes

CASE 200

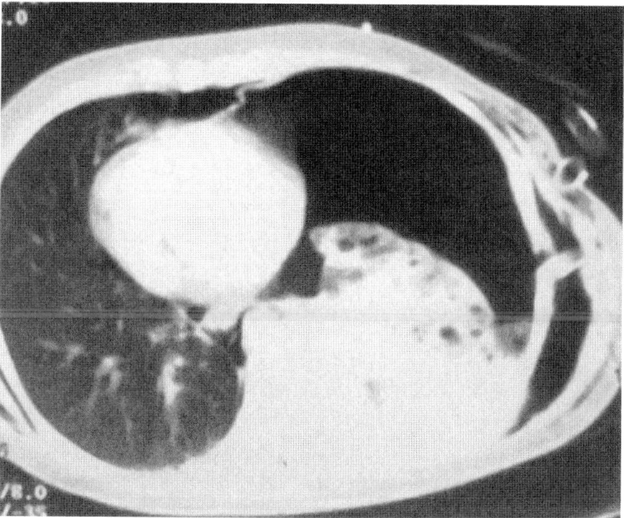

You are shown an image of a blunt trauma patient.

1. What is the diagnosis?
2. What is the location most frequently seen in this type of injury?
3. What are two proposed mechanisms producing this injury?
4. Why won't a chest tube necessarily help in treating this pathology?

CASE 200

Fallen Lung (Complete Mainstem Bronchus Tear) and Tension Pneumothorax

1. Fallen lung, severely contused lung, and tension pneumothorax.
2. Within 2.5 cm of the carina.
3. A sudden increase in intraluminal pressure against a closed glottis, and shearing force created by rapid deceleration between the more fixed carina and more mobile or flexible mainstem bronchus.
4. Air leaks into the pleural space from the torn bronchus as quickly as it is suctioned by the chest tube.

References

Karmy-Jones R, Avansino J, Stern EJ: CT of blunt tracheal rupture, *AJR Am J Roentgenol* 180:1670, 2003.

Kumpe DA, Oh KS, Wyman SM: A characteristic pulmonary finding in unilateral complete bronchial transection, *AJR Am J Roentgenol* 110:704–706, 1970.

Cross-Reference

Emergency Radiology: THE REQUISITES, pp 66–69.

Comment

Tears or fractures of the airways occur in approximately 1.5% of blunt chest trauma cases, and 80% are within 2.5 cm of the carina. Given the high-energy impact required to cause this injury, there are associated fractures to the upper ribs, clavicle, and sternum in about 40% of patients sustaining tracheobronchial injuries. Pneumomediastinum is seen in about 60% and pneumothorax in 70% of cases by chest radiography. Diffuse and progressive subcutaneous air is also a hallmark of the presentation. The two major hypotheses of main airway rupture are sudden increase in intraluminal pressure against a closed glottis, and shearing force created by sudden deceleration between the more fixed carina and more mobile or flexible mainstem bronchus.

In specific cases of major bronchial injury other findings can include air surrounding the bronchus; a sharply angled, tapered, and an occluded bronchus; and, with tearing of the mediastinal pleura, a persistent pneumothorax or tension pneumothorax despite adequate chest tube location in pleural space and suction. On occasion, if the advential tissue around a bronchus remains intact, a fibrin plug/hematoma or mediastinal soft tissue can occlude an air leak initially.

When there is complete disruption of a mainstem bronchus and other anchoring attachments, the lung falls into a gravity-dependent position posteriorly, laterally, or inferiorly depending on the patient's position, creating the "fallen lung" sign described by Kumpe in 1970. In a typical pneumothorax the lung collapses medially toward the hilum. If on radiography of an upright patient the superior margin of the lung projects below the level of the upper lobe bronchus takeoff, the diagnosis of complete mainstem bronchus transection can be made confidently. Radiography and computed tomography are usually diagnostic, but bronchoscopy can be used in equivocal cases. Bronchial stenosis is a potential complication of delayed treatment by surgical reanastomosis.

Notes

G

H